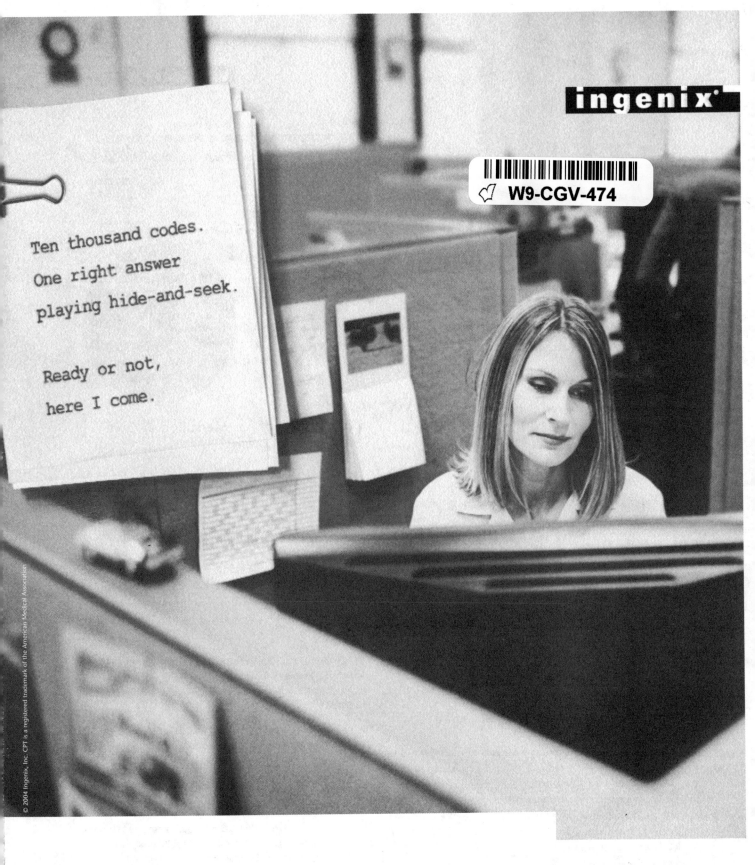

ingenix

W9-CGV-474

Ten thousand codes.
One right answer
playing hide-and-seek.

Ready or not,
here I come.

With more products, in more formats, Ingenix helps you find the answers to your coding questions.

You're a sleuth. You're a detective. In a word, you're a coder. And every day you work hard tracking down answers. Reimbursement depends on it. Ingenix has tools that can help. We have a breadth of coding products, including a complete suite of ICD-9-CM, HCPCS, CPT® and DRG source solutions. And they come in whatever format works best for you—Web-based tools, books, desktop software, CDs and binders. If you are searching for training tools, benchmarking and pricing information, we have that too. So when you're looking for answers, look to Ingenix. We're simplifying the complex business of health care.

To purchase call 1-800-INGENIX.
Or visit www.ingenixonline.com

SAVE MORE and qualify for REWARDS when you order at IngenixOnline.com.

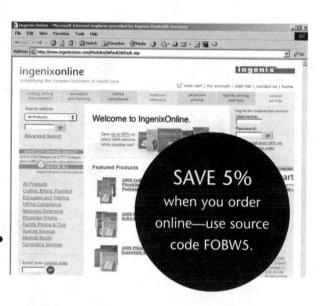

SAVE 5% when you order online—use source code FOBW5.

- Get rewards for every $500 you spend at Ingenix Online with our **e-Smart** program**

- Find what you're looking for—in less time with **enhanced basic and advanced search** capability

- Experience a **quick, hassle-free purchase process** with streamlined checkout options

- Create and maintain your own **Wish List**

- Quickly sign-up for **Ingenix Insights**—our e-alert showcasing coding, billing and reimbursement case study and analysis

- Sign-up for free 30-day trials to **e-Coding and e-Billing/Payment solutions**

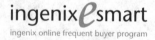

ingenix online frequent buyer program

Get rewards when you order online.

Ingenix e-Smart is a program designed to reward our best Ingenix Online customers. If you are a registered online customer and qualify to participate**, all you have to do is use the returning customer checkout option for your web purchases every time you shop online. We keep track of your purchases. Once you reach $500, we send you a FREE product—it's that easy!

If you are not yet registered, go to IngenixOnline.com and register right away so we can get you started with the Ingenix e-Smart program.

Are you part of our Medallion or Gold Medallion programs?

Ingenix Online has enhanced options for you, for a hassle-free, streamlined purchase and account management experience!

To view your enhanced online account options, simply register with us at IngenixOnline.com. You will then be able to easily place orders for items already reflecting your 2005 Price List discounts, get access to your purchase history, track shipments, change your profile, manage your address book and much more.

(*) 5% offer valid online, cannot be combined with any other offer and is not applicable to Partner, Medallion and Gold Medallion accounts with an established price list. Bookstore products, package items and conferences not included.

(**) Offer valid only for Ingenix customers who are NOT part of Medallion, Gold Medallion or Partner Accounts programs. You must be registered at Ingenix Online to have your online purchases tracked for rewards purposes. Shipping charges and taxes still apply and cannot be used for rewards. E-smart reward offers valid online only.

100% Money Back Guarantee:
If our merchandise* ever fails to meet your expectations, please contact our Customer Service Department toll-free at 1.800.INGENIX (464.3649), option 1, for an immediate response.
*Software: Credit will be granted for unopened packages only.

CPT is a registered trademark of the American Medical Association.

Make the Right Coding Decisions the First Time!

Encoder Pro Professional

Item No.: 2717

Available: Now

$499.95*

*Call for multi-user pricing.

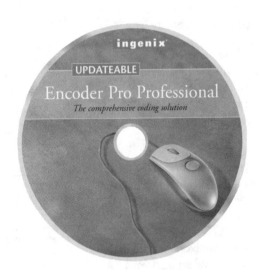

Improve your reimbursement and your staff's productivity by increasing coding efficiency and accuracy. Powered by the CodeLogic™ Search Engine, you and your coders get lightning fast search results that return relevant code edit content; allowing your staff to make speedy and accurate code selection.

- **Exclusive—Easily search all three code sets simultaneously.** Powerful Code Lookup across CPT®, HCPCS, and ICD-9-CM code sets with Ingenix Code Logic™ Search Engine. Search using multiple lay terms, acronyms, abbreviations, and even misspelled words.

- **Exclusive—Enhance your understanding of procedures with easy-to-understand Ingenix lay descriptions.**

- **Stay in compliance with quarterly releases of Medicare's national and local coverage determinations.** Receive quarterly updates to Medicare coverage guidelines.

- **Reference coding rules and billing combinations for procedures and services and their commercially acceptable modifiers.**

- **Quickly check your selected code for proper reporting.** Access Ingenix references and Medicare color code edits for instant validation on gender, age, unbundles, and more.

- **Customize your coding experience.** Use sticky notes and bookmarks to help you set reminders and establish relationships among codes.

Four simple ways to place an order.

Call

1.800.ingenix (464.3649), option 1. Mention source code FOBA5 when ordering.

Mail

PO Box 27116
Salt Lake City, UT 84127-0116
With payment and/or purchase order.

Fax

801.982.4033
With credit card information and/or purchase order.

Click

www.ingenixonline.com
Save 5% when you order online today—use source code FOBW5.

ingenix esmart
ingenix online frequent buyer program

GET REWARDS FOR SHOPPING ONLINE!
To find out more, visit IngenixOnline.com

E-Smart program available only to Ingenix customers who are not part of Medallion, Gold Medallion or Partner Accounts programs. You must be registered at Ingenix Online to have your online purchases tracked for rewards purposes. Shipping charges and taxes still apply and cannot be used for rewards. Offer valid online only.

100% Money Back Guarantee

If our merchandise* ever fails to meet your expectations, please contact our Customer Service Department toll-free at 1.800.ingenix (464.3649), option 1 for an immediate response.

*Software: Credit will be granted for unopened packages only.

Customer Service Hours

7:00 am - 5:00 pm Mountain Time
9:00 am - 7:00 pm Eastern Time

Shipping and Handling

no. of items	fee
1	$10.95
2-4	$12.95
5-7	$14.95
8-10	$19.95
11+	Call

ingenix

FOBA5

Order Form

Information

Customer No. _____ Contact No. _____

Source Code _____

Contact Name _____

Title _____ Specialty _____

Company _____

Street Address _____

City — NO PO BOXES, PLEASE _____ State _____ Zip _____

Telephone ( ) _____ Fax ( ) _____
IN CASE WE HAVE QUESTIONS ABOUT YOUR ORDER

E-mail _____ @ _____
REQUIRED FOR ORDER CONFIRMATION AND SELECT PRODUCT DELIVERY.

Ingenix respects your right to privacy. We will not sell or rent your e-mail address or fax number to anyone outside Ingenix and its business partners. If you would like to remove your name from Ingenix promotion, please call 1.800.ingenix (464.3649), option 1.

Product

Item No.	Qty	Description	Price	Total

Subtotal _____

UT, OH, & VA residents, please add applicable   Sales tax _____

(See chart on the left)   Shipping & handling charges _____
All foreign orders, please call for shipping costs

Total _____

Payment

○ Please bill my credit card   ○ MasterCard   ○ VISA   ○ Amex   ○ Discover

Card No. | | | | | | | | | | | | | | | | | | | Expires _____
MONTH   YEAR

Signature _____

○ Check enclosed, made payable to: Ingenix, Inc.   ○ Please bill my office

Purchase Order No. _____
ATTACH COPY OF PURCHASE ORDER

FOBA5

ingenix

HCPCS Level II
Professional

2005

16th edition

Publisher's Notice

The Ingenix *2005 HCPCS* is designed to be an accurate and authoritative source of information about this government coding system. Every effort has been made to verify the accuracy of the listings, and all information is believed reliable at the time of publication. Absolute accuracy cannot be guaranteed, however. This publication is made available with the understanding that the publisher is not engaged in rendering legal or other services that require a professional license. If you identify a correction or wish to share information, please email the Ingenix customer service department at customerservice@ingenix.com or fax us at 801.982.4033.

Acknowledgments

Brad Ericson, MPC, *Product Manager*
Lynn Speirs, *Senior Director, Publishing Services*
Sheri Poe Bernard, CPC, *Senior Product Director*
Kristin Hodkinson, RHIT, CPC, CPC-H, CIC, *Clinical/Technical Editor*
Wendy McConkie, CPC, CPC-H, *Clinical/Technical Editor*
Karen Kacher, RN, CPC, *Clinical/Technical Editor*
Regina Magnani, RHIT, *Clinical/Technical Editor*
Jean Parkinson, *Project Editor*
Kerrie Hornsby, *Desktop Publishing Manager*
Gregory Kemp, *Desktop Publishing Specialist*

Continuing Education Units for AAPC Certified Members

This publication has prior approval by the American Academy of Professional Coders for continuing education units. Granting of prior approval in no way constitutes endorsement by AAPC of the publication content nor the publisher. Instructions to submit CEUs are available at www.aapc.com/education/ceus/ceus.html

Technical Editors

Kristin Hodkinson, RHIT, CPC, CPC-H, CIC
Clinical/Technical Editor

Ms. Hodkinson has more than 10 years of experience in the health care profession including commercial insurance payers, health information management, and patient accounts. She has extensive background in both the professional and technical components of CPT/HCPCS and ICD-9-CM coding. Her areas of expertise include interventional radiology and cardiology, hospital chargemaster, and the Outpatient Prospective Payment System (OPPS). She recently served as the APC coordinator for a health care system in Florida. She is a member of the American Academy of Professional Coders (AAPC) and the American Health Information Management Association (AHIMA).

Wendy McConkie, CPC, CPC-H
Clinical/Technical Editor

Ms. McConkie has more than 20 years of experience in the health care field. She has extensive background in CPT/HCPCS and ICD-9-CM coding. She served several years as a coding consultant. Her areas of expertise include physician and hospital CPT coding assessments, chargemaster reviews, and the Outpatient Prospective Payment System (OPPS). She is a member of the American Academy of Professional Coders (AAPC).

Regina Magnani, RHIT
Clinical/Technical Editor

Ms. Magnani has 25 years of experience in the health care industry in both health information management and patient financial services. Her areas of expertise include patient financial services, CPT/HCPCS and ICD-9-CM coding, the Outpatient Prospective Payment System (OPPS), and chargemaster development and maintenance. She is an active member of the Healthcare Financial Management Association (HFMA), the American Health Information Management Association (AHIMA), and the American Association of Heathcare Administrative Management (AAHAM).

Karen Kachur, RN, CPC
Clinical/Technical Editor

Ms. Kachur is a Clinical/Technical Editor for Ingenix with expertise in CPT/HCPCS and ICD-9-CM coding, in addition to physician billing, compliance, and fraud and abuse. Prior to joining Ingenix, she worked for many years as a staff RN in a variety of clinical settings including medicine, surgery, intensive care, psychiatry, and geriatrics. Ms Kachur has served as assistant director of a hospital utilization management and quality assurance department. She also has extensive experience as a nurse reviewer for Blue Cross/Blue Shield.

Sheri Poe Bernard, CPC
Senior Product Director

Ms. Bernard has contributed to the development of coding products for Ingenix for more than 12 years, and her areas of expertise include ICD-9-CM and ICD-10 coding systems. A member of the National Advisory Board of the American Academy of Professional Coders, Ms. Bernard chairs its committee on ICD-10, and is a nationally-recognized speaker on ICD-10 coding systems. Prior to joining Ingenix, Ms. Bernard was a journalist specializing in business and medical writing and editing.

Introduction

HCPCS (pronounced "hick-picks") is the acronym for the Healthcare Common Procedure Coding System. This system is a uniform method for health care providers and medical suppliers to report professional services, procedures, and supplies. Prior to the development of HCPCS in 1983, there was no uniform system for coding a procedure, service, or supply for reimbursement.

Blue Cross/Blue Shield created and required use of its own coding system; many other insurance companies created their own method of coding physician services and procedures. States also developed codes for Medicaid and workers' compensation programs. The dental profession also developed codes. All contribute to HCPCS Level II development and maintenance. Despite the addition and subtraction of codes over the code set's history, the Centers for Medicare and Medicaid Services, (CMS) has maintained the intentions of HCPCS, which is to accomplish the following:

- Meet the operational needs of Medicare/Medicaid
- Coordinate government programs by uniform application of CMS policies
- Allow providers and suppliers to communicate their services in a consistent manner
- Ensure the validity of profiles and fee schedules through standardized coding
- Enhance medical education and research by providing a vehicle for local, regional, and national utilization comparisons

Ingenix's HCPCS Level II products are compiled to facilitate the coding of supplies and services provided by physicians, therapists, home health, outpatient departments, and other caregivers. The second level of HCPCS Level II includes such a broad spectrum of services and supplies—from patient transport to ostomy supplies, from chemotherapy drugs to durable medical equipment, and from new technologies to surgical procedures—it's often referred to as the "catch-all code system." Chapters differ by service, and some are specifically for use by dentists, Blue Cross, outpatient prospective payment system hospitals, and Medicaid.

The dynamic nature of the code set, which must be updated frequently to better serve various providers and payers, makes coding HCPCS Level II codes a difficult chore. Ingenix helps coders with a number of features, including:

- All the official HCPCS Level II codes and descriptions
- Ingenix expert coding tips and annotations
- New, changed, and deleted codes
- Medicare rules indicated by icon and color coding
- Medicare manual references and actual excerpts
- Ambulatory surgery center (ASC) group and ambulatory payment classification (APC) status codes
- Codes payable under the DMEPOS fee schedule
- Codes not payable under the SNF fee schedule
- *AHA Coding Clinic* citations
- Age and sex edits
- Quantity alerts for codes requiring that attention be paid to the number of items used
- Modifiers
- An enhanced index and table of drugs
- Illustrations
- Choice of formats

In addition, *HCPCS Level II Professional* customers may subscribe to an email service to receive special reports when information in this book changes. Contact customer service at (800) INGENIX, option 1 to sign up.

Additional Copies

Contact the customer service department toll free at 1.800.INGENIX (464.3649), option 1 or access www.ingenixonline.com via your computer.

Use of Official Sources

Our HCPCS books are based on the CMS official 2005 update releases of HCPCS Level II codes, descriptions, and other relevant data. Other sources of information from which HCPCS codes and their usage are gleaned include CMS's hospital Outpatient Prospective Payment System (OPPS), *Medicare Carriers Manual (MCM), Coverage Issues Manual (CIM), Publication 100* sections, the Medicare physician fee schedule, and ASC rules.

Proprietary information in our HCPCS books includes annotations, age and sex edits, coding tips, an enhanced index and drug table, and other useful features.

Effective Dates for 2005

This new HCPCS Level II product is effective for dates of service beginning January 1, 2005. A three-month grace period no longer applies to changed and discontinued HCPCS codes in 2005. Carriers will no longer accept both 2005 changed and discontinued codes and valid 2005 codes from physicians, suppliers, and providers. Changes that occur quarterly also do not have a grace period. Ingenix offers an updateable HCPCS product for codes that are posted by CMS after November 1, 2004.

This 2005 HCPCS Level II includes additions, changes, and deletions released by CMS before November 2004 via the agency's public use files. Appropriate alterations have been made based on CMS program memos and transmittals, the October and November 2004 HCPCS temporary national coding decisions for 2005 documents, and the addendum B of the outpatient prospective payment system (OPPS) update of November 2004; these are noted to promote accurate coding.

Because of the unstable nature of HCPCS Level II codes, everything has been done to include the latest information available at print time. Unfortunately, HCPCS Level II codes, their descriptions, and other related information change throughout the year. Consult the patient's payer and the CMS Website to confirm the status of any HCPCS Level II code. The existence of a code does not imply coverage under any given payment plan.

What to Do if You Have Questions

If you have any questions, call our customer service department toll-free at 1.800.INGENIX (464.3649), option 1.

If you have comments on the content of this book, please email them to customerservice@ingenix.com or fax them to (801) 982-2783.

HCPCS Levels of Codes

The nearly 5,000 HCPCS Level II national codes represent just one part of a larger, three-level coding system called HCPCS.

Each of the three HCPCS levels is a unique coding system. The levels I, II, and III are also known by the names shown here with the level numbers.

Level I—CPT

HCPCS Level I is the American Medical Association's *Physician's Current Procedural Terminology* (CPT®). The Level I codes include five-digit codes and two-digit modifiers, both with descriptive terms for reporting services performed by health care providers. Level I codes and modifiers are described in detail in the CPT book. The AMA released its first edition of the CPT code book in 1966 with the intention of simplifying the reporting of procedures or services rendered by physicians or health care providers under their supervision. CPT is a registered trademark of the American Medical Association.

Category I Procedures are grouped within six major sections: evaluation and management (E/M), anesthesiology, surgery, radiology, pathology and laboratory, and medicine. The major sections are divided into subsections according to body part, service, or diagnosis (e.g., mouth, amputation, or septal defect). Alpha-numeric Category II and Category III sections follow.

Category II codes end with an F and help track Performance Measures. Category III codes are developed to track emerging technology, services, and procedures. These codes end with a T.

Level II—HCPCS National Codes

The CPT book does not contain all the codes needed to report medical services and supplies, and CMS developed the second level of codes-those found in this book. In contrast to the five-digit codes found in Level I, national codes consist of one alphabetic character (a letter between A and V), followed by four digits. (All D codes are copyright by the American Dental Association.) They are grouped by the type of service or supply they represent and are updated annually by CMS with input from private insurance companies. Level II codes are required for reporting most medical services and supplies provided to Medicare and Medicaid patients and by most private payers.

Level II of HCPCS also contains modifiers, which are either alphanumeric or two letters in the range from A1 to VP. National modifiers can be used with all levels of HCPCS codes. The appendixes include a complete listing of Level II modifiers. Some Level II modifiers can be used with CPT codes.

The permanent national codes serve the important function of providing a standardized coding system that is managed jointly by private and public insurers. It supplies a predictable set of uniform codes that provides a stable environment for claims submission and processing.

Level III—Local Codes

The HCPCS Level III codes are just one part of a larger three-level coding system that became a two-level coding system. The Health Insurance Portability and Accountability Act (HIPAA) required that there be standardized procedure coding. To meet this requirement, all unapproved HCPCS Level III codes/modifiers were eliminated by December 31, 2003, except in rare cases.

To compensate for the loss in local reporting, a greater number of codes are available on the national level. For example, since 2000 there has been 47 percent increase in the number of Level II codes, owing in part to the increasing number of codes recently added.

Organization

The Ingenix 2005 *HCPCS Level II Professional* contains mandated changes and new codes for use as of January 1, 2005. Deleted codes have also been indicated and cross-referenced to active codes when possible. New codes have been added to the appropriate sections, eliminating the time-consuming step of looking in two places for a code. However, keep in mind that the information in this book is a reproduction of the 2005 HCPCS; additional information on coverage issues may have been provided to carriers after publication. All carriers periodically update their systems and records throughout the year. If this book does not agree with your carrier, it is either because of a mid-year update or correct, or a specific regional policy.

To make this year's HCPCS book even more useful, we included codes noted in addendum B of the November 2005 OPPS update as published in the *Federal Register* and from program memorandums through 2005 that include codes not discussed in other CMS documents. The sources for these codes are noted in blue beneath the description.

Index

Since HCPCS is organized by code number rather than by service or supply name, the index enables the coder to locate any code without looking through individual ranges of codes. Just look up the medical or surgical supply, service, orthotic, prosthetic, or generic or brand name drug in question to find the appropriate codes. This index also refers to many of the brand names by which these items are known.

Table of Drugs and Cross-Referencing

Our HCPCS provides three ways to cross-reference from brand name to generic drugs. In the listing of codes, brand name items are included after the generic name. The brand names listed are examples only and may not include all products available for that type of drug. Our table of drugs lists A codes, several C codes, all J codes, a few K codes, many S codes, and several Q codes under generic drug names with amount, route of administration, and code numbers. Brand name drugs are also listed in the table with a reference to the appropriate generic drug.

Color-coded Coverage Instructions

The Ingenix HCPCS Level II code book provides colored symbols for each coverage and reimbursement instruction. A legend to these symbols is provided on the bottom of each two-page spread.

Red Color Bar	Codes that are not covered by or are invalid for Medicare are covered by a red bar. The pertinent *Coverage Issues Manual* (CIM) and *Pub 100 Medicare Carriers Manual* (MCM) reference numbers are also given explaining why a particular code is not covered. These numbers refer to appendix 4, where we have listed the Medicare references.
Yellow Color Bar	Issues that are left to "carrier discretion" are covered with a yellow bar. Contact the carrier for specific coverage information on those codes.
Blue Color Bar	A blue bar for "special coverage instructions" over a code means that special coverage instructions apply to that code. These special instructions are also typically given in the form of CIM and MCM reference numbers. The appendixes provide the full text of the cited CIM and MCM references.
☑	Many codes in HCPCS report quantities that may not coincide with quantities available in the marketplace. For instance, a HCPCS code for a surgical mask reports 20 masks, but the product is generally sold in a box of 100; "5" must be indicated in the quantity box on the CMS claim form to ensure proper reimbursement. This symbol indicates that care should be taken to verify quantities in this code.

Your 2005 *HCPCS Level II Professional* uses the AMA's CPT code book conventions to indicate new, revised, and deleted codes.

- A black circle (●) precedes a new code.
- A black triangle (▲) precedes a code with revised terminology or rules.
- A circle (○) precedes a reinstated code.
- Codes deleted from the 2005 active codes appear with a strike-out.

Remember that beginning 2005 there is no 90-day grace period to implement these changes.

Notes

A few of the subsections, headings, or codes have special instructions that apply only to them. The term "NOTE" sometimes, but not always, is used to identify these instructions. Some notes are found following the subsection, heading, or code to which they apply. Others appear as part of a description in a heading or code, separated by a comma or dash or placed within parentheses.

Unlisted Procedures

CMS does not use consistent terminology when a code for a specific procedure is not listed. The code description may include any of the following terms: unlisted, not otherwise classified (NOC), unspecified, unclassified, other, and miscellaneous. When coding this type of procedure, check with your Medicare carrier in case a specific HCPCS Level III code is available. If one is not available, the appropriate unlisted procedure code should be used and a special report should be submitted with the claim.

Age and Sex Edits

Age and sex edits help identify supplies and procedures Medicare and commercial payers may consider appropriate for a patient of a certain age or gender. Icons to the right of the code description are intuitive and keyed at the bottom of each page. Here are some examples:

P	Pediatrics:	Years 0 – 10
A	Adult:	Years 11 – 99
M	Maternity:	Years 12 – 50
I	Infant:	Months 0 – 12

Gender is indicated by the following icons:

♀   Female

♂   Male

ASC Groupings
Codes designated as being paid by ASC groupings are denoted in the HCPCS Level II code book by the group number.

APC Status Indicators

[A]-[Y] *APC Status Indicators*
Status indicators identify how individual HCPCS Level II codes are paid or not paid under the OPPS. The same status indicator is assigned to all the codes within an APC. Consult the payer or resource to learn which CPT codes fall within various APCs. Status indicators for HCPCS and their definitions are below:

[A]   Indicates services that are paid under some other method such as the DMEPOS fee schedule or the physician fee schedule

Indicates codes not allowed or paid under OPPS

[C]   Indicates inpatient services that are not paid under the OPPS

[E]   Indicates services for which payment is not allowed under the OPPS. In some instances, the service is not covered by Medicare. In other instances, Medicare does not use the code in question but does use another code to describe the service

[F]   Indicates corneal tissue acquisition costs, which are paid separately

[G]   Indicates a current drug or biological for which payment is made under the transitional pass-through

[H]   Indicates a device for which payment is made under the transitional pass-through

[K]   Indicates non-pass-through drugs and biologicals. Effective July 1, 2001, copayments for these items and the service of the administration of the items are aggregated and may not exceed the inpatient hospital deductible.

[L]   Indicates influenza or pneumococcal pneumonia vaccine paid as of reasonable cost with no deductable or coinsurance

[N]   Indicates services that are incidental, with payment packaged into another service or APC group

[P]   Indicates services paid only in partial hospitalization programs

[S]   Indicates significant procedures for which payment is allowed under the hospital OPPS but to which the multiple procedure reduction does not apply

[T]   Indicates surgical services for which payment is allowed under the hospital OPPS. Services with this payment indicator are the only ones to which the multiple procedure payment reduction applies.

[V]   Indicates medical visits for which payment is allowed under the hospital OPPS

[X]   Indicates ancillary services for which payment is allowed under the hospital OPPS

[Y]   Indicates nonimplantable durable medical equipment (DME) that are billed by providers other than home health agencies to the DMERC

ර්   Use this icon to identify when to consult the CMS DMEPOS for payment of this durable medical item in your area

⊘   Certain items and services are not covered under the Skilled Nursing Facility Prospective Payment System (SNFPPS). Use this icon to identify those codes before you bill

MED: This notation precedes an instruction pertaining to this code in the Centers for Medicare and Medicaid Services' (CMS) new Publication 100 (Pub 100) electronic manual or in a National Coverage Decision (NCD). These CMS sources, formerly called the Medicare Carriers Manual (MCM) and Coverage Issues Manual (CIM), present the rules for submitting these services to the federal government or its contractors and are included in the appendix of this book

AHA: Beginning this year, we include *American Hospital Association Coding Clinic for HCPCS* citations.

Appendixes
The following is a list of the appendixes in the Ingenix HCPCS Level II code book.

Appendix 1: Modifiers
Under certain situations, procedures have been altered by a specific circumstance. Modifiers are required to adequately report the procedure. Appendix 1 contains an introduction and a complete listing of modifiers used with HCPCS Level II codes.

Appendix 2: Abbreviations and Acronyms
A complete list of all abbreviations and acronyms for the current year is provided in a summary format.

Appendix 3: Table of Drugs
The brand names are listed in alphabetical order and will refer to the appropriate specific generic drug for correct code assignment by route of administration and dosage.

Appendix 4: Medicare References
To make it easier to understand the coverage issues associated with certain codes, we have provided the coverage guidelines for HCPCS Level II codes using the manuals published by CMS.

Appendix 5: HCPCS Codes for which CPT Codes Should be Reported
Some HCPCS codes are to be reported using another code. Use this appendix to find out which ones are affected.

Appendix 6: New, Changed, Deleted, and Reinstated HCPCS Codes for 2005
This appendix lists all new, changed, deleted, and reinstated HCPCS codes as of November 8, 2004, effective January 1, 2005.

ELIMINATION OF THE 90-DAY GRACE PERIOD
Effective January 1, 2005, Medicare providers will no longer have a 90-day grace period to use discontinued CPT codes for services rendered in the first 90 days after the new codes become effective. Use of such codes to bill services provided after the date on which the codes are discontinued will cause claims to be returned and not paid. This change is due to the standardized code set provisions under the Health Insurance Portability and Accountability Act (HIPAA), which requires providers to use the medical code set that is valid at the time the service is provided.

How to Use HCPCS Level II

Coders should keep in mind, however, that the insurance companies and government do not base payment solely on what was done for the patient. They need to know why the services were performed. In addition to using the HCPCS coding system for procedures and supplies, coders must also use the ICD-9-CM coding system to denote the diagnosis. This book will not discuss ICD-9-CM codes, which can be found in a current ICD-9-CM code book for diagnosis codes. To locate a HCPCS Level II code, follow these steps:

1. Identify the services or procedures the patient received.

   Example:

   Patient administered PSA exam.

2. Look up the appropriate term in the index.

   Example:

   > **Screening**
   > prostate

   Coding Tip: Coders who are unable to find the procedure or service in the index can look in the table of contents for the type of procedure or device to narrow the code choices. Also, coders should remember to check the unlisted procedure guidelines for additional choices.

3. Assign a tentative code.

   Example:

   Codes G0103

   Coding Tip: To the right of the terminology, there may be a single code or multiple codes, a cross-reference or an indication that the code has been deleted. Tentatively assign all codes listed.

4. Locate the code or codes in the appropriate section. When multiple codes are listed in the index, be sure to read the narrative of all codes listed to find the appropriate code based on the service performed.

   Example:

   > G0103   Prostate cancer screening; prostate specific antigen
   > test (PSA), total

5. Check for color bars, symbols, notes, and references.

   Example:

   > Ⓐ   G0103   Prostate cancer screening; prostate specific antigen
   > test (PSA), total   ♂
   > **MED: 100-3, 210.1; 100-4, 18, 50**

6. Review the appendixes for the reference definitions and other guidelines for coverage issues that apply.

7. Determine whether any modifiers should be used.

8. Assign the code.

   Example:

   The code assigned is G0103.

Coding Standards

Levels of Use
Coders may find that the same procedure is coded at two or even three levels. Which code is correct? There are certain rules to follow if this should occur.

When both a CPT and a HCPCS Level II code have virtually identical narratives for a procedure or service, the CPT code should be used. If, however, the narratives are not identical (for example, the CPT code narrative

is generic, whereas the HCPCS Level II code is specific), the Level II code should be used.

Be sure to check for a national or local code when a CPT code description contains an instruction to include additional information, such as describing specific medication. For example, when billing Medicare or Medicaid for supplies, avoid using CPT code 99070, supplies and materials (except spectacles), provided by the physician over and above those usually included with the office visit or other services rendered (list drugs, trays, supplies, or materials provided). There are many HCPCS Level II codes that specify supplies in more detail.

Special Reports
Submit a special report with the claim when a new, unusual, or variable procedure is provided or a modifier is used. Include the following information:

- A copy of the appropriate report (e.g., operative, x-ray), explaining the nature, extent, and need for the procedure
- Documentation of the medical necessity of the procedure
- Documentation of the time and effort necessary to perform the procedure

Developing and Maintaining HCPCS Codes
Ingenix does not develop or maintain HCPCS Level II codes. The federal government does.

Any supplier or manufacturer can submit a request for coding modification to the HCPCS Level II national codes. A document explaining the HCPCS modification process, as well as a detailed format for submitting a recommendation for a modification to HCPCS Level II codes, is available on the HCPCS website at http://cms.hhs.gov/medicare/hcpcs/default.asp. Besides the information requested in this format, a requestor should also submit any additional descriptive material, including the manufacturer's product literature and information that is believed would be helpful in furthering CMS's understanding of the medical features of the item for which a coding modification is being recommended. The HCPCS coding review process is an ongoing continuous process.

The review cycle runs from April 2nd through the following April 1st. Requests may be submitted at any time throughout the year. Requests that are received and complete by April 1st of the current year will be considered for inclusion in the next annual update (January 1st of the following year). Requests received on or after April 2nd, and requests received earlier that require additional evaluation, will be included in a later HCPCS update. There are three types of coding modifications to the HCPCS that can be requested as below:

- That a code be added when there is not a distinct code that describes a product, a code may be requested (1) if the FDA allows the product to be marketed in the United States, (2) the product has been on the market for at least 6 months, and (3) the product represents 3 percent or more of the outpatient use for that type of product in the national market.

  NOTE: If a request for a new code is approved, the addition of a new HCPCS codes does not mean that the item is necessarily covered by Medicare. Whether an item identified by a new code is covered is determined by the Medicare law, regulations, and medical review policies and not by the assignment of a code.

- That the language used to describe an existing code be changed. When there is an existing code, a recommendation to modify the code can be made when an interested party believes that the descriptor for the code needs to be modified to provide a better description of the category of products represented by the code.

- That an existing code be deleted. When an existing code becomes obsolete or is duplicative of another code, a request can be made to delete the code.

During any time in which there is no currently existing code to describe a product, a miscellaneous code or not otherwise classified code can be used. The use of a miscellaneous code permits a claims history to be established for an item that can be used to support the need for a national permanent code. Also, CMS maintains that any code in HCPCS can be used by a provider to report a service or supply, but payment will not be guaranteed.

Requests for coding modifications should be sent to the following address:

Alpha-Numeric HCPCS Coordinator
Center for Medicare Management
Centers for Medicare and Medicaid Services
C5-08-27
7500 Security Boulevard
Baltimore, MD 21244-1850

HCPCS Workgroup

The CMS/HCPCS Workgroup reviews recommendations for coding modifications that are submitted to CMS using the process described above. The HCPCS Workgroup is an internal workgroup that is comprised of representatives of the major components of CMS, the Veterans Administration, the Medicaid State agencies, and the SADMERC. The SADMERC participates on the workgroup as a representative for the four DMERCs.

When a recommendation for a modification to the HCPCS is received at CMS, it is reviewed at a regularly scheduled meeting of the HCPCS Workgroup. Ordinarily, the HCPCS Workgroup meets monthly. After considering a coding request, the HCPCS Workgroup decides what recommendation CMS will make to the HCPCS National Panel regarding whether the coding request warrants a change to the national permanent codes. It may also establish a temporary Medicare national code pending National Panel action. The Workgroup's recommendations to the National Panel ordinarily fall into one of the following categories:

1. **Add a Code**

   There is no existing code that matches the item or service described in the coding request and data indicate that there will be sufficient claims activity to warrant the need for a new code. This recommendation is not made when there is already an existing code that describes an item or service that is essentially equivalent to the item or service for which a new code has been requested. In addition, this recommendation is not made if the item or service is not primarily diagnostic or therapeutic in nature or if it represents a professional health care service that would fall under Level I of the HCPCS.

   In those cases in which the HCPCS Workgroup decides to recommend to the National Panel that a new code be established, the Workgroup also considers whether the coding request warrants the establishment of a temporary code. A temporary code would be assigned when it is necessary for the efficient operation of the Medicare/Medicaid programs that an item be assigned a separate code without waiting for the next annual update for national permanent codes.

2. **Use an Existing Code that Describes the Item or Service**

   There is an existing code that matches the item described in the coding request. For the efficiency of the HCPCS, the workgroup does not recommend separate codes for like products, that is, like products should fit within the same code.

3. **Use an Existing Code for Miscellaneous Items or Services**

   A miscellaneous code should be used to describe the item identified in the coding request. This recommendation is made when there is no existing code that matches the item described in the coding request but the HCPCS Workgroup expects that so few claims will be submitted for the item that a separate code is not warranted. For example, the request may be for a code for an item that is not covered by Medicare.

4. **Revise an Existing Code**

   An existing code descriptor should be revised to better describe the category of items or services it represents.

5. **Delete an Existing Code**

   An existing code should be deleted because it no longer serves a useful purpose.

   Based on the nature of the coding request, any one or a combination of the above recommendations could be made in response to a request for a change in the HCPCS.

Evaluating HCPCS Coding Requests

The HCPCS workgroup applies the following criteria to determine whether there is a demonstrated need for a new or modified code or the need to remove a code:

- When an existing code adequately describes the item in a coding request, then no new or modified code is established. An existing code adequately describes an item in a coding request when the existing code describes products with the following:
  - Functions similar to the item in the coding request.
  - No significant therapeutic distinctions from the item in the coding request.

- When an existing code describes products that are almost the same in function with only minor distinctions from the item in the coding request, the item in the coding request may be grouped with that code and the code descriptor modified to reflect the distinctions.

- A code is not established for an item that is used only in the inpatient setting or for an item that is not diagnostic or therapeutic in nature.

- A new or modified code is not established for an item unless the FDA allows the item to be marketed.

- There must be sufficient claims activity or volume, as evidenced by 6 months of marketing activity, so that the adding of a new or modified code enhances the efficiency of the system and justifies the administrative burden of adding or modifying a code.

- An item must be used at least 3 percent of the time or more in outpatient settings as opposed to inpatient settings.

- The determination to remove a code is based on the consideration of whether a code is obsolete (for example, products no longer are used, other more specific codes have been added) or duplicative and no longer useful (for example, new codes are established that better describe items identified by existing codes).

- In developing its recommendations for the National Panel, the HCPCS Workgroup uses the criteria mentioned above. In deciding upon a recommendation, the workgroup does not include cost as a factor.

National Panel

The National Panel has been in existence since the 1980's, and is responsible for managing the standardized, national HCPCS Level II permanent codes. Temporary codes are managed by CMS or other insurers to meet their particular program needs. While we are only one member of the National Panel, our staff manages the administrative process for maintaining HCPCS Level II codes. We receive all of the requests for modifications to the coding system, we make these requests available to the other Panel members, and chair the National Panel meetings that are held to discuss and make decisions regarding these requests.

The National Panel is responsible for making the final decisions pertaining to additions, deletions, and modifications to the HCPCS codes. The National Panel jointly reviews all requests for coding changes and makes final decisions regarding the annual update to the national codes. Changes to the permanent codes are not approved unless there is a unanimous vote in favor of the change by all three members of the Panel. The Panel sends letters to those who requested coding modifications to inform them of the Panel's decision regarding their coding requests. The decision letters include the following types of responses:

- As indicated by the enclosure to this letter, a change to the national codes has been approved that reflects, completely or in part, your coding request. (Approximately 65 percent of the requesters receive this type of response.)

- our request for a coding modification to this year's update has not been approved because the scope of your request necessitates that additional consideration be given to your request before the Panel reaches a final decision.

- Your reported sales volume was insufficient to support your request for a modification to the national codes. To determine whether there is sufficient sales volume to warrant a permanent code, we ask requestors to submit 6 months of the most recent sales volume.

- Your request for a new national code has not been approved because there already is an existing permanent or temporary code that describes your product.

- Your request for a code has not been approved because your product is not used by health care providers for diagnostic or therapeutic purposes.

- Your request for a code has not been approved because the code you requested is for capital equipment.

- Your request for a code has not been approved because your product is an integral part of another service and payment for that service includes payment for your product; therefore, your product may not be billed separately to Medicare.
- Your request for a modification to the language that describes the current code has not been approved because it does not improve the code descriptor.
- Your request for a new code has not been approved because your product is not primarily medical in nature (for example, generally not useful in the absence of an illness or injury).
- Your request for a code has not been approved because your product is used exclusively in the inpatient hospital setting.

Decision letters also inform the requestors that they may contact their Medicare contractor for assistance in answering any coding questions pertaining to Medicare. A requestor who is dissatisfied with the Panel's decision may submit a new request asking the Panel to reconsider and re-evaluate the code request. At that time, the requestor should include new information or additional explanations to support the request. This is not an appeal process per se, but an entirely new submission asking for a coding change, which we believe is an even more complete avenue of appeal.

HCPCS/Medicare Website

To provide information to suppliers and manufacturers regarding the HCPCS coding system, CMS has a Medicare HCPCS website. CMS's website, http://cms.hhs.gov/medicare/hcpcs/default.asp lists all of the current HCPCS codes, an alphabetical index of HCPCS codes by type of service or product, and an alphabetical table of drugs for which there are Level II codes. The website also includes a copy of the agenda for the upcoming National Panel meetings. Interested parties can submit comments regarding the agenda items to the National Panel by sending an email to CMS through this website. These comments are included as part of the National Panel's review as it considers the coding requests.

2 Load, hook prosthesis, L6795

3-in-1 composite commode, E0164

A

Abarelix, J0128

Abbokinase, J3364, J3365

Abscess, incision and drainage, D7510-D7520

Abciximab, J0130

Abdomen/abdominal
dressing holder/binder, A4462
pad, low profile, L1270

Abdominal binder
elastic, A4462

Abduction
control, each L2624
pillow, E1399
rotation bar, foot, L3140-L3170

Ablation
renal tumors, S2090-S2091

Abortion, S2260-S2267

Absorption dressing, A6251-A6256

Abutments
for implants, D6056-D6057
retainers for resin bonded "Maryland bridge," D6545

Access system, A4301

Accession of tissue, dental, D0472-D0474

Accessories
ambulation devices, E0153-E0159
artificial kidney and machine (see also ESRD), E1510-E1699
beds, E0271-E0280, E0305-E0326
wheelchairs, E0950-E1001, E1050-E1298, K0001-K0108

AccuChek
blood glucose meter, E0607
test strips, box of 50, A4253

Accu Hook, prosthesis, L6790

Accurate
prosthetic sock, L8420-L8435
stump sock, L8470-L8485

Acetate concentrate for hemodialysis, A4708

Acetazolamide sodium, J1120

Acetylcysteine, inhalation solution, J7608

Achromycin, J0120

Acid concentrate for hemodialysis, A4709

ACTH, J0800

Acthar, J0800

Actimmune, J9216

Action neoprene supports, L1825

Action Patriot manual wheelchair, K0004

Action Xtra, Action MVP, Action Pro-T, manual wheelchair, K0005

Active Life
convex one-piece urostomy pouch, A4421
flush away, A5051
one-piece
drainable custom pouch, A5061
pre-cut closed-end pouch, A5051
stoma cap, A5055

Acyclovir, Q4075
sodium, S0071

Adalimumab, J0135

Adaptor
neurostimulator, C1883
pacing lead, C1883

Addition
cushion AK, L5648
cushion BK, L5646
harness upper extremity, L6675-L6676
wrist, flexion, extension, L6620

Adenocard, J0150

Adenosine, J0150-J0152

Adhesive
barrier, C1765
catheter, A4364
disc or foam pad, A5126
medical, A4364
Nu-Hope
1 oz bottle with applicator, A4364
3 oz bottle with applicator, A4364
ostomy, A4364
pads, A6203-A6205, A6212-A6214, A6219-A6221, A6237-A6239, A6245-A6247, A6254-A6256
remover, A4365, A4455
support, breast prosthesis, A4280
tape, A4450, A4452
tissue, G0168

Adjunctive services, dental, D9220-D9310

Adjustabrace™ 3, L2999

Adjustment, bariatric band, S2083

Administration, medication, T1502
direct observation, H0033

Adoptive immunotherapy, S2107

Admission, direct, for chest pain, G0263

Adrenal transplant, S2103

Adrenalin, J0170

Adriamycin, J9000

Adrucil, J9190

AdvantaJet, A4210

AFO, E1815, E1830, L1900-L1990, L4392, L4396

Agalsidase beta, J0180, S0159

A-hydroCort, J1720

Aimsco Ultra Thin syringe, 1 cc or 1/2 cc, each, A4206

Air ambulance (see also **Ambulance**)

Air bubble detector, dialysis, E1530

Aircast, L4350-L4380

Air fluidized bed, E0194

Airlife Brand Misty-Neb nebulizer, E0580

Air pressure pad/mattress, E0186, E0197

AirSep, E0601

Air travel and nonemergency transportation, A0140

Aircast air stirrup ankle brace, L1906

Akineton, J0190

Alarm, pressure, dialysis, E1540

Alatrofloxacin mesylate, J0200

Albumarc, P9041

Albumin, human, P9041

Albuterol
administered through DME, J7611, J7613
with ipratropium bromide, J7616

Alcohol
abuse service, H0047
pint, A4244
testing, H0048
wipes, A4245

Aldesleukin, J9015

Aldomet, J0210

Aldurazyme, J1931, S0158

Alefacept, J0215
intramuscular, C9212
intravenous C9211

Alemtuzumab, J9010
injection, S0088

Alferon N, J9215

Algiderm, alginate dressing, A6196-A6199

Alginate dressing, A6196-A6199

Alglucerase, J0205

Algosteril, alginate dressing, A6196-A6199

Alimta, J9305

Alkaban-AQ, J9360

Alkaline battery for blood glucose monitor, A4254

Alkeran, J8600

Allkare protective barrier wipe, box of 100, A5119

Allogenic cord blood harvest, S2140

Allograft
small intestine and liver, S2053
soft dental tissue, D4275

Alpha 1-proteinase inhibitor, human, J0256

Alteplase recombinant, J2997

Alternating pressure mattress/pad, E0180, E0181, E0277
pump, E0182

Alternative communication device, i.e., communication board, E1902

Anchor, screw, C1713

Avastin, J9035, S0116

Alveoloplasty, D7310, D7320, D7321
with extraction(s), D7311

Alveolus, fracture, D7770

Amalgam, restoration, dental, D2140-D2161

Amantadine hydrochloride, G9017

Ambulance, A0021-A0999
air, A0436
disposable supplies, A0382-A0398
oxygen, A0422
response, treatment, no transport, T2006

Ambulation device, E0100-E0159

Ambulation stimulator
spinal cord injured, K0600

Amcort, J3302

A-methaPred, J2920, J2930

Amevive, C9211, C9212

Amifostine, J0207

Amikacin sulfate, S0072

Aminaid, enteral nutrition, B4154

Aminocaproic acid, S0017

Aminophylline/Aminophyllin, J0280

Aminolevulinic acid, topical, J7308

Amiodarone hydrochloride, J0282

Amitriptyline HCl, J1320

Amirosyn-RF, parenteral nutrition, B5000

Ammonia N-13
diagnostic imaging agent, A9526

Ammonia test paper, A4774

Amobarbital, J0300

Amphocin, J0285

Amphotericin B, J0285
cholesterol sulfate, J0288
lipid complex, J0287
liposome, J0289

Ampicillin sodium, J0290
sodium/sulbactam sodium, J0295

Amputee
adapter, wheelchair, E0959
prosthesis, L5000-L7510, L7520, L7900, L8400-L8465
stump sock, L8470
wheelchair, E1170-E1190, E1200

Amygdalin, J3570

Amytal, J0300

Anabolin LA 100, J2320-J2322

Analgesia, dental, D9230, D9241, D9242
non-intravenous conscious sedation, D9248

Anastrozole, S0170

Ancef, J0690

Andrest 90-4, J0900

Andro-Cyp, J1070-J1080

Andro-Estro 90-4, J0900

Androgyn L.A., J0900

Andro L.A. 200, J3130

Androlone
-D 100, J2321

Andronaq
-LA, J1070

Andronate
-100, J1070
-200, J1080

Andropository 100, J3120

Andryl 200, J3130

Anectine, J0330

Anergan (25, 50), J2550

Anesthesia
dental, D9210-D9221
dialysis, A4736-A4737

Angiography
coronary arteries S8093
digital subtraction, S9022
Iliac artery, C0278
magnetic resonance, C8901-C8914, C8918-C8920
reconstruction, G0288
renal artery, G0275

Anistreplase, J0350

Ankle-foot orthosis (AFO; *see also*
Orthopedic shoe, and tibia), L1900-L1990, L2106-L2116
Dorsiwedge Night Splint, L4398 or A4570 or L2999
Specialist™
Ankle Foot Orthosis, L1930
Tibial Pre-formed Fracture Brace, L2116
Surround™ Ankle Stirrup Braces with Floam™, L1906

Anterior-posterior orthosis
lateral orthosis, L0520, L0560-L0565, L0700, L0710

Antibiotic home infusion therapy, S9494-S9504

Antibody testing, HIV-1, S3645

Anticeptic
chlorhexidine, A4248

Anticoagulation clinic, S9401

Antiemetic drug, prescription
oral, Q0163-Q0181
rectal, K0416

Antifungal home infusion therapy, S9494-9504

Anti-hemophilic factor (Factor VIII), J7190-J7192

Anti-inhibitors, J7198

Anti-neoplastic drug, NOC, J9999

Antispas, J0500

Antithrombin III, J7197

Antiviral home infusion therapy, S9494-S9504

Anzemet, J1260

Apexification, dental, D3351-D3353

Apicoectomy, dental, D3410-D3426

A.P.L., J0725

Apnea monitor, E0618-E0619
electrodes, A4556
lead wires, A4557
with recording feature, E0619

Appliance
cleaner, A5131
orthodontic,
fixed, D8220
removable, D8210
removal, D7997
pneumatic, E0655-E0673

Apomorphine hydrochloride, S0167

Aprepitant, J8501

Apresoline, J0360

Aprotinin, Q2003

AquaMEPHYTON, J3430

AquaPedic sectional gel flotation, E0196

Aqueous
shunt, L8612
sterile, J7051

Ara-C, C9422

Aralen, J0390

Aramine, J0380

Aranesp, Q0137

Arbutamine HCl, J0395

Arch support, L3040-L3100

Aredia, C9411, J2430

Argatroban, C9121

Argyle Sentinel Seal chest drainage unit, E0460

Aristocort
forte, J3302
intralesional, J3302

Aristospan
Intra-articular, J3303
Intralesional, J3303

Arm
sling
deluxe, A4565
mesh cradle, A4565
universal
arm, A4565
elevator, A4565
wheelchair, E0973

Arrestin, J3250

Arrow, power wheelchair, K0014

Arsenic trioxide, J9017

Arthrocentesis, dental, D7870

Arthroplasty, dental, D7865

Arthroscopy
knee
harvest of cartilage, S2112
removal loose body, FB, G0289
shoulder
with capsulorrhaphy, S2300

Arthroscopy, dental, D7872-D7877

Arthrotomy, dental, D7860

Artificial
kidney machines and accessories (*see also* Dialysis), E1510-E1699
larynx, L8500

Asparaginase, J9020

Aspart insulin, S5551

Aspiration, bone marrow, G0364

Assessment
audiologic, V5008-V5020
family, H1011
geriatric, S0250
mental health, H0031
nursing, G0264
speech, V5362-V5364

Assertive community treatment, H0039-H0040

Assistive listening device, V5268-V5274
alerting device, V5269
cochlear implant assistive device, V5273
TDD, V5272
telephone amplifier, V5268
television caption decoder, V5271

Assisted living, T2030-T2031

Asthma
education, S9441
observation for, G0244

Astramorph, J2275

Atgam, J7504

Ativan, J2060

Atropine
inhalation solution
concentrated, J7635
unit dose, J7636
sulfate, J0460

Attends, adult diapers, A4335

Audiologic assessment, V5008-V5020

Audiometry, S0618

Auricular prosthesis, D5914, D5927

Aurothioglucose, J2910

Autoclix lancet device, A4258

Auto-Glide folding walker, E0143

Autolance lancet device, A4258

Autolet lancet device, A4258

Autolet Lite lancet device, A4258

Autolet Mark II lancet device, A4258

Autoplex T, J7198

Avonex, J1825

Azacitidine, C9218. S0168

Azathioprine, J7500, J7501
parenteral, C9436

Azithromycin
injection, J0456

Aztreonam, S0073

B

Babysitter, child of parents in treatment, T1009

Back supports, L0700-L0960

Baclofen, J0475, J0476
intrathecal refill kit, C9008, C9009
intrathecal screening kit, C9007
per 2000 mcg
refill kit, C9009

Bacterial sensitivity study, P7001

Bactocill, J2700

Bag
drainage, A4357
irrigation supply, A4398
spacer, for metered dose inhaler, A4627
urinary, A4358, A5112

BAL in oil, J0470

Balken, fracture frame, E0946

Bandage
- compression
  - high, A6452
  - light, A6448-A6450
  - medium, A6451
- conforming, AA6442-A6447
- Orthoflex elastic plastic bandages, A4580
- padding, A6441
- self-adherent, A6453-A6455
- Specialist Plaster bandages, A4580

Banflex, J2360

Bariatric
- bed, E0302-E0304
- surgery, S2082, S2083

Barium enema, G0106
- cancer screening, G0120

Barrier
- 4 x 4, A4372
- adhesion, C1765
- with flange, A4373

Baseball finger splint, A4570

Basiliximab, Q2019

Bath chair, E0240

Bathtub
- chair, E0240
- heat unit, E0249
- stool or bench, E0245
- transfer bench, E0247, E0248
- transfer rail, E0246
- wall rail, E0241, E0242

Battery, L7360, L7364
- blood glucose monitor, A4254
- charger, L7362, L7366
- cochlear implant device
  - alkaline, L8622
  - lithium, L2620
  - zinc, L8621
- hearing device, V5266
- infusion pump, A4632
- lithium, L7367
  - charger, L7368
- replacement
  - ear pulse generator, A4638
  - external defibrillator, K0607
  - external infusion pump, K0601-K0605
  - TENS, A4630
  - ventilator, A4611-A4613

Bayer chemical reagent strips, box of 100 glucose/ketone urine test strips, A4250

BCG live, intravesical, J9031

BCW 600, manual wheelchair, K0007

BCW Power, power wheelchair, K0014

BCW recliner, manual wheelchair, K0007

B-D alcohol swabs, box, A4245

B-D disposable insulin syringes, up to 1cc, per syringe, A4206

B-D lancets, per box of 100, A4258

Bebax, foot orthosis, L3160

Becaplermin gel, S0157

Becker, hand prosthesis
- Imperial, L6840
- Lock Grip, L6845
- Plylite, L6850

Bed
- air fluidized, E0194
- accessory, E0315
- cradle, any type, E0280
- drainage bag, bottle, A4357, A5102
- extra size for bariatric patients, E0302-E0304
- hospital, E0250-E0270
  - full electric, home care, without mattress, E0297
  - manual, without mattress, E0293
  - safety enclosure frame/canopy, E0316

Bed — *continued*
- hospital — *continued*
  - semi-electric, without mattress, E0295
  - pan, E0275, E0276
    - Moore, E0275
  - rail, E0305, E0310
  - safety enclosure frame/canopy, hospital bed, E0316

Behavior management, dental care, D9920

Behavioral health, H0002-H0030
- day treatment, H2013
- per hour, H2012

Bell-Horn
- prosthetic shrinker, L8440-L8465

Belt
- adapter, A4421
- extremity, E0945
- Little Ones Sur-Fit pediatric, A4367
- ostomy, A4367
- pelvic, E0944
- wheelchair, E0978

Bena-D (10, 50), J1200

Benadryl, J1200

Benahist (10, 50), J1200

Ben-Allergin-50, J1200

Bench, bathtub (*see also* **Bathtub**), E0245

Benesch boot, L3212-L3214

Benoject (-10, -50), J1200

Bentyl, J0500

Benztropine, J0515

Berkeley shell, foot orthosis, L3000

Berubigen, J3420

Betadine, A4246
- swabs/wipes, A4247

Betalin 12, J3420

Betameth, J0704

Betamethasone, J7622-J7624
- acetate and betamethasone sodium phosphate, J0702
- sodium phosphate, J0704

Betaseron, J1830

Bethanechol chloride, J0520

Bevacizumab, J9035, S0116

Bicarbonate concentration for hemodialysis, A4706-A4707

Bicillin, Bicillin C-R, Bicillin C-R 900/300, and Bicillin L-A, J0530-J0580

BiCNU, J9050

Bifocal, glass or plastic, V2200-V2299

Bilirubin (phototherapy) light, E0202

Binder
- extremity, nonelastic, A4465
- lumbar-sacral-orthosis (LSO), A4462

Biofeedback device, E0746

Bio Flote alternating air pressure pump, pad system, E0181, E0182

Biologic materials, dental, D4265

Biologics, unclassified, J3590

Biopsy
- bone marrow with aspiration, G0364
- hard tissue, dental, D7285
- soft tissue, dental, D7286
- transepithelial brush, D7288

Biperiden lactate, J0190

Birth control pills, S4993

Birthing classes, S9436-S9439, S9442

Bite disposable jaw locks, E0700

Bitewing radiographs, D0270-D0277

Bitolterol mesylate, inhalation solution
- concentrated, J7628
- unit dose, J7629

Bivalirudin, J0583

Bleaching, dental
- external, per arch, D9972
- external, per tooth, D9973
- internal, per tooth, D9974

Blenoxane, J9040

Bleomycin sulfate, C9417, J9040

Blood
- Congo red, P2029
- glucose monitor, A4258, E0607
  - with voice synthesizer, E2100
  - with integrated lancing system, E2101
- glucose test strips, A4253
- leak detector, dialysis, E1560
- leukocyte poor, P9016
- mucoprotein, P2038
- pressure equipment, A4660, A4663, A4670
- pump, dialysis, E1620
- strips, A4253
- supply, P9010-P9022
- testing supplies, A4770
- transfusion, home, S9538
- tubing, A4750, A4755
  - leukocytes reduced, P9051-P9056
  - CMV-negative, P9051, P9053, P9055

Bock, hand prosthesis, L6875, L6880

Bock Dynamic, foot prosthesis, L5972

Bock, Otto (*see* **Otto Bock**)

Body jacket
- scoliosis, L1300, L1310

Body sock, L0984

Body wrap
- foam positioners, E0191
- therapeutic overlay, E0199

Bond or cement, ostomy, skin, A4364

Bone replacement graft, dental, D7953

Bone tissue excision, dental, D7471-D7490

Boot
- pelvic, E0944
- surgical, ambulatory, L3260
- walking
  - non-pneumatic, L4386
  - pneumatic, L4360

Bortezomib, J9041

Boston type spinal orthosis, L1200

Botulinum toxin
- type A, J0585
- type B, J0587

Brachytherapy
- cesium 131, C2633
- gold 198 C1716
- HA
  - 103, C2635
  - 125, C2634
- high dose rate iridium 192, C1717
- iodine 125, C1718
- linear P-10, C2636
- needle, C1715
- non-high dose rate iridium 192, C1719
- palladium 103, C1720
- radioelements, Q3001
- source, C1716-C1720, C2616
- yttrium 90, C2616

Brake attachment, wheeled walker, E0159

Breas PV10, E0601

Breast
  exam (with pelvic exam), G0101
  mammography, G0202-G0206
  milk processing, T2101
  prosthesis, L8000-L8035, L8600
    adhesive skin support, A4280
  pump, E0602-E0604
    supplies, A4281-A4286

Breathing circuit, A4618

Brethine, J3105

Bricanyl subcutaneous, J3105

Bridge
  recement, D6930
  repair, by report, D6980

Brompheniramine maleate, J0945

Broncho-Cath endobronchial tubes, with CPAP system, E0601

Bruxism appliance, D9940

Buck's, traction
  frame, E0870
  stand, E0880

Budesonide, J7626, J7633

Bulb for therapeutic light box, A4634

Bumetanide, S0171

Bupivicaine, S0020

Buprenorphine hydrochloride, J0592

Bupropion HCl, S0106

Burn garment, A6501, A6512

Bus, nonemergency, A0110

Busulfan, injection, C1178

Butorphanol tartrate, J0595
  nasal spray, S0012

C

Cabergoline, Q2001

Caffeine citrate, J0706

Calcimar, J0630

Calcitonin-salmon, J0630

Calcitrol, S0161, J0636

Calcium
  disodium edetate, J0600
  disodium versenate, J0600
  EDTA, J0600
  gluconate, J0610
  glycerophosphate and calcium lactate, J0620
  lactate and calcium glycerophosphate, J0620
  leucovorin, J0640

Calibrator solution, A4256

Calphosan, J0620

Camisole, post mastectomy, S8460

Camping therapy, T2036-T2037

Camptosar, J9206

Canavan disease, genetic test, S3851

Cancer screening
  breast exam, G0101
  barium enema, G0122
  cervical exam, G0101
  colorectal, G0104-G0106, G0120-G0122, G0328
  prostate, G0102-G0103

Cane, E0100, E0105
  accessory, A4636, A4637
  Easy-Care quad, E0105
  quad canes, E0105
  Quadri-Poise, E0105
  wooden canes, E0100

Canister
  disposable, used with suction pump, A7000
  non-disposable, used with suction pump, A7001

Cannula
  fistula, set (for dialysis), A4730
  nasal, A4615
  tracheostomy, A4623

Canolith, repositioning, S9092

Capecitabine, oral, J8520, J8521

Carbocaine with Neo-Cobefrin, J0670

Carbon filter, A4680

Carboplatin, J9045

Cardiac event, recorder implantable, C1764, E0616

Cardiokymography, Q0035

Cardiovascular services, M0300-M0301

Cardioverter-defibrillator, C1721, C1722, C1882

Cardioverter defibrillator pulse generator, G0297
  dual chamber
    insertion, G0300
    repositioning, G0300
  single chamber
    insertion, G0298-G0299

Carelet safety lancet, A4258

Carex
  adjustable bath/shower stool, E0245
  aluminum crutches, E0114
  cane, E0100
  folding walker, E0135
  shower bench, E0245

Carmus bischl nitro, C9437

Carmustine, J9050

Carnitor, J1955

Case management, T1016-T1017
  per month, T2022

Casec, enteral nutrition, B4155

Cash, spinal orthosis, L0370

Caspofungin acetate, J0637

Cast
  dental diagnostic study models, D0470
  diagnostic, dental, D0470
  gauntlet, Q4013-Q4016
  hand restoration, L6900-L6915
  hip spica, Q4025-Q4028
  long arm, Q4005-Q4008
  materials, special, A4590
  padding, (not separately reimbursable from the casting procedure or casting supplies codes)
    Delta-Rol™ Cast Padding
    Sof-Rol™ Cast Padding
    Specialist™ 100 Cotton Cast Padding
    Specialist™ Cast Padding
  plaster, A4580
  post and core, dental, D2952
    each additional, D2953
  short arm, Q4009-Q4012
  shoulder, Q4003-Q4004
  supplies, A4580, A4590, Q4050
    Delta-Cast™ Elite™ Casting Material, A4590
    Delta-Lite™ Conformable Casting Tape, A4590
    Delta-Lite™ C-Splint™ Fibreglass Immobilizer, A4590
    Delta-Lite™ "S" Fibreglass Casting Tape, A4590
    Flashcast™ Elite™ Casting Material, A4590
    Orthoflex™ Elastic Plaster Bandages, A4580
    Orthoplast™ Splints (and Orthoplast™ II Splints), A4590

Cast — *continued*
  supplies — *continued*
    Specialist™ J-Splint™ Plaster Roll Immobilizer
    Specialist™ Plaster Bandages, A4580
    Specialist™ Plaster Roll Immobilizer, A4580
    Specialist™ Plaster Splints, A4580
  thermoplastic, L2106, L2126

Caster, wheelchair, E0997, E0998, K0099

Catheter, A4300-A4365
  anchoring device, A4333, A4334
    percutaneous, A5200
  balloon, C1727
  brachytherapy, C1728
  cap, disposable (dialysis), A4860
  drainage, C1729
  electrophysiology, C2630
  diagnostic, C1730, C1731
    ablation, C1732, C1733
  external collection device, A4326-A4330, A4348
  guiding, C1887
  hemodialysis, C1750, C1752
  implantable access, A4301
  implantable intraspinal, E0785
  indwelling, A4338-A4346
  infusion, C1752
  insertion tray, A4354
  intermittent, with insertion supplies, A4353
  intracardiac echocardiography, C1759
  intradiscal, C1754
  intraspinal, C1755
  intravascular ultrasound, C1753
  irrigation supplies, A4355
  lubricant, A4332
  male, A4349
  non-vascular balloon dilatation, C1726
  occlusion, C2628
  oropharyngeal suction, A4628
  pacing, transesophageal, C1756
  suprapubic, cystoscopic, C2627
  thrombectomy, embolectomy, C1757
  pleural, A7042
  tracheal suction, A4605, A4624
  transluminal
    angioplasty
      laser, C1885
      nonlaser, C1725
    atherectomy
      directional, C1714
      rotational, C1724
  ureteral, C1758

CBC, G0306-G0307

Cefadyl, J0710

Cefazolin sodium, J0690

Cefepime HCl, J0692

Cefizox, J0715

Cefotaxime sodium, J0698

Cefotetan disodium, S0074

Cefoxitin, J0694

Ceftazidime, J0713

Ceftizoxime sodium, J0715

Ceftriaxone sodium, J0696

Ceftoperazone, S0021

Cefuroxime sodium, J0697

Celestone phosphate, J0704

Cellular therapy, M0075

Cel-U-Jec, J0704

Cement, ostomy, A4364

Cenacort
  A-40, J3301
  Forte, J3302

Centrifuge, for dialysis, E1500

Cephalin flocculation, blood, P2028

Cephalothin sodium, J1890

Cephapirin sodium, J0710

Ceredase, J0205

Cerezyme, J1785

Certified nurse assistant, S9122

Cerubidine, J9150

Cerumen removal, G0268

Cervical
collar, L0120, L0130, L0140, L0150
halo, L0810-L0830
head harness/halter, E0942
helmet, L0100, L0110
Softop, leather protective, L0110
orthosis, L0100-L0200
traction equipment, not requiring frame,
E0855

Cervical cap contraceptive, A4261

**Cervical-thoracic-lumbar-sacral orthosis
(CTLSO)**, L0700, L0710, L1000

Cetuximab, J9055

Chair
adjustable, dialysis, E1570
bathtub, E0240
lift, E0627
rollabout, E1031
shower or bath, E0240
sitz bath, E0160-E0162

Challenger manual wheelchair, K0009

Champion 1000 manual wheelchair,
K0004

Champion 30000, manual wheelchair,
K0005

Chealamide, J3520

Chelation therapy, M0300
home infusion, administration, S9355

CheckMate Plus blood glucose monitor,
E0607

Chemical endarterectomy, M0300

Chemistry and toxicology tests, P2028-
P3001

Chemodenervation, vocal cord, S2341

Chemotherapy
antineoplastic
hormonal, G0356
non-hormonal, G0355
assessment
fatigue, G9029-G9032
nausea and vomiting, G9021-G9024
pain, G9025-G9028
dental, D4381
drug, oral, not otherwise classified,
J8999
drugs (*see also* **drug by name**), J9000-
J9999
home infusion, continous, S9325-S9379,
S9494-S9497
infusion, G0359-G0362

**Chemstrip bG, box of 50 blood glucose
test strips**, A4253

**Chemstrip K, box of 100 ketone urine
test strips**, A4250

**Chemstrip UGK, box of 100 glucose/
ketone urine test strips**, A4250

Chest pain, observation for, G0244

Chest shell (cuirass), E0457

Chest wrap, E0459

CHF, observation for, G0244

Childbirth class, S9442
cesarean birth, S9438
Lamaze, S9436
preparation, S9436
refresher, S9437
VBAC (vaginal birth after cesarean), S9439

Childcare, T2026-T2027

Childcare, parents in treatment, T1009

Chin
cup, cervical, L0150
strap (for CPAP device), A7036

Chlorambucil, S0172

Chloramphenicol sodium succinate,
J0720

Chlordiazepoxide HCl, J1990

Chlorhexidine, A4248

Chloromycetin sodium succinate, J0720

Chloroprocaine HCl, J2400

Chloroquine HCl, J0390

Chlorothiazide sodium, J1205

Chlorpromazine HCl, J3230, Q0171-
Q0172

Chondrocyte cell harvest, arthroscopic,
S2112

Chopart prosthetic
ankle, L5050, L5060
below knee, L5100

Chorex (-5, -10), J0725

Chorignon, J0725

Chorionic gonadotropin, J0725

Choron 10, J0725

Chromic phosphate, Q3011

Chronimed Comfort insulin infusion set
23", A4230
43", A4230

Chux's, A4554

Cida
exostatic cervical collar, L0140, L0150
form fit collar, L0120

Cidofovir, J0740

Cilastatin sodium, imipenem, J0743

Cimetidine hydrochloride, S0023

Cisplatin, J9060, J9062
powder or solution, C9418

Ciprofloxacin, J0744

Cladribine, C9419, J9065

Claforan, J0698

Clamp
external urethral, A4356

Classes, S9441-S9446
asthma, S9441
birthing, S9442
lactation, S9443

Clavicle
splint, L3650, L3660
support
2-buckle closure, L3660
4-buckle closure, L3660

Cleaning solvent, Nu-Hope
4 oz bottle, A4455
16 oz bottle, A4455

Cleanser, wound, A6260

Cleft palate, feeder, S8265

Clindamycin phosphate, S0077

Clonidine, J0735

Closure device, vascular, C1760

Clozapine, S0136

Clevis, hip orthosis, L2570, L2600, L2610

Clinic visit/encounter, T1015
multidisciplinary, child services, T1025

Clinical trials
lodging costs, S9994
meals, S9996
phase II, S9990
phase III, S9991

Clinical trials — *continued*
service, S9988
transportation costs, S9992

Clotting time tube, A4771

Clubfoot wedge, L3380

Cobaltous chloride, C9013

Cobex, J3420

Cochlear implant
battery
alkaline, L8622
lithium L8620
headset, L8615
microphone, L8616
transmitter cable, L8618
transmitting coil, L8617
zinc, L8621

Cochlear prosthetic implant, L8614
replacement, L8619

Codeine phosphate, J0745

Codimal-A, J0945

Cogentin, J0515

Coil, imaging, C1770

Colchicine, J0760

Colistimethate sodium, J0770

Collagen
implant, urinary tract, L8603
skintest, Q3031
wound dressing, A6021-A6024

Collar, cervical
contour (low, standard), L0120
multiple, post, L0180-L0200
nonadjust (foam), L0120
Philly™ One-piece™ extrication collar,
L0150
tracheotomy, L0172
Philadelphia™ tracheotomy cervical
collar, L0172
traction, E0942
Turtle Neck safety collars, E0942

**Collection microorganisms for culture
and sensitivity**, D0415

Colonoscopy, cancer screening
patient at high risk, G0105
patient not at high risk, G0121

Coloplast
closed pouch, A5051
drainable pouch, A5061
closed, A5054
small, A5063
skin barrier
4 x 4, A4362
6 x 6, A5121
8 x 8, A5122
stoma cap, A5055

Coly-Mycin M, J0770

Coma stimulation, S9056

**Combined connective tissue and double
pedicle graft, dental**, D4276

Combo-Seat universal raised toilet seat,
E0244

Commode, E0160-E0169
"3-in-1" Composite, E0164
Economy VersaGuard Coated, E0164
lift, E0625
pail, E0167
seat, wheelchair, E0968

Communication board, E1902

Compa-Z, J0780

Compazine, J0780

Composite dressing, A6203-A6205

Compressed gas system, E0424-E0480,
L3902

Compression
burn garment, A6501-A6512
stockings, L8100-L8239

Compression bandage
high, A6452
light, A6448
medium, A6451

Compressogrip prosthetic shrinker, L8440-L8465

Compressor, E0565, E0570, E0650-E0652

Concentrator
oxygen, E1390, E1391

Condom
male, A4267
female, A4268

Conductive
garment (for TENS), E0731
paste or gel, A4558

Conductivity meter (for dialysis), E1550

Condylectomy, D7840

Conforming bandage, A6442-A6447

Congenital torticollis orthotic, L0112

Congo red, blood, P2029

Connector bar, dental, D6920
dental implant, supported, D6055

Conscious sedation, dental, D9241-D9242

Consultation
dental slides, D0484
biopsy, D0485

Consultation, dental, D9210

Contact layer, A6206-A6208

Contact lens, S0500, S0512-S0514, V2500-V2599

Continent device, A5081, A5082

Continuous positive airway pressure (CPAP) device, E0601
chin strap, A7036
face mask, A7030-A7031
filter, A7038-A7039
headgear, A7035
nasal application accessories, A7032-A7034
oral interface, A7044
tubing, A7037

Contraceptive
cervical cap, A4261
condom
male, A4267
female, A4268
diaphragm, A4266
foam, A4269
gel, A4269
hormone patch, J7304
intrauterine, copper, J7300
Levonorgestrel, implants and supplies, A4260
pills, S4993
spermacide, A4269
vaginal ring, J7303

Contracts, maintenance, ESRD, A4890

Contrast material
injection during MRI, A4643
low osmolar, A4644-A4646

Controlyte, enteral nutrition, B4155

Coordinated care fee, G9009-G9012

Cophene-B, J0945

Coping, D2975

Coping, dental, D6975

Copying fee, medical records, S9981-S9982

Core buildup, dental, D2950, D6973

Corgonject-5, J0725

Corn, trim or remove, S0390

Corneal tissue processing, V2785

Coronary artery bypass surgery, direct
with coronary arterial grafts, only
single, S2205
two grafts, S2206
with coronary arterial and venous grafts
single, each, S2208
two arterial and single venous, S2209
with coronary venous grafts, only
single, S2207

Coronoidectomy, dental, D7991

Corset, spinal orthosis, L0970-L0976

Corticotropin, J0800

Cortrosyn, J0835

Corvert, J1742

Cosmegen, J9120

Cosyntropin, J0835

Cotranzine, J0780

Cough stimulation device, E0482

Counseling
end of life, S0257
for control of dental disease, D1310, D1320

Cover, wound
alginate dressing, A6196-A6198
foam dressing, A6209-A6214
hydrocolloid dressing, A6234-A6239
hydrogel dressing, A6242-A6248
specialty absorptive dressing, A6251-A6256

CPAP (continuous positive airway pressure) device, E0601
chin strap, A7036
exhalation port, A7045
face mask, A7030-A7031
headgear, A7035
humidifier, E0561-E0562
nasal application accessories, A7032-A7034
oral interface, A7044
supplies, E0470-E0472, E0561-E0562
tubing, A7037

Cradle, bed, E0280

Creation
anal lesions by radiofrequency, C9716

Crisis intervention, H2011, T2034

Criticare HN, enteral nutrition, B4153

Cromolyn sodium, inhalation solution, unit dose, J7631

Crown
abutment supported, D6094, D6194
additional construction, D2971
as retainer for FPD, D6720-D6792
composite resin, D2390
implant/abutment supported, D6058-D6067
implant/abutment supported retainer for FPD, D6720-D6792
indirect resin based composite, D6710
individual restoration, D2710-D2799
lengthening, D4249
prefabricated, D2930-D2933
provisional, D2799
recementation, D2920
repair, D2980
resin-based composite, D2712, D2710
stainless steel, D2934
titanium, D2794, D6794

Crutch
substitute
lower leg platform, E0118

Crutches, E0110-E0116
accessories, A4635-A4637, K0102
aluminum, E0114
articulating, spring assisted, E0117

Crutches — *continued*
forearm, E0111
Ortho-Ease, E0111
underarm, other than wood, pair, E0114
Quikfit Custom Pack, E0114
Red Dot, E0114
underarm, wood, single, E0113
Ready-for-use, E0113
wooden, E0112

Cryoprecipitate, each unit, P9012

Cryopreservation of cells, G0265

Cryosurgery
renal tumors, S2090-S2091

Crysticillin (300 A.S., 600 A.S.), J2510

CTLSO, L1000-L1120, L0700, L0710

Cubicin, J0878

Cuirass, E0457

Culture sensitivity study, P7001

Curasorb, alginate dressing, A6196-A6199

Curettage, apical, perpendicular, D3410-D3426

Cushion
decubitus care, E0190
positioning, E0190

Cushion, wheelchair, E0977
AK addition, L5648
BK addition, L5646

Customized item (in addition to code for basic item), S1002

Custom Masterhinge™ Hip Hinge 3, L2999

Cyanocobalamin cobalt, C1079, Q3012

Cycler
disposable set, A4671

Cycler dialysis machine, E1594

Cyclophosphamide, C9420, J9070-J9092
lyophilized, C9421, J9093-J9097
oral, J8530

Cyclosporine, C9438, J7502, J7515, J7516

Cylinder tank carrier, K0104

Cystourethroscopy
for uretereral calculi, S2070

Cytarabine, C9422, J9110

Cytarabine liposome, J9098

Cytarabine 100, J9100

CytoGam, J0850

Cytologic
sample collection, dental, D7287
smears, dental, D0480

Cytomegalovirus immune globulin (human), J0850

Cytopathology, screening, G0123, G0124, G0141, G0143-G0148

Cytosar-U, C9422, J9100

Cytovene, J1570

Cytoxan, J8530, J9070-J9097

D

Darbepoetin alpha
ESRD, Q4054
non-ESRD, Q0137

Dacarbazine, C9423, J9130, J9140

Daclizumab, J7513

Dactinomycin, J9120

Dalalone, J1100

Dalfopristin, J2270

Dalteparin sodium, J1645

Daptomycin, J0878

Darbepoetin alpha, J0880
  ESRD Q4054
  non-ESRD Q0137

Daunorubicin, C9424

Daunorubicin citrate, J9151
  HCl, J9150

DaunoXome, J9151

DDAVP, J2597

Debridement
  endodontic, D3221
  periodontal, D4355

Decadron, J1100

Decadron-LA, J1094

Decadron Phosphate, J1100

Deca-Durabolin, J2320-J2322

Decaject, J1100

Decaject-LA, J1094

Decalcification procedure, D0475

Decolone
  -50, J2320
  -100, J2321

De-Comberol, J1060

Decompression, disk, S2348

Decompression, vertebral axial, S9090

Decubitus care equipment, E0180-E0199
  cushion or pillow, E0190
  mattress
    AquaPedic Sectional Gel Flotation, E0196
    Iris Pressure Reduction/Relief, dry, E0184
    PressureGuard II, air, E0186
    TenderFlo II, E0187
    TenderGel II, E0196
  pressure pads, overlays, E0197-E0199
    Body Wrap, E0199
    Geo-Matt, E0199
    Iris, E0199
    PressureKair, E0197
    Richfoam Convoluted and Flat, E0199
  pressure pads, with pumps, E0180, E0181
    Bio Flote, E0181
    KoalaKair, E0181
  protectors
    Heel or elbow, E0191
      Body Wrap Foam Positioners, E0191
      Pre-Vent, E0191
  pump, E0182
    Bio Flote, E0182
    Pillo, E0182
    TenderCloud, E0182

Deferoxamine mesylate, J0895

Dehist, J0945

Dehydroergotamine mesylate, J1110

Deionizer, water purification system, E1615

Deladumone (OB), J0900

Delatest, J3120

Delatestadiol, J0900

Delatestryl, J3120, J3130

Delestrogen, J0970

Delivery/set-up/dispensing, A9901

Delta-Cortef, J7510

Delta-Cast™ Elite™ Casting Material, A4590

Delta-Lite™ Conformable Casting Tape, A4590

Delta-Lite™ C-Splint™ Fibreglass Immobilizer, A4590

Delta-Lite™ "S" Fibreglass Casting Tape, A4590

Delta-Net™ Orthopaedic Stockinet, (not separately reimbursable from the casting procedure or casting supplies codes)

Delta-Rol™ Cast Padding, (not separately reimbursable from the casting procedure or casting supplies codes)

Deltasone, J7506

Deluxe item (list in addition to code for basic item), S1001

Demadex, J3265

Demerol HCl, J2175

Demonstration project
  chemotherapy assessment, G9021-G9024
  low vision therapist, G9036
  occupational therapist, G9034
  orientation and mobility specialist, G9035
  rehabilitation teacher, G9037

Dennis Browne, foot orthosis, L3140, L3150

Dentures (removable)
  adjustments, D5410-D5422
  complete, D5110-D5140
  overdenture, D5860-D5861
  partial, D5211-D5281
    mandibular, D5226
    maxillary, D5225
  precision attachment, D5862
  rebase, D5710-D5721
  reline, D5730-D5761
  repairs, D5510, D5520, D5610-D5650
  temporary, D5810-D5821

DepAndro
  100, J1070
  200, J1080

Dep-Androgyn, J1060

DepMedalone
  40, J1030
  80, J1040

Depo-estradiol cypionate, J1000

Depogen, J1000

Depoject, J1030, J1040

Depo
  -Medrol, J1020, J1030, J1040
  -Provera, J1051, J1055
  -Testadiol, J1060
  -Testosterone, J1070, J1080

Depopred
  -40, J1030
  -80, J1040

Depotest, J1070, J1080

Depotestogen, J1060

Derata injection device, A4210

Dermagraft, C9201

Dermal tissue
  human origin, J7342, J7350

Desensitizing medicament, dental, D9910

Desensitizing resin, dental, D9911

Desferal mesylate, J0895

Desmopressin acetate, J2597

Detector, blood leak, dialysis, E1560

Device
  joint, C1776
  ocular, C1784
  retrieval, C1773
  tissue localization and excision, C1819
  urinary incontinence repair, C1771, C2631

DeVilbiss
  9000D, E0601
  9001D, E0601

Dexacen-4, J1100

Dexamethasone
  acetate, J1094
  inhalation solution
    concentrated, J7637
    unit dose, J7638
  oral, S0173
  sodium phosphate, J1100

Dexasone, J1100

Dexferrum (iron dextran), J1750

Dexone, J1100

Dexrazoxane HCl, C9410, J1190

Dextran, J7100, J7110

Dextroamphetamine sulfate, S0160

Dextrose, S5010-S5014
  saline (normal), J7042
  water, J7060, J7070

Dextrostick, A4772

D.H.E. 45, J1110

Diabetes
  alcohol swabs, per box, A4245
  battery for blood glucose monitor, A4254
  bent needle set for insulin pump infusion, A4231
  blood glucose monitor, E0607
    with integrated lancer, E2101
    with voice synthesizer, E2100
  blood glucose test strips, box of 50, A4253
  injection device, needle-free, A4210
  insulin, J1817
  insulin pump, external, E0784
  lancet device, A4258
  lancets, box of 100, A4259
  non needle cannula for insulin infusion, A4232
  retinal exam, S3000
  shoe inserts, A5502-A5511, K0628, K0629
  syringe, disposable
    box of 100, S8490
    each, A4206
  urine glucose/ketone test strips, box of 100, A4250

Diabetic management program
  E/M of sensory neuropathy, G0246-G0247
  follow-up visit to MD provider, S9141
  follow-up visit to non-MD provider, S9140
  foot care, G0247
  group session, S9455
  insulin pump initiation, S9145
  nurse visit, S9460

Diagnostic
  dental services, D0100-D0999
  radiology services, D0210-D0340

Diagnostic imaging agent
  ammonia N-13, A9526
  I-131 tositumomab, A9533
  sodium iodide I-131 A9528, A9531

Dialet lancet device, A4258

Dialysate
  concentrate additives, A4765
  peritoneal dialysis solution, A4720-A4726, A4766
  solution, A4728
  testing solution, A4760

Dialysis
  access system, C1881
  air bubble detector, E1530
  anesthetic, A4736-A4737
  bath conductivity, meter, E1550
  blood leak detector, E1560
  centrifuge, E1500

Dialysis — *continued*
cleaning solution, A4674
concentrate
acetate, A4708
acid, A4709
bicarbonate, A4706-A4707
drain bag/bottle, A4911
emergency treatment, G0257
equipment, E1510-E1702
extension line, A4672-A4673
filter, A4680
fluid barrier, E1575
heating pad, E0210
hemostats, E1637
infusion pump, E1520
home equipment repair, A4890
mask, surgical, A4928
peritoneal, A4300, A4643, A4714-A4726,
A4766 E1592, E1594
clamps, E1634
pressure alarm, E1540
scale, E1639
shunt, A4740
supplies, A4656-A4927
surgical mask, A4928
syringe, A4657
tourniquet, A4929
unipuncture control system, E1580

Dialyzer, artificial kidney, A4690

Diamox, J1120

Diaper service, T4538

Diaphragm, contraceptive, A4266

Diazepam, J3360

Diazoxide, J1730

Dibent, J0500

Didanosine, S0137

Didronel, J1436

Dietary education, S9449, S9452

Dietary planning, dental nutrition, D1310

Diethylstilbestrol, C9439
diphosphate, J9165

Diflucan injection, J1450

Digital subtraction angiography, S9022

Digoxin, J1160

Dihydrex, J1200

Dihydroergotamine mesylate, J1110

Dilantin, J1165

Dilaudid, J1170

Dilomine, J0500

Dilor, J1180

Dimenhydrinate, J1240

Dimercaprol, J0470

Dimethyl sulfoxide (DMSO), J1212

Dinate, J1240

Dioval (XX, 40), J0970, J1380, J1390

Diphenacen-50, J1200

Diphenhydramine HCl, J1200, Q0163

Dipyridamole, J1245

Disarticulation
lower extremities, prosthesis, L5000-
L5999
upper extremities, prosthesis, L6000-
L6692

Discoloration, dental, removal, D9970

Disease management program, S0317

Disetronic
glass cartridge syringe for insulin pump,
each, A4232
H-Tron insulin pump, E0784
insulin infusion set with bent needle,
with or without wings, each, A4231

Diskard head halter, E0940

Disk decompression, lumbar, S2348

Diskectomy, lumbar, S2350, S2351
single interspace, S2350

Disotate, J3520

Di-Spaz, J0500

Dispensing service, hearing aid, V5269

Disposable
diapers, A4335
supplies, ambulance, A0382-A0398
underpads, A4554

Ditate-DS, J0900

Diuril sodium, J1205

D-med 80, J1040

DMSO, J1212

DNA analysis, S3840
fecal, S3890

Dobutamine HCl, J1250

Dobutrex, J1250

Docetaxel, J9170

Dolasetron mesylate, J1260, Q0180
oral, S0174

Dolophine HCl, J1230

Dome, J9130
and mouthpiece (for nebulizer), A7016

Dommanate, J1240

Don-Joy
cervical support collar, L0150
deluxe knee immobilizer, L1830
rib belt, L0210
wrist forearm splint, L3984

Dopamine HCl, Q4076

Dornase alpha, inhalation solution, unit dose, J7639

Donor cadaver
harvesting multivisceral organs, with
allografts, S2055

Dornix Plus, E0601

Dorrance prosthesis
hand, L6825
hook, L6700-L6780

Dorsiwedge™ Night Splint, A4570, L2999,
L4398

Double bar
AK, knee-ankle-foot orthosis, L2020,
L2030
BK, ankle-foot orthosis, L1990

Doxercalciferol, J1270

Doxil, J9001

Doxorubicin HCl, C9415, J9000

Drainage
bag, A4357, A4358, A4911
board, postural, E0606
bottle, A5102, A4911

Dramamine, J1240

Dramanate, J1240

Dramilin, J1240

Dramocen, J1240

Dramoject, J1240

Dressing (*see also* **Bandage**), A6021-A6404
alginate, A6196-A6199
composite, A6200-A6205
contact layer, A6206-A6208
film, A6257-A6259
foam, A6209-A6215
gauze, A6216-A6230, A6402-A6404
holder/binder, A4462
hydrocolloid, A6234-A6241
hydrogel, A6242-A6249
specialty absorptive, A6251-A6256

Dressing — *continued*
tape, A4450, A4452
transparent film, A6257-A6259
tubular, K0620

Dronabinol, Q0167-Q0168

Droperidol, J1790
and fentanyl citrate, J1810

Dropper, A4649

Drugs (*see also* **Table of Drugs**)
administered through a metered dose
inhaler, J3535
chemotherapy, J8999-J9999
dental
injection, D9610
other, D9910
disposable delivery system, 5 ml or less
per hour, A4306
disposable delivery system, 50 ml or
greater per hour, A4305
immunosuppressive, J7500-J7599
infusion supplies, A4221, A4222, A4230-
A4232
injections (see also drug name), J0120-
J8999
not otherwise classified, J3490, J7599,
J7699, J7799, J8499, J8999,
J9999
prescription, oral, J8499, J8999

Drugs or biologicals, unclassified, C9399

Dry pressure pad/mattress, E0184,
E0199

Dry socket, localized osteitis, D9930

DTIC-Dome, C9423, J9130

Dunlap
heating pad, E0210
hot water bottle, E0220

Duo-Gen L.A., J0900

Duolock curved tail closures, A4421

Durable medical equipment (DME),
E0100-E1830, K codes

Duracillin A.S., J2510

Duraclon, J0735

Duragen (-10, -20, -40), J0970, J1380,
J1390

Duralone
-40, J1030
-80, J1040

Duramorph, J2275

Duratest
-100, J1070
-200, J1080

Duratestrin, J1060

Durathate-200, J3130

Durr-Fillauer
cervical collar, L0140
Pavlik harness, L1620

Dymenate, J1240

Dyphylline, J1180

E

Ear wax removal, G0268

Easy Care
folding walker, E0143
quad cane, E0105

ECG
initial Medicare exam, G0366-G0368

Echosclerotherapy, S2202

Economy VersaGuard coated commode,
E0164

Economy knee splint, L1830

ECWP, G0279, G0280

Edetate
  calcium disodium, J0600
  edetate disodium, J3520

Education
  asthma, S9441
  birthing, S9436-S9439, S9442
  diabetes, S9145
  exercise, S9451
  family planning, individualized
      programs, school based, T1018
  infant safety, S9447
  lactation, S9443
  Lamaze, S9436
  parenting, S9444
  smoking cessation, S9453
  stress management, S9454
  weight management, S9449

Efalizumab, S0162

Eggcrate dry pressure pad/mattress, E0184, E0199

Elastic support, L8100-L8230

Elastoplast adhesive tape, A4454, A6265

Elavil, J1320

Elbow
  brace, universal rehabilitation, L3720
  disarticulation, endoskeletal, L6450
  Masterhinge™ Elbow Brace 3, L3999
  orthosis (EO), E1800, L3700-L3740
  protector, E0191

Electric stimulator supplies, A4595

Electrical work, dialysis equipment, A4870

Electrodes, per pair, A4556

Electrohydraulic shockwave therapy
  plantar fasciitis, C9721
  tennis elbow, C9720

Electromagnetic therapy, G0295, G0329

Electron beam computed tomography, S8092

Electron microscopy – diagnostic, D0481

Elevating leg rest, K0195

Elevator, air pressure, heel, E0370

Eloxatin, C9205

Elliot's B solution, Q2002

Elspar, J9020

Embolization, protection system, C1884
  for tumor destruction, S2095

Embryo
  cryopreserved transferred, S4037
  monitor/store cryopreserved, S4040

Emergency dental treatment, D9430

EMG, E0746

Eminase, J0350

Enameloplasty, D9971

Enbrel, J1438

Encounter, clinic, T1015

End of life care planning, S0257

Endarterectomy, chemical, M0300

Endodontic procedures, D3110-D3999

Endoscope sheath, A4270

Endoscopy, upper GI, S2215

Endoskeletal system, addition, L5925, L5984

Enema
  bag, reusable, A4458
  barium, G0106
  cancer screening, G0120

Enovil, J1320

Enoxaparin sodium, J1650

Enrich, enteral nutrition, B4150

Ensure, enteral nutrition, B4150
  HN, B4150
  Plus, B4152
  Plus HN, B4152
  powder, B4150

Enteral
  administration services, feeding, S9340-S9343
  feeding supply kit (syringe) (pump)
      (gravity), B4034-B4036
  fiber or additive, B4104
  formulae, B4150-B4162
      electrolytes, B4102, B4103
      for metabolic disease, B4157
      intact nutrients, B4149, B4150, B4152
      pediatric, B4158-B4162
  gastronomy tube, B4086
  nutrition infusion pump (with alarm)
      (without), B9000, B9002
  supplies, not otherwise classified, B9998

Epinephrine, J0170

Epiribicin HCl, J9178

Epoetin alpha, Q4055
  for non-ESRD use, Q0136

Epoprostenol, J1325
  dilutant, sterile, S0155
  infusion pump, K0455

Equilibration, dental, D9951-D9952

Erbitux, J9055

Ergonovine maleate, J1330

Ertapenem sodium, J1335

Erythromycin lactobionate, J1364

ESRD (End Stage Renal Disease; *see also* **Dialysis)**
  bundle demo/basic, G9013
      expanded, G9014
  counseling or assessment, G0308-G0319
      home dialysis, G0320-G0327
  machines and accessories, E1510-E1699
  plumbing, A4870
  services, E1510-E1699, G0308-G0327
  supplies, A4656-A4927

Estra-D, J1000

Estradiol, J1000, J1060
  cypionate and testosterone cypionate, J1060
  L.A., J0970, J1380, J1390
  L.A. 20, J0970, J1380, J1390
  L.A. 40, J0970, J1380, J1390
  valerate and testosterone enanthate, J0900

Estra-L (20, 40), J0970, J1380, J1390

Estra-Testrin, J0900

Estro-Cyp, J1000

Estrogen conjugated, J1410

Estroject L.A., J1000

Estrone (5, Aqueous), J1435

Estronol, J1435
  -L.A., J1000

Ethanolamine oleate, Q2007

Ethyol, J0207

Etidronate disodium, J1436

Etopophos, J9181, J9182
  oral, J8560

Etoposide, C9414, C9425, J9181, J9182
  oral, J8560

Evaluation
  comprehensive, multi-discipline, H2000
  dental, D0120-D0180
  team for handicapped, T1024

Everone, J3120, J3130

Exactech lancet device, A4258

Examination
  breast and pelvic, G0101
  initial Medicare, G0344
  oral, D0120-D0160

Excision, tissue localization, C1819

Exercise
  class, S9451
  equipment, A9300

Exo-Static overdoor traction unit, E0860

Exostosis (tuberosity) removal
  lateral, D7471
  osseous tuberosity, D7485
  reduction of fibrous tuberosity, D7972

External
  ambulatory infusion pump, E0781, E0784
  counterpulsation, G0166
  power, battery components, L7360-L7499
  power, elbow, L7191
  urinary supplies, A4356-A4359

External defibrillator
  battery replacement, K0607
  electrode replacement, K0609
  garment replacement, K0608

Extracorporeal shock wave therapy (ECWP), G0279, G0280

Extractions, D7111-D7140
  surgical, D7210-D7250

Extraoral films, D0250, D0260

Extremity belt/harness, E0945

Eye
  lens (contact) (spectacle), S0500-S0514, V2100-V2615
  pad, A6410-A6411
  patch, A6410-A6411
  prosthetic, V2623-V2629
  service (miscellaneous), V2700-V2799

E-ZJect Lite Angle lancets, box of 100, A4259

E-ZJect disposable insulin syringes, up to 1 cc, per syringe, A4206

E-Z-lets lancet device, A4258

E-Z Lite wheelchair, E1250

F

Fabrazyme, J0180, S0159

Face tent, oxygen, A4619

Factor VIII, anti-hemophilic factor, J7190-J7192

Factor IX, anti-hemophilic factor, J7193-J7195

Factrel, J1620

Family stabilization, S9482

Famotidine, S0028

Fecal
  occult blood test, G0107

Fee, coordinated care, G9009-G9012

Fentanyl citrate, J3010
  and droperidol, J1810

Fern test, Q0114

Fertility services
  donor service (sperm or embryo), S4025
  in vitro fertilization, S4013-S4022
  ovulation induction, S4042
  sperm procurement, S4026, S4030-S4031

Fetal surgery, repair teratoma, S2405

Fiberotomy, dental, transeptal, D7291

Filgrastim (G-CSF), J1440, J1441

Filler, wound
  alginate, A6199
  foam, A6215

Filler, wound — *continued*
  hydrocolloid, A6240-A6241
  hydrogel, A6248
  not elsewhere classified, A6261, A6262

Film
  dressing, A6257-A6259
  radiographic, dental, D0210-D0340

Filter
  carbon, A4680
  CPAP device, A7038-A7039
  dialysis carbon, A4680
  ostomy, A4368
  tracheostoma, A4481
  vena cava, C1880

Finasteride, S0138

Finger
  baseball splint, A4570
  fold-over splint, A4570
  four-pronged splint, A4570

Fisher & Paykel HC220, E0601

Fistula
  cannulation set, A4730
  oroantral, D7260
  salivary, D7983

Fitness club membership, S9970

Fixed partial dentures (bridges), retainers
  crowns, D6720-D6792
  inlay/onlay, D6545-D6615
  implant/abutment support, D6068-D6077
  pontics, D6221-D6252
  recementation, D6930
  repair, D6980
  resin bonded, D6545

Flap, gingival, D4240, D4241

Flashcast™ Elite™ casting material, A4590

Flexoject, J2360

Flexon, J2360

Flipper, dental prosthesis, D5820-D5821

Flolan, J1325

Flowmeter, E0440, E0555, E0580

Flow rate meter, peak, A4614

Floxuridine, C9426, J9200

Fluconazole, injection, J1450

Fludara, J9185

Fludarabine phosphate, J9185

Fluid barrier, dialysis, E1575

Flunisolide, J7641

Fluoride
  custom tray/gel carrier, D5986
  dispensing for home use, D9630
  topical, D1201-D1205

Fluorine-18 fluorodeoxyglucose imaging, S8085

Fluorouracil, J9190

Fluphenazine decanoate, J2680

Flutamide, S0175

Flutter device, S8185

Fluvestrant, J9395

Foam
  dressing, A6209-A6215
  pad adhesive, A5126

Folding walker, E0135, E0143

Fold-over finger splint, A4570

Folex, J9260
  PFS, J9260

Foley catheter, A4312-A4316, A4338-A4346

Follitropin
  beta, S0128

Follutein, J0725

Fomepizole, Q2008

Fomivirsen sodium, intraocular, J1452

Fondaparinux sodium, J1652

Food supplement, S9434

Food thickener, B4100

Foot, care, routine, S0390, G0247

Foot, cast boot
  Specialist™ Closed-Back Cast Boot, L3260
  Specialist™ Gaitkeeper™ Boot, L3260
  Specialist™ Open-Back Cast Boot, L3260
  Specialist™ Toe Insert for Specialist™ Closed-Back Cast Boot and Specialist™ Health/Post Operative Shoe, A9270

Foot, insoles/heel cups
  Specialist™ Heel Cups, L3485
  Specialist™ Insoles, L3510

Foot, soles
  Masterfoot™ Walking Cast Sole, L3649
  Solo™ Cast Sole, L3540

Footdrop splint, L4398

Footplate, E0175, E0970

Footwear, orthopedic, L3201-L3265

Forearm crutches, E0110, E0111

Fortaz, J0713

Forteo, J3110

Fortex, alginate dressing, A6196-A6199

Foscarnet sodium, J1455

Foscavir, J1455

Fosphenytoin, Q2009

Fosphenytoin sodium, S0078

Foster care, H0041-H0042

Four Poster, fracture frame, E0946

Four-pronged finger splint, A4570

Fracture
  bedpan, E0276
  frame, E0920, E0930, E0946-E0948
  orthosis, L2108-L2136, L2106-L2136, L3980-L3986
  orthotic additions, L3995
  Specialist™ Pre-Formed Humeral Fracture Brace, L3980

Fractures, dental, treatment
  alveolus, D7670, D7770
  malar/zygomatic arch
    incision, D7650-D7660
    surgical incision, D7750-D7760
  mandible
    compound closed reduction, D7740
    compound open reduction, D7730
    simple closed reduction, D7640
    simple open reduction, D7630
  maxilla
    compound closed reduction, D7720
    compound open reduction, D7710
    simple closed reduction, D7620
    simple open reduction, D7610

Fragmin, J1645

Frame
  meaning spectacles, V2020, V2025
    sales tax, S9999
  safety, for hospital bed, E0316

FreAmine HBC, parenteral nutrition, B5100

Frejka, hip orthosis, L1600
  replacement cover, L1610

Frenectomy/frenotomy (frenulectomy), D7960

Frenuloplasty, D7963

FUDR, J9200

Fulvestrant, J9395

Fungizone, J0285

Furomide MD, J1940

Furosemide, J1940

G

Gadolinium, A4647

Gait trainer
  pediatric
    anterior, E8002
    posterior, E8000
    upright, E8001

Gallium Ga-67, Q3002

Gallium nitrate, J1457

Gamastan, J1460

Gamma globulin, J1460

Gamulin RH, J2790

Ganciclovir
  implant, J7310
  sodium, J1570

Ganirelix acetate, S0132

Garamycin, J1580

Gas system
  compressed, E0424, E0425
  gaseous, E0430, E0431, E0441, E0443
  liquid, E0434-E0440, E0442, E0444

Gastric
  band, S2082
  band adjustment, S2083
  restrictive procedure/laparoscopic, S2082

Gastric electrical stimulation device, implantation, S2213

Gastric suction pump, E2000

Gastrostomy/jejunostomy tubing, B4086

Gastrostomy tube, B4086

Gatifloxacin, J1590

Gaucher disease, genetic test, S3848

Gauze, A6216-A6230, A6266
  impregnated, A6222-A6230, A6266
  nonimpregnated, A6216, A6221, A6402
  pads, A6216-A6230, A6402-A6404
    Johnson & Johnson, A6402
    Kendall, A6402
    Moore, A6402

Gefitinib, J8565

Gel
  conductive, A4558
  pressure pad, E0185, E0196
  sheet, dermal or epidermal, A6025

Gemcitabine HCl, J9201

Gemtuzumab ozogamicin, J9300

GemZar, J9201

Genetic testing, S3818-S3853

Genmould™ Creamy Plaster, A4580

Gentamicin (sulfate), J1580

Gentran, J7100, J7110

Geo-Matt
  therapeutic overlay, E0199

Geronimo PR, power wheelchair, K0011

Gerval Protein, enteral nutrition, B4155

Gestational home visit
  for diabetes, S9214
  for hypertension, S9211
  for preeclampsia, S9213

GIFT, S4013

Gingiva, pericoronal, removal, D7971

Gingival flap D4240, D4241

Gingivectomy/gingivoplasty, D4210-D4211

Glass ionomer (resin restoration), D2330-D2394

Glasses
air conduction, V5070
binaural, V5120-V5150
bone conduction, V5080
frames, V2020, V2025
hearing aid, V5150, V5190, V5230
lens, V2100-V2499, V2610, V2718, V2730, V2755, V2770, V2780

Glatiramer acetate, J1595

Glaucoma screening, G0117-G0118

Global fee, urgent care center, S9083

Gloves
dialysis, A4927
non-sterile, A4927
sterile, A4930

Glucagon HCl, J1610

Glucometer
II blood glucose meter, E0607
II blood glucose test strips, box of 50, A4253
3 blood glucose meter, E0607
3 blood glucose test strips, box of 50, A4253

Glucose
monitor device, continuous, noninvasive, S1030-S1031
test strips, A4253, A4772

Glukor, J0725

Gluteal pad, L2650

Glycopyrrolate, inhalation solution
concentrated, J7642
unit dose, J7643

Gold
foil dental, D2340-D2430
sodium thiomalate, J1600

Gomco
aspirators, E0600

Gonadorelin HCl, C9435, J1620

Gonic, J0725

Goserelin acetate implant (see also Implant), J9202

Grab bar, trapeze, E0910, E0940

Grade-aid, wheelchair, E0974

Gradient pressure aids, S8421-S8429

Graftjacket
Reg Matrix. C9221
SftTis, C9222

Graft
vascular, C1768

Graft, dental
bone replacement, D4263-D4264
maxillofacial soft/hard tissue, D7955
ridge augmentation, D7950
soft tissue and pedicle, G4276
soft tissue, D4270-D4273

Granisetron HCl, J1626, Q0166, S0091

Gravity traction device, E0941

Gravlee jet washer, A4470

Greissing, foot prosthesis, L5978

Guide wire, C1769

Guided tissue regeneration, dental, D4266-D4267

Guilford multiple-post collar, cervical orthosis, L0190

Gynogen, J1380, J1390
L.A. (10, 20, 40), J0970, J1380, J1390

H

H-Tron Plus insulin pump, E0784

H. Weniger finger orthosis
cock-up splint, L3914
combination Oppenheimer
with
knuckle bender no. 13, L3950
reverse knuckle no. 13B, L3952
composite elastic no. 10, L3946
dorsal wrist no. 8, L3938
with outrigger attachment no. 8A, L3940
finger extension, with clock spring no. 5, L3928
finger extension, with wrist support no. 5A, L3930
finger knuckle bender no. 11, L3948
knuckle bender splint type no. 2, L3918
knuckle bender, two segment no. 2B, L3922
knuckle bender with outrigger no. 2, L3920
Oppenheimer, L3924
Palmer no. 7, L3936
reverse knuckle bender no. 9, L3942
with outrigger no. 9A, L3944
safety pin, modified no. 6A, L3934
safety pin, spring wire no. 6, L3932
spreading hand no. 14, L3954
Thomas suspension no. 4, L3926

Haberman Feeder, S8265

Habilitation, T2012-T2021

Hair analysis (excluding arsenic), P2031

Haldol, J1630
decanoate (-50, -100), J1631

Hallus-valgus dynamic splint, L3100

Hallux prosthetic implant, L8642

Haloperidol, J1630
decanoate, J1631

Halo procedures, L0810-L0860

Halter, cervical head, E0942

Hand restoration, L6900-L6915
partial prosthesis, L6000-L6020
orthosis (WHFO), E1805, E1825, L3800-L3805, L3900-L3954
rims, wheelchair, E0967

Handgrip (cane, crutch, walker), A4636

Harness, E0942, E0944, E0945

Harvest
bone marrow, G0267
multivisceral organs, cadaver donor, S2055
peripheral stem cell, G0267, S2150

Harvey arm abduction orthosis, L3960

Health club membership, S9970

Hearing devices, L8614, V5008-V5299
accessories/supplies, V5267
analog, V5242-V5251
battery, V5266
digital, V5250-V5261
dispensing fee, V5241
ear mold/insert, V5264-V5265
ear impression, V5275

Heat
application, E0200-E0239
lamp, E0200, E0205
pad, E0210, E0215, E0217, E0218, E0238, E0249
units, E0239
Hydrocollator, mobile, E0239
Thermalator T-12-M, E0239

Heater (nebulizer), E1372

Heating pad, Dunlap, E0210
for peritoneal dialysis, E0210

Heel
elevator, air, E0370
loop/holder, E0951
pad, L3480, L3485
protector, E0191
shoe, L3430-L3485
stabilizer, L3170

Helicopter, ambulance (see also Ambulance), A0431

Helmet
cervical, L0100, L0110
with face guard, E0701

Hematopoietic hormone administration, S9537

Hemalet lancet device, A4258

Hemin, Q2011

Hemi-wheelchair, E1083-E1086

Hemipelvectomy prosthesis, L5280

Hemisection, dental, D3920

Hemodialysis
acetate concentrate, A4708
acid solution, A4709
bicarbonate concentrate, A4706-A4707
drain bag/bottle, A4911
catheter, C1750, C1752
machine, E1590
mask, surgical, A4928
protamine sulfate, A4802
surgical mask, A4928
tourniquet, A4929

Hemodialyzer, portable, E1635

Hemofil M, J7190

Hemophilia clotting factor, J7190-J7199

Hemostats, for dialysis, E1637

Hemostix, A4773

Heparin
infusion pump (for dialysis), E1520
lock flush, J1642
sodium, J1644

HepatAmine, parenteral nutrition, B5100

Hepatic-aid, enteral nutrition, B4154

Hepatitis B immune globulin, C9105

Hep-Lock (U/P), J1642

Herceptin, J9355

Hexadrol phosphate, J1100

Hexalite, A4590

Hexior power wheelchair, K0014

High Frequency chest wall oscillation equipment, A7025-A7026, E0483

High risk area requiring escort, S9381

Hip
Custom Masterhinge™ Hip Hinge 3, L2999
disarticulation prosthesis, L5250, L5270
Masterhinge™ Hip Hinge 3, L2999
orthosis (HO), L1600-L1686

Hip-knee-ankle-foot orthosis (HKAFO), L2040-L2090

Histaject, J0945

Histerone (-50, -100), J3140

Histrelin acetate, Q2020

HIV-1 antibody testing, S3645

HKAFO, L2040-L2090

HN2, J9230

Holder
heel, E0951
toe, E0952

Hole cutter tool, A4421

Hollister
belt adapter, A4421
closed pouch, A5051, A5052
colostomy/ileostomy kit, A5061
drainable pouches, A5061
    with flange, A5063
medical adhesive, A4364
pediatric ostomy belt, A4367
remover, adhesive, A4455
stoma cap, A5055
skin barrier, A4362, A5122
skin cleanser, A4335
skin conditioning creme, A4335
skin gel protective dressing wipes, A5119
stoma cap, A5055
two-piece pediatric ostomy system,
    A5054, A5063, A5073
urostomy pouch, A5071, A5072

Home health
aide, S9122, T1030-T1031
    home health setting, G0156
care
    certified nurse assistant, S9122,
        T1021
    home health aide, S9122, T1021
    nursing care, S9122-S9124, T1030-
        T1031
    re-certification, G0179-G0180
gestational
    assessment, T1028
    delivery suppies, S8415
    diabetes, S9214
    hypertension, S9211
    pre-eclampsia, S9213
    preterm labor, S9208-S9209
hydration therapy, S9373-S9379
infusion therapy, S9325-S9379, S9494-
    S9497, S9537-S9810
nursing services, S9212-S9213
postpartum hypertension, S9212
services of
    clinical social worker, G0155
    occupational therapist, G0152
    physical therapist, G0151
    skilled nurse, G0154
    speech/language pathologist, G0153
transfusion, blood products, S9538
wound care, S9097

Home uterine monitor, S9001

Hosmer
baby mitt, L6870
child hand, mechanical, L6872
forearm lift, assist unit only, L6635
gloves, above hands, L6890, L6895
hand prosthesis, L6868
hip orthotic joint, post-op, L1685
hook
    with
        neoprene fingers, #8X, L6740
        neoprene fingers, #88X, L6745
        plastisol, #10P, L6750
    #5, L6705
    #5X, L6710
    #5XA, L6715
    child, L6755, L6765
    small adult, L6770
    stainless steel #8, L6735
        with neopren, L6780
    work, #3, L6700
        for use with tools, #7, L6725
        with lock, #6, L6720
        with wider opening, L6730
passive hand, L6868
soft, passive hand, L6865

Hospice
care, S9126, T2041-T2046
evaluation and counseling services, G0337
referral visit, S0255

Hospital call, **dental**, D9420

Hot water bottle, E0220

H-Tron insulin pump, E0784

Houdini security suit, E0700

House call, **dental**, D9410

Housing, **supported**, H0043-H0044

Hoyer patient lifts, E0621, E0625, E0630

Hudson
adult multi-vent venturi style mask,
    A4620
nasal cannula, A4615
oxygen supply tubing, A4616
UC-BL type shoe insert, L3000

Humalog, J1815, J1817, S5550

Human insulin, J1815, J1817

Human serum albumin with octafluoropropane, C9202

Humidifier, E0550-E0560
water chamber, A7046

Humira, J0135

Humulin insulin, J1815, J1817

Hyaluronidase, J3470

Hyate, J7191

Hybolin
decanoate, J2321

Hycamtin, J9350

Hydralazine HCl, J0360

Hydrate, J1240

Hydration therapy, S9373-S9379

Hydration with intravenous infusion,
G0345, G0346

Hydraulic patient lift, E0630

Hydrocollator, E0225, E0239

Hydrocolloid dressing, A6234-A6241

Hydrocortisone
acetate, J1700
sodium phosphate, J1710
sodium succinate, J1720

Hydrocortone
acetate, J1700
phosphate, J1710

Hydrogel dressing, A6242-A6248

Hydromorphone, J1170, S0092

Hydroxyurea, S0176

Hydroxyzine HCl, J3410
pamoate, Q0177-Q0178

Hylan G-F 20, J7320

Hyoscyamine sulfate, J1980

Hyperbaric oxygen chamber, **topical**, A4575

Hyperstat IV, J1730

Hypertonic saline solution, J7130

Hypo-Let lancet device, A4258

Hypothermia
intragastric, M0100

HypRho-D, J2790

Hyrexin-50, J1200

Hyzine-50, J3410

I

I&D
ntraoral, D7511, D7521

I-131 sodium iodide
capsule, C9402-C9405

Ibutilide fumarate, J1742

Ice cap or collar, E0230

Idamycin, J9211

Idarubicin HCl, C9429, J9211

Ifex, J9208

Ifosfamide, C9427, J9208

IL-2, J9015

Iletin insulin, J1815, J1817, S5552

Ilfeld, **hip orthosis**, L1650

Images, **oral/facial**, D0350

Imaging coil, **MRI**, C1770

Imatinib, S0088

Imiglucerase, J1785

Imitrex, J3030

Immune globulin IV, J1563, J1564

Immunofluorescence
direct, D0482
indirect, D0483

Immunosuppressive drug, **not otherwise classified**, J7599

Impacted tooth, **removal**, D7220-D7241

Impaction
tooth, treatment, D7283

Implant
access system, A4301
aqueous shunt, L8612
auditory device
    brainstem, S2235
    middle ear, S2230
breast, L8600
cochlear, L8614, L8619
collagen, urinary tract, L8603
contraceptive, A4260
dental
    chin, D7995
    endodontic, D3460
    endosteal/endosseous, D6010
    eposteal/subperiosteal, D6040
    facial, D7995
    maintenance, D6080
    other implant service, D6053-6079
    supported prosthetics, D6053-D6079
        removal, D6100
        repair, D6090, D6095
    transosteal/tensosseous, D6050
ganciclovir, J7310
gastric electrical stimulation device,
    S2213
gastric stimulation, S2213
goserelin acetate, J9202
hallux, L8642
infusion pump, E0782, E0783
injectable bulking agent, urinary tract,
    L8606
joint, L8630, L8641, L8658
lacrimal duct, A4262, A4263
levonorgestral, A4260
maintenance procedures, D6080, D6100
maxillofacial, D5913-D5937
metacarpophalangeal joint, L8630
metatarsal joint, L8641
neurostimulator, pulse generator or
    receiver, E0755, E0756
Norplant, A4260
not otherwise specified, L8699
ocular, L8610
ossicular, L8613
osteogenesis stimulator, E0749
percutaneous access system, A4301
removal, dental, D6100
repair, dental, D6090
vascular access portal, A4300
vascular graft, L8670
yttrium 90, S2095
Zoladex, J9202

Implantation/reimplantation, **tooth**,
D7270
intentional reimplantation, D3470

Impregnated gauze dressing, A6222-A6230

Imuran, J7500, J7501

Inapsine, J1790

Incontinence
adult
    brief or diaper, T4521-T4524
    pull-on protection, T4525-T4528

Incontinence — *continued*
appliances and supplies, A4310, A4534, A5051-A5093, A5102-A5114, A5119-A5200
disposable/liner, T4535
garment, A4520
pediatric
brief or diaper, T4529-T4530
pull-on protection, T4531-T4532
reusable
diaper or brief, T4539
pull-on protection, T4536
treatment system, E0740
underpad
disposable, T4541, T4542
reusable, T4537, T4540
youth
brief or diaper, T4533
pull-on protection, T4534

Inderal, J1800

Indium 111
capromab pendetide, A9507
ibritumomab tiuxetan, A9522
oxyguinoline, C1091
pentetate disodium, C1092
satumomab pendetide, A4642

Infant safety, CPR, training, S9447

Infed, J1750

Infergen, J9212

Infliximab injection, J1745

Infusion, G0258
catheter, C1752
pump, C1772, C2626
ambulatory, with administrative equipment, E0781
epoprostenol, K0455
heparin, dialysis, E1520
implantable, E0782, E0783
implantable, refill kit, A4220
insulin, E0784
mechanical, reusable, E0779, E0780
nonprogrammable, C1891
supplies, A4221, A4222, A4230-A4232
Versa-Pole IV, E0776
supplies, A4222, A4223
therapy, home, S9347, S9497-S9504

Inhalation solution (*see also* drug name), J7608-J7799

Initial
ECG, Medicare, G0366-G0368
physical exam, Medicare, G0344

Injectable bulking agent, urinary tract, L8606

Injection (*see also* drug name), J0120-J7506
busulfan, C1178
contrast material, during MRI, A4643
dental service, D9610, D9630
IM or subcutaneous, G0351
inert substance, into UGI, C9704
IV push, G0353, G0354
metatarsal neuroma, S2135
procedure
sacroiliac joint, G0254-G0260
supplies for self-administered, A4211

Injection adjustment, bariatric band, S2083

Inlay, dental
fixed partial denture retainers
metallic, D6545-D6615
porcelain/ceramic, D6548-D6609
metallic, D2510-D2530
porcelain/ceramic, D2610-2630
recement inlay, D2910
intentional replantation, D3470, D7270
resin-based composite, D2650-D2652
titanium, D6624

Innovar, J1810

Insert
convex, for ostomy, A5093
diabetic, for shoe, A5501-A5511

Insertion
inert substance, into UGI, C9704
tray, A4310-A4316

In-situ tissue hybridization, D0479

Insulin, J1815, J1817
delivery device other than pump, S5565-S5571
home infusion administration, S9353
intermediate acting, S5552
long acting, S5553
NPH, S5552, J1815
rapid onset, S5550-S5551

Insulin pump, external, E0784

Intal, J7631

Integra, C9206

Interdigital neuritis injection, S2135

Intergrilin injection, J1327

Interferon
Alfa, J9212-J9215
Alfacon-1, J9212
Beta-1a, J1825, Q3025-Q3026
Beta-1b, J1830
Gamma, J9216
home injection, S9559

Intermittent
peritoneal dialysis system, E1592
positive pressure breathing (IPPB) machine, E0500

Interphalangeal joint, prosthetic implant, L8658

Interscapular thoracic prosthesis
endoskeletal, L6570
upper limb, L6350-L6370

Intrafallopian transfer
complete cycle, gamete, S4013
complete cycle, zygote, S4014
donor egg cycle, S4023
incomplete cycle, S4017

Intraocular lenses, C1780, V2630-V2632, Q1001-Q1005
new technology
category 1, Q1001
category 2, Q1002
category 3, Q1003
category 4, Q1004
category 5, Q1005

Intraoral radiographs, D0210-D0240

Intrauterine device
copper contraceptive, J7300
other, S4989
Progestacert, S4989

Intravaginal culture, S4036

Intravenous infusion
hydration, G0345, G0346
therapeutic, diagnostic, G0347-G0350

Intravenous push, G0353, G0354, G0357, G0358

Intravenous sedation/analgesia, dental
first 30 minutes, D9241
each additional 15 minutes, D9242

Introducer sheath
guiding, C1766, C1892, C1893
other than guiding, C1984, C2629

Intron A, J9214

Iodine I-123, A9516

Iodine I-131
albumin, A9524
iobenguane sulfate, A9508
sodium iodide, A9517

Iodine swabs/wipes, A4247

IPD
system, E1592

IPPB machine, E0500

Ipratropium bromide
inhalation solution, unit dose, J7644

Iressa, J8565

Irinotecan, J9206

Iris Preventix pressure relief/reduction mattress, E0184

Iris therapeutic overlays, E0199

IRM ankle-foot orthosis, L1950

Irodex, J1750

Iron
dextran, J1750
sucrose, J1756

Irrigation
implanted access device, G0363

Irrigation/evacuation system, bowel
control unit, E0350
disposable supplies for, E0352

Irrigation supplies, A4320, A4322, A4355, A4397-A4400
Surfit
irrigation sleeve, A4397
night drainage container set, A5102
Visi-flow irrigator, A4398, A4399

Islet cell transplant
laparoscopy, G0342
laparotomy, G0343
percutaneous, G0341

Isocaine HCl, J0670

Isocal, enteral nutrition, B4150
HCN, B4152

Isoetharine
inhalation solution
concentrated, J7648
unit dose, J7649

Isolates, B4150, B4152

Isoproterenol HCl, inhalation solution
concentrated, J7658
unit dose, J7659

Isotein, enteral nutrition, B4153

Isuprel, J7658-J7659

Itraconazole, J1835

IUD, J7300

IV pole, E0776, K0105

J

J-cell battery, replacement for blood glucose monitor, A4254

Jace tribrace, L1832

Jacket
scoliosis, L1300, L1310

Jenamicin, J1580

Johnson's orthopedic wrist-hand cock-up splint, L3914

Johnson's thumb immobilizer, L3800

Joint device, C1776

K

Kabikinase, J2995

Kaleinate, J0610

Kaltostat, alginate dressing, A6196-A6199

Kanamycin sulfate, J1840, J1850

Kantrex, J1840, J1850

Kartop Patient Lift, toilet or bathroom (*see also* Lift), E0625

Keflin, J1890

Kefurox, J0697

Kefzol, J0690

Kenaject -40, J3301

Kenalog (-10,-40), J3301

Keratectomy photorefractive, S0810

Keratoprosthesis, C1818

Kestrone-5, J1435

Keto-Diastix, box of 100 glucose/ketone urine test strips, A4250

Ketorolac thomethamine, J1885

Key-Pred
-25,-50, J2650

K-Flex, J2360

Kidney
ESRD supply, A4656-A4927
system, E1510
wearable artificial, E1632

Kilovolt imaging, C9722

Kingsley gloves, above hands, L6890

Kits
enteral feeding supply (syringe) (pump) (gravity), B4034-B4036
fistula cannulation (set), A4730
parenteral nutrition, B4220-B4224
surgical dressing (tray), A4550
tracheostomy, A4625

Klebcil, J1840, J1850

Knee
Adjustabrace™ 3, L2999
disarticulation, prosthesis, L5150-L5160
immobilizer, L1830
joint, miniature, L5826
Knee-O-Prene™ Hinged Knee Sleeve, L1810
Knee-O-Prene™ Hinged Wraparound Knee Support, L1810
orthosis (KO), E1810, L1800-L1880
locks, L2405-L2425
Masterbrace™ 3, L2999
Masterhinge Adjustabrace™ 3, L2999
Performance Wrap™ (KO), L1825

Knee-ankle-foot orthosis (KAFO), L2000-L2039, L2126-L2136

Knee-O-Prene™ Hinged Knee Sleeve, L1810

Knee-O-Prene™ Hinged Wraparound Knee Support, L1810

KnitRite
prosthetic
sheath, L8400-L8415
sock, L8420-L8435
stump sock, L8470-L8485

KoalaKair mattress overlay, with pump, E0180

Kodel clavicle splint, L3660

Kogenate, J7192

Konakion, J3430

Konyne-HT, J7194

K-Y Lubricating Jelly, A4402, A4332

Kyphoplasty, C9718, C9719, S2362-S2362

Kyphosis pad, L1020, L1025

Kytril, J1626

L

Labor care (not resulting in delivery), S4005

Laboratory tests
chemistry, P2028-P2038
microbiology, P7001
miscellaneous, P9010-P9615, Q0111-Q0115
toxicology, P3000-P3001, Q0091

Lacrimal duct implant
permanent, A4263
temporary, A4262

Lactated Ringer's infusion, J7120

LAE 20, J0970, J1380, J1390

Laetrile, J3570

Lancet, A4258, A4259

Lanoxin, J1160

Laparoscopy, bariatric band, S2082

Laronidase, J1931, S0158

Laryngectomy
tube, A7520-A7522

Larynx, artificial, L8500

Laser
application, S8948
assisted uvulopalatoplasty (LAUP) S2080
in situ keratomileusis, S0800
myringotomy, S2225
vaporation, prostate, C9713

Laser skin piercing device, for blood collection, E0620
replacement lens, A4257

Lasix, J1940

LAUP, S2080

Lead
adaptor
neurostimulator, C1883
pacing, C1883
cardioverter, defibrillator, C1777, C1895, C1896
environmental, home evaluation, T1029
neurostimulator, C1778
neurostimulator/test kit, C1897
pacemaker, C1779, C1898, C1899

Lederle, J8610

LeFort
I osteotomy, D7946-D7947
II osteotomy, D7948-D7949
III osteotomy, D7948-D7949

Leg
bag, A4358, A5112
extensions for walker, E0158
Nextep™ Contour™ Lower Leg Walker, L2999
Nextep™ Low Silhouette™ Lower Leg Walkers, L2999
rest, elevating, K0195
rest, wheelchair, E0990
strap, A5113, A5114, K0038, K0039

Legg Perthes orthosis, L1700-L1755

Lens
aniseikonic, V2118, V2318
contact, V2500-V2599
deluxe feature, V2702
eye, S0504-S0508, S0580-S0590, V2100-V2615, V2700-V2799
intraocular, C1780, V2630-V2632
low vision, V2600-V2615
mirror coating, V2761
occupational multifoca, V2786
polarization, V2762
polycarbonate, V2784
progressive, V2781
skin piercing device, replacement, A4257
tint, V2744
addition, V2745

Lente insulin, J1815, S5552

Lenticular lens
bifocal, V2221
single vision, V2121
trifocal, V2321

Lepirudin, Q2021

Lerman Minerva spinal orthosis, L0174

Lesions, surgical excision, dental, D7410-D7465

Leucovorin calcium, J0640

Leukocyte
poor blood, each unit, P9016

Leuprolide acetate, C9430, J9217, J9218, J1950

Leuprolide acetate implant, J9219

Leustat, C9419

Leustatin, J9065

Levalbuterol
administered through DME, J7612, J7614
with ipratropium bromide, J7617

Levamisole HCl, S0177

Levaquin I.U., J1956

Levine, stomach tube, B4086

Levocarnitine, J1955

Levo-Dromoran, J1960

Levofloxacin, J1956

Levonorgestrel, contraceptive implants and supplies, A4260, J7302

Levorphanol tartrate, J1960

Librium, J1990

Lice infestation treatment, A9180

Lidocaine HCl for intravenous infusion, J2001

Lifescan lancets, box of 100, A4259

Lifestand manual wheelchair, K0009

Lifestyle modification program, coronary heart disease, S0340-S0342

Lift
combination, E0637
patient, and seat, E0621-E0635
Hoyer
Home Care, E0621
Partner All-Purpose, hydraulic, E0630
Partner Power Multifunction, E0625
shoe, L3300-L3334
standing frame system, E0638

Lift-Aid patient lifts, E0621

Light box, E0203

Lincocin, J2010

Lincomycin HCl, J2010

Lioresal, J0475, C9009

Liquaemin sodium, J1644

Lispro insulin, S5551

Lithium battery for blood glucose monitor, A4254

Lithrotripsy, gallstones, S9034

Little Ones
drainable pouch, A5063
mini-pouch, A5054
one-piece custom drainable pouch, A5061
one-piece custom urostomy pouch, A5071
pediatric belt, A4367
pediatric urine collector, A4335
urostomy pouch, transparent, A5073

Lively, knee-ankle-foot orthosis, L2038

LMD, 10%, J7100

Lobectomy, lung, donor, S2061

Localized osteitis, dry socket, D9110, D9930

Lodging
NOS, S9976
recipient, escort nonemergency transport, A0180, A0200
transplant-related, S9975

Lomustine, S0178

Lonalac powder, enteral nutrition, B4150

Lorazepam, J2060

Lovenox, J1650

Low osmolar contrast
100-199 mgs iodine, A6444
200-299 mgs iodine, A4645
300-399 mgs iodine, A4646

Lower limb, prosthesis, addition, L5968

LPN services, T1003

Lubricant, A4332, A4402

Lufyllin, J1180

Lumbar
orthosis, K0634-K0636
pad, L1030, L1040
-sacral orthosis (LSO), K0637-K0649

Luminal sodium, J2560

Lung volume reduction surgery services, G0302-G0305

Lunelle, J1056

Lupron, J9218
depot, J1950

LVRS services, G0302-G0305

Lymphedema therapy, S8950

Lymphocyte immune globulin, J7504, J7511

M

Madamist II medication compressor/nebulizer, E0570

Magnacal, enteral nutrition, B4152

Magnesium sulphate, J3475

Magnetic
resonance angiography, C8901-C8914, C8918-C8920
resonance imaging, low field, S8042
source imaging, S8035

Maintenance contract, ESRD, A4890

Malar bone, fracture repair, D7650, D7750, D7760

Malibu cervical turtleneck safety collar, L0150

Malocclusion correction, D8010-D8999

Mammogram
computer analysis, S8075

Mammography, G0202-G0206

Management
disease, S0317

Mandible, fracture, D7630-D7640, D7730-D7740

Mannitol, J2150

Mapping
topographic brain, S8040
vessels, G0365

Marmine, J1240

Maryland bridge (resin-bonded fixed prosthesis)
pontic, D6210-D6252
retainer/abutment, D6545

Mask
oxygen, A4620
surgical, for dialysis, A4928

Mastectomy
bra, L8002
camisole, S8460
form, L8020
prosthesis, L8000-L8039, L8600
sleeve, L8010

Masterbrace™ 3, L2999

Masterfoot™ Walking Cast Sole, L3649

Masterhinge Adjustabrace™ 3, L2999

Masterhinge™ Elbow Brace 3, L3999

Masterhinge™ Hip Hinge 3, L2999

Masterhinge™ Shoulder Brace 3, L3999

Mattress
air pressure, E0186, E0197
alternating pressure, E0277
pad, Bio Flote, E0181
pad, KoalaKair, E0181
AquaPedic Sectional, E0196
decubitus care, E0196
dry pressure, E0184
flotation, E0184
gel pressure, E0196
hospital bed, E0271, E0272
non-powered, pressure reducing, E0373
Iris Preventix pressure relief/reduction, E0184
Overlay, E0371-E0372
TenderFlor II, E0187
TenderGel II, E0196
water pressure, E0187, E0198
powered, pressure reducing, E0277

Maxilla, fracture, D7610-D7620, D7710-D7720

Maxillofacial dental procedures, D5911-D5999

MCP, multi-axial rotation unit, L5986

MCT Oil, enteral nutrition, B4155

Meals
adults in treatment, T1010
per diem NOS, S9977

Mechlorethamine HCl, J9230

Medialization material for vocal cord, C1878

Medical and surgical supplies, A4206-A6404

Medical conference, S0220-S0221

Medical food, S9435

Medical records copying fee, S9981-S9982

Medicare "welcome"
ECG, G0366-G0368
physical, G0344

Medi-Jector injection device, A4210

MediSense 2 Pen blood glucose monitor, E0607

Medralone
40, J1030
80, J1040

Medrol, J7509

Medroxyprogesterone acetate, J1055
with estradiol cypionate, J1056

Mefoxin, J0694

Megestrol acetate, S0179

Melphalan HCl, J9245
oral, J8600

Menotropins, S0122

Mental health
assessment, H0031
hospitalization, H0035
peer services, H0038
self-help, H0038
service plan, H0032
services, NOS, H0046
supportive treatment, H0026-H0037

Mepergan (injection), J2180

Meperidine, J2175
and promethazine, J2180

Mepivacaine HCl, J0670

Mercaptopurine, S0108

Meritene, enteral nutrition, B4150
powder, B4150

Meropenem, J2185

Mesh, C1781

Mesna, C9428, J9209

Mesnex, C9428, J9209

Metabolism error, food supplement, S9434

Metacarpophalangeal joint prosthesis, L8630

Metaproterenol
inhalation solution
concentrated, J7668
unit dose, J7669

Metaraminol bitartrate, J0380

Metatarsal joint, prosthetic implant, L8641

Metatarsal neuroma injection, S2135

Meter, bath conductivity, dialysis, E1550

Methacholine chloride, J7674

Methadone, S0109

Methadone HCl, J1230

Methergine, J2210

Methocarbamol, J2800

Methotrexate, oral, J8610
sodium, J9250, J9260

Methyldopate HCl, J0210

Methylergonovine maleate, J2210

Methylprednisolone
acetate, J1020-J1040
oral, J7509
sodium succinate, J2920, J2930

Metoclopramide HCl, J2765

Metronidazole, S0030

Meunster Suspension, socket prosthesis, L6110

Miacalcin, J0630

Microabrasion, enamel, D9970

Microbiology test, P7001

Midazolam HCl, J2250

Micro-Fine
disposable insulin syringes, up to 1 cc, per syringe, A4206
lancets, box of 100, A4259

Microcapillary tube, A4651
sealant, A4652

Microlipids, enteral nutrition, B4155

Microspirometer, S8190

Mileage, ambulance, A0380, A0390

Milk, breast
processing, T2101

Milrinone lactate, J2260

Milwaukee spinal orthosis, L1000

Minerva, spinal orthosis, L0700, L0710

Mini-bus, nonemergency transportation, A0120

Minimed
3 cc syringe, A4232
506 insulin pump, E0784
insulin infusion set with bent needle wings, each, A4231
Sof-Set 24" insulin infusion set, each, A4230

Minoxidil, S0139

Miscellaneous, A9150-A9600

Mitomycin, C9432 , J9280-J9291

Mitoxana, C9427

Mitoxantrone HCl, J9293

Mobilite hospital beds, E0293, E0295, E0297

Moducal, enteral nutrition, B4155

Moisture exchanger for use with invasive mechanical ventilation, A4483

Moisturizer, skin, A6250

Monarc-M, J7190

Monitor
apnea, E0618
blood glucose, E0607
Accu-Check, E0607
Tracer II, E0607
blood pressure, A4670
pacemaker, E0610, E0615
ventilator, E0450

Monoclonal antibodies, J7505

Monoject disposable insulin syringes, up to 1 cc, per syringe, A4206

Monojector lancet device, A4258

Morcellator, C1782

Morphine sulfate, J2270, J2271, S0093
sterile, preservative-free, J2275

Moulage, facial, D5911-D5912

Mouth exam, athletic, D9941

Mouthpiece (for respiratory equipment), A4617

Moxifloxacin, J2280

M-Prednisol-40, J1030
-80, J1040

MRI
contrast material, A4643
low field, S8042

Mucoprotein, blood, P2038

Multifetal pregnancy reduction, ultrasound guidance, S8055

Multiple post collar, cervical, L0180-L0200

Multipositional patient support system, E0636

Muscular dystrophy, genetic test, S3853

Muse, J0275

Mutamycin, J9280

Mycophenolate mofetil, J7517

Mycophenolic acid, J7518

Mylotarg, J9300

Myochrysine, J1600

Myolin, J2360

Myotonic muscular dystrophy, genetic test, S3853

Myringotomy, S2225

N

Nafcillin sodium, S0032

Nail trim, G0127, S0390

Nalbuphine HCl, J2300

Naloxone HCl, J2310

Nandrobolic L.A., J2321

Nandrolone
decanoate, J2320-J2322

Narrowing device, wheelchair, E0969

Narcan, J2310

Nasahist B, J0945

Nasal
application device (for CPAP device), A7032-A7034
vaccine inhalation, J3530

Nasogastric tubing, B4081, B4082

Navelbine, J9390

ND Stat, J0945

Nebcin, J3260

Nebulizer, E0570-E0585
aerosol compressor, E0571
aerosol mask, A7015
aerosols, E0580
Airlife Brand Misty-Neb, E0580
Power-Mist, E0580
Up-Draft Neb-U-Mist, E0580
Up-Mist hand-held nebulizer, E0580
compressor, with, E0570
Madamist II medication
compressor/nebulizer, E0570
Pulmo-Aide compressor/nebulizer, E0570
Schuco Mist nebulizer system, E0570
corrugated tubing
disposable, A7010, A7018
non-disposable, A7011
distilled water, A7018
drug dispensing fee, E0590
filter
disposable, A7013
non-disposable, A7014
heater, E1372
large volume
disposable, prefilled, A7008
disposable, unfilled, A7007
not used with oxygen
durable glass, A7017
pneumatic, administration set, A7003, A7005, A7006
pneumatic, nonfiltered, A7004
portable, E0570
small volume, E0574
spacer or nebulizer, S8100
with mask, S8101
ultrasonic, dome and mouthpiece, A7016
ultrasonic, reservoir bottle
non-disposable, A7009
water, A7018
water collection device large volume
nebulizer, A7012
distilled water, A7018

NebuPent, J2545

Needle, A4215
any size, A4656
brachytherapy, C1715
non-coring, A4212
with syringe, A4206-A4209

Negative pressure wound therapy
canister set, A6551
dressing set, A6550
pump, E2402

Nembutal sodium solution, J2515

Neocyten, J2360

Neo-Durabolic, J2320-J2322

Neomax knee support, L1800

Neoplasms, dental, D7410-D7465

Neoquess, J0500

Neosar, J9070-J9092

Neostigmine methylsulfate, J2710

Neo-Synephrine, J2370

NephrAmine, parenteral nutrition, B5000

Nesacaine MPF, J2400

Nesiritide, J2324

NETT pulmonary rehabilitation
education
skills
group, G0111
individual, G0110
nutritional guidance
initial, G0112
subsequent, G0113
psychological testing, G0115
psychosocial consultation, G0114
psychosocial counseling, G0116

Neulasta, J2505

Neumega, J2355

Neurolysis
foot, S2135

Neuromuscular stimulator, E0745
ambulation of spinal cord injured, K0600

Neuro-Pulse, E0720

Neurostimulator
generator, C1767
implantable
pulse generator, E0756
receiver, E0757
lead, C1778
patient programmer, C1787, E0754
receiver and/or transmitter, C1816

Neutrexin, J3305

Newington
Legg Perthes orthosis L1710
mobility frame, L1500

Newport Lite hip orthosis, L1685

Nextep™ Contour™ Lower Leg Walker, L2999

Nextep™ Low Silhouette™ Lower Leg Walkers, L2999

Nicotine
gum, S4995
patches, S4990-S4991

Niemann-Pick disease, genetic test, S3849

Nightguard, D9940

Nipent, J9268

Nitric oxide, for hypoxic respiratory failure in neonate, S1025

Nitrogen mustard, J9230

Nitrous oxide, dental analgesia, D9230

Nonchemotherapy drug, oral, J8499

Noncovered services, A9270, G0293-G0294

Nonemergency transportation, A0080-A0210

Nonimpregnated gauze dressing, A6216, A6221, A6402, A6404

Nonintravenous conscious sedation, dental, D9248

Nonprescription drug, A9150

Nonthermal pulsed high frequency radiowaves treatment device, E0761

Nordryl, J1200

Norflex, J2360

Norplant System contraceptive, A4260

Northwestern Suspension, socket prosthesis, L6110

Not otherwise classified drug, J3490, J7599, J7699, J7799, J8499, J8999, J9999, Q0181

Novantrone, J9293

Novo Nordisk insulin, J1815, J1817

Novo Seven, Q0187

NPH insulin, J1815, S5552

Nubain, J2300

NuHope
adhesive, 1 oz bottle with applicator, A4364
adhesive, 3 oz bottle with applicator, A4364
cleaning solvent, 4 oz bottle, A4455
cleaning solvent, 16 oz bottle, A4455
hole cutter tool, A4421

Numorphan H.P., J2410

Nursing care, in home
  licensed practical nurse, S9124
  registered nurse, S9123

Nursing home visit, dental, D9410

Nursing services, S9211-S9212, T1000-T1004

Nutri-Source, enteral nutrition, B4155

Nutrition
  counseling
    dental, D1310, D1320
    dietary, S9452
  enteral infusion pump, B9000, B9002
  enteral formulae, B4150-B41625
  parenteral infusion pump, B9004, B9006
  parenteral solution, B4164-B5200

Nutritional counseling, dietition visit, S9470

NYU, hand prosthesis, child, L6872

O

Observation care for CHF, chest pain or asthma, G0244

Obturator prosthesis
  definitive, D5932
  dental
    postsurgical, D5932
    refitting, D5933
    surgical, D5931
  interim, D5936
  surgical, D5931

Occipital/mandibular support, cervical, L0160

Occlusal
  adjustment, dental, D9951-D9952
  guard, dental, D9940
  orthotic device, D7877

Occlusion/analysis, D9950

Occlusion device placement, G0264

Ocular device, C1784

Occupational multifocal lens, V2786

Occupational therapist
  home health setting, G0152

Occupational therapy, S9129

Octafluoropropane with human serum albumin, C9202

Octreotide
  intramuscular form, J2353
  subcutaneous or intravenous form, J2354

Ocular prosthetic implant, L8610

Oculinum, J0585

Odansetron HCl, J2405, Q0179

Odontoplasty (enameloplasty), D9971

Office service, M0064

Offobock cosmetic gloves, L6895

O-Flex, J2360

Ofloxacin, S0034

Ohio Willow
  prosthetic sheath
    above knee, L8410
    below knee, L8400
    upper limb, L8415
  prosthetic sock, L8420-L8435
  stump sock, L8470-L8485

Olanzapine, S0166

Omalizumab, J2357, S0107

Omnipen-N, J0290

Oncaspar, J9266

Oncoscint, A4642

Oncovin, J9370

Ondanestron HCl, S0181

One-Button foldaway walker, E0143

One Touch
  Basic blood glucose meter, E0607
  Basic test strips, box of 50, A4253
  Profile blood glucose meter, E0607

Onlay, dental
  fixed partial denture retainer, metallic, D6602, D6615
  metallic, D2542-D2544
  porcelain/ceramic, D2642-D2644
  resin-based composite, D2662, D2664
  titanium, D6634

O & P Express
  above knee, L5210
  ankle-foot orthosis with bilateral uprights, L1990
  anterior floor reaction orthosis, L1945
  below knee, L5105
  elbow disarticulation, L6200
  hip disarticulation, L5250
  hip-knee-ankle-foot orthosis, L2080
  interscapular thoracic, L6370
  Legg Perthes orthosis, Scottish Rite, L1730
  Legg Perthes orthosis, Patten, L1755
  knee-ankle-foot orthosis, L2000, L2010, L2020, L2036
  knee disarticulation, L5150, L5160
  partial foot, L5000, L5020
  plastic foot drop brace, L1960
  supply/accessory/service, L9900

Oppenheimer, wrist-hand-finger orthosis, L3924

Operculectomy, D7971

Oprelvekin, J2355

Osteotomy, periacetabular, S2115

Oral and maxillofacial surgery, D7111-D7999

Oral disease
  test for detection, D0431
  test for susceptibility, D0421

Oral examination, D0120-D0160

Oral hygiene instruction, D1330

Oral interpreter or sign language services, T1013

Oral orthotic treatment for sleep apnea, S8260

Oral pathology
  accession of tissue, D0472-D0474
  bacteriologic studies, D0415
  cytology, D0480
  other oral pathology procedures, D0502

Oraminic II, J0945

Orcel, C9200

Organ donor procurement, S2152

Ormazine, J3230

Oropharyngeal suction catheter, A4628

Orphenadrine, J2360

Orphenate, J2360

Orthodontics, D8000-D8999

Ortho-Ease forearm crutches, E0111

Orthoflex™ Elastic Plaster Bandages, A4580

Orthoguard hip orthosis, L1685

Orthomedics
  ankle-foot orthosis, L1900
  pediatric hip abduction splint, L1640
  plastic foot drop brace, L1960
  single axis shoe insert, L2180
  ultralight airplane arm abduction splint, L3960
  upper extremity fracture orthosis
    combination, L3986
    humeral, L3980
    radius/ulnar, L3982

Orthomerica
  below knee test socket, L5620
  pediatric hip abduction splint, L1640
  plastic foot drop brace, L1960
  single axis shoe insert, L2180
  upper extremity fracture orthosis
    humeral, L3980
    radius/ulnar, L3982
  wrist extension cock-up, L3914

Orthopedic devices, E0910-E0948
  cervical
    Diskard head halters, E0942
    Turtle Neck safety collars, E0942

Orthopedic shoes
  arch support, L3040-L3100
  footwear, L3201-L3265
  insert, L3000-L3030
  lift, L3300-L3334
  miscellaneous additions, L3500-L3595
  positioning device, L3140-L3170
  transfer, L3600-L3649
  wedge, L3340-L3420

Orthoplast™ Splints (and Orthoplast™ II Splints), A4590

Orthotic additions
  carbon graphite lamination, L2755
  cervical congenital torticollis, L0112
  electric lock, L6638
  electronic elbow with microprocessor, L7181
  endoskeletal knee-shin system, L5848
    with microprocessor, L5856, L5857
  fracture, L2180-L2192, L3995
  halo, L0860
  heavy duty feature, L5995
  lock mechanism for elbow, L6698
  lower extremity, L2200-L2999, L5781-L5782, L5646-L5648, L5984
  ratchet lock, L2430
  replacement strap, L4002
  rocker bottom for ankle, L2232
  scoliosis, L1010-L1120, L1210-L1290
  shoe, L3300-L3595, L3649
  shoulder lock, L6646-L6648
  socket insert for elbow, L6694-L6697
  spinal, L0970-L0999
  suspension sleeve for knee, L5685
  upper extremity joint, L3956
  upper limb, L3810-L3890, L3970-L3974, L3995
  vacuum pump, L5781-L5782

Orthotic appliance, D7880

Orthotic devices
  ankle-foot (see also **Orthopedic shoes**), E1815, E1830, L1900-L1990, L2108-L2116, L3160
  anterior-posterior, L0530
  anterior-posterior-lateral, L0700, L0710
  cervical, L0100-L0200
  cervical-thoracic-lumbar-sacral, L0700, L0710
  congenital trorticollis, L0112
  elbow, E1800, L3700-L3740
  fracture, L3980-L3986
  halo, L0810-L0830
  hand, E1805, E1825, L3800-L3805, L3900-L3954
  hip, L1600-L1686
  hip-knee-ankle-foot, L2040-L2090
  interface material, E1820
  knee, E1810, L1800-L1880
  knee-ankle-foot, L2000-L2038, L2126-L2136
  Legg Perthes, L1700-L1755
  lumbar, K0634-K0636
  lumbar-sacral, K0634-K0649
  lumbar-sacral, hip, femur, L1690
  multiple post collar, L0180-L0200
  not otherwise specified, L0999, L1499, L2999, L3999, L5999, L7499, L8039, L8239
  pneumatic splint, L4350-L4380
  repair or replacement, L4000-L4210

Orthotic devices — *continued*
  replace soft interface material, L4392-L4394
  sacroiliac, K0630-K0633
  scoliosis, L1000, L1200, L1300-L1499
  shoe, *see* **Orthopedic shoes**
  shoulder, L3650-L3675
  shoulder-elbow-wrist-hand, L3960-L3969
  spinal, cervical, L0100-L0200
  thoracic, L0210
  thoracic-hip-knee-ankle, L1500-L1520
  toe, L1830
  transfer (shoe orthosis), L3600-L3640
  walking splint, nonpneumatic, L4386
  wrist-hand-finger, E1805, E1825, L3800-L3805, L3900-L3954

Or-Tyl, J0500

Oseltamivir phosphate, G9019

Osmolite, enteral nutrition, B4150
  HN, B4150

Osseous dental surgery, graft, D4260-D4264

Ossicula prosthetic implant, L8613

Osteitis, localized, dry socket, D9930

Osteogenic stimulator, E0747-E0749, E0760

Osteoplasty, D7940

Osteotomy
  dental, D7941-D7945
  segmented/subapical, D7944

Ostomy
  absorbant material, A4422
  accessories, A5093
  adhesive remover wipes, A4365
  appliance belt, A4367
  filter, A4368
  irrigation supply, A4398, A4399
  pediatric one-piece system, A5061, A5062
  pediatric two-piece drainable pouch, A5063
  pouch, A4416-A4420, A4423-A4434
    drainable, A4413
    pediatric, A5061-5062
  skin barrier, A4414-A4415
    extended wear, A4407-A4410
    paste, A4405-A4406
  vent, A4366

Otto Bock prosthesis
  battery, six volt, L7360
  battery charger, six volt, L7362
  electronic greifer, L7020, L7035
  electronic hand, L7010, L7025
  hook adapter, L6628
  lamination collar, L6629
  pincher tool, L6810
  wrist, L6629, L7260

Overdenture, D5860-D5861

Overlay, mattress, E0371-E0373

Ovulation induction, S4042

Owens & Minor
  cervical collar, L0140
  cervical helmet, L0120

Oxacillin sodium, E0445
  probe, A4606

Oxaliplatin, C9205, J9263

Oximeter, S8105

Oxi-Uni-Pak, E0430

Oxygen
  ambulance, A0422
  chamber, hyperbaric, topical, A4575
  concentrator, E1390, E1391
  gaseous, S8120
  liquid, S8121
  mask, A4620
  medication supplies, A4611-A4627

Oxygen — *continued*
  portable, E0443-E0444
  rack/stand, E1355
  regulator, E1353
  respiratory equipment/supplies, A4611-A4627, E0424-E0480
    Argyle Sentinel seal chest drainage unit, E0460
    Oxi-Uni-Pak, E0430
  supplies and equipment, E0425-E0444, E0455, E1353-E1406
  tent, E0455
  tubing, A4616
  water vapor enriching system, E1405, E1406

Oxymorphone HCl, J2410

Oxytetracycline HCl, J2460

Oxytocin, J2590

P

Pacemaker
  dual chamber
    non-rate responsive, C2619
    rate responsive, C1785
  lead, C1779, C1898, C1899
  monitor, E0610, E0615
  other than single or dual chamber, C2621
  single chamber
    non rate responsive, C2620
    rate responsive, C1786

Pacer manual wheelchair, K0003

Packing strips, A6407

Paclitaxel, C9431, J9265

Pad
  abdominal, L1270
  adhesive, A6203-A6205, A6212-A6214, A6219-A6221, A6237-A6239, A6245-A6247, A6254-A6256
  alginate, A6196-A6199
  alternating pressure, E0180, E0181
  arm, K0019
  asis, L1250
  condylar, L2810
  crutch, A4635
  gel pressure, E0185, E0196
  gluteal L2650
  gradient pressure pads, S8421-S8429
  heating, E0210, E0215, E0217, E0238, E0249
  heel, L3480, L3485
  knee, L1858
  kyphosis, L1020, L1025
  lumbar, L1030, L1040, L1240
  nonadhesive (dressing), A6209-A6211, A6216-A6218, A6222-A6224, A6228-A6230, A6234-A6236, A6242-A6244
  orthotic device interface, E1820
  replacement, infrared heat system, A4639
  rib gusset, L1280
  sheepskin, E0188, E0189
  shoe, L3430-L3485
  stabilizer, L3170
  sternal, L1050
  thoracic, L1060, L1260
  torso support, L0960
  triceps, L6100
  trocanteric, L1290
  truss, L8320, L8330
  water circulating, cold, with pump, E0218
  water circulating, heat, with pump, E0217
  water circulating, heat, unit, E0249
  water pressure, E0198

Padden Shoulder Immobilizer, L3670

Pail, for use with commode chair, E0167

Palicizumab RSV IgM, C9003

Palmer, wrist-hand-finger orthosis, L3936

Palonosetron HCl, J2469

Pamidronate disodium, C9411, J2430

Pan, for use with commode chair, E0167

Pantoprazole sodium, C9113, S0164

Papanicolaou (Pap) screening smear, P3000, P3001, Q0091

Papaverine HCl, J2440

Paraffin, A4265
  bath unit, E0235

Paragard T 380-A, IUD, J7300

Paramagnetic contrast material, (Gadolinium), A4647

Paramedic intercept, S0208

Paranasal sinus ultrasound, S9024

Paraplatin, J9045

Parapodium, mobility frame, L1500

Parenteral nutrition
  administration kit, B4224
  home infusion therapy, S9364-S9368
  pump, B9004, B9006
  solution, B4164-B5200
  supplies, not otherwise classified, B9999
  supply kit, B4220, B4222

Parenting class, S9444
  infant safety, S9447

Paricalcitol, J2501

Parking fee, nonemergency transport, A0170

Partial dentures
  fixed
    implant/adjustment-supported retainers, D6068-D6077
    pontic, D6210-D6252
    retainers, D6545-D6792
  removable, D5211-D5281

PASRR, T2010-T2011

Paste, conductive, A4558

Patient lift, E0625, E0637, E0639, E0640

Pathology and laboratory tests, miscellaneous, P9010-P9615

Patten Bottom, Legg Perthes orthosis, L1755

Pavlik harness, hip orthosis, L1650

Peak flow meter, S8110
  portable, S8096

Pediatric hip abduction splint
  Orthomedics, L1640
  Orthomerica, L1640

Pediculosis treatment, A9180

PEFR, peak expiratory flow rate meter, A4614

Pegfilgastrim, J2505

Pegademase bovine, Q2012

Pegaspargase, J9266

Peg-L-asparaginase, J9266

Pelvic and breast exam, G0101

Pelvic belt/harness/boot, E0944

Pemetrexed, J9305

Penicillin G
  benzathine and penicillin G procaine, J0530-J0580
  potassium, J2540
  procaine, aqueous, J2510

Penlet lancet device, A4258

Penlet II lancet device, A4258

Pentamidine isethionate, J2545, S0080

Pentastarch, Q2013

Pentazocine HCl, J3070

Pentobarbital sodium, J2515

Pentostatin, J9268

Percussor, E0480

Percutaneous
access system, A4301

Perflexane lipic microspheres, C9203

Perflutren lipid microsphere, C9112

Performance Wrap™ (KO), L1825

Periapical service, D3410-D3470

Periodontal procedures, D4000-D4999

Periradicular/apicoectomy, D3410-D3426

Perlstein, ankle-foot orthosis, L1920

Permapen, J0560-J0580

Peroneal strap, L0980

Peroxide, A4244

Perphenazine, J3310, Q0175-Q0176

Persantine, J1245

Personal care services, T1019-T1020

Pessary, A4561-A4562

PET imaging
brain imaging, G0336
breast, G0252-G0254
cervical, G0330
colorectal, G0213-G0215
esophageal, G0226-G0228
lung, G0125, G0210-G0212
lymphoma, G0220-G0222
metabolic bain imaging, G0229-G0230
myocardial perfusion, G0030-G0047
ovarian, G0331
regional, G0125, G0223-G0225, G0234
thyroid, G0296
whole body, G0125, G0210-G0228, G0230-G0234

Pfizerpen, J2540
A.S., J2510

PGE₁, J0270

Phamacologicals, dental, D9610, D9630

Pharmacy services, S9430

Pharmaplast disposable insulin syringes, per syringe, A4206

Phelps, ankle-foot orthosis, L1920

Phenazine (25, 50), J2550

Phenergan, J2550

Phenobarbital sodium, J2560

Phentolamine mesylate, J2760

Phenylephrine HCl, J2370

Phenytoin sodium, J1165

Philadelphia™ tracheotomy cervical collar, L0172

Philly™ One-piece™ Extrication collar, L0150

pHisoHex solution, A4246

Photofrin, J9600

Photographs, dental, diagnostic, D0350

Phototherapy
home visit service (Bili-Lite), S9098
keratectomy (PKT), S0812
light, E0202

Physical exam for college, S0622

Physical therapy, S8990
shoulder stretch device, E1841

Physical therapy/therapist
home health setting, G0151, S9131

Phytonadione, J3430

Pillo pump, E0182

Pillow
abduction, E1399
decubitus care, E0190
positioning, E0190

Pin retention, per tooth, D2951

Pinworm examination, Q0113

Piperacillin sodium, S0081

Pit and fissure sealant, D1351

Pitocin, J2590

Planing, dental root, D0350

Plasma
frozen, P9058-P9060
multiple donor, pooled, frozen, P9023
protein fraction, P9048
single donor, fresh frozen, P9017

Plastazote, L3002, L3252, L3253, L3265, L5654-L5658

Plaster
bandages
Orthoflex™ Elastic Plaster Bandages, A4580
Specialist™ Plaster Bandages, A4580
Genmould™ Creamy Plaster, A4580
Specialist™ J-Splint™ Plaster Roll Immobilizer, A4580
Specialist™ Plaster Roll Immobilizer, A4580
Specialist™ Plaster Splints, A4580

Platelet
concentrate, each unit, P9019
rich plasma, each unit, P9020

Platelets, P9032-P9040, P9052-P9053

Platform, for home blood glucose monitor, A4255

Platform attachment
forearm crutch, E0153
walker, E0154

Platinol, J9060, J9062

Pleural catheter, A7042
drainage bottle, A7043

Plenaxis, J0128

Plicamycin, J9270

Plumbing, for home ESRD equipment, A4870

Pneumatic
appliance, E0655-E0673, L4350-L4380
compressor, E0650-E0652, E0675
splint, L4350-L4380
tire, wheelchair, E0953

Pneumatic nebulizer
administration set
small volume
filtered, A7006
non-filtered, A7003
non-disposable, A7005
small volume, disposable, A7004

Pneumococcal conjugate vaccine, S0195

Polaris, E0601

Polaris Lt, E0601

Polocaine, J0670

Polycillin-N, J0290

Polycose, enteral nutrition,
liquid, B4155
powder, B4155

Poly-l-lactic acid, S0196

Pontic
indirect resin based composite, D6205
titanium, D6214

Pontics, D5281, D6210-D6252

Poor blood, each unit, P9016

Porfimer, J9600

Pork insulin, J1815, J1817

Port
indwelling, C1788

Portable
equipment transfer, R0070-R0076
hemodialyzer system, E1635
nebulizer, E0570
x-ray equipment, Q0092

Portagen Powder, enteral nutrition, B4150

Posey restraints, E0700

Positive airway pressure device supply, A7046

Post-coital examination, Q0115

Post and core, dental, D2952-D2954, D2957, D6970-D6972, D6976-D6977

Post, removal, dental, D2955

Postural drainage board, E0606

Potassium
chloride, J3480
hydroxide (KOH) preparation, Q0112

Pouch
Active Life convex one-piece urostomy, A4421
closed, A4387, A5052
drainable, A4388-A4389, A5061
fecal collection, A4330
Little Ones Sur-fit mini, A5054
ostomy, A4375-A4378, A4387-A4391, A5051-A5054, A5061-A5063, A4416-A4420, A4423-A4434
pediatric, drainable, A5061
Pouchkins pediatric ostomy system, A5061, A5062, A5073
Sur-Fit, drainable, A5063
urinary, A4379-A4383, A4391, A5071-A5073
urosotomy, A5073

Power mist nebulizer, E0580

Pralidoxime chloride, J2730

Precision attachment, dental, D5862, D6950

Precision, enteral nutrition
HN, B4153
Isotonic, B4153

Predalone-50, J2650

Predcor (-25, -50), J2650

Predicort-50, J2650

Prednisolone
acetate, J2650
oral, J7506, J7510

Prednisone, J7506

Predoject-50, J2650

Prefabricated crown, D2930-D2933

Prefabricated post and core, dental, D2954, D6972
each additional (same tooth), D2957, D6977

Pregnancy care, H1000-H1005

Pregnyl, J0725

Premarin IV, J1410

Premium knee sleeve, L1830

Prenatal care, H1000-H1005

Preparatory prosthesis, L5510-L5595

Prescription drug, (*see also* **Table of Drugs**) J3490, J8499
chemotherapy, J8999, J9999
nonchemotherapy, J8499

Pressure
alarm, dialysis, E1540
pad, E0180-E0199

PressureGuard II, E0186

PressureKair mattress overlay, E0197

Prestige blood glucose monitor, E0607

Pre-Vent heel & elbow protector, E0191

Prevention, developmental delay, H2037

Preventive
dental procedures, D1110-D1550
foot care, S0390

Preventive health Medicare
ECG, G0366-G0368
exam, G0344

Primacor, J2260

Primaxin, J0743

Priscoline HCl, J2670

Probe
cryoablation, C2618
oximeter, A4606
percutaneous lumbar discectomy, C2614

Procainamide HCl, J2690

Procarbazine HCl, S0182

Processing
breast milk, T2101

Prochlorperazine, J0780, Q0164-Q0165
oral, S0183

Procrit, Q0136

Procurement, organ donor, S2152

Procuren, S9055

Profasi HP, J0725

Profilnine Heat-Treated, J7194

Progesterone, J2675

Prograf, J7507

Prolastin, J0256

Proleukin, J9015

Prolixin decanoate, J2680

Prolotherapy, M0076

Promazine HCl, J2950

Promethazine HCl, J2550, Q0169-Q0170

Promethazine and meperdine, J2180

Promix, enteral nutrition, B4155

Pronation/supination device, forearm,
E1802

Pronestyl, J2690

Propac, enteral nutrition, B4155

Prophylaxis, dental, D1110, D1120

Proplex (-T and SX-T), J7194

Propranolol HCl, J1800

Prorex (-25, -50), J2550

Prostaglandin E₁, J0270

Prostaphlin, J2700

Prostate
laser vaporation, C9713

Prosthesis
adhesive, used for facial
remover, A4365
auricular, D5914
breast, C1789, L8000-L8035, L8600
cranial, D5924
dental, fixed, D6210-D6999
dental, removable, D5110-D5899
eye, L8610, V2623-V2629
finger joint, L8659
fitting, L5400-L5460, L6380-L6388
grasper, L6881
hand, L6000-L6020
hemifacial, L8044
implants, L8600-L8699
larynx, L8500, L8505
lower extremity, L5700-L5999, L8642
mandibular resection, D5934-D5935
maxiofacial, provided by a nonphysician,
L8040-L8048

Prosthesis — *continued*
metacarpal, L8631
midfacial, L8041
miscellaneous service, L8499
nasal septal, L8047
obturator, D5931-D5933, D5936
ocular, D5916
orbital, D5915
palatal, D5954-D5959
partial facial, L8046
penile
inflatable, C1813
non-inflatable, C2622
repair, K0449, L7520
repair or modification, maxillofacial,
L8048-L8049
socks (shrinker, sheath, stump sock),
L8400-L8480
tracheoesophageal, L8511-L8514
tracheoesophageal gelatin capsule,L8515
tracheostomy speaking, L8501
unspecified maxillofacial, L8048
upper extremity, L6000-L6915
urinary sphincter, C1815
vacuum erection system, L7900

Prosthetic additions
lower extremity, L5610-L5999
upper extremity, L6600-L7274

Prosthetic shrinker, L8440-L8465

Prosthodontic procedures
fixed, D6210-D6999
implant-supported, D6055-D6079
maxillofacial, D5911-D5999
pediatric partial denture, D6985
removable, D5110-D5999

Prostigmin, J2710

Prostin VR Pediatric, J0270

Protamine sulfate, J2720, A4802

Protectant, skin, A6250

Protector, heel or elbow, E0191

Protirelin, J2725

Protonix, S0164

Protopam chloride, J2730

Provisional, dental
retainer crown (FPD), D6793
single crown, D2799

Prozine-50, J2950

Psychiatric care, H0036-H0037, H2013-
H2014

PTK, S0812

Pulmo-Aide compressor
nebulizer, E0570

Pulp cap, D3110, D3120

Pulp capping, D3110, D3120

Pulp sedation, D2940

Pulp vitality test, D0460

Pulpal debridement, D3221

Pulpal therapy, on primary teeth,
D3230, D3240

Pulpotomy, D3220
vitality test, D0460

Pulse generator,
ear E2120
battery, A4638

Pump
alternating pressure pad, E0182
ambulatory infusion, E0781
ambulatory insulin, E0784
Bio Flote alternating pressure pad,
E0182
blood, dialysis, E1620
breast, E0602-E0604
supplies, A4281-A4286
Broncho-Cath endobronchial tubes, with
CPAP, E0601

Pump — *continued*
enteral infusion, B9000, B9002
supply, K0552
gastric suction, E2000
Gomco lightweight mobile aspirator,
E0600
Gomco portable aspirator, E0600
heparin infusion, E1520
implantable infusion, E0782, E0783
implantable infusion, refill kit, A4220
infusion
non-programmable, C1891, C2626
supplies, A4230-A4232
insulin, external, E0784
instruction, S9145
negative pressure wound therapy, E2402
parenteral infusion, B9004, B9006,
K0455
Pillo alternating pressure pad, E0182
speech aid, D5952-D5953, D5960
suction
CPAP, E0601
gastric, E2000
portable, E0600
TenderCloud alternating pressure pad,
E0182
water circulating pad, E0217, E0218,
E0236

Purification system, E1610, E1615

Purified pork insulin, J1815, J1817

Pyeloscopy
for ureteral calculi, S2070

Pyridoxine HCl, J3415

Quad cane, E0105

Quadri-Poise canes, E0105

Quelicin, J0330

Quick Check blood glucose test strips,
box of 50, A4253

Quick release restraints, E0700

Quikfit crutch, E0114

Quik-Fold Walkers, E0141, E0143

Quinoprestin, J2770

R

Rack/stand, oxygen, E1355

Radiation, dental
carrier, D5983
cone locator, D5985
shield, D5984

Radiation therapy, intraoperative, S8049

Radioelements for brachytherapy, Q3001

Radiofrequency transmitter, sacral root
neurostimulator, replacement,
E0759

Radiograph, dental, D0210-D0340

Radioimmunoscintigraphy, S8080

Radiology service, R0070-R0076

Radiopharmaceutical
ammonia N-13, A9526
cobaltous chloride, C9013
diagnostic imaging agent, A4641, A4642,
A9500-A9505, C1080
I-131 tositumomab, A9533-A9534,
C1080, C1081
indium I-111
ibitumomab tiuxetan, C1082
satumomab pendetide, A4642
sodium iodide I-131, A9528-A9531
technetium Tc 99m
albumin aggregated, A9519
arcitumomab, C1122
depreotide, A9511
disofenin, A9510
exametazime, A9521
glucepatate, Q3006
mebrofenin, A9513
medronate, A9503

Radiopharmaceutical — *continued*
　technetium Tc 99m — *continued*
　　mertiatide, Q3005
　　oxidronate, Q3009
　　pentetate, A9515
　　pertechnetate, A9512
　　pyrophosphate, A9515
　　sestamibi, A9500
　　sulfur colloid, A9520
　　tetrofosmin, A9502
　　vicisate, Q3003
　therapeutic, A9600, C0181, C1083
　yttrium 90 ibritumomab tiuxetan, C1083

Rail
　bathtub, E0241, E0242, E0246
　bed, E0305, E0310
　toilet, E0243

Rancho hip action, hip orthosis, L1680

Range of motion device
　shoulder, E1841

Raptiva, S0162

Rasburicase, J2783

Rascal, power wheelchair, K0010

Ready-For-Use wooden crutches, E0113

Reassessment, nutrition therapy, G0270-
　G0271

Recement
　cast or prefabricated post and core,
　　D2915
　crown, D2920
　inlay, D2910

Recombinant
　ankle splints, L4392-L4398
　DNA insulin, J1815, J1817

Recombinate, J7192

Red blood cells, P9038-P9040

Red blood cells, each unit, P9021, P9022

Red Dot
　crutches, E0114
　folding walkers, E0135, E0143

Redisol, J3420

Reflux treatment, S2215

Regitine, J2760

Reglan, J2765

Regular insulin, J1815

Regulator, oxygen, E1353

Rehabilitation
　vestibular, S9476

Rehabilitation program, H2001

Rehabilitation service
　juveniles, H2033
　mental health clubhouse, H2030-H2031
　psychosocial, H2017-H2018
　substance abuse, H2034-H2036
　supported employment, H2023-H2024

Rehabilitation teacher, G9037

Reimplantation, dental
　accidentally evulsed, D7270
　intentional, D3470

Relefact TRH, J2725

Relenza, G9018

Remicade, J1745

RemRes, E0601

REMStar, E0601

Renacidin, Q2004

RenAmin, parenteral nutrition, B5000

Renu, enteral nutrition, B4150

ReoPro, TRH, J0130

Repair
　contract, ERSD, A4890

Repair — *continued*
　dental, D2980, D3351-D3353, D5510-
　　D5630, D6090, D6980, D7852,
　　D7955
　diaphragmatic hernia, S2400
　durable medical equipment, E1340
　hearing aid, V5014, V5336
　home dialysis equipment, A4890
　occlusal guard, dental, D9942
　orthotic, L4000-L4130
　prosthetic, L7500, L7510, L7520
　skilled technical, E1340

Replacement
　battery, A4254, A4630
　　ear pulse generator, A4638
　handgrip for cane, crutch, walker A4636
　ostomy filters, A4421
　tip for cane, crutch, walker, A4637
　underarm pad for crutch, A4635

Repositioning device, mandibular, S8262

Rep-Pred
　40, J1030
　80, J1040

ResCap headgear, A7035

Reservoir
　metered dose inhaler, A4627

Residential care, T2032-T2033

Resin dental restoration, D2330-D2394

Resipiradyne II Plus pulmonary
　function/ventilation monitor,
　E0450

ResMed Sb Elite, E0601

RespiGam, J1565

Respiratory syncytial virus immune
　globulin, J1565

Respiratory therapy, G0237-G0238

Respite care, T1005
　in home, S9125
　not in home, H0045

Restorations, dental
　amalgam, D2140-D2161
　gold foil, D2410-D2430
　resin-based composite, D2330-D2394
　inlay/onlay, D2510-D2664, D6600-
　　D6615

Restorative dental work, D2330-D2999

Restorative injection, face, S0196

Restraint
　any type, E0710
　belts
　　Posey, E0700
　　Secure-All, E0700
　Bite disposable jaw locks, E0700
　body holders
　　Houdini security suit, E0700
　　Quick Release, one piece, E0700
　　Secure-All, one piece, E0700
　　System2 zippered, E0700
　　UltraCare vest-style
　　　with sleeves, E0700
　hand
　　Secure-All finger control mit, E0700
　limb holders
　　Posey, E0700
　　Quick Release, E0700
　　Secure-All, E0700
　pelvic
　　Secure-All, E0700

Retail therapy item, miscellaneous,
　T1999

Retainers, dental
　fixed partial denture, D6545-D6792
　implant/abutment supported, D6068-
　　D6077
　orthodontic, D8680

Retinal device, intraoperative, C1784

Retinal exam for diabetes, S3000

Retinal tamponade, C1814

Retinoblastoma, genetic test, S3841

Retrieval device, insertable, C1773

Retrograde dental filling, D3430

Rhesonativ, J2790

Rheumatrex, J8610

Rho(D) immune globulin, human, J2790,
　J2792
　minidose, J2788

RhoGAM, J2790

Rib belt
　thoracic, L0210, L0220
　Don-Joy, L0210

Rice ankle splint, L1904

Richfoam convoluted & flat overlays,
　E0199

Ride Lite 200, Ride Lite 9000, manual
　wheelchair, K0004

Ridge augmentation/sinus lift, dental,
　D7950

Rimantadine HCl, G9020

Rimso, J1212

Ringer's lactate infusion, J7120

Ring, ostomy, A4404

Risperidone, long acting, J2794

Rituxan, J9310

Rituximab, J9310

Riveton, foot orthosis, L3140, L3150

RN services, T1002

Road Savage power wheelchair, K0011

Road Warrior power wheelchair, K0011

Robaxin, J2800

Robin-Aids, prosthesis
　hand, L6855, L6860
　partial hand, L6000-L6020

Rocephin, J0696

Rocking bed, E0462

Rollabout chair, E1031

Root canal therapy, D3310-D3353

Root planning and scaling, dental,
　D4341

Root removal, dental, D7140, D7250

Root resection/amputation, dental,
　D3450

Ropivacaine hydrochloride, J2795

RSV immune globulin, J1565

Rubex, J9000

Rubramin PSC, J3420

Sabre power wheelchair, K0011

Sacral nerve stimulation test
　lead, each, A4290

Sacroiliac orthosis, K0630-K0633

Safe, hand prosthesis, L5972

Safety
　enclosure frame/canopy, for hospital
　　bed, E0316
　equipment, E0700
　eyeglass frames, S0516
　vest, wheelchair, E0980

Saline, A4216-A4217
　hypertonic, J7130
　solution, J7030-J7051

Saliva test, hormone level
　during menopause, S3650
　preterm labor risk, S3652

Salivary gland excision, D7983

Samarium Sm-153 lexidronamm, A9605

Sam Brown, Legg Perthes orthosis,
　L1750

Sansibar Plus, E0601

Saquinavir, S0140

Sargramostim (GM-CSF), J2820

Satumomab pendetide, A4642

Scale, for dialysis, E1639

Schuco
　mist nebulizer system, E0570
　vac aspirator, E0600

Scintimammography, S8080

Scleral lens bandage, S0515

Scoliosis, L1000, L1200, L1300-L1499
　additions, L1010-L1120, L1210-L1290

Scott ankle splint, canvas, L1904

Scott-Craig, stirrup orthosis, L2260

Scottish-Rite, Legg Perthes orthosis,
　L1730

Screening
　cervical or vaginal, G0101
　colorectal cancer, G0104-G0107, G0120-
　　G0122
　digital rectal, annual, S0605
　glaucoma, G0117-G0118
　gynecological
　　established patient, S0612
　　new patient, S0610
　newborn metabolic, S3620
　ophthalmological, including refraction
　　established patient, S0621
　　new patient, S0620
　preadmission, T2010-T2011
　proctoscopy, S0601
　program participation, T1023
　prostate
　　digital, rectal, G0102
　　prostate specific antigen test (PSA),
　　　G0103

Screw, anchor, C1713

Sealant
　dental, D1351
　pulmonary, liquid, C2615
　skin, A6250
　tooth, D1351

Seat
　attachment, walker, E0156
　insert, wheelchair, E0992
　lift (patient), E0621, E0627-E0629

Seattle Carbon Copy II, foot prosthesis,
　L5976

Secure-All
　restraints, E0700
　universal pelvic traction belt, E0890

Sedation, dental
　deep, D9220-D9221
　intravenous, conscious, D9241-D9242
　non-intravenous, D9248

Sedative filling, dental, D2940

Selestoject, J0704

Semilente insulin, J1815

Sensitivity study, P7001

Septal defect implant system, C1817

Sequestrectomy, dental, D7550

Sermorelin acetate, Q2014

Serum clotting time tube, A4771

SEWHO, L3960-L3974

Sexa, G0130

Sheepskin pad, E0188, E0189

Sheath
　introducer
　　guiding, C1766, C1892, C1893
　　other than guiding, C1984, C2629

Shoes
　arch support, L3040-L3100
　for diabetics, A5500-A5508
　insert, L3000-L3030
　　for diabetics, A5511
　lift, L3300-L3334
　miscellaneous additions, L3500-L3595
　orthopedic (*see* **Orthopedic shoes**),
　　L3201-L3265
　positioning device, L3140-L3170
　post-operative
　　Specialist™ Health/Post Operative
　　　Shoe, A9270
　transfer, L3600-L3649
　wedge, L3340-L3485

Shoulder
　abduction positioner, L3999
　braces, L3999
　　Masterhinge™ Shoulder Brace 3,
　　　L3999
　disarticulation, prosthetic, L6300-L6320,
　　L6550
　orthosis (SO), L3650-L3675
　　elastic shoulder immobilizer, L3670
　　Padden Shoulder Immobilizer, L3670
　　Sling and Swathe, L3670
　　Velpeau Sling Immobilizer, L3670
　spinal, cervical, L0100-L0200

Shoulder-elbow-wrist-hand orthosis
　(SEWHO), L3960-L3969

Shower chair, E0240

Shunt accessory for dialysis, A4740
　aqueous, L8612

Sialodochoplasty, D7982

Sialolithotomy, D7980

Sialography, D0310

Sickle cell anemia, genetic test, S3850

Sierra wrist flexion unit, L6805

Sigmoidoscopy, cancer screening,
　G0104, G0106

Sign language or oral interpreter
　services, T1013

Sildenafil citrate, S0090

Silenzio Elite, E0601

Single bar "AK," ankle-foot orthosis,
　L2000, L2010

Single bar "BK," ankle-foot orthosis,
　L1980

Sinus lift, dental, D7950

Sinusol-B, J0945

Sinusotomy, in dentistry, D7560

Sirolimus, J7520

Sitz bath, E0160-E0162

Skilled nurse, G0128
　home health setting, G0154

Skin
　barrier, ostomy, A4362, A4369, A4385
　bond or cement, ostomy, A4364
　gel protective dressing wipes, A5119
　sealant, protectant, moisturizer, A6250

Sling, A4565
　axilla, L1010
　Legg Perthes, L1750
　lumbar, L1090
　patient lift, E0621, E0630, E0635
　pelvic, L2580
　Sam Brown, L1750
　SEWHO, L3969
　trapezius, L1070

Sling and Swathe, orthosis (SO), L3670

Smoking cessation program, S9075

SO, vest type abduction retrainer, L3675

Social worker
　home health setting, G0155
　nonemergency transport, A0160
　visit in home, S9127

Sock
　body sock, L0984
　prosthetic sock, L8420-L8435, L8480,
　　L8485
　stump sock, L8470-L8485

Sodium
　chloride injection, J2912
　chromate Cr-51, C9000, C9102
　ferric gluconate in sucrose, J2916
　hyaluronate, J7317
　iothalamate I-125, C9103
　succinate, J1720

Sodium hyaluronate, C9220, C9413

Sodium iodide I-131
　diagnostic imaging agent A9528, A9531
　therapeutic agent, A9530

Sickle cell anemia, genetic test, S3850

Sof-Rol™ Cast Padding, (not separately
　reimbursable from the casting
　procedure or casting supplies codes)

Soft Touch lancets, box of 100, A4259

Softclix lancet device, A4258

Softop helmet, L0110

Soft Touch II lancet device, A4258

Solganal, J2910

Solo Cast Sole, L3540

Solo LX, E0601

Solu-Cortef, J1720

Solu-Medrol, J2920, J2930

Solurex, J1100

Solurex LA, J1100

Solution
　calibrator, A4256
　dialysate, A4760, A4728
　enteral formulae, B4150-B4155
　parenteral nutrition, B4164-B5200

Somatrem, J2940

Somatropin, J2941

S.O.M.I. brace, L0190, L0200

S.O.M.I. multiple-post collar, cervical
　orthosis, L0190

Sorbent cartridge, ESRD, E1636

Sorbsan, alginate dressing, A6196-A6198

Source
　brachytherapy
　　gold 198, C1716
　　iodine 125, C1718
　　non-high dose rate iridium 192,
　　　C1719
　　palladium 103, C1720
　　yttrium 90, C2616

Spacer
　interphalangeal joint, L8658

Space maintainer, dental, D1510-D1550

Sparine, J2950

Spasmoject, J0500

Specialist™ Ankle Foot Orthosis, L1930

Specialist™ Closed-Back Cast Boot,
　L3260

Specialist™ 100 Cotton Cast Padding,
　(not separately reimbursable from the
　casting procedure or casting supplies
　codes)

Specialist™ Cast Padding, (not separately
　reimbursable from the casting
　procedure or casting supplies codes)

Specialist™ Gaitkeeper™ Boot, L3260

Specialist™ Health/Post Operative Shoe, A9270

Specialist™ Heel Cups, L3485

Specialist™ Insoles, L3510

Specialist™ J-Splint™ Plaster Roll Immobilizer, A4580

Specialist™ Open-Back Cast Boot, L3260

Specialist™ Orthopaedic Stockinet, (not separately reimbursable from the casting procedure or casting supplies codes)

Specialist™ Plaster Bandages, A4580

Specialist™ Plaster Roll Immobilizer, A4580

Specialist™ Plaster Splints, A4580

Specialist™ Pre-Formed Humeral Fracture Brace, L3980

Specialist™ Pre-Formed Ulnar Fracture Brace, L3982

Specialist™ Thumb Orthosis, L3800

Specialist™ Tibial Pre-formed Fracture Brace, L2116

Specialist™ Toe Insert for Specialist™ Closed-Back Cast Boot and Specialist™ Health/Post Operative Shoe, A9270

Specialist™ Wrist/Hand Orthosis, L3999

Specialist™ Wrist-Hand-Thumb-orthosis, L3999

Specialty absorptive dressing, A6251-A6256

Spectacles, S0504-S0510, S0516-S0518

Spectinomycin HCl, J3320

Speech aid
    pediatric, D5952
    adult, D5953

Speech and language pathologist
    home health setting, G0153

Speech assessment, V5362-V5364
    speech generating device
        software, E2511
        supplies, E2500-E2599

Speech therapy, S9128

Spenco shoe insert, foot orthosis, L3001

Sperm procurement, S4026, S4030-S4031
    donor service, S4025

Sphygmomanometer/blood pressure, A4660

Spinal orthosis
    Boston type, L1200
    cervical, L0100-L0200
    cervical-thoracic-lumbar-sacral orthosis (CTLSO), L0700, L0710, L1000
    halo, L0810-L0830
    Milwaukee, L1000
    multiple post collar, L0180-L0200
    scoliosis, L1000, L1200, L1300-L1499
    torso supports, L0970-L0999

Spirometer, electronic, S8190

Splint, A4570, L3100, L4350-L4380
    ankle, L4392-L4398, S8451
    digit, prefabricated, S8450
    dynamic, E1800, E1805, E1810, E1815
    elbow, S8452
    footdrop, L4398
    long arm, Q4017-Q4020
    long leg, Q4041-Q4044
    Orthoplast™ Splints (and Orthoplast™ II Splints), A4590
    pneumatic, L4350
    short arm, Q4021-Q4024

Splint — *continued*
    short leg, Q4045-Q4046
    Specialist™ Plaster Splints, A4580
    supplies, Q4051
    Thumb-O-Prene™ Splint, L3999
    toad finger, A4570
    wrist, S8451
    Wrist-O-Prene™ Splint, L3800

Splinting, dental
    commissure, D5987
    provisional, D4320-D4321
    surgical, D5988

Spoke protectors, each, K0065

Sports supports hinged knee support, L1832

Stainless steel crown, D2930-D2931, D2933

Stains
    immunohistochemical, D0478
    microorganisms, D0476
    not for microorganisms, D0477

Standing frame system, E0638

Star Lumen tubing, A4616

Steeper, hand prosthesis, L6868, L6873

Sten, foot prosthesis, L5972

Stent
    coated
        with delivery system, C1874
        without delivery system, C1875
    in dentistry, D5982
    non-coated, non-covered
        with delivery system, C1876
        without delivery system, C1877
    non-coronary
        temporary, C2617, C2625

Stent placement, transcatheter
    intracoronary, G0290-G0291

Stereotactic radiosurgery, G0242-G0243, G0251
    planning, G0338
    therapy, G0339, G0340

Sterile cefuroxime sodium, J0697

Sterile water, A4216-A4217

Stilphostrol, J9165

Stimulated intrauterine insemination, S4035

Stimulation
    electrical, G0281-G0283
    electromagnetic, G0295

Stimulation, gastric electrical implant, S2213

Stimulators
    cough, device, E0482
    electric, supplies, A4595
    neuromuscular, E0744, E0745
    osteogenesis, electrical, E0747-E0749
    salivary reflex, E0755
    ultrasound, E0760

Stocking
    Delta-Net™ Orthopaedic Stockinet, (not separately reimbursable from the casting procedure or casting supplies codes)
    gradient compression, L8100-L8239
    Specialist™ Orthopaedic Stockinet, (not separately reimbursable from the casting procedure or casting supplies codes)

Stoma
    cap, A5055
    catheter, A5082
    cone, A4399
    plug, A5081

Stomach tube, B4083

Stomahesive
    skin barrier, A4362, A5122
    sterile wafer, A4362
    strips, A4362

Storm Arrow power wheelchair, K0014

Storm Torque power wheelchair, K0011

Streptase, J2995

Streptokinase, J2995

Streptomycin sulfate, J3000

Streptozocin, J9320

Stress breaker, in dentistry, D6940

Stress management class, S9454

Strip(s)
    blood, A4253
    glucose test, A4253, A4772
    Nu-Hope
        adhesive, 1 oz bottle with applicator, A4364
        adhesive, 3 oz bottle with applicator, A4364
    urine reagent, A4250

Strontium 89 chloride, A9600, C9401

Study, gastrointestinal fat absorption, S3708

Stump sock, L8470-L8485

Stylet, A4212

Sublimaze, J3010

Substance abuse treatment, T1006-T1012
    childcare during, T1009
    couples counseling, T1006
    family counseling, T1006
    meals during, T1010
    skills development, T1012
    treatment plan, T1007

Succinylcholine chloride, J0330

Sucostrin, J0330

Suction pump
    portable, E0600

Sulfamethoxazole and trimethoprim, S0039

Sullivan
    CPAP, E0601

Sumacal, enteral nutrition, B4155

Sumatriptan succinate, J3030

Sunglass frames, S0518

Sunbeam moist/dry heat pad, E0215

Supplies
    infection control NOS, S8301

Supply/accessory/service, A9900

Support
    arch, L3040-L3090
    cervical, L0100-L0200
    elastic, L8100-L8239
    spinal, L0970-L0999
    vaginal, A4561-A4562

Supported housing, H0043-H0044

Supra crestal fibrotomy, D7291

Supreme bG Meter, E0607

SureStep blood glucose monitor, E0607

Sur-Fit/Active Life tail closures, A4421

Sur-Fit
    closed-end pouch, A5054
    disposable convex inserts, A5093
    drainable pouch, A5063
    flange cap, A5055
    irrigation sleeve, A4397
    urostomy pouch, A5073

Sure-Gait folding walker, E0141, E0143

Sure-Safe raised toilet seat, E0244

Surgery
oral, D7111-D7999
stereotactic, G0251

Surgical
ambulatory center, in dentistry, D9420
boot, L3208-L3211
mask, for dialysis, A4928
stocking, A4490-A4510
suite procedure, S0206
supplies, miscellaneous, A4649
tray, A4550

Suturing, complicated, in dentistry, D7911-D7912

Sus-Phrine, J0170

Sustacal, enteral nutrition, B4150
HC, B4152

Sustagen Powder, enteral nutrition, B4150

Swabs, betadine or iodine, A4247

Swanson, wrist-hand-finger orthosis, L3910

Swede, ACT, Cross, or Elite manual wheelchair, K0005

Swede Basic F# manual wheelchair, K0004

Swedish knee orthosis, L1850

Swivel adaptor, S8186

Synkayvite, J3430

Synovectomy, D7854

Syntocinon, J2590

Synvise, J7320

Syringe, A4213
dialysis, A4657
insulin, box of 100, S8490
with needle, A4206-A4209

System2 zippered body holder, E0700

Sytobex, J3420

T

Tables, bed, E0274, E0315

Tachdijan, Legg Perthes orthosis, L1720

Tacrine hydrochloride, S0014

Tacrolimus, oral, J7507

Talwin, J3070

Tamoxifen citrate, S0187

Tamponade
retinal, C1814

Tape
non waterproof, A4450
waterproof, A4452

Tarabine PFS, C9422

Taxi, nonemergency transportation, A0100

Taxol, C9431

Taxotere, J9170

Tay-Sachs, genetic test, S3847

Tazidime, J0713
multiple-post collar, cervical orthosis, L0190

Tc 99m fanolesomab, C1093

Technitium Tc 99
albumin aggregated, A9519
arcitumomab, C1122
depreotide, A9511
disofenin, A9510
exametazime, A9521
glucepatate, Q3006
mebrofenin, A9513
medronate, A9503
mertiatide, Q3005
oxidronate, Q3009

Technitium Tc 99 — *continued*
pentetate, A9515
pertechretate, A9512
pyrophosphate, A9514
sestamibi, A9500
sulfur colloid, A9520
tetrofosmin, A9502
vicisate, Q3003

Technol
Colles splint, L3986
wrist and forearm splint, L3906

TEEV, J0900

Telehealth tranmission, T1014

Telemonitoring, for CHF, equipment rental, S9109

Television
amplifier, V5270
caption decoder, V5271

Temozolomide, J8700

Temporomandibular joint (TMJ)
radiographs, D0320-D0321
treatment, D7810-D7899

TenderCloud electric air pump, E0182

TenderFlo II, E0187

TenderGel II, E0196

Tenderlet lancet device, A4258

Tenecteplase, J3100

Teniposide, Q2017

TENS, A4595, E0720-E0749
Neuro-Pulse, E0720

Tent, oxygen, E0455

Terbutaline
inhalation solution
concentrated, J7680
unit dose, J7681
sulfate, J3105

Teriparatide, J3110

Terminal devices, L6700-L6895

Terramycin IM, J2460

Terumo disposable insulin syringes, up to 1 cc, per syringe, A4206

Test materials, home monitoring, G0249

Testadiate-Depo, J1080

Testaqua, J3140

Testa-C, J1080

Test-Estra-C, J1060

Test-Estro Cypionates, J1060

Testex, J3150

Testoject
-50, J3140
-LA, J1070, J1080

Testone
LA 100, J3120
LA 200, J3130

Testosterone
aqueous, J3140
cypionate and estradiol cypionate, J1060
enanthate and estradiol valerate, J0900, J3120, J3130
pellet, S0189
propionate, J3150
suspension, J3140

Testradiate, J0900

Testradiol 90/4, J0900

Testrin PA, J3120, J3130

Tetanus immune globulin, human, J1670

Tetracycline, J0120

Thalassemia, genetic test
alpha, S3845
hemoglobin E beta, S3846

Thallous chloride Tl 201, A9505, C9400

Theelin aqueous, J1435

Theophylline, J2810

TheraCys, J9031

Therapeutic
agent, A4321
procedures, respiratory, G0239

Therapeutic radiopharmaceutical
I-131 tositumomab, A9534
sodium iodide I-131, A9530

Therapy
lymphedema, S8950
nutrition, reassessment, G0270-G0271
respiratory, G0237-G0239

Thermalator T-12-M, E0239

Thermometer
oral, A4931
rectal, A4932

Thiamine HCl, J3411

Thickener, food, B4100

Thiethylperazine maleate, Q0174

Thinning solvent, NuHope, 2 oz bottle, A4455

Thiotepa, C9433, J9340

Thomas
heel wedge, foot orthosis, L3465, L3470
suspension, wrist-hand-finger orthosis, L3926

Thoracic-hip-knee-ankle (THKO), L1500-L1520
Big Hug, L1510
Chameleon, L1510
Easy Stand, L1500
Little Hug, L1510
Tristander, L1510

Thoracic-lumbar-sacral orthosis (TLSO)
scoliosis, L1200-L1290

Thoracic orthosis, L0210

Thorazine, J3230

Thumb
immobilizer, Johnson's, L3800
Specialist™ Thumb Orthosis, L3800

Thumb-O-Prene™ Splint, L3999

Thymoglobulin, J7511

Thymol turbidity, blood, P2033

Thypinone, J2725

Thyrotropin, J3240
alpha, J3240

Thytropar, J3240

Tibia
Specialist™ Tibial Pre-formed Fracture Brace, L2116
Toad finger splint, A4570

Ticarcillin disodium and clavulanate potassium, S0040

Tice BCG, J9031

Ticon, J3250

Tigan, J3250

Tiject-20, J3250

Tinzaparin sodium, J1655

Tip (cane, crutch, walker) replacement, A4637

Tire, wheelchair, E0996, E0999, E1000

Tirofiban HCl, J3246

Tissue
conditioning, dental, D5850-D5851
connective
human, C1762
non-human, C1763
dermal and epidermal, J7340

Tissue — *continued*
epidermal and dermal, J7340
excision of hyperplastic, dental, D7970
human origin, J7344
localization and excision device, C1819
marker, C1879
non-human, J7343

TLSO, L0450-L0490, L1200-L1290

Tobacco counseling, D1320

Tobramycin
inhalation solution, J7682
sulfate, J3260
unit dose, J7682

Toe
holder, E0952
Specialist™ Toe Insert for Specialist™
Closed-Back Cast Boot and
Specialist™ Health/Post Operative
Shoe, A9270

Toilet
transfer bench, E0247-E0248

Toilet accessories, E0167-E0175, E0243,
E0244, E0625
raised toilet seat, E0244
Combo-Seat Universal, E0244
Moore, E0244
Sure-Safe, E0244
transfer bench, E0247, E0248

Tolazoline HCl, J2670

Toll, non-emergency transport, A0170

Tomographic radiograph, dental, D0322

Tooth, natural
caries susceptibility test, D0425
impacted, removal, D7220-D7241
intentional reimplantation, D3470
pulp vitality test, D0460
reimplantation, evulsed tooth, D7270
surgical exposure, D7280
surgical repositioning, D7290
transplantation, D7272

Topical hyperbaric oxygen chamber,
A4575

Topographic brain mapping, S8040

Topotecan, J9350

Toradol, J1885

Toronto, Legg Perthes orthosis, L1700

Torsemide, J3265

Torso support, L0790-L0999

Torus, removal of
mandibularis, D7473
palatinus, D7472

Totacillin-N, J0290

Total Universal Buck's Boot, E0870

TPN, home infusion therapy, S9364-
S9368

Tourniquet, for dialysis, A4929

Tracer blood glucose
meter, E0607
strips, box of 50, A4253

Tracer II Diabetes Care System, E0607

Tracer Wheelchairs, E1240, E1250,
E1260, E1270, E1280, E1285, E1290,
E1295

Tracheal suction catheter, A4624

Tracheoesophageal prosthesis supplies,
L8511-L8514

Tracheostoma
adhesive disc, A7506
filter, A7504
filter holder, A7503, A7507, A7509
housing, A7505, A7508
replacement diaphragm, faceplate,
A7502
valve, A7501

Tracheostomy
care kit, A4629
filter, A4481
mask, A7525
speaking valve, L8501
supplies, A4623-A4626, A4628, A4629,
S8189, A7523-A7526
tube, A7520-A7522

Tracheotomy, in dentistry, D7990

Traction equipment, E0840-E0948
cervical equipment
not requiring frame, E0855
stand or frame, E0849
extremity, E0870, E0880
Total Universal Buck's Boot, E0870
head harness/halter, cervical, E0942
occipital-pull head halter, E0942
overdoor, cervical, E0860
Exo-Static, E0860
pelvic, E0890, E0900
Secure-All universal, belt, E0890

Training
child development, T1027
diabetes, G0108, G0109
home care, S5108-S5109
INR monitoring device, G0248
medication, H0034
skills, H2014

Tramacal, enteral nutrition, B4154

Trancyte, C9123

**Transcutaneous electrical nerve
stimulator (TENS)**, E0720-E0749

Transducer protector, dialysis, E1575

Transfer board or device, E0972

Transfer (shoe orthoses), L3600-L3640

Transfusion, blood products, at home,
S9538

**Transmitter, external, for
neurostimultor, sacral root**, E0759

Transparent film (for dressing), A6257-
A6259

Transplant
autologous chondrocyte, J7330
bone marrow, allogeneic, S2150
islet cell, G0341-G0343
islet cell tissue, allogeneic, S2102
multivisceral organs, S2054
pancreas/kidney, S2065
small intestine and liver allografts,
S2053
tooth, D7272

Transport chair, E1037-E1038
heavy weight, E1039

Transportation
ALS, Q3019-Q3020
ambulance, A0021-A0999
corneal tissue, V2785
EKG (portable), R0076
extra attendent, A0424
handicapped, A0130
nonemergency, A0080-A0210, Q3020,
T2001-T2005, T2049
mileage, S0215
parking fees, A0170
service, including ambulance, A0021-
A0999
taxi, nonemergency, A0100
toll, nonemergency, A0170
volunteer, nonemergency, A0080, A0090
waiting time, T2007
x-ray (portable), R0070, R0075

Trapeze bar, E0910, E0940

Traum-aid, enteral nutrition, B4154

Travasorb, enteral nutrition, B4150
Hepatic, B4154
HN, B4153
MCT, B4154
Renal, B4154

Traveler manual wheelchair, K0001

Tray
insertion, A4310-A4316, A4354
irrigation, A4320
surgical (see also kits), A4550
wheelchair, E0950

Treprostinil, Q4077
sodium, S0114

Tretinoin, S0117

Triam-A, J3301

Triamcinolone
acetonide, J3301
diacetate, J3302
hexacetonide, J3303
inhalation solution
concentrated, J7683
unit dose, J7684

Trifupromazine HCl, J3400

Trifocal, glass or plastic, V2300-V2399

Trigeminal division block anesthesia,
D9212

Tri-Kort, J3301

Trilafon, J3310

Trilog, J3301

Trilone, J3302

Trim nails, G0127

Trimethobenzamide HCl, J3250, Q0173

Trimetrexate glucoronate, J3305

Triptorelin pamoate, J3315

Trismus appliance, D5937

Trobicin, J3320

Trovan, J0200

Truform prosthetic shrinker, L8440-
L8465

Truss, L8300-L8330

Tub
transfer bench, E0247-E0248

Tube/Tubing
anchoring device, A5200
blood, A4750, A4755
chest
drain valve, A7040
drainage container, A7041
CPAP device, A7037
gastrostomy, B4086
irrigation, A4355
microcapillary, calibrated, A4651
sealant, A4652
nasogastric, B4081, B4082
oxygen, A4616
serum clotting time, A4771
stomach, B4083
suction pump, each, A7002
tire, K0064, K0068, K0078, K0091,
K0093, K0095, K0097
tracheostomy or larygotomy plug, A7527
urinary drainage, A4331

Tumor
infiltrating lymphocyte therapy, S2107
oral, removal, dentistry, D7440-D7465

Tumor destruction
embolization, S2095
renal, S2090-S2091

**Turbinate somnoplasty coagulating
electrode**, C1322

Turtle Neck safety collars, E0942

U

Ulcers
electromagnetic therapy, G0329

Ultra Blood Glucose
monitor, E0607
test strips, box of 50, A4253

UltraCare vest-style body holder, E0700
Ultrafast computed tomography, S8092
Ultrafine disposable insulin syringes, per syringe, A4206
Ultralente insulin, J1815
Ultrasound
  aerosol generator, E0574
  guidance for multifetal pregnancy reduction, S8055
  paranasal sinus, S9024
Ultraviolet light-therapy
  bulb, A4633
  cabinet, E0691-E0694
  system panel, E0691-E693
Ultrazine-10, J0780
Unasyn, J0295
Unclassified drug, J3490
Underpads, disposable, A4554
Unilet lancet device, A4258
Unipuncture control system, dialysis, E1580
Unistik lancet device, A4258
Universal
  remover for adhesives, A4455
  socket insert
    above knee, L5694
    below knee, L5690
  telescoping versarail bed rail, E0310
Up-Draft Neb-U-Mist, E0580
Upper extremity addition, locking elbow, L6693
Upper extremity fracture orthosis, L3980-L3999
Upper limb prosthesis, L6000-L7499
Urea, J3350
Ureaphil, J3350
Urecholine, J0520
Ureterostomy supplies, A4454-A4590
Ureteroscopy
  for ureteral calculi, S2070
Urethral suppository, Alprostadil, J0275
Urgent care, S9088
  global fee, S9083
Urinal, E0325, E0326
Urinary
  catheter, A4324-A4325, A4338-A4346, A4351-A4353
  catheter irrigation, A4321
  collection and retention (supplies), A4310-A4359, K0407, K0408, K0410, K0411
  incontinence supplies, A4310-A4421, A4423-A4434, A4521-A4538, A5051-A5093, A5102-A5114, A5119-A5200
  leg bag, A5105, A5112
  tract implant, collagen, L8603
  incontinence repair device, C1771, C2631
Urine
  collector, A4335
  sensitivity study, P7001
  tests, A4250
Urofollitropin, Q2018
Urokinase, J3364, J3365
Urostomy pouch, A5073
USMC
  hinged Swedish knee cage, L1850
  universal knee immobilizer, L1830
Uvulopalatoplasty, laser assisted, S2080
U-V lens, V2755

V

Vabra aspirator, A4480
Vaccination, administration
  hepatitis B, G0010
  influenza virus, G0008
  pneumococcal, G0009
Vacuum erection system, L7900
Vaginal
  contraceptive ring, J7303
Valergen (10, 20, 40), J0970, J1380, J1390
Valertest No. 1, 2, J0900
Valium, J3360
Valrubicin, J9357
Valstar, J9357
Vancocin, J3370
Vancoled, J3370
Vancomycin HCl, J3370
Vaporizer, E0605
Vascular
  catheter (appliances and supplies), A4300-A4306
  closure device, C1760
  synthetic, L8670
Velban, J9360
Velcade, J9041
V Elite, E0601
Vent
  ostomy, A4366
Velosulin, J1815
Velpeau Sling Immobilizer, L3670
Velban, J9360
Veneers, dental, D2960-D2962
Ventilator
  battery, A4611-A4613
  moisture exchanger, disposable, A4483
  negative pressure, E0460
  pressure support, E0463, E0464
  pressure with flow triggering, E0454
  volume control, E0450, E0461
  volume, stationary or portable, E0450, E0483
Ventilator tray
  wheelchair, E1029-E1030
Ventolin, J7618-J7619
VePesid, J8560, J9181, J9182
Versa-Pole IV pole, E0776
Versed, J2250
Vertebral axial decompression, S9090
Verteporfin, J3395, J3396
Vesprin, J3400
Vest, safety, wheelchair, E0980
Vestibuloplasty, D7340-D7350
Vestibular rehabilitation, S9476
V-Gan (25, 50), J2550
Vidaza, C9218, S0168
Vinblastine sulfate, J9360
Vincasar PFS, J9370
Vincristine sulfate, J9370-J9380
Vinorelbine tartrate, J9390
Viral culture, D0416
Visi wheelchair tray, E0950
Visi-flow
  irrigation, A4367, A4397, A4398, A4399, A4402, A4421
  stoma cone, A4399

Vision Record wheelchair, K0005
Vision service, S0500-S0592, V2020-V2799
Visit, home nurse, T1030-T1031
Vistaject, J3410
Vistaril, J3410
Vistide, J0740
Vitajet, A4210
Vital HN, enteral nutrition, B4153
Vitamin
  multiple, A9153
  single, A9152
  supplement in ESRD, S0194
Vitamin B_{12} cyanocobalamin, J3420
Vitamin B_{17}, J3570
Vitamin K, J3430
Vitrasert, J7310
Vivonex, enteral nutrition
  HN, B4153
  T.E.N., B4153
Vocal cord
  chemodenervation, S2341
  medialization material, implantable, C1878
Von Hippel-Lindau disease, genetic test, S3842
Von Rosen, hip orthosis, L1630
Von Willebrand factor complex, Q2022
Voriconazole, J3465
Vortex power wheelchair, K0014
VPlus, E0601

W

Walker, E0130-E0144
  accessories, A4636, A4637
  attachments, E0153-E0159
  enclosed with wheels, E0144
  folding
    Auto-Glide, E0143
    Easy Care, E0143
    framed with wheels, E0144
    heavy duty
      with wheels, E0148
      without wheels, E0149
    heavy duty, multiple braking system, E0141
    One-Button, E0143
    Quik-Fold, E0141, E0143
    Red Dot, E0135, E0143
    Sure-Gait, E0141, E0143
Water
  ambulance, A0429
  distilled (for nebulizer), A7018
  for nebulizer, A7018
  pressure pad/mattress, E0187, E0198
  purification system (ESRD), E1610, E1615
  softening system (ESRD), E1625
  sterile, A4712, A4216-A4217
  treated, A4714
Water chamber
  humidifier, A7046
Wedge, positioning, E0190
Wedges, shoe, L3340-L3420
Wehamine, J1240
Wehdryl, J1200
Weight management class, S9449
Wellcovorin, J0640
Wet mount, Q0111
Wheel attachment, rigid pickup walker, E0155

Wheelchair, E0950-E1298, K0001-K0108
  accessories, E0950-E1001, E1065,
      E2203-E2399
    elevating leg rest, E0990
      handrim, E2205
        power seating system, E1019,
          E1021
        wheel lock, E2206
    seat support base, E2618
    tray, E0950
      Visi, E0950
  amputee, E1170-E1200
  bearings, any type, K0452
  component or accessory, NOS, K0108
  cushion
    back, E2291, E2293, E2605, E2606,
        E2608-E2617, E2620, E2621
      custom, E2609
    seat, E2610
      general, E2601, E2602
      positioning, E2605, E2606, E2607
      replacement cover, E2619
      skin protection, E2603, E2604,
          E2607
  heavy-duty
    shock absorber, E1015-E1016
    Tracer, E1280, E1285, E1290, E1295
  lightweight, E1240-E1270
    EZ Lite, E1250
    Tracer, E1240, E1250, E1260, E1270
  manual, adult, E1161
    accessories, E2201-E2204, E2300-
        E2399
  motorized, E1210-E1213
  narrowing device, E0969
  pediatric, E1229, E1231-E1238
    back
      contoured, E2293
      planar, E2291
    modification, E1011
    power, E1239
    seat
      contoured, E2294
      planar, E2292
  power, accessories, E2300-E2399
    gear box, E2369
    motor and gear box, E2370
    motor, E2368
  reclining back, E1014
  residual limb support, E1020
  seat or back cushion, K0669
  specially sized, E1220-E1230
  support, E1020
  tire, E0996, E0999, E1000
  transfer board or device, E0972
  transport chair, E1037-E1038
  van, nonemergency, A0130, S0209
WHFO, with inflatable air chamber,
    L3807

Whirlpool equipment, E1300-E1310
WHO, wrist extension, L3914
Wig, S8095
Win RhoSD, J2792
Wipes, A4245, A4247
  Allkare protective barrier, A5119
Wire, guide, C1769
WIZZ-ard manual wheelchair, K0006
Wound
  cleanser, A6260
  cover
    alginate dressing, A6196-A6198
    collagen dressing, A6021-A6024
    foam dressing, A6209-A6214
    hydrocolloid dressing, A6234-A6239
    hydrogel dressing, A6242-A6248
    packing strips, A6407
    specialty absorptive dressing, A6251-
        A6256
      warming card, E0232
    warming device, E0231
      non-contact warming cover, A6000
  dental, D7910-D7912
  electrical stimulation, E0769
  filler
    alginate, A6199
    foam, A6215
    hydrocolloid, A6240-A6241
    hydrogel, A6242-A6248
    not elsewhere classified, A6261-A6262
  healing
    other growth factor preparation,
        S9055
    Procuren, S9055
  packing strips, A6407
  pouch, A6154
    warming device, E0231
      cover, A6000
      warming card, E0232
  therapy
    negative pressure
      supplies, A6550-A6551
Wrap
  abdominal aneurysm, M0301
Wrist
  brace, cock-up, L3908
  disarticulation prosthesis, L6050, L6055
  hand/finger orthosis (WHFO), E1805,
      E1825, L3800-L3954
  Specialist™ Pre-Formed Ulnar Fracture
      Brace, L3982
  Specialist™ Wrist/Hand Orthosis, L3999
  Specialist™ Wrist-Hand-Thumb-orthosis,
      L3999
  Splint, lace-up, L3800
  Wrist-O-Prene™ Splint, L3800

Wycillin, J2510
Wydase, J3470

X

Xcaliber power wheelchair, K0014
Xenon Xe-133, Q3004
Xolair, J2357
X-ray
  dental implant, D6190
X-ray equipment, portable, Q0092,
    R0070, R0075

Y

Y set tubing for peritoneal dialysis,
    A4719
Yttrium 90
  ibritumomab tiuxeton, A9523
  microsphere
    brachytherapy, C2616
    procedure, S2095

Z

Zanamivir, G9018
Zantac, J2780
Zalcitabine, S0141
Zenapax, J7513
Zetran, J3360
Zidovudine, J3485
ZIFT, S4014
Zinacef, J0697
Zinecard, C9410, J1190
Ziprasidone mesylate, J3486
Zithromax
  I.V., J0456
  oral, Q0144
Zofran, J2405
Zoladex, J9202
Zoledronic acid, J3487
Zolicef, J0690
Zosyn, J2543
Zygomatic arch, fracture treatment,
    D7650, D7660, D7750, D7760
Zyprexa, S0166
Zyvok, J2020

TRANSPORTATION SERVICES INCLUDING AMBULANCE *A0000–A0999*

This code range includes ground and air ambulance, nonemergency transportation (taxi, bus, automobile, wheelchair van), and ancillary transportation-related fees.

Ambulance Origin and Destination modifiers used with Transportation Service codes are single-digit modifiers used in combination in boxes 12 and 13 of CMS form 1491. The first digit indicates the transport's place of origin, and the destination is indicated by the second digit. The modifiers most commonly used are:

D   Diagnostic or therapeutic site other than 'P' or 'H'

E   Residential, domiciliary, custodial facility (nursing home, not skilled nursing facility)

G   Hospital-based dialysis facility (hospital or hospital-related)

H   Hospital

I   Site of transfer (for example, airport or helicopter pad) between types of ambulance

J   Non-hospital-based dialysis facility

N   Skilled nursing facility (SNF)

P   Physician's office (includes HMO non-hospital facility, clinic, etc.)

R   Residence

S   Scene of accident or acute event

X   Intermediate stop at physician's office enroute to the hospital (includes HMO non-hospital facility, clinic, etc.) Note: Modifier X can only be used as a designation code in the second position of a modifier.

See Q3019, Q3020, and S0215. For Medicaid, see T codes and T modifiers.

Claims for transportation services fall under the jurisdiction of the local carrier.

E	**A0021**	Ambulance service, outside state per mile, transport (Medicaid only)
E	**A0080**	Non-emergency transportation, per mile — vehicle provided by volunteer (individual or organization), with no vested interest
E	**A0090**	Non-emergency transportation, per mile — vehicle provided by individual (family member, self, neighbor) with vested interest
E	**A0100**	Non-emergency transportation; taxi
E	**A0110**	Non-emergency transportation and bus, intra- or interstate carrier
E	**A0120**	Non-emergency transportation: mini-bus, mountain area transports, or other transportation systems
E	**A0130**	Non-emergency transportation: wheelchair van
E	**A0140**	Non-emergency transportation and air travel (private or commercial), intra- or interstate
E	**A0160**	Non-emergency transportation: per mile — caseworker or social worker
E	**A0170**	Transportation ancillary: parking fees, tolls, other
E	**A0180**	Non-emergency transportation: ancillary: lodging — recipient
E	**A0190**	Non-emergency transportation: ancillary: meals — recipient
E	**A0200**	Non-emergency transportation: ancillary: lodging — escort
E	**A0210**	Non-emergency transportation: ancillary: meals — escort
A	**A0225**	Ambulance service, neonatal transport, base rate, emergency transport, one way
A	**A0380**	BLS mileage (per mile) See code(s): A0425
A	**A0382**	BLS routine disposable supplies
A	**A0384**	BLS specialized service disposable supplies; defibrillation (used by ALS ambulances and BLS ambulances in jurisdictions where defibrillation is permitted in BLS ambulances)
A	**A0390**	ALS mileage (per mile) See code(s): A0425
A	**A0392**	ALS specialized service disposable supplies; defibrillation (to be used only in jurisdictions where defibrillation cannot be performed by BLS ambulances)
A	**A0394**	ALS specialized service disposable supplies; IV drug therapy
A	**A0396**	ALS specialized service disposable supplies; esophageal intubation
A	**A0398**	ALS routine disposable supplies

WAITING TIME TABLE

	UNITS		TIME
1	1/2	to	1 hr.
2	1	to	11/2 hrs.
3	11/2	to	2 hrs.
4	2	to	21/2 hrs.
5	21/2	to	3 hrs.
6	3	to	31/2 hrs.
7	31/2	to	4 hrs.
8	4	to	41/2 hrs.
9	41/2	to	5 hrs.
10	5	to	51/2 hrs.

A	**A0420**	Ambulance waiting time (ALS or BLS), one-half (1/2) hour increments ⊘
A	**A0422**	Ambulance (ALS or BLS) oxygen and oxygen supplies, life sustaining situation ⊘
A	**A0424**	Extra ambulance attendant, ground (ALS or BLS) or air (fixed or rotary winged); (requires medical review) ⊘ Pertinent documentation to evaluate medical appropriateness should be included when this code is reported.
A	**A0425**	Ground mileage, per statute mile
A	**A0426**	Ambulance service, advanced life support, non-emergency transport, level 1 (ALS 1)
A	**A0427**	Ambulance service, advanced life support, emergency transport, level 1 (ALS 1 — emergency)
A	**A0428**	Ambulance service, basic life support, non-emergency transport (BLS)
A	**A0429**	Ambulance service, basic life support, emergency transport (BLS — emergency)
A	**A0430**	Ambulance service, conventional air services, transport, one way (fixed wing)
A	**A0431**	Ambulance service, conventional air services, transport, one way (rotary wing)
A	**A0432**	Paramedic intercept (PI), rural area, transport furnished by a volunteer ambulance company which is prohibited by state law from billing third party payers

A   **A0433**   Advanced life support, level 2 (ALS 2)

A   **A0434**   Specialty care transport (SCT)

A   **A0435**   Fixed wing air mileage, per statute mile

A   **A0436**   Rotary wing air mileage, per statute mile

E   **A0800**   Ambulance transport provided between the hours of 7 p.m. and 7 a.m.

E   **A0888**   Non-covered ambulance mileage, per mile (e.g., for miles traveled beyond closest appropriate facility) ⊘
MED: 100-2, 10, 20

A   **A0999**   Unlisted ambulance service ⊘
Determine if an alternative HCPCS Level II or a CPT code better describes the service being reported. This code should be used only if a more specific code is unavailable.
MED: 100-2, 10, 10.1; 100-2, 10, 20

MEDICAL AND SURGICAL SUPPLIES *A4000–A8999*

This section covers a wide variety of medical, surgical, and some durable medical equipment (DME) related supplies and accessories. DME-related supplies, accessories, maintenance, and repair required to ensure the proper functioning of this equipment is generally covered by Medicare under the prosthetic devices provision.

MISCELLANEOUS SUPPLIES

These codes are to be filed with the Medicare local carrier, unless otherwise noted (if incident to a physicians' services, not separately billable) unless they represent incidental services or supplies which are referred to the DME regional carrier.

E ☑ **A4206** Syringe with needle, sterile 1 cc, each ⊘
This code specifies a 1 cc syringe but is also used to report 3/10 cc or 1/2 cc syringes.

E ☑ **A4207** Syringe with needle, sterile 2 cc, each ⊘

E ☑ **A4208** Syringe with needle, sterile 3 cc, each ⊘

E ☑ **A4209** Syringe with needle, sterile 5 cc or greater, each ⊘

E   **A4210** Needle-free injection device, each ⊘
Sometimes covered by commercial payers with preauthorization and physician letter stating need (e.g., for insulin injection in young children).
MED: 100-3, 280.1

B   **A4211** Supplies for self-administered injections ⊘
When a drug that is usually injected by the patient (e.g., insulin or calcitonin) is injected by the physician, it is excluded from Medicare coverage unless administered in an emergency situation (e.g., diabetic coma).
MED: 100-2, 15, 50

B   **A4212** Non-coring needle or stylet with or without catheter

E   **A4213** Syringe, sterile, 20 cc or greater, each ⊘

E   **A4215** Needles only, sterile, any size, each ⊘

A ☑ **A4216** Sterile water/saline, 10 ml ⅃⊘
MED: 100-2, 15, 50

A ☑ **A4217** Sterile water/saline, 500 ml ⅃⊘
MED: 100-2, 15, 50

N   **A4220** Refill kit for implantable infusion pump ⊘
Implantable infusion pumps are covered by Medicare for 5-FUdR therapy for unresected liver or colorectal cancer and for opioid drug therapy for intractable pain. They are not covered by Medicare for heparin therapy for thromboembolic disease. Report drugs separately.
MED: 100-3, 280.14

Y   **A4221** Supplies for maintenance of drug infusion catheter, per week (list drug separately) ⅃⊘

▲ Y   **A4222** Infusion supplies for external drug infusion pump, per cassette or bag (list drugs separately) ⅃⊘

● ☑ **A4223** Infusion supplies not used with external infusion pump, per cassette or bag (list drugs separately)

Y ☑ **A4230** Infusion set for external insulin pump, non-needle cannula type ⊘
Covered by some commercial payers as ongoing supply to preauthorized pump.
MED: 100-3, 280.14

Y ☑ **A4231** Infusion set for external insulin pump, needle type ⊘
Covered by some commercial payers as ongoing supply to preauthorized pump.
MED: 100-3, 280.14

Y ☑ **A4232** Syringe with needle for external insulin pump, sterile, 3 cc ⊘
Covered by some commercial payers as ongoing supply to preauthorized pump.
MED: 100-3, 280.14

E ☑ **A4244** Alcohol or peroxide, per pint ⊘

E ☑ **A4245** Alcohol wipes, per box ⊘

E ☑ **A4246** Betadine or PhisoHex solution, per pint ⊘

E ☑ **A4247** Betadine or iodine swabs/wipes, per box ⊘

N ☑ **A4248** Chlorhexidine containing antiseptic, 1 ml ⊘

E ☑ **A4250** Urine test or reagent strips or tablets (100 tablets or strips) ⊘
MED: 100-2, 15, 110

Note: Codes A4253–A4256 are for home blood glucose monitors. For supplies for End Stage Renal Disease (ESRD)/dialysis, see codes A4651–A4929. (Some codes in this range do not specify ESRD/dialysis, verify coverage with your carrier). For DME items for ESRD, see codes E1500–E1699.

Y ☑ **A4253** Blood glucose test or reagent strips for home blood glucose monitor, per 50 strips ⅃⊘
Medicare covers glucose strips for diabetic patients using home glucose monitoring devices prescribed by their physicians. Medicare jurisdiction: DME regional carrier.
MED: 100-3, 40.2

Y ☑ **A4254** Replacement battery, any type, for use with medically necessary home blood glucose monitor owned by patient, each ⅃⊘
Medicare covers glucose strips for diabetic patients using home glucose monitoring devices prescribed by their physicians. Medicare jurisdiction: DME regional carrier.
MED: 100-3, 40.2

Y ☑ **A4255** Platforms for home blood glucose monitor, 50 per box ⅃⊘
Some Medicare carriers cover monitor platforms for diabetic patients using home glucose monitoring devices prescribed by their physicians. Medicare jurisdiction: DME regional carrier. Some commercial payers also provide this coverage to non-insulin dependent diabetics.
MED: 100-3, 40.2

Reference chart

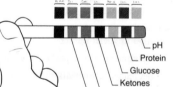

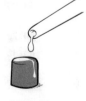

Dipstick urinalysis: The strip is dipped and color-coded squares are read at timed intervals (e.g., pH immediately; ketones at 15 sec., etc.). Results are compared against a reference chart

Tablet reagents turn specific colors when urine droplets are placed on them

Special Coverage Instructions   Noncovered by Medicare   Carrier Discretion   ☑ Quantity Alert   ● New Code   ○ Reinstated Code   ▲ Revised Code

2 — A Codes   A Adult   M Maternity   P Pediatrics   I Infant   A-Y APC Status Indicator   *2005 HCPCS*

Y   **A4256**   **Normal, low, and high calibrator solution/chips** &bnacc;ø
Some Medicare carriers cover calibration solutions or chips for diabetic patients using home glucose monitoring devices prescribed by their physicians. Medicare jurisdiction: DME regional carrier. Some commercial payers also provide this coverage to non-insulin dependent diabetics.

MED: 100-3, 40.2

Y ☑ **A4257**   **Replacement lens shield cartridge for use with laser skin piercing device, each**   &bnacc;ø

Y ☑ **A4258**   **Spring-powered device for lancet, each**   &bnacc;ø
Some Medicare carriers cover lancing devices for diabetic patients using home glucose monitoring devices prescribed by their physicians. Medicare jurisdiction: DME regional carrier. Some commercial payers also provide this coverage to non-insulin dependent diabetics.

MED: 100-3, 40.2

Y ☑ **A4259**   **Lancets, per box of 100**   &bnacc;ø
Medicare covers lancets for diabetic patients using home glucose monitoring devices prescribed by their physicians. Medicare jurisdiction: DME regional carrier. Some commercial payers also provide this coverage to non-insulin dependent diabetics.

MED: 100-3, 40.2

E   **A4260**   **Levonorgestrel (contraceptive) implants system, including implants and supplies**   ♀ø
Covered by some commercial payers. Always report concurrent to the implant procedure. Use this code for Norplant.

E   **A4261**   **Cervical cap for contraceptive use**   ♀ø

N ☑ **A4262**   **Temporary, absorbable lacrimal duct implant, each**   ø
Always report concurrent to the implant procedure.

N ☑ **A4263**   **Permanent, long-term, nondissolvable lacrimal duct implant, each**
Always report concurrent to the implant procedure.

Y ☑ **A4265**   **Paraffin, per pound**   &bnacc;ø
Medicare jurisdiction: DME regional carrier.

MED: 100-3, 280.1

E   **A4266**   **Diaphragm for contraceptive use**   ♀

E ☑ **A4267**   **Contraceptive supply, condom, male, each**

E ☑ **A4268**   **Contraceptive supply, condom, female, each**   ♀

E ☑ **A4269**   **Contraceptive supply, spermicide (e.g., foam, gel), each**   A

A ☑ **A4270**   **Disposable endoscope sheath, each**   ø

A   **A4280**   **Adhesive skin support attachment for use with external breast prosthesis, each**   A♀&bnacc;

E   **A4281**   **Tubing for breast pump, replacement**   M♀

E   **A4282**   **Adapter for breast pump, replacement**   M♀

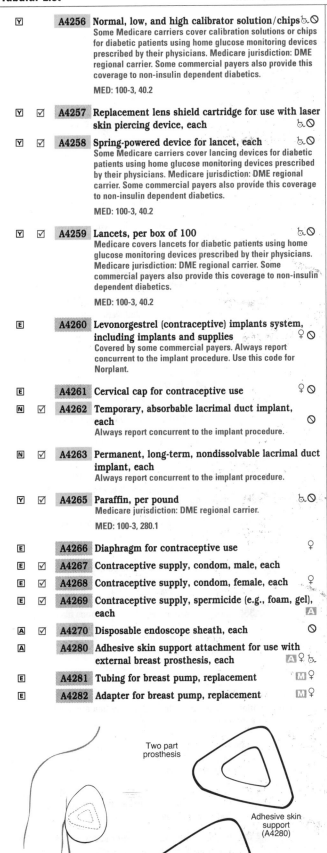

Two part prosthesis

Adhesive skin support (A4280)

Any of several breast prostheses fits over skin support

A4301

Needle access

Implanted reservoir under refill injection

Catheter   Body of reservoir and pump

Swan-Ganz catheter

Monitoring device

Tip with balloon

Detail of tapered tip and balloon

Markings along catheter measure depth of insertion

A4300

Ports

Junction divider

E   **A4283**   **Cap for breast pump bottle, replacement**   M♀

E   **A4284**   **Breast shield and splash protector for use with breast pump, replacement**   M♀

E   **A4285**   **Polycarbonate bottle for use with breast pump, replacement**   M♀

E   **A4286**   **Locking ring for breast pump, replacement**   M♀

B ☑ **A4290**   **Sacral nerve stimulation test lead, each**
AHA: 1Q, '02, 9

VASCULAR CATHETERS

N   **A4300**   **Implantable access catheter, (e.g., venous, arterial, epidural subarachnoid, or peritoneal, etc.) external access**
MED: 100-2, 15, 120

N   **A4301**   **Implantable access total catheter, port/reservoir (e.g., venous, arterial, epidural, subarachnoid, peritoneal, etc.)**   ø

A   **A4305**   **Disposable drug delivery system, flow rate of 50 ml or greater per hour**   ø

A   **A4306**   **Disposable drug delivery system, flow rate of 5 ml or less per hour**   ø

INCONTINENCE APPLIANCES AND CARE SUPPLIES
Covered by Medicare when the medical record indicates incontinence is permanent, or of long and indefinite duration.

Medicare claims fall under the jurisdiction of the DME regional carrier for a permanent condition, and under the local carrier when provided in the physician's office for a temporary condition.

A   **A4310**   **Insertion tray without drainage bag and without catheter (accessories only)**   &bnacc;
MED: 100-2, 15, 120

A   **A4311**   **Insertion tray without drainage bag with indwelling catheter, Foley type, two-way latex with coating (Teflon, silicone, silicone elastomer or hydrophilic, etc.)**   &bnacc;
MED: 100-2, 15, 120

A   **A4312**   **Insertion tray without drainage bag with indwelling catheter, Foley type, two-way, all silicone**   &bnacc;
MED: 100-2, 15, 120

A   **A4313**   **Insertion tray without drainage bag with indwelling catheter, Foley type, three-way, for continuous irrigation**   &bnacc;
MED: 100-2, 15, 120

| Special Coverage Instructions | Noncovered by Medicare | Carrier Discretion | ☑ Quantity Alert | ● New Code | ○ Reinstated Code | ▲ Revised Code |

2005 HCPCS   ♀ Female Only   ♂ Male Only   **1-9** ASC Groups   MED: Pub 100/NCD Reference   &bnacc; DMEPOS Paid   ø SNF Excluded   **A Codes — 3**

Medical and Surgical Supplies

A4314 — A4359

[A] **A4314** Insertion tray with drainage bag with indwelling catheter, Foley type, two-way latex with coating (Teflon, silicone, silicone elastomer or hydrophilic, etc.)
MED: 100-2, 15, 120

[A] **A4315** Insertion tray with drainage bag with indwelling catheter, Foley type, two-way, all silicone
MED: 100-2, 15, 120

[A] **A4316** Insertion tray with drainage bag with indwelling catheter, Foley type, three-way, for continuous irrigation
MED: 100-2, 15, 120

[A] **A4320** Irrigation tray with bulb or piston syringe, any purpose
MED: 100-2, 15, 120

[A] **A4321** Therapeutic agent for urinary catheter irrigation
MED: 100-2, 15, 120

[A] ☑ **A4322** Irrigation syringe, bulb or piston, each
MED: 100-2, 15, 120

~~A4324~~ ~~Male external catheter, with adhesive coating, each~~
See code(s): A4349

~~A4325~~ ~~Male external catheter, with adhesive strip, each~~
See code(s): A4349

[A] ☑ **A4326** Male external catheter specialty type with integral collection chamber, each ♂

[A] ☑ **A4327** Female external urinary collection device; metal cup, each ♀
MED: 100-2, 15, 120

[A] ☑ **A4328** Female external urinary collection device; pouch, each ♀
MED: 100-2, 15, 120

[A] ☑ **A4330** Perianal fecal collection pouch with adhesive, each
MED: 100-2, 15, 120

[A] ☑ **A4331** Extension drainage tubing, any type, any length, with connector/adaptor, for use with urinary leg bag or urostomy pouch, each
MED: 100-2, 15, 120

▲ [A] ☑ **A4332** Lubricant, individual sterile packet, each
MED: 100-2, 15, 120

[A] ☑ **A4333** Urinary catheter anchoring device, adhesive skin attachment, each
MED: 100-2, 15, 120

[A] ☑ **A4334** Urinary catheter anchoring device, leg strap, each

[A] **A4335** Incontinence supply; miscellaneous ⊘
MED: 100-2, 15, 120

[A] ☑ **A4338** Indwelling catheter; Foley type, two-way latex with coating (Teflon, silicone, silicone elastomer, or hydrophilic, etc.), each
MED: 100-2, 15, 120

[A] ☑ **A4340** Indwelling catheter; specialty type, (e.g., Coude, mushroom, wing, etc.), each
MED: 100-2, 15, 120

[A] ☑ **A4344** Indwelling catheter, Foley type, two-way, all silicone, each

Normal anatomy anterior view — Left ureter, Ureteral orifice, Urethra, Urethral sphincter, Spongiosal muscles

Side view — Urachus, Peritoneum, Left ureter, Pubic bone, Urogenital diaphragm, Foley-style indwelling catheter (A4344-A4346)

Multiple port indwelling catheters allow for irrigation and drainage

[A] ☑ **A4346** Indwelling catheter; Foley type, three-way for continuous irrigation, each
MED: 100-2, 15, 120

~~A4347~~ ~~Male external catheter with or without adhesive, with or without anti-reflux device, per dozen~~

[A] **A4348** Male external catheter with integral collection compartment, extended wear, each (e.g., 2 per month) ♂
MED: 100-2, 15, 120

● ☑ **A4349** Male external catheter, with or without adhesive, disposable, each
MED: 100-2, 15, 120

[A] ☑ **A4351** Intermittent urinary catheter; straight tip, with or without coating (Teflon, silicone, silicone elastomer, or hydrophilic, etc.), each
MED: 100-2, 15, 120

[A] ☑ **A4352** Intermittent urinary catheter; coude (curved) tip, with or without coating (Teflon, silicone, silicone elastomeric, or hydrophilic, etc.), each
MED: 100-2, 15, 120

[A] ☑ **A4353** Intermittent urinary catheter, with insertion supplies
MED: 100-2, 15, 120

[A] **A4354** Insertion tray with drainage bag but without catheter
MED: 100-2, 15, 120

[A] ☑ **A4355** Irrigation tubing set for continuous bladder irrigation through a three-way indwelling Foley catheter, each
MED: 100-2, 15, 120

EXTERNAL URINARY SUPPLIES

Medicare claims fall under the jurisdiction of the DME regional carrier for a permanent condition, and under the local carrier when provided in the physician's office for a temporary condition.

[A] ☑ **A4356** External urethral clamp or compression device (not to be used for catheter clamp), each
MED: 100-2, 15, 120

[A] ☑ **A4357** Bedside drainage bag, day or night, with or without anti-reflux device, with or without tube, each
MED: 100-2, 15, 120

[A] ☑ **A4358** Urinary drainage bag, leg or abdomen, vinyl, with or without tube, with straps, each
MED: 100-2, 15, 120

[A] ☑ **A4359** Urinary suspensory without leg bag, each
MED: 100-2, 15, 120

| Special Coverage Instructions | Noncovered by Medicare | Carrier Discretion | ☑ Quantity Alert | ● New Code | ○ Reinstated Code | ▲ Revised Code |

4 — A Codes   [A] Adult   [M] Maternity   [P] Pediatrics   [I] Infant   [A]-[Y] APC Status Indicator   **2005 HCPCS**

OSTOMY SUPPLIES

Medicare claims fall under the jurisdiction of the DME regional carrier for a permanent condition, and under the local carrier when provided in the physician's office for a temporary condition.

A ☑ **A4361** Ostomy faceplate, each ⚬
MED: 100-2, 15, 120

A ☑ **A4362** Skin barrier; solid, four by four or equivalent; each ⚬
MED: 100-2, 15, 120

A ☑ **A4364** Adhesive, liquid, or equal, any type, per oz. ⚬
MED: 100-2, 15, 120

A ☑ **A4365** Adhesive remover wipes, any type, per 50 ⚬
MED: 100-2, 15, 120

A ☑ **A4366** Ostomy vent, any type, each ⚬

A ☑ **A4367** Ostomy belt, each ⚬
MED: 100-2, 15, 120

A ☑ **A4368** Ostomy filter, any type, each ⚬

A ☑ **A4369** Ostomy skin barrier, liquid (spray, brush, etc.), per oz ⚬
MED: 100-2, 15, 120

A ☑ **A4371** Ostomy skin barrier, powder, per oz ⚬
MED: 100-2, 15, 120

A ☑ **A4372** Ostomy skin barrier, solid 4 x 4 or equivalent, with built-in convexity, each ⚬
MED: 100-2, 15, 120

A ☑ **A4373** Ostomy skin barrier, with flange (solid, flexible or accordion), with built-in convexity, any size, each ⚬
MED: 100-2, 15, 120

A ☑ **A4375** Ostomy pouch, drainable, with faceplate attached, plastic, each ⚬
MED: 100-2, 15, 120

A ☑ **A4376** Ostomy pouch, drainable, with faceplate attached, rubber, each ⚬
MED: 100-2, 15, 120

A ☑ **A4377** Ostomy pouch, drainable, for use on faceplate, plastic, each ⚬
MED: 100-2, 15, 120

A ☑ **A4378** Ostomy pouch, drainable, for use on faceplate, rubber, each ⚬
MED: 100-2, 15, 120

A ☑ **A4379** Ostomy pouch, urinary, with faceplate attached, plastic, each ⚬
MED: 100-2, 15, 120

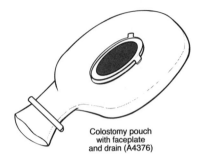

Colostomy pouch
with faceplate
and drain (A4376)

A ☑ **A4380** Ostomy pouch, urinary, with faceplate attached, rubber, each ⚬⊘
MED: 100-2, 15, 120

A ☑ **A4381** Ostomy pouch, urinary, for use on faceplate, plastic, each ⚬
MED: 100-2, 15, 120

A ☑ **A4382** Ostomy pouch, urinary, for use on faceplate, heavy plastic, each ⚬
MED: 100-2, 15, 120

A ☑ **A4383** Ostomy pouch, urinary, for use on faceplate, rubber, each ⚬
MED: 100-2, 15, 120

A ☑ **A4384** Ostomy faceplate equivalent, silicone ring, each ⚬
MED: 100-2, 15, 120

A ☑ **A4385** Ostomy skin barrier, solid 4 x 4 or equivalent, extended wear, without built-in convexity, each ⚬
MED: 100-2, 15, 120

A ☑ **A4387** Ostomy pouch, closed, with barrier attached, with built-in convexity (one piece), each ⚬
MED: 100-2, 15, 120

A ☑ **A4388** Ostomy pouch, drainable, with extended wear barrier attached, (one piece), each ⚬
MED: 100-2, 15, 120

A ☑ **A4389** Ostomy pouch, drainable, with barrier attached, with built-in convexity (one piece), each ⚬
MED: 100-2, 15, 120

A ☑ **A4390** Ostomy pouch, drainable, with extended wear barrier attached, with built-in convexity (1 piece), each ⚬⊘
MED: 100-2, 15, 120

A ☑ **A4391** Ostomy pouch, urinary, with extended wear barrier attached (1 piece), each ⚬
MED: 100-2, 15, 120

A ☑ **A4392** Ostomy pouch, urinary, with standard wear barrier attached, with built-in convexity (1 piece), each ⚬
MED: 100-2, 15, 120

A ☑ **A4393** Ostomy pouch, urinary, with extended wear barrier attached, with built-in convexity (1 piece), each ⚬
MED: 100-2, 15, 120

A ☑ **A4394** Ostomy deodorant for use in ostomy pouch, liquid, per fluid oz. ⚬

A ☑ **A4395** Ostomy deodorant for use in ostomy pouch, solid, per tablet ⚬
MED: 100-2, 15, 120

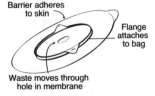

Barrier adheres to skin

Flange attaches to bag

Waste moves through hole in membrane

Faceplate flange
and skin barrier
combination
(A4373)

Special Coverage Instructions   Noncovered by Medicare   Carrier Discretion   ☑ Quantity Alert   ● New Code   ○ Reinstated Code   ▲ Revised Code

2005 HCPCS   ♀ Female Only   ♂ Male Only   **1**-**9** ASC Groups   MED: Pub 100/NCD Reference   ⚬ DMEPOS Paid   ⊘ SNF Excluded   **A Codes — 5**

A4396 Ostomy belt with peristomal hernia support
MED: 100-2, 15, 120

A4397 Irrigation supply; sleeve, each
MED: 100-2, 15, 120

A4398 Ostomy irrigation supply; bag, each
MED: 100-2, 15, 120

A4399 Ostomy irrigation supply; cone/catheter, including brush
MED: 100-2, 15, 120

A4400 Ostomy irrigation set
MED: 100-2, 15, 120

A4402 Lubricant, per oz.
MED: 100-2, 15, 120

A4404 Ostomy ring, each
MED: 100-2, 15, 120

A4405 Ostomy skin barrier, non-pectin based, paste, per oz.
MED: 100-2, 15, 120

A4406 Ostomy skin barrier, pectin-based, paste, per oz.
MED: 100-2, 15, 120

A4407 Ostomy skin barrier, with flange (solid, flexible, or accordion), extended wear, with built-in convexity, 4 x 4 in. or smaller, each
MED: 100-2, 15, 120

A4408 Ostomy skin barrier, with flange (solid, flexible or accordion), extended wear, with built-in convexity, larger than 4 x 4 in., each
MED: 100-2, 15, 120

A4409 Ostomy skin barrier, with flange (solid, flexible or accordion), extended wear, without built-in convexity, 4 x 4 in. or smaller, each
MED: 100-2, 15, 120

A4410 Ostomy skin barrier, with flange (solid, flexible or accordion), extended wear, without built-in convexity, larger than 4 x 4 in., each
MED: 100-2, 15, 120

A4413 Ostomy pouch, drainable, high output, for use on a barrier with flange (2 piece system), with filter, each
MED: 100-2, 15, 120

A4414 Ostomy skin barrier, with flange (solid, flexible or accordion), without built-in convexity, 4 x 4 in. or smaller, each
MED: 100-2, 15, 120

A4415 Ostomy skin barrier, with flange (solid, flexible or accordion), without built-in convexity, larger than 4 x 4 in., each
MED: 100-2, 15, 120

A4416 Ostomy pouch, closed, with barrier attached, with filter (one piece), each

A4417 Ostomy pouch, closed, with barrier attached, with built-in convexity, with filter (one piece), each

A4418 Ostomy pouch, closed; without barrier attached, with filter (one piece), each

A4419 Ostomy pouch, closed; for use on barrier with non-locking flange, with filter (two piece), each

A4420 Ostomy pouch, closed; for use on barrier with locking flange (two piece), each

A4421 Ostomy supply; miscellaneous
Determine if an alternative HCPCS Level II or a CPT code better describes the service being reported. This code should be used only if a more specific code is unavailable.
MED: 100-2, 15, 120

A4422 Ostomy absorbent material (sheet/pad/crystal packet) for use in ostomy pouch to thicken liquid stomal output, each
MED: 100-2, 15, 120

A4423 Ostomy pouch, closed; for use on barrier with locking flange, with filter (two piece), each

A4424 Ostomy pouch, drainable, with barrier attached, with filter (one piece), each

A4425 Ostomy pouch, drainable; for use on barrier with non-locking flange, with filter (two piece system), each

A4426 Ostomy pouch, drainable; for use on barrier with locking flange (two piece system), each

A4427 Ostomy pouch, drainable; for use on barrier with locking flange, with filter (two piece system), each

A4428 Ostomy pouch, urinary, with extended wear barrier attached, with faucet-type tap with valve (one piece), each

A4429 Ostomy pouch, urinary, with barrier attached, with built-in convexity, with faucet-type tap with valve (one piece), each

A4430 Ostomy pouch, urinary, with extended wear barrier attached, with built-in convexity, with faucet-type tap with valve (one piece), each

A4431 Ostomy pouch, urinary; with barrier attached, with faucet-type tap with valve (one piece), each

A4432 Ostomy pouch, urinary; for use on barrier with non-locking flange, with faucet-type tap with valve (two piece), each

A4433 Ostomy pouch, urinary; for use on barrier with locking flange (two piece), each

A4434 Ostomy pouch, urinary; for use on barrier with locking flange, with faucet-type tap with valve (two piece), each

ADDITIONAL MISCELLANEOUS SUPPLIES

A4450 Tape, non-waterproof, per 18 sq. in.
See also code A4452.
MED: 100-2, 15, 120

A4452 Tape, waterproof, per 18 sq. in.
See also code A4450.
MED: 100-2, 15, 120

A4455 Adhesive remover or solvent (for tape, cement or other adhesive), per oz.
MED: 100-2, 15, 120

A4458 Enema bag with tubing, reusable

A4462 Abdominal dressing holder, each
Dressings applied by a physician are included as part of the professional service. Surgical dressings obtained by the patient to perform homecare as prescribed by the physician are covered.
MED: 100-2, 15, 100

A4465 Nonelastic binder for extremity

Special Coverage Instructions   Noncovered by Medicare   Carrier Discretion   ☑ Quantity Alert   ● New Code   ○ Reinstated Code   ▲ Revised Code

6 — A Codes   A Adult   M Maternity   P Pediatrics   I Infant   A-Y APC Status Indicator   *2005 HCPCS*

E		A4670	Automatic blood pressure monitor ⊘

MED: 100-3, 20.19; 100-4, 8, 130; 100-4, 8, 70; 100-4, 8, 80; 100-4, 8, 90; 100-4, 8, 90.1; 100-4, 8, 90.3.2

B	☑	A4671	Disposable cycler set used with cycler dialysis machine, each ⊘

MED: 100-4, 8, 130; 100-4, 8, 70; 100-4, 8, 80; 100-4, 8, 90; 100-4, 8, 90.1; 100-4, 8, 90.3.2

B	☑	A4672	Drainage extension line, sterile, for dialysis, each⊘

MED: 100-4, 8, 130; 100-4, 8, 70; 100-4, 8, 80; 100-4, 8, 90; 100-4, 8, 90.1; 100-4, 8, 90.3.2

B		A4673	Extension line with easy lock connectors, used with dialysis ⊘

MED: 100-4, 8, 130; 100-4, 8, 70; 100-4, 8, 80; 100-4, 8, 90; 100-4, 8, 90.1; 100-4, 8, 90.3.2

B	☑	A4674	Chemicals/antiseptics solution used to clean/sterilize dialysis equipment, per 8 oz ⊘

MED: 100-4, 8, 130; 100-4, 8, 70; 100-4, 8, 80; 100-4, 8, 90; 100-4, 8, 90.1; 100-4, 8, 90.3.2

A	☑	A4680	Activated carbon filter for hemodialysis, each ⊘

MED: 100-3, 230.7; 100-4, 8, 130; 100-4, 8, 70; 100-4, 8, 80; 100-4, 8, 90; 100-4, 8, 90.1; 100-4, 8, 90.3.2

A	☑	A4690	Dialyzer (artificial kidneys), all types, all sizes, for hemodialysis, each ⊘

MED: 100-4, 8, 130; 100-4, 8, 70; 100-4, 8, 80; 100-4, 8, 90; 100-4, 8, 90.1; 100-4, 8, 90.3.2

A	☑	A4706	Bicarbonate concentrate, solution, for hemodialysis, per gallon ⊘

MED: 100-4, 8, 130; 100-4, 8, 70; 100-4, 8, 80; 100-4, 8, 90; 100-4, 8, 90.1; 100-4, 8, 90.3.2

A	☑	A4707	Bicarbonate concentrate, powder, for hemodialysis, per packet ⊘

MED: 100-4, 8, 130; 100-4, 8, 70; 100-4, 8, 80; 100-4, 8, 90; 100-4, 8, 90.1; 100-4, 8, 90.3.2

A	☑	A4708	Acetate concentrate solution, for hemodialysis, per gallon ⊘

MED: 100-4, 8, 130; 100-4, 8, 70; 100-4, 8, 80; 100-4, 8, 90; 100-4, 8, 90.1; 100-4, 8, 90.3.2

A	☑	A4709	Acid concentrate, solution, for hemodialysis, per gallon ⊘

MED: 100-4, 8, 130; 100-4, 8, 70; 100-4, 8, 80; 100-4, 8, 90; 100-4, 8, 90.1; 100-4, 8, 90.3.2

A	☑	A4714	Treated water (deionized, distilled, or reverse osmosis) for peritoneal dialysis, per gallon ⊘

MED: 100-3, 230.7; 100-4, 8, 130; 100-4, 8, 70; 100-4, 8, 80; 100-4, 8, 90; 100-4, 8, 90.1; 100-4, 8, 90.3.2

A		A4719	Y set tubing for peritoneal dialysis ⊘

MED: 100-4, 8, 130; 100-4, 8, 70; 100-4, 8, 80; 100-4, 8, 90; 100-4, 8, 90.1; 100-4, 8, 90.3.2

A	☑	A4720	Dialysate solution, any concentration of dextrose, fluid volume greater than 249 cc, but less than or equal to 999 cc, for peritoneal dialysis ⊘

MED: 100-4, 8, 130; 100-4, 8, 70; 100-4, 8, 80; 100-4, 8, 90; 100-4, 8, 90.1; 100-4, 8, 90.3.2

A	☑	A4721	Dialysate solution, any concentration of dextrose, fluid volume greater than 999 cc, but less than or equal to 1999 cc, for peritoneal dialysis ⊘

MED: 100-4, 8, 130; 100-4, 8, 70; 100-4, 8, 80; 100-4, 8, 90; 100-4, 8, 90.1; 100-4, 8, 90.3.2

A	☑	A4722	Dialysate solution, any concentration of dextrose, fluid volume greater than 1999 cc, but less than or equal to 2999 cc, for peritoneal dialysis ⊘

MED: 100-4, 8, 130; 100-4, 8, 70; 100-4, 8, 80; 100-4, 8, 90; 100-4, 8, 90.1; 100-4, 8, 90.3.2

A	☑	A4723	Dialysate solution, any concentration of dextrose, fluid volume greater than 2999 cc, but less than or equal to 3999 cc, for peritoneal dialysis ⊘

MED: 100-4, 8, 130; 100-4, 8, 70; 100-4, 8, 80; 100-4, 8, 90; 100-4, 8, 90.1; 100-4, 8, 90.3.2

A	☑	A4724	Dialysate solution, any concentration of dextrose, fluid volume greater than 3999 cc, but less than or equal to 4999 cc, for peritoneal dialysis ⊘

MED: 100-4, 8, 130; 100-4, 8, 70; 100-4, 8, 80; 100-4, 8, 90; 100-4, 8, 90.1; 100-4, 8, 90.3.2

A	☑	A4725	Dialysate solution, any concentration of dextrose, fluid volume greater than 4999 cc, but less than or equal to 5999 cc, for peritoneal dialysis ⊘

MED: 100-4, 8, 130; 100-4, 8, 70; 100-4, 8, 80; 100-4, 8, 90; 100-4, 8, 90.1; 100-4, 8, 90.3.2

A	☑	A4726	Dialysate solution, any concentration of dextrose, fluid volume greater than 5999 cc ⊘

MED: 100-4, 8, 130; 100-4, 8, 70; 100-4, 8, 80; 100-4, 8, 90; 100-4, 8, 90.1; 100-4, 8, 90.3.2

B	☑	A4728	Dialysate solution, non-dextrose containing, 500 ml ⊘

A	☑	A4730	Fistula cannulation set for hemodialysis, each ⊘

MED: 100-4, 8, 130; 100-4, 8, 70; 100-4, 8, 80; 100-4, 8, 90; 100-4, 8, 90.1; 100-4, 8, 90.3.2

A	☑	A4736	Topical anesthetic, for dialysis, per gm ⊘

MED: 100-4, 8, 130; 100-4, 8, 70; 100-4, 8, 80; 100-4, 8, 90; 100-4, 8, 90.1; 100-4, 8, 90.3.2

A	☑	A4737	Injectable anesthetic, for dialysis, per 10 ml ⊘

MED: 100-4, 8, 130; 100-4, 8, 70; 100-4, 8, 80; 100-4, 8, 90; 100-4, 8, 90.1; 100-4, 8, 90.3.2

A		A4740	Shunt accessory, for hemodialysis, any type ⊘

Medicare jurisdiction: DME regional carrier.

MED: 100-4, 8, 130; 100-4, 8, 70; 100-4, 8, 90; 100-4, 8, 90.1; 100-4, 8, 90.3.2

A	☑	A4750	Blood tubing, arterial or venous, for hemodialysis, each ⊘

MED: 100-4, 8, 130; 100-4, 8, 70; 100-4, 8, 80; 100-4, 8, 90; 100-4, 8, 90.1; 100-4, 8, 90.3.2

A		A4755	Blood tubing, arterial and venous combined, for hemodialysis, each ⊘

MED: 100-4, 8, 130; 100-4, 8, 70; 100-4, 8, 80; 100-4, 8, 90; 100-4, 8, 90.1; 100-4, 8, 90.3.2

A	☑	A4760	Dialysate solution test kit, for peritoneal dialysis, any type, each ⊘

MED: 100-4, 8, 130; 100-4, 8, 70; 100-4, 8, 80; 100-4, 8, 90; 100-4, 8, 90.1; 100-4, 8, 90.3.2

A	☑	A4765	Dialysate concentrate, powder, additive for peritoneal dialysis, per packet ⊘

MED: 100-4, 8, 130; 100-4, 8, 70; 100-4, 8, 80; 100-4, 8, 90; 100-4, 8, 90.1; 100-4, 8, 90.3.2

A		A4766	Dialysate concentrate, solution, additive for peritoneal dialysis, per 10 ml ⊘

MED: 100-4, 8, 130; 100-4, 8, 70; 100-4, 8, 80; 100-4, 8, 90; 100-4, 8, 90.1; 100-4, 8, 90.3.2

A		A4770	Blood collection tube, vacuum, for dialysis, per 50 ⊘

MED: 100-4, 8, 130; 100-4, 8, 70; 100-4, 8, 80; 100-4, 8, 90; 100-4, 8, 90.1; 100-4, 8, 90.3.2

A	☑	A4771	Serum clotting time tube, for dialysis, per 50 ⊘

MED: 100-4, 8, 130; 100-4, 8, 70; 100-4, 8, 80; 100-4, 8, 90; 100-4, 8, 90.1; 100-4, 8, 90.3.2

Special Coverage Instructions | Noncovered by Medicare | Carrier Discretion | ☑ Quantity Alert | ● New Code | ○ Reinstated Code | ▲ Revised Code

2005 HCPCS | ♀ Female Only | ♂ Male Only | 1-9 ASC Groups | MED: Pub 100/NCD Reference | ♿ DMEPOS Paid | ⊘ SNF Excluded | A Codes — 9

Medical and Surgical Supplies

A4670 — A4771

Medical and Surgical Supplies

A4772 — A5200

A ☑ **A4772** Blood glucose test strips, for dialysis, per 50 ⊘
MED: 100-4, 8, 130; 100-4, 8, 70; 100-4, 8, 80; 100-4, 8, 90; 100-4, 8, 90.1; 100-4, 8, 90.3.2

A ☑ **A4773** Occult blood test strips, for dialysis, per 50 ⊘
MED: 100-4, 8, 130; 100-4, 8, 70; 100-4, 8, 80; 100-4, 8, 90; 100-4, 8, 90.1; 100-4, 8, 90.3.2

A ☑ **A4774** Ammonia test strips, for dialysis, per 50 ⊘
MED: 100-4, 8, 130; 100-4, 8, 70; 100-4, 8, 80; 100-4, 8, 90; 100-4, 8, 90.1; 100-4, 8, 90.3.2

A ☑ **A4802** Protamine sulfate, for hemodialysis, per 50 mg ⊘
MED: 100-4, 8, 130; 100-4, 8, 70; 100-4, 8, 80; 100-4, 8, 90; 100-4, 8, 90.1; 100-4, 8, 90.3.2

A ☑ **A4860** Disposable catheter tips for peritoneal dialysis, per 10 ⊘
MED: 100-4, 8, 130; 100-4, 8, 70; 100-4, 8, 80; 100-4, 8, 90; 100-4, 8, 90.1; 100-4, 8, 90.3.2

A **A4870** Plumbing and/or electrical work for home hemodialysis equipment ⊘
MED: 100-4, 8, 130; 100-4, 8, 70; 100-4, 8, 80; 100-4, 8, 90; 100-4, 8, 90.1; 100-4, 8, 90.3.2

A **A4890** Contracts, repair and maintenance, for hemodialysis equipment ⊘
MED: 100-2, 15, 110.2

A ☑ **A4911** Drain bag/bottle, for dialysis, each ⊘

A **A4913** Miscellaneous dialysis supplies, not otherwise specified ⊘
Pertinent documentation to evaluate medical appropriateness should be included when this code is reported. Determine if an alternative HCPCS Level II or a CPT code better describes the service being reported. This code should be used only if a more specific code is unavailable.

A ☑ **A4918** Venous pressure clamp, for hemodialysis, each ⊘

A ☑ **A4927** Gloves, non-sterile, per 100 ⊘

A ☑ **A4928** Surgical mask, per 20 ⊘
For ESRD see also codes A4650-A4999

A **A4929** Tourniquet for dialysis, each ⊘

A **A4930** Gloves, sterile, per pair ⊘

A **A4931** Oral thermometer, reusable, any type, each ⊘

E **A4932** Rectal thermometer, reusable, any type, each

ADDITIONAL OSTOMY SUPPLIES
Medicare claims fall under the jurisdiction of the DME regional carrier, unless otherwise noted.

A ☑ **A5051** Ostomy pouch, closed; with barrier attached (one piece), each ♿
MED: 100-2, 15, 120

A ☑ **A5052** Ostomy pouch, closed; without barrier attached (one piece), each ♿
MED: 100-2, 15, 120

A ☑ **A5053** Ostomy pouch, closed; for use on faceplate, each ♿
MED: 100-2, 15, 120

A ☑ **A5054** Ostomy pouch, closed; for use on barrier with flange (two piece), each ♿
MED: 100-2, 15, 120

A **A5055** Stoma cap ♿
MED: 100-2, 15, 120

A ☑ **A5061** Ostomy pouch, drainable; with barrier attached, (one piece), each ♿

A ☑ **A5062** Ostomy pouch, drainable; without barrier attached (one piece), each ♿
MED: 100-2, 15, 120

A ☑ **A5063** Ostomy pouch, drainable; for use on barrier with flange (two piece system), each ♿
MED: 100-2, 15, 120

A ☑ **A5071** Ostomy pouch, urinary; with barrier attached (one piece), each ♿
MED: 100-2, 15, 120

A ☑ **A5072** Ostomy pouch, urinary; without barrier attached (one piece), each ♿
MED: 100-2, 15, 120

A ☑ **A5073** Ostomy pouch, urinary; for use on barrier with flange (two piece), each ♿
MED: 100-2, 15, 120

A **A5081** Continent device; plug for continent stoma ♿
MED: 100-2, 15, 120

A **A5082** Continent device; catheter for continent stoma ♿
MED: 100-2, 15, 120

A **A5093** Ostomy accessory; convex insert ♿
Medicare jurisdiction: local carrier.
MED: 100-2, 15, 120

ADDITIONAL INCONTINENCE APPLIANCES/SUPPLIES
Medicare claims fall under the jurisdiction of the DME regional carrier, unless otherwise noted.

A ☑ **A5102** Bedside drainage bottle, with or without tubing, rigid or expandable, each ♿
MED: 100-2, 15, 120

A **A5105** Urinary suspensory; with leg bag, with or without tube ♿
MED: 100-2, 15, 120

A **A5112** Urinary leg bag; latex ♿
MED: 100-2, 15, 120

A ☑ **A5113** Leg strap; latex, replacement only, per set ♿
MED: 100-2, 15, 120

A ☑ **A5114** Leg strap; foam or fabric, replacement only, per set ♿
MED: 100-2, 15, 120

SUPPLIES FOR EITHER INCONTINENCE OR OSTOMY APPLIANCES
For additional skin barrier codes see new codes A4405–A4415.

▲ A ☑ **A5119** Skin barrier, wipes or swabs, per box 50 ♿
MED: 100-2, 15, 120

A ☑ **A5121** Skin barrier; solid, 6 x 6 or equivalent, each ♿
MED: 100-2, 15, 120

A ☑ **A5122** Skin barrier; solid, 8 x 8 or equivalent, each ♿
MED: 100-2, 15, 120

A **A5126** Adhesive or non-adhesive; disk or foam pad ♿
MED: 100-2, 15, 120

A ☑ **A5131** Appliance cleaner, incontinence and ostomy appliances, per 16 oz ♿
MED: 100-2, 15, 120

A **A5200** Percutaneous catheter/tube anchoring device, adhesive skin attachment ♿
MED: 100-2, 15, 120

Special Coverage Instructions   Noncovered by Medicare   Carrier Discretion   ☑ Quantity Alert   ● New Code   ○ Reinstated Code   ▲ Revised Code

10 — A Codes   A Adult   M Maternity   P Pediatrics   I Infant   A-Y APC Status Indicator   **2005 HCPCS**

DIABETIC SHOES, FITTING, AND MODIFICATIONS

According to Medicare, documentation from the prescribing physician must certify the diabetic patient has one of the following conditions: peripheral neuropathy with evidence of callus formation; history of preulcerative calluses; history of ulceration; foot deformity; previous amputation; or poor circulation. The footwear must be fitted and furnished by a podiatrist, pedorthist, orthotist, or prosthetist.

Y ☑ **A5500** For diabetics only, fitting (including follow-up) custom preparation and supply of off-the-shelf depth-inlay shoe manufactured to accommodate multi-density insert(s), per shoe
MED: 100-2, 15, 140

Y ☑ **A5501** For diabetics only, fitting (including follow-up) custom preparation and supply of shoe molded from cast(s) of patient's foot (custom molded shoe), per shoe
MED: 100-2, 15, 140

Y ☑ **A5503** For diabetics only, modification (including fitting) of off-the-shelf depth-inlay shoe or custom molded shoe with roller or rigid rocker bottom, per shoe
MED: 100-2, 15, 140

Y ☑ **A5504** For diabetics only, modification (including fitting) of off-the-shelf depth-inlay shoe or custom molded shoe with wedge(s), per shoe
MED: 100-2, 15, 140

Y ☑ **A5505** For diabetics only, modification (including fitting) of off-the-shelf depth-inlay shoe or custom molded shoe with metatarsal bar, per shoe
MED: 100-2, 15, 140

Y ☑ **A5506** For diabetics only, modification (including fitting) of off-the-shelf depth-inlay shoe or custom molded shoe with off-set heel(s), per shoe
MED: 100-2, 15, 140

Y ☑ **A5507** For diabetics only, not otherwise specified modification (including fitting) of off-the-shelf depth-inlay shoe or custom molded shoe, per shoe
MED: 100-2, 15, 140

Y ☑ **A5508** For diabetics only, deluxe feature of off-the-shelf depth-inlay shoe or custom-molded shoe, per shoe ⊘
MED: 100-2, 15, 140

E **A5509** For diabetics only, direct formed, molded to foot with external heat source (i.e., heat gun) multiple density insert(s), prefabricated, per shoe
MED: 100-2, 15, 140

E **A5510** For diabetics only, direct formed, compression molded to patient's foot without external heat source, multiple-density insert(s) prefabricated, per shoe
MED: 100-2, 15, 140

E **A5511** For diabetics only, custom-molded from model of patient's foot, multiple density insert(s), custom-fabricated, per shoe
MED: 100-2, 15, 140

DRESSINGS

Medicare claims for A6021–A6404 fall under the jurisdiction of the local carrier if the supply or accessory is used for an implanted prosthetic device (e.g., pleural catheter) or implanted DME (e.g., infusion pump). Medicare claims for other uses of A6021–A6404 fall under the jurisdiction of the DME regional carrier. The jurisdiction for Medicare claims containing all other codes falls to the DME regional carrier, unless otherwise noted.

E **A6000** Non-contact wound warming wound cover for use with the non-contact wound warming device and warming card ⊘
MED: 100-2, 16, 20

A ☑ **A6010** Collagen based wound filler, dry form, per gram of collagen ⅃
MED: 100-2, 15, 100

A ☑ **A6011** Collagen based wound filler, gel/paste, per gram of collagen ⅃
MED: 100-2, 15, 100

A ☑ **A6021** Collagen dressing, pad size 16 sq. in. or less, each ⅃
MED: 100-2, 15, 100

A ☑ **A6022** Collagen dressing, pad size more than 16 sq. in. but less than or equal to 48 sq. in., each ⅃
MED: 100-2, 15, 100

A ☑ **A6023** Collagen dressing, pad size more than 48 sq. in., each ⅃
MED: 100-2, 15, 100

A ☑ **A6024** Collagen dressing wound filler, per 6 in. ⅃
MED: 100-2, 15, 100

E ☑ **A6025** Gel sheet for dermal or epidermal application, (e.g., silicone, hydrogel, other), each ⊘

A ☑ **A6154** Wound pouch, each ⅃
MED: 100-2, 15, 100

A ☑ **A6196** Alginate or other fiber gelling dressing, wound cover, pad size 16 sq. in. or less, each dressing ⅃
MED: 100-2, 15, 100

A ☑ **A6197** Alginate or other fiber gelling dressing, wound cover, pad size more than 16 sq. in. but less than or equal to 48 sq. in., each dressing ⅃
MED: 100-2, 15, 100

A ☑ **A6198** Alginate or other fiber gelling dressing, wound cover, pad size more than 48 sq. in., each dressing
MED: 100-2, 15, 100

A ☑ **A6199** Alginate or other fiber gelling dressing, wound filler, per 6 in. ⅃
MED: 100-2, 15, 100

A ☑ **A6200** Composite dressing, pad size 16 sq. in. or less, without adhesive border, each dressing ⅃
MED: 100-2, 15, 100

A ☑ **A6201** Composite dressing, pad size more than 16 sq. in. but less than or equal to 48 sq. in., without adhesive border, each dressing ⅃
MED: 100-2, 15, 100

A ☑ **A6202** Composite dressing, pad size more than 48 sq. in., without adhesive border, each dressing ⅃
MED: 100-2, 15, 100

A ☑ **A6203** Composite dressing, pad size 16 sq. in. or less, with any size adhesive border, each dressing ⅃
MED: 100-2, 15, 100

A ☑ **A6204** Composite dressing, pad size more than 16 sq. in. but less than or equal to 48 sq. in., with any size adhesive border, each dressing ⅃
MED: 100-2, 15, 100

A ☑ **A6205** Composite dressing, pad size more than 48 sq. in., with any size adhesive border, each dressing
MED: 100-2, 15, 100

A ☑ **A6206** Contact layer, 16 sq. in. or less, each dressing
MED: 100-2, 15, 100

| Special Coverage Instructions | Noncovered by Medicare | Carrier Discretion | ☑ Quantity Alert | ● New Code | ○ Reinstated Code | ▲ Revised Code |

2005 HCPCS   ♀ Female Only   ♂ Male Only   **1-9** ASC Groups   MED: Pub 100/NCD Reference   ⅃ DMEPOS Paid   ⊘ SNF Excluded   **A Codes — 11**

Medical and Surgical Supplies

A6207 — A6242

A ☑ **A6207** Contact layer, more than 16 sq. in. but less than or equal to 48 sq. in., each dressing
MED: 100-2, 15, 100

A ☑ **A6208** Contact layer, more than 48 sq. in., each dressing
MED: 100-2, 15, 100

A ☑ **A6209** Foam dressing, wound cover, pad size 16 sq. in. or less, without adhesive border, each dressing
MED: 100-2, 15, 100

A ☑ **A6210** Foam dressing, wound cover, pad size more than 16 sq. in. but less than or equal to 48 sq. in., without adhesive border, each dressing
MED: 100-2, 15, 100

A ☑ **A6211** Foam dressing, wound cover, pad size more then 48 sq. in., without adhesive border, each dressing
MED: 100-2, 15, 100

A ☑ **A6212** Foam dressing, wound cover, pad size 16 sq. in. or less, with any size adhesive border, each dressing
MED: 100-2, 15, 100

A ☑ **A6213** Foam dressing, wound cover, pad size more than 16 sq. in. but less than or equal to 48 sq. in., with any size adhesive border, each dressing
MED: 100-2, 15, 100

A ☑ **A6214** Foam dressing, wound cover, pad size more than 48 sq. in., with any size adhesive border, each dressing
MED: 100-2, 15, 100

A ☑ **A6215** Foam dressing, wound filler, per gram
MED: 100-2, 15, 100

A ☑ **A6216** Gauze, non-impregnated, non-sterile, pad size 16 sq. in. or less, without adhesive border, each dressing
MED: 100-2, 15, 100

A ☑ **A6217** Gauze, non-impregnated, non-sterile, pad size more than 16 sq. in. but less than or equal to 48 sq. in., without adhesive border, each dressing
MED: 100-2, 15, 100

A ☑ **A6218** Gauze, non-impregnated, non-sterile, pad size more than 48 sq. in., without adhesive border, each dressing
MED: 100-2, 15, 100

A ☑ **A6219** Gauze, non-impregnated, pad size 16 sq. in. or less, with any size adhesive border, each dressing
MED: 100-2, 15, 100

A ☑ **A6220** Gauze, non-impregnated, pad size more than 16 sq. in. but less than or equal to 48 sq. in., with any size adhesive border, each dressing
MED: 100-2, 15, 100

A ☑ **A6221** Gauze, non-impregnated, pad size more than 48 sq. in., with any size adhesive border, each dressing
MED: 100-2, 15, 100

A ☑ **A6222** Gauze, impregnated with other than water, normal saline, or hydrogel, pad size 16 sq. in. or less, without adhesive border, each dressing
MED: 100-2, 15, 100

A ☑ **A6223** Gauze, impregnated with other than water, normal saline, or hydrogel, pad size more than 16 sq. in. but less than or equal to 48 sq. in., without adhesive border, each dressing
MED: 100-2, 15, 100

A ☑ **A6224** Gauze, impregnated with other than water, normal saline, or hydrogel, pad size more than 48 sq. in., without adhesive border, each dressing
MED: 100-2, 15, 100

A ☑ **A6228** Gauze, impregnated, water or normal saline, pad size 16 sq. in. or less, without adhesive border, each dressing
MED: 100-2, 15, 100

A ☑ **A6229** Gauze, impregnated, water or normal saline, pad size more than 16 sq. in. but less than or equal to 48 sq. in., without adhesive border, each dressing
MED: 100-2, 15, 100

A ☑ **A6230** Gauze, impregnated, water or normal saline, pad size more than 48 sq. in., without adhesive border, each dressing
MED: 100-2, 15, 100

A ☑ **A6231** Gauze, impregnated, hydrogel, for direct wound contact, pad size 16 sq. in. or less, each dressing
MED: 100-2, 15, 100

A ☑ **A6232** Gauze, impregnated, hydrogel, for direct wound contact, pad size greater than 16 sq. in., but less than or equal to 48 sq. in., each dressing
MED: 100-2, 15, 100

A ☑ **A6233** Gauze, impregnated, hydrogel for direct wound contact, pad size more than 48 sq. in., each dressing
MED: 100-2, 15, 100

A ☑ **A6234** Hydrocolloid dressing, wound cover, pad size 16 sq. in. or less, without adhesive border, each dressing
MED: 100-2, 15, 100

A ☑ **A6235** Hydrocolloid dressing, wound cover, pad size more than 16 sq. in. but less than or equal to 48 sq. in., without adhesive border, each dressing
MED: 100-2, 15, 100

A ☑ **A6236** Hydrocolloid dressing, wound cover, pad size more than 48 sq. in., without adhesive border, each dressing
MED: 100-2, 15, 100

A ☑ **A6237** Hydrocolloid dressing, wound cover, pad size 16 sq. in. or less, with any size adhesive border, each dressing
MED: 100-2, 15, 100

A ☑ **A6238** Hydrocolloid dressing, wound cover, pad size more than 16 sq. in. but less than or equal to 48 sq. in., with any size adhesive border, each dressing
MED: 100-2, 15, 100

A ☑ **A6239** Hydrocolloid dressing, wound cover, pad size more than 48 sq. in., with any size adhesive border, each dressing
MED: 100-2, 15, 100

A ☑ **A6240** Hydrocolloid dressing, wound filler, paste, per fluid oz.
MED: 100-2, 15, 100

A ☑ **A6241** Hydrocolloid dressing, wound filler, dry form, per gram
MED: 100-2, 15, 100

A ☑ **A6242** Hydrogel dressing, wound cover, pad size 16 sq. in. or less, without adhesive border, each dressing
MED: 100-2, 15, 100

Special Coverage Instructions   Noncovered by Medicare   Carrier Discretion   ☑ Quantity Alert   ● New Code   ○ Reinstated Code   ▲ Revised Code

12 — A Codes   A Adult   M Maternity   P Pediatrics   I Infant   A-Y APC Status Indicator   *2005 HCPCS*

A ☑ **A6243** Hydrogel dressing, wound cover, pad size more than 16 sq. in. but less than or equal to 48 sq. in., without adhesive border, each dressing ♿
MED: 100-2, 15, 100

A ☑ **A6244** Hydrogel dressing, wound cover, pad size more than 48 sq. in., without adhesive border, each dressing ♿
MED: 100-2, 15, 100

A ☑ **A6245** Hydrogel dressing, wound cover, pad size 16 sq. in. or less, with any size adhesive border, each dressing ♿
MED: 100-2, 15, 100

A ☑ **A6246** Hydrogel dressing, wound cover, pad size more than 16 sq. in. but less than or equal to 48 sq. in., with any size adhesive border, each dressing ♿
MED: 100-2, 15, 100

A ☑ **A6247** Hydrogel dressing, wound cover, pad size more than 48 sq. in., with any size adhesive border, each dressing ♿
MED: 100-2, 15, 100

A ☑ **A6248** Hydrogel dressing, wound filler, gel, per fluid oz. ♿
MED: 100-2, 15, 100

A **A6250** Skin sealants, protectants, moisturizers, ointments, any type, any size
Surgical dressings applied by a physician are included as part of the professional service. Surgical dressings obtained by the patient to perform homecare as prescribed by the physician are covered.
MED: 100-2, 15, 100

A ☑ **A6251** Specialty absorptive dressing, wound cover, pad size 16 sq. in. or less, without adhesive border, each dressing ♿
MED: 100-2, 15, 100

A ☑ **A6252** Specialty absorptive dressing, wound cover, pad size more than 16 sq. in. but less than or equal to 48 sq. in., without adhesive border, each dressing ♿
MED: 100-2, 15, 100

A ☑ **A6253** Specialty absorptive dressing, wound cover, pad size more than 48 sq. in., without adhesive border, each dressing ♿
MED: 100-2, 15, 100

A ☑ **A6254** Specialty absorptive dressing, wound cover, pad size 16 sq. in. or less, with any size adhesive border, each dressing ♿
MED: 100-2, 15, 100

A ☑ **A6255** Specialty absorptive dressing, wound cover, pad size more than 16 sq. in. but less than or equal to 48 sq. in., with any size adhesive border, each dressing ♿
MED: 100-2, 15, 100

A ☑ **A6256** Specialty absorptive dressing, wound cover, pad size more than 48 sq. in., with any size adhesive border, each dressing ♿
MED: 100-2, 15, 100

A ☑ **A6257** Transparent film, 16 sq. in. or less, each dressing ♿
Surgical dressings applied by a physician are included as part of the professional service. Surgical dressings obtained by the patient to perform homecare as prescribed by the physician are covered. Use this code for Polyskin, Tegaderm, and Tegaderm HP.
MED: 100-2, 15, 100

A ☑ **A6258** Transparent film, more than 16 sq. in. but less than or equal to 48 sq. in., each dressing ♿
Surgical dressings applied by a physician are included as part of the professional service. Surgical dressings obtained by the patient to perform homecare as prescribed by the physician are covered.
MED: 100-2, 15, 100

A ☑ **A6259** Transparent film, more than 48 sq. in., each dressing ♿
Surgical dressings applied by a physician are included as part of the professional service. Surgical dressings obtained by the patient to perform homecare as prescribed by the physician are covered.
MED: 100-2, 15, 100

A **A6260** Wound cleansers, any type, any size ⊘
Surgical dressings applied by a physician are included as part of the professional service. Surgical dressings obtained by the patient to perform homecare as prescribed by the physician are covered.
MED: 100-2, 15, 100

A ☑ **A6261** Wound filler, gel/paste, per fluid oz., not elsewhere classified
Surgical dressings applied by a physician are included as part of the professional service. Surgical dressings obtained by the patient to perform homecare as prescribed by the physician are covered.
MED: 100-2, 15, 100

A ☑ **A6262** Wound filler, dry form, per gram, not elsewhere classified
MED: 100-2, 15, 100

A ☑ **A6266** Gauze, impregnated, other than water, normal saline, or zinc paste, any width, per linear yard ♿
Surgical dressings applied by a physician are included as part of the professional service. Surgical dressings obtained by the patient to perform homecare as prescribed by the physician are covered.
MED: 100-2, 15, 100

A ☑ **A6402** Gauze, non-impregnated, sterile, pad size 16 sq. in. or less, without adhesive border, each dressing ♿
Surgical dressings applied by a physician are included as part of the professional service. Surgical dressings obtained by the patient to perform homecare as prescribed by the physician are covered.
MED: 100-2, 15, 100

A ☑ **A6403** Gauze, non-impregnated, sterile, pad size more than 16 sq. in. but less than or equal to 48 sq. in., without adhesive border, each dressing ♿
Surgical dressings applied by a physician are included as part of the professional service. Surgical dressings obtained by the patient to perform homecare as prescribed by the physician are covered.
MED: 100-2, 15, 100

A ☑ **A6404** Gauze, non-impregnated, sterile, pad size more than 48 sq. in., without adhesive border, each dressing
MED: 100-2, 15, 100

☑ **A6407** Packing strips, non-impregnated, up to two in. in width, per linear yard ♿

A ☑ **A6410** Eye pad, sterile, each ♿
MED: 100-2, 15, 100

A ☑ **A6411** Eye pad, non-sterile, each ♿
MED: 100-2, 15, 100

E ☑ **A6412** Eye patch, occlusive, each

A ☑ **A6441** Padding bandage, non-elastic, non-woven/non-knitted, width greater than or equal to 3 in. and less than 5 in., per yard ♿

Medical and Surgical Supplies

A6442 — A7012

A ☑ **A6442** Conforming bandage, non-elastic, knitted/woven, non-sterile, width less than 3 in., per yard ⅃

A ☑ **A6443** Conforming bandage, non-elastic, knitted/woven, non-sterile, width greater than or equal to 3 in. and less than 5 in., per yard ⅃

A ☑ **A6444** Conforming bandage, non-elastic, knitted/woven, non-sterile, width greater than or equal to 5 in., per yard ⅃

A ☑ **A6445** Conforming bandage, non-elastic, knitted/woven, sterile, width less than 3 in., per yard ⅃

A ☑ **A6446** Conforming bandage, non-elastic, knitted/woven, sterile, width greater than or equal to 3 in. and less than 5 in., per yard ⅃

A ☑ **A6447** Conforming bandage, non-elastic, knitted/woven, sterile, width greater than or equal to 5 in., per yard ⅃

A ☑ **A6448** Light compression bandage, elastic, knitted/woven, width less than 3 in., per yard ⅃

A ☑ **A6449** Light compression bandage, elastic, knitted/woven, width greater than or equal to 3 in. and less than 5 in., per yard ⅃

A ☑ **A6450** Light compression bandage, elastic, knitted/woven, width greater than or equal to 5 in., per yard ⅃

A ☑ **A6451** Moderate compression bandage, elastic, knitted/woven, load resistance of 1.25 to 1.34 foot pounds at 50 percent maximum stretch, width greater than or equal to 3 in. and less than 5 in., per yard ⅃

A ☑ **A6452** High compression bandage, elastic, knitted/woven, load resistance greater than or equal to 1.35 foot pounds at 50 percent maximum stretch, width greater than or equal to 3 in. and less than five in., per yard ⅃

A ☑ **A6453** Self-adherent bandage, elastic, non-knitted/non-woven, width less than 3 in., per yard ⅃

A ☑ **A6454** Self-adherent bandage, elastic, non-knitted/non-woven, width greater than or equal to 3 in. and less than 5 in., per yard ⅃

A ☑ **A6455** Self-adherent bandage, elastic, non-knitted/non-woven, width greater than or equal to 5 in., per yard ⅃

A ☑ **A6456** Zinc paste impregnated bandage, non-elastic, knitted/woven, width greater than or equal to 3 in. and less than 5 in., per yard ⅃

A **A6501** Compression burn garment, bodysuit (head to foot), custom fabricated ⅃
MED: 100-2, 15, 100

A **A6502** Compression burn garment, chin strap, custom fabricated ⅃
MED: 100-2, 15, 100

A **A6503** Compression burn garment, facial hood, custom fabricated ⅃
MED: 100-2, 15, 100

A **A6504** Compression burn garment, glove to wrist, custom fabricated ⅃
MED: 100-2, 15, 100

A **A6505** Compression burn garment, glove to elbow, custom fabricated ⅃
MED: 100-2, 15, 100

A **A6506** Compression burn garment, glove to axilla, custom fabricated ⅃
MED: 100-2, 15, 100

A **A6507** Compression burn garment, foot to knee length, custom fabricated ⅃
MED: 100-2, 15, 100

A **A6508** Compression burn garment, foot to thigh length, custom fabricated ⅃
MED: 100-2, 15, 100

A **A6509** Compression burn garment, upper trunk to waist including arm openings (vest), custom fabricated ⅃
MED: 100-2, 15, 100

A **A6510** Compression burn garment, trunk, including arms down to leg openings (leotard), custom fabricated ⅃
MED: 100-2, 15, 100

A **A6511** Compression burn garment, lower trunk including leg openings (panty), custom fabricated ⅃
MED: 100-2, 15, 100

A **A6512** Compression burn garment, not otherwise classified
MED: 100-2, 15, 100

Y ☑ **A6550** Dressing set for negative pressure wound therapy electrical pump, stationary or portable, each ⅃

Y ☑ **A6551** Canister set for negative pressure wound therapy electrical pump, stationary or portable, each ⅃

Y ☑ **A7000** Canister, disposable, used with suction pump, each ⅃⊘
Medicare jurisdiction: DME regional carrier.

Y ☑ **A7001** Canister, non-disposable, used with suction pump, each ⅃⊘
Medicare jurisdiction: DME regional carrier.

Y **A7002** Tubing, used with suction pump, each ⅃⊘
Medicare jurisdiction: DME regional carrier.

Y **A7003** Administration set, with small volume nonfiltered pneumatic nebulizer, disposable ⅃⊘
Medicare jurisdiction: DME regional carrier.

Y **A7004** Small volume nonfiltered pneumatic nebulizer, disposable ⅃⊘
Medicare jurisdiction: DME regional carrier.

Y **A7005** Administration set, with small volume nonfiltered pneumatic nebulizer, non-disposable ⅃⊘
Medicare jurisdiction: DME regional carrier.

Y **A7006** Administration set, with small volume filtered pneumatic nebulizer ⅃⊘
Medicare jurisdiction: DME regional carrier.

Y **A7007** Large volume nebulizer, disposable, unfilled, used with aerosol compressor ⅃⊘
Medicare jurisdiction: DME regional carrier.

Y **A7008** Large volume nebulizer, disposable, prefilled, used with aerosol compressor ⅃⊘
Medicare jurisdiction: DME regional carrier.

Y **A7009** Reservoir bottle, non-disposable, used with large volume ultrasonic nebulizer ⅃⊘
Medicare jurisdiction: DME regional carrier.

Y ☑ **A7010** Corrugated tubing, disposable, used with large volume nebulizer, 100 feet ⅃⊘
Medicare jurisdiction: DME regional carrier.

Y ☑ **A7011** Corrugated tubing, non-disposable, used with large volume nebulizer, 10 feet ⊘

Y **A7012** Water collection device, used with large volume nebulizer ⅃⊘
Medicare jurisdiction: DME regional carrier.

Special Coverage Instructions   Noncovered by Medicare   Carrier Discretion   ☑ Quantity Alert   ● New Code   ○ Reinstated Code   ▲ Revised Code

14 — A Codes   A Adult   M Maternity   P Pediatrics   I Infant   A-Y APC Status Indicator   **2005 HCPCS**

Ⓨ   **A7013** Filter, disposable, used with aerosol compressor ℥⊘
Medicare jurisdiction: DME regional carrier.

Ⓨ   **A7014** Filter, non-disposable, used with aerosol compressor or ultrasonic generator ℥⊘
Medicare jurisdiction: DME regional carrier.

Ⓨ   **A7015** Aerosol mask, used with DME nebulizer ℥⊘
Medicare jurisdiction: DME regional carrier.

Ⓨ   **A7016** Dome and mouthpiece, used with small volume ultrasonic nebulizer ℥⊘
Medicare jurisdiction: DME regional carrier.

Ⓨ   **A7017** Nebulizer, durable, glass or autoclavable plastic, bottle type, not used with oxygen ℥⊘
Medicare jurisdiction: DME regional carrier.
MED: 100-3, 280.1

Ⓨ ☑ **A7018** Water, distilled, used with large volume nebulizer, 1000 ml ℥⊘
Medicare jurisdiction: DME regional carrier.

Ⓨ ☑ **A7025** High frequency chest wall oscillation system vest, replacement for use with patient owned equipment, each ℥

Ⓨ ☑ **A7026** High frequency chest wall oscillation system hose, replacement for use with patient owned equipment, each ℥

Ⓨ ☑ **A7030** Full face mask used with positive airway pressure device, each ℥

Ⓨ ☑ **A7031** Face mask interface, replacement for full face mask, each ℥

Ⓨ ☑ **A7032** Replacement cushion for nasal application device, each ℥

Ⓨ   **A7033** Replacement pillows for nasal application device, pair ℥

Ⓨ   **A7034** Nasal interface (mask or cannula type) used with positive airway pressure device, with or without head strap ℥

Ⓨ   **A7035** Headgear used with positive airway pressure device ℥

Ⓨ   **A7036** Chinstrap used with positive airway pressure device ℥

Ⓨ   **A7037** Tubing used with positive airway pressure device ℥

Ⓨ   **A7038** Filter, disposable, used with positive airway pressure device ℥

Ⓨ   **A7039** Filter, non disposable, used with positive airway pressure device ℥

●   **A7040** One way chest drain valve

●   **A7041** Water seal drainage container and tubing for use with implanted chest tube

Ⓐ   **A7042** Implanted pleural catheter, each ℥

Ⓐ   **A7043** Vacuum drainage bottle and tubing for use with implanted catheter ℥

Ⓨ   **A7044** Oral interface used with positive airway pressure device, each ℥

●   **A7045** Exhalation port with or without swivel used with accessories for positive airway devices, replacement only
MED: 100-3, 230.17

Ⓨ ☑ **A7046** Water chamber for humidifier, used with positive airway pressure device, replacement, each ℥⊘
MED: 100-3, 230.17

Ⓐ ☑ **A7501** Tracheostoma valve, including diaphragm, each ℥⊘
Medicare jurisdiction: DME regional carrier.
MED: 100-2, 15, 120

Ⓐ ☑ **A7502** Replacement diaphragm/faceplate for tracheostoma valve, each ℥
Medicare jurisdiction: DME regional carrier.
MED: 100-2, 15, 120

Ⓐ ☑ **A7503** Filter holder or filter cap, reusable, for use in a tracheostoma heat and moisture exchange system, each ℥
Medicare jurisdiction: DME regional carrier.
MED: 100-2, 15, 120

Ⓐ ☑ **A7504** Filter for use in a tracheostoma heat and moisture exchange system, each ℥
Medicare jurisdiction: DME regional carrier.
MED: 100-2, 15, 120

Ⓐ ☑ **A7505** Housing, reusable without adhesive, for use in a heat and moisture exchange system and/or with a tracheostoma valve, each ℥
Medicare jurisdiction: DME regional carrier.
MED: 100-2, 15, 120

Ⓐ ☑ **A7506** Adhesive disc for use in a heat and moisture exchange system and/or with tracheostoma valve, any type each ℥
Medicare jurisdiction: DME regional carrier.
MED: 100-2, 15, 120

Ⓐ ☑ **A7507** Filter holder and integrated filter without adhesive, for use in a tracheostoma heat and moisture exchange system, each ℥
Medicare jurisdiction: DME regional carrier.
MED: 100-2, 15, 120

Ⓐ ☑ **A7508** Housing and integrated adhesive, for use in a tracheostoma heat and moisture exchange system and/or with a tracheostoma valve, each ℥
Medicare jurisdiction: DME regional carrier.
MED: 100-2, 15, 120

Ⓐ ☑ **A7509** Filter holder and integrated filter housing, and adhesive, for use as a tracheostoma heat and moisture exchange system, each ℥
Medicare jurisdiction: DME regional carrier.
MED: 100-2, 15, 120

Ⓐ ☑ **A7520** Tracheostomy/laryngectomy tube, non-cuffed, polyvinylchloride (PVC), silicone or equal, each ℥

Ⓐ ☑ **A7521** Tracheostomy/laryngectomy tube, cuffed, polyvinylchloride (PVC), silicone or equal, each ℥

Ⓐ ☑ **A7522** Tracheostomy/laryngectomy tube, stainless steel or equal (sterilizable and reusable), each ℥

Ⓐ ☑ **A7523** Tracheostoma shower protector, each

Ⓐ ☑ **A7524** Tracheostoma stent/stud/button, each ℥

Ⓐ ☑ **A7525** Tracheostomy mask, each ℥

Ⓐ ☑ **A7526** Tracheostomy tube collar/holder, each ℥

● ☑ **A7527** Tracheostomy/laryngectomy tube plug/stop, each

Special Coverage Instructions   Noncovered by Medicare   Carrier Discretion   ☑ Quantity Alert   ● New Code   ○ Reinstated Code   ▲ Revised Code

2005 HCPCS   ♀ Female Only   ♂ Male Only   **1-9** ASC Groups   **MED:** Pub 100/NCD Reference   ℥ DMEPOS Paid   ⊘ SNF Excluded   **A Codes — 15**

ADMINISTRATIVE, MISCELLANEOUS & INVESTIGATIONAL *A9000–A9999*

This section of codes reports items such as nonprescription drugs, noncovered items/services, exercise equipment and, most notably, radiopharmaceutical diagnostic imaging agents.

B **A9150** Nonprescription drug ⊘
Medicare jurisdiction: local carrier.

● ☑ **A9152** Single vitamin/mineral/trace element, oral, per dose, not otherwise specified

● ☑ **A9153** Multiple vitamins, with or without minerals and trace elements, oral, per dose, not otherwise specified

● **A9180** Pediculosis (lice infestation) treatment, topical, for administration by patient/caretaker

E **A9270** Noncovered item or service ⊘
Medicare jurisdiction: local or DME regional carrier.
MED: 100-2, 16, 20

E **A9280** Alert or alarm device, not otherwise classified ⊘

E **A9300** Exercise equipment ⊘
MED: 100-2, 15, 110.1; 100-3, 280.1

K ☑ **A9500** Supply of radiopharmaceutical diagnostic imaging agent, technetium Tc 99m sestamibi, per dose
Use this code for Cardiolite. Medicare jurisdiction: local carrier.
MED: 100-4, 12, 70; 100-4, 13, 20; 100-4, 13, 90

K ☑ **A9502** Supply of radiopharmaceutical diagnostic imaging agent, technetium Tc 99m tetrofosmin, per unit dose
Medicare jurisdiction: local carrier.
MED: 100-4, 12, 70; 100-4, 13, 20; 100-4, 13, 90

N ☑ **A9503** Supply of radiopharmaceutical diagnostic imaging agent, technetium Tc 99m, medronate, up to 30 millicurie
Medicare jurisdiction: local carrier.
MED: 100-4, 12, 70; 100-4, 13, 20; 100-4, 13, 90
AHA: 2Q, '02, 9

N **A9504** Supply of radiopharmaceutical diagnostic imaging agent, technetium Tc 99m apcitide
Medicare jurisdiction: local carrier.
MED: 100-4, 12, 70; 100-4, 13, 20; 100-4, 13, 90
AHA: 4Q, '01, 5; 2Q, '02, 9

N ☑ **A9505** Supply of radiopharmaceutical diagnostic imaging agent, thallous chloride Tl-201, per millicurie
Medicare jurisdiction: local carrier.
MED: 100-4, 12, 70; 100-4, 13, 20; 100-4, 13, 90
AHA: 2Q, '02, 9

K ☑ **A9507** Supply of radiopharmaceutical diagnostic imaging agent, indium In-III capromab pendetide, per dose
Medicare jurisdiction: local carrier.
MED: 100-4, 12, 70; 100-4, 13, 20; 100-4, 13, 90

K ☑ **A9508** Supply of radiopharmaceutical diagnostic imaging agent, iobenguane sulfate I-131, per 0.5 millicurie
AHA: 2Q, '02, 9

N ☑ **A9510** Supply of radiopharmaceutical diagnostic imaging agent, technetium Tc 99m disofenin, per vial

K ☑ **A9511** Supply of radiopharmaceutical diagnostic imaging agent, technetium Tc 99m, Depreotide, per millicurie
AHA: 2Q, '02, 9

N ☑ **A9512** Supply of radiopharmaceutical diagnostic imaging agent, technetium Tc 99m pertechnetate, per mci

N ☑ **A9513** Supply of radiopharmaceutical diagnostic imaging agent, technetium Tc 99m mebrofenin, per mci

N ☑ **A9514** Supply of radiopharmaceutical diagnostic imaging agent, technetium Tc 99m pyrophosphate, per mci

N ☑ **A9515** Supply of radiopharmaceutical diagnostic imaging agent, technetium Tc 99m pentetate, per mci

N ☑ **A9516** Supply of radiopharmaceutical diagnostic imaging agent, I-123 sodium iodide capsule, per 100 uci

K ☑ **A9517** Supply of radiopharmaceutical therapeutic imaging agent, I-131 sodium iodide capsule, per mci ⊘

N ☑ **A9519** Supply of radiopharmaceutical diagnostic imaging agent, technetium Tc 99m macroaggregated albumin, per mci

N ☑ **A9520** Supply of radiopharmaceutical diagnostic imaging agent, technetium Tc 99m sulfur colloid, per mci

K ☑ **A9521** Supply of radiopharmaceutical diagnostic imaging agent, technetium Tc 99m exametazine, per dose

B ☑ **A9522** Supply of radiopharmaceutical diagnostic imaging agent, indium 111 ibritumomab tiuxetan, per mci
MED: 100-4, 12, 70; 100-4, 13, 20; 100-4, 13, 90
AHA: 2Q, '03, 8

B ☑ **A9523** Supply of radiopharmaceutical therapeutic imaging agent, yttrium 90 ibritumomab tiuxetan, per mci
MED: 100-4, 12, 70; 100-4, 13, 20; 100-4, 13, 90
AHA: 2Q, '03, 8

K ☑ **A9524** Supply of radiopharmaceutical diagnostic imaging agent, iodinated I-131 serum albumin, 5 microcuries
MED: 100-4, 12, 70; 100-4, 13, 20; 100-4, 13, 90

E ☑ **A9525** Supply of low or iso-osmolar contrast material, 10 mg of iodine

K ☑ **A9526** Supply of radiopharmaceutical diagnostic imaging agent, ammonia N-13, per dose
MED: 100-3, 220.6

K ☑ **A9528** Supply of radiopharmaceutical diagnostic agent, I-131 sodium iodide capsule, per millicurie

K ☑ **A9529** Supply of radiopharmaceutical diagnostic agent, I-131 sodium iodide solution, per millicurie

K ☑ **A9530** Supply of radiopharmaceutical therapeutic agent, I-131 sodium iodide solution, per millicurie

N ☑ **A9531** Supply of radiopharmaceutical diagnostic agent, I-131 sodium iodide, per microcurie (up to 100 microcuries)

N ☑ **A9532** Supply of radiopharmaceutical therapeutic agent, iodinated I-125, serum albumin, 5 microcuries

B ☑ **A9533** Supply of radiopharmaceutical diagnostic imaging agent, I-131 tositumomab, per millicurie

B ☑ **A9534** Supply of radiopharmaceutical therapeutic imaging agent, I-131 tositumomab, per millicurie

K ☑ **A9600** Supply of therapeutic radiopharmaceutical, strontium 89 chloride, per millicurie
Medicare jurisdiction: local carrier.
AHA: 2Q, '02, 9

K ☑ **A9605** Supply of therapeutic radiopharmaceutical, samarium Sm-153 lexidronamm, 50 millicuries
AHA: 2Q, '02, 9

Special Coverage Instructions   Noncovered by Medicare   Carrier Discretion   ☑ Quantity Alert   ● New Code   ○ Reinstated Code   ▲ Revised Code

16 — A Codes   **A** Adult   **M** Maternity   **P** Pediatrics   **I** Infant   **A-Y** APC Status Indicator   *2005 HCPCS*

[N]   A9699   Supply of radiopharmaceutical therapeutic imaging agent, not otherwise classified

[E]   A9700   Supply of injectable contrast material for use in echocardiography, per study
MED: 100-4, 12, 30.4

AHA: 4Q, '01, 5

[A]   A9900   Miscellaneous DME supply, accessory, and/or service component of another HCPCS code   ⊘
Medicare jurisdiction: local carrier if implanted DME; if other, regional carrier.

[A]   A9901   DME delivery, set up, and/or dispensing service component of another HCPCS code   ⊘
Medicare jurisdiction: local carrier if implanted DME; if other, regional carrier.

[Y]   A9999   Miscellaneous DME supply or accessory, not otherwise specified   ⊘

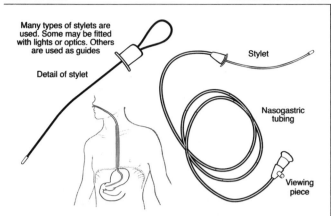

Many types of stylets are used. Some may be fitted with lights or optics. Others are used as guides

Detail of stylet

Stylet

Nasogastric tubing

Viewing piece

ENTERAL AND PARENTERAL THERAPY *B4000–B9999*
This section includes codes for supplies, formulae, nutritional solutions, and infusion pumps.

ENTERAL FORMULAE AND ENTERAL MEDICAL SUPPLIES
Certification of medical necessity is required for coverage. Submit a revision to the certification of medical necessity if the patient's daily volume changes by more than one liter; if there is a change in infusion method; or if there is a change from premix to home mix or parenteral to enteral therapy.

Ⓐ **B4034** Enteral feeding supply kit; syringe, per day ⊘
MED: 100-2, 15, 120; 100-3, 180.2; 100-4, 20, 100.2.2; 100-4, 20, 100.2.2.3

Ⓐ **B4035** Enteral feeding supply kit; pump fed, per day ⊘
MED: 100-2, 15, 120; 100-3, 180.2; 100-4, 20, 100.2.2; 100-4, 20, 100.2.2.3

Ⓐ **B4036** Enteral feeding supply kit; gravity fed, per day ⊘
MED: 100-2, 15, 120; 100-3, 180.2; 100-4, 20, 100.2.2; 100-4, 20, 100.2.2.3

Ⓐ **B4081** Nasogastric tubing with stylet ⊘
MED: 100-2, 15, 120; 100-3, 180.2; 100-4, 20, 100.2.2; 100-4, 20, 100.2.2.3

Ⓐ **B4082** Nasogastric tubing without stylet ⊘
MED: 100-2, 15, 120; 100-3, 180.2; 100-4, 20, 100.2.2; 100-4, 20, 100.2.2.3

Ⓐ **B4083** Stomach tube — Levine type ⊘
MED: 100-2, 15, 120; 100-3, 180.2; 100-4, 20, 100.2.2; 100-4, 20, 100.2.2.3

Ⓐ **B4086** Gastrostomy/jejunostomy tube, any material, any type, (standard or low profile), each ⊘

Ⓔ **B4100** Food thickener, administered orally, per oz.

● ☑ **B4102** Enteral formula, for adults, used to replace fluids and electrolytes (e.g., clear liquids), 500 ml = 1 unit
MED: 100-3, 180.2

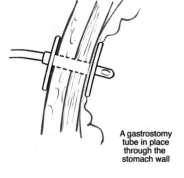

A gastrostomy tube in place through the stomach wall

● ☑ **B4103** Enteral formula, for pediatrics, used to replace fluids and electrolytes (e.g., clear liquids), 500 ml = 1 unit
MED: 100-3, 180.2

● ☑ **B4104** Additive for enteral formula (e.g., fiber)
MED: 100-3, 180.2

● ☑ **B4149** Enteral formula, blenderized natural foods with intact nutrients, includes proteins, fats, carbohydrates, vitamins and minerals, may include fiber, administered through an enteral feeding tube, 100 calories = 1 unit
MED: 100-2, 15, 120; 100-3, 180.2; 100-4, 20, 100.2.2; 100-4, 20, 100.2.2.3

▲ Ⓐ **B4150** Enteral formula, nutritionally complete with intact nutrients, includes proteins, fats, carbohydrates, vitamins and minerals, may include fiber, administered through an enteral feeding tube, 100 calories = 1 unit ⊘
Use this code for Enrich, Ensure, Ensure HN, Ensure Powder, Isocal, Lonalac Powder, Meritene, Meritene Powder, Osmolite, Osmolite HN, Portagen Powder, Sustacal, Renu, Sustagen Powder, Travasorb.

MED: 100-2, 15, 120; 100-3, 180.2; 100-4, 20, 100.2.2; 100-4, 20, 100.2.2.3

~~B4151~~ ~~Enteral formulae, category I: natural intact protein/protein isolates, administered through an enteral feeding tube, 100 calories = 1 unit~~

▲ Ⓐ **B4152** Enteral formula, nutritionally complete, calorically dense (equal to or greater than 1.5 kcal/ml) with intact nutrients, includes proteins, fats, carbohydrates, vitamins and minerals, may include fiber, administered through an enteral feeding tube, 100 calories = 1 unit ⊘
Use this code for Magnacal, Isocal HCN, Sustacal HC, Ensure Plus, Ensure Plus HN.

MED: 100-2, 15, 120; 100-3, 180.2; 100-4, 20, 100.2.2; 100-4, 20, 100.2.2.3

▲ Ⓐ **B4153** Enteral formula, nutritionally complete, hydrolyzed proteins (amino acids and peptide chain), includes fats, carbohydrates, vitamins and minerals, may include fiber, administered through an enteral feeding tube, 100 calories = 1 unit ⊘
Use this code for Criticare HN, Vivonex t.e.n. (Total Enteral Nutrition), Vivonex HN, Vital (Vital HN), Travasorb HN, Isotein HN, Precision HN, Precision Isotonic.

MED: 100-2, 15, 120; 100-3, 180.2; 100-4, 20, 100.2.2; 100-4, 20, 100.2.2.3

▲ Ⓐ **B4154** Enteral formula, nutritionally complete, for special metabolic needs, excludes inherited disease of metabolism, includes altered composition of proteins, fats, carbohydrates, vitamins and/or minerals, may include fiber, administered through an enteral feeding tube, 100 calories = 1 unit ⊘
Use this code for Hepatic-aid, Travasorb Hepatic, Travasorb MCT, Travasorb Renal, Traum-aid, Tramacal, Aminaid.

MED: 100-2, 15, 120; 100-3, 180.2; 100-4, 20, 100.2.2; 100-4, 20, 100.2.2.3

Enteral and Parenteral Therapy

B4155 — B4224

▲ Ⓐ **B4155** Enteral formula, nutritionally incomplete/modular nutrients, includes specific nutrients, carbohydrates (e.g., glucose polymers), proteins/amino acids (e.g., glutamine, arginine), fat (e.g., medium chain triglycerides) or combination, administered through an enteral feeding tube, 100 calories = 1 unit ⊘
Use this code for Propac, Gerval Protein, Promix, Casec, Moducal, Controlyte, Polycose Liquid or Powder, Sumacal, Microlipids, MCT Oil, Nutri-source.
MED: 100-2, 15, 120; 100-3, 180.2; 100-4, 20, 100.2.2; 100-4, 20, 100.2.2.3

~~**B4156** Enteral formulae; category VI; standardized nutrients, administered through an enteral feeding tube, 100 calories = 1 unit~~

● ☑ **B4157** Enteral formula, nutritionally complete, for special metabolic needs for inherited disease of metabolism, includes proteins, fats, carbohydrates, vitamins and minerals, may include fiber, administered through an enteral feeding tube, 100 calories = 1 unit
MED: 100-3, 180.2

● ☑ **B4158** Enteral formula, for pediatrics, nutritionally complete with intact nutrients, includes proteins, fats, carbohydrates, vitamins and minerals, may include fiber and/or iron, administered through an enteral feeding tube, 100 calories = 1 unit
MED: 100-3, 180.2

● ☑ **B4159** Enteral formula, for pediatrics, nutritionally complete soy based with intact nutrients, includes proteins, fats, carbohydrates, vitamins and minerals, may include fiber and/or iron, administered through an enteral feeding tube, 100 calories = 1 unit
MED: 100-3, 180.2

● ☑ **B4160** Enteral formula, for pediatrics, nutritionally complete calorically dense (equal to or greater than 0.7 kcal/ml) with intact nutrients, includes proteins, fats, carbohydrates, vitamins and minerals, may include fiber, administered through an enteral feeding tube, 100 calories = 1 unit
MED: 100-3, 180.2

● ☑ **B4161** Enteral formula, for pediatrics, hydrolyzed/amino acids and peptide chain proteins, includes fats, carbohydrates, vitamins and minerals, may include fiber, administered through an enteral feeding tube, 100 calories = 1 unit
MED: 100-3, 180.2

● ☑ **B4162** Enteral formula, for pediatrics, special metabolic needs for inherited disease of metabolism, includes proteins, fats, carbohydrates, vitamins and minerals, may include fiber, administered through an enteral feeding tube, 100 calories = 1 unit
MED: 100-3, 180.2

PARENTERAL NUTRITION SOLUTIONS AND SUPPLIES

Ⓐ **B4164** Parenteral nutrition solution; carbohydrates (dextrose), 50% or less (500 ml = 1 unit) — home mix ⊘
MED: 100-2, 15, 120; 100-3, 180.2; 100-4, 20, 100.2.2; 100-4, 20, 100.2.2.3

Ⓐ **B4168** Parenteral nutrition solution; amino acid, 3.5%, (500 ml = 1 unit) — home mix ⊘
MED: 100-2, 15, 120; 100-3, 180.2; 100-4, 20, 100.2.2; 100-4, 20, 100.2.2.3

Ⓐ **B4172** Parenteral nutrition solution; amino acid, 5.5% through 7%, (500 ml = 1 unit) — home mix ⊘
MED: 100-2, 15, 120; 100-3, 180.2; 100-4, 20, 100.2.2; 100-4, 20, 100.2.2.3

Ⓐ **B4176** Parenteral nutrition solution; amino acid, 7% through 8.5%, (500 ml = 1 unit) — home mix ⊘
MED: 100-2, 15, 120; 100-3, 180.2; 100-4, 20, 100.2.2; 100-4, 20, 100.2.2.3

Ⓐ **B4178** Parenteral nutrition solution; amino acid, greater than 8.5% (500 ml = 1 unit) — home mix ⊘
MED: 100-2, 15, 120; 100-3, 180.2; 100-4, 20, 100.2.2; 100-4, 20, 100.2.2.3

Ⓐ **B4180** Parenteral nutrition solution; carbohydrates (dextrose), greater than 50% (500 ml = 1 unit) — home mix ⊘
MED: 100-2, 15, 120; 100-3, 180.2; 100-4, 20, 100.2.2; 100-4, 20, 100.2.2.3

Ⓐ **B4184** Parenteral nutrition solution; lipids, 10% with administration set (500 ml = 1 unit) ⊘
MED: 100-2, 15, 120; 100-3, 180.2; 100-4, 20, 100.2.2; 100-4, 20, 100.2.2.3

Ⓐ **B4186** Parenteral nutrition solution; lipids, 20% with administration set (500 ml = 1 unit) ⊘
MED: 100-2, 15, 120; 100-3, 180.2; 100-4, 20, 100.2.2; 100-4, 20, 100.2.2.3

Ⓐ ☑ **B4189** Parenteral nutrition solution; compounded amino acid and carbohydrates with electrolytes, trace elements, and vitamins, including preparation, any strength, 10 to 51 grams of protein - premix ⊘
MED: 100-2, 15, 120; 100-3, 180.2; 100-4, 20, 100.2.2; 100-4, 20, 100.2.2.3

Ⓐ ☑ **B4193** Parenteral nutrition solution; compounded amino acid and carbohydrates with electrolytes, trace elements, and vitamins, including preparation, any strength, 52 to 73 grams of protein - premix ⊘
MED: 100-2, 15, 120; 100-3, 180.2; 100-4, 20, 100.2.2; 100-4, 20, 100.2.2.3

Ⓐ ☑ **B4197** Parenteral nutrition solution; compounded amino acid and carbohydrates with electrolytes, trace elements and vitamins, including preparation, any strength, 74 to 100 grams of protein - premix ⊘
MED: 100-2, 15, 120; 100-3, 180.2; 100-4, 20, 100.2.2; 100-4, 20, 100.2.2.3

Ⓐ ☑ **B4199** Parenteral nutrition solution; compounded amino acid and carbohydrates with electrolytes, trace elements and vitamins, including preparation, any strength, over 100 grams of protein - premix ⊘
MED: 100-2, 15, 120; 100-3, 180.2; 100-4, 20, 100.2.2; 100-4, 20, 100.2.2.3

Ⓐ **B4216** Parenteral nutrition; additives (vitamins, trace elements, heparin, electrolytes) — home mix, per day ⊘
MED: 100-2, 15, 120; 100-3, 180.2; 100-4, 20, 100.2.2; 100-4, 20, 100.2.2.3

Ⓐ **B4220** Parenteral nutrition supply kit; premix, per day ⊘
MED: 100-2, 15, 120; 100-3, 180.2; 100-4, 20, 100.2.2; 100-4, 20, 100.2.2.3

Ⓐ **B4222** Parenteral nutrition supply kit; home mix, per day ⊘
MED: 100-2, 15, 120; 100-3, 180.2; 100-4, 20, 100.2.2; 100-4, 20, 100.2.2.3

Ⓐ **B4224** Parenteral nutrition administration kit, per day ⊘
MED: 100-2, 15, 120; 100-3, 180.2; 100-4, 20, 100.2.2; 100-4, 20, 100.2.2.3

| Special Coverage Instructions | Noncovered by Medicare | Carrier Discretion | ☑ Quantity Alert | ● New Code | ○ Reinstated Code | ▲ Revised Code |

20 — B Codes   Ⓐ Adult   Ⓜ Maternity   Ⓟ Pediatrics   Ⓘ Infant   Ⓐ-☑ APC Status Indicator   *2005 HCPCS*

Ⓐ **B5000** Parenteral nutrition solution; compounded amino acid and carbohydrates with electrolytes, trace elements, and vitamins, including preparation, any strength, renal — Amirosyn RF, NephrAmine, RenAmine — premix ⊘
Use this code for Amirosyn-RF, NephrAmine, RenAmin.

MED: 100-2, 15, 120; 100-3, 180.2; 100-4, 20, 100.2.2; 100-4, 20, 100.2.2.3

Ⓐ **B5100** Parenteral nutrition solution; compounded amino acid and carbohydrates with electrolytes, trace elements, and vitamins, including preparation, any strength, hepatic — FreAmine HBC, HepatAmine — premix ⊘
Use this code for FreAmine HBC, HepatAmine.

MED: 100-2, 15, 120; 100-3, 180.2; 100-4, 20, 100.2.2; 100-4, 20, 100.2.2.3

Ⓐ **B5200** Parenteral nutrition solution; compounded amino acid and carbohydrates with electrolytes, trace elements, and vitamins, including preparation, any strength, stress — branch chain amino acids — premix ⊘
MED: 100-2, 15, 120; 100-3, 180.2; 100-4, 20, 100.2.2; 100-4, 20, 100.2.2.3

ENTERAL AND PARENTERAL PUMPS
Submit documentation of the need for the infusion pump. Medicare will reimburse for the simplest model that meets the patient's needs.

Ⓐ **B9000** Enteral nutrition infusion pump — without alarm ⊘
MED: 100-2, 15, 120; 100-3, 180.2; 100-4, 20, 100.2.2; 100-4, 20, 100.2.2.3

Ⓐ **B9002** Enteral nutrition infusion pump — with alarm ⊘
MED: 100-2, 15, 120; 100-3, 180.2; 100-4, 20, 100.2.2; 100-4, 20, 100.2.2.3

Ⓐ **B9004** Parenteral nutrition infusion pump, portable ⊘
MED: 100-2, 15, 120; 100-3, 180.2; 100-4, 20, 100.2.2; 100-4, 20, 100.2.2.3

Ⓐ **B9006** Parenteral nutrition infusion pump, stationary ⊘
MED: 100-2, 15, 120; 100-3, 180.2; 100-4, 20, 100.2.2; 100-4, 20, 100.2.2.3

Ⓐ **B9998** NOC for enteral supplies ⊘
MED: 100-2, 15, 120; 100-3, 180.2; 100-4, 20, 100.2.2; 100-4, 20, 100.2.2.3

Ⓐ **B9999** NOC for parenteral supplies ⊘
Determine if an alternative HCPCS Level II or a CPT code better describes the service being reported. This code should be used only if a more specific code is unavailable.

MED: 100-2, 15, 120; 100-3, 180.2; 100-4, 20, 100.2.2; 100-4, 20, 100.2.2.3

| Special Coverage Instructions | Noncovered by Medicare | Carrier Discretion | ☑ Quantity Alert | ● New Code | ○ Reinstated Code | ▲ Revised Code |

2005 HCPCS ♀ Female Only ♂ Male Only ❶-❾ ASC Groups MED: Pub 100/NCD Reference ⅙ DMEPOS Paid ⊘ SNF Excluded **B Codes — 21**

OUTPATIENT PPS *C1000–C9999*

This section reports drugs, biologicals, and devices eligible for transitional pass-through payments for hospitals, and for items classified in new-technology ambulatory payment classifications (APCs) under the outpatient prospective payment system. These supplies can be billed in addition to the APC for ambulatory surgery center services when billing APCs to Medicare. Similar to all reimbursement requirements, Medicare makes transitional pass-through payments for a device only in conjunction with a procedure for its implantation or insertion. Consequently, a device will be considered medically necessary and eligible for a transitional pass-through payment only if the associated procedure is also medically necessary and payable under the outpatient prospective payment system.

CMS established categories for determining transitional pass-through payment devices, effective April 1, 2001, to meet the requirements of the Medicare, Medicaid, and SCHIP Benefits Improvement and Protection Act (BIPA). These new codes are also in the C series of HCPCS and are exclusively for use in billing for transitional pass-through payments. The introduction of categories does not affect payment methods. The transitional pass-through payment for a device will continue to be based on the charge on the individual bill, reduced to cost, and subject to a deduction that represents the cost of similar devices already included in the APC payment rate.

Each item previously determined to qualify fits in one of these categories. Other items may be billed using the category codes, even though CMS has not qualified them on an item-specific basis, as long as they:

- Meet the definition of a device that qualifies for transitional pass-through payments and other requirements and definitions

- Are described by the long descriptor associated with an active category code assigned by CMS

- Correlate with the definitions of terms and other general explanations issued by CMS to accompany coding assignments in this or subsequent instructions

- Have been approved by the Food and Drug Administration, if required. Some investigational devices have received an FDA investigational device exemption and may qualify

- Are considered reasonable and necessary for the diagnosis or treatment of an illness or injury

- Are an integral part of the procedure

- Are used for one patient only, are single use, come in contact with human tissue, and are surgically implanted or inserted. They may or may not remain with the patient when the patient is released from the hospital

- Cannot be taken as a depreciation, such as equipment, instruments, apparatuses, or implements

- Are not supplies used during the service or procedure, other than radiological site markers

- Are not materials such as biological or synthetics that are used to replace human skin

Future program memorandums will announce any new categories CMS develops. Keep in mind that the qualification of a device for transitional pass-through payments is temporary.

K ☑ **C1079** **Supply of radiopharmaceutical diagnostic imaging agent, cyanocobalamin Co-57/58, per 0.5 millicurie**

○ K ☑ **C1080** **Supply of radiopharmaceutical diagnostic imaging agent, I-131 tositumomab, per dose**

○ K ☑ **C1081** **Supply of radiopharmaceutical therapeutic imaging agent, I-131 tositumomab, per dose**

○ K ☑ **C1082** **Supply of radiopharmaceutical diagnostic imaging agent, indium 111 ibritumomab tiuxetan, per dose**

○ K ☑ **C1083** **Supply of radiopharmaceutical therapeutic imaging agent, yttrium 90 ibritumomab tiuxetan, per dose**

~~C1088~~ ~~Laser optic treatment system, Indigo Laseroptic Treatment System~~

K ☑ **C1091** **Supply of radiopharmaceutical diagnostic imaging agent, indium 111 oxyquinoline, per 0.5 millicurie** ⊘

K ☑ **C1092** **Supply of radiopharmaceutical diagnostic imaging agent, indium 111 pentetate, per 0.5 millicurie** ⊘

● **C1093** **Supply of radiopharmaceutical diagnostic imaging agent, technetium Tc 99m fanolesomab, per dose (10-20 mci)**

K **C1122** **Supply of radiopharmaceutical diagnostic imaging agent, technetium Tc 99m arcitumomab, per vial** ⊘

K ☑ **C1178** **Injection, busulfan, per 6 mg** ⊘
Use this code for Busulfex.

K **C1200** **Supply of radiopharmaceutical diagnostic imaging agent, technetium Tc 99m sodium glucoheptonate, per vial** ⊘

K **C1201** **Supply of radiopharmaceutical diagnostic imaging agent, technetium Tc 99m succimer, per vial** ⊘

S **C1300** **Hyperbaric oxygen under pressure, full body chamber, per 30 minute interval** ⊘

● K **C1305** **Graftskin, per 44 square centimeters** ⊘
AHA: 2Q, '02, 10

○ N **C1713** **Anchor/screw for opposing bone-to-bone or soft tissue-to-bone (implantable)**
AHA: 1Q, '01, 5; 3Q, '02, 5

○ N **C1714** **Catheter, transluminal atherectomy, directional**
AHA: 1Q, '01, 5; 3Q, '02, 5; 4Q, '03, 8

○ N **C1715** **Brachytherapy needle**
AHA: 1Q, '01, 5; 3Q, '02, 5

▲ H **C1716** **Brachytherapy source, gold 198, per source** ⊘
AHA: 1Q, '01, 5; 3Q, '02, 5

▲ H **C1717** **Brachytherapy source, high dose rate iridium 192, per source**
AHA: 1Q, '01, 5; 3Q, '02, 5

▲ H **C1718** **Brachytherapy source, iodine 125, per source** ⊘
AHA: 1Q, '01, 5; 3Q, '02, 5; 1Q, '04, 2

▲ H **C1719** **Brachytherapy source, non-high dose rate iridium 192, per source** ⊘
AHA: 1Q, '01, 5; 3Q, '02, 5

▲ H **C1720** **Brachytherapy source, palladium 103, per source** ⊘
AHA: 1Q, '01, 5; 3Q, '02, 5; 1Q, '04, 2

● N **C1721** **Cardioverter-defibrillator, dual chamber (implantable)**
AHA: 1Q, '01, 5; 3Q, '02, 5

○ N **C1722** **Cardioverter-defibrillator, single chamber (implantable)**
AHA: 1Q, '01, 5; 3Q, '02, 5

○ N **C1724** **Catheter, transluminal atherectomy, rotational**
AHA: 1Q, '01, 5; 3Q, '02, 5; 4Q, '03, 8

○ N **C1725** **Catheter, transluminal angioplasty, non-laser (may include guidance, infusion/perfusion capability)**
AHA: 1Q, '01, 5; 3Q, '02, 5; 4Q, '03, 8

○ N **C1726** **Catheter, balloon dilatation, non-vascular**
AHA: 1Q, '01, 5; 3Q, '02, 5

○ N **C1727** **Catheter, balloon tissue dissector, non-vascular (insertable)**
AHA: 1Q, '01, 5; 3Q, '02, 5

Special Coverage Instructions   Noncovered by Medicare   Carrier Discretion   ☑ Quantity Alert   ● New Code   ○ Reinstated Code   ▲ Revised Code

2005 HCPCS   ♀ Female Only   ♂ Male Only   **1-9** ASC Groups   **MED:** Pub 100/NCD Reference   ♿ DMEPOS Paid   ⊘ SNF Excluded   **C Codes — 23**

Outpatient PPS

C1728 — C1818

○ Ⓝ **C1728** Catheter, brachytherapy seed administration
AHA: 1Q, '01, 5; 3Q, '02, 5

○ Ⓝ **C1729** Catheter, drainage
AHA: 1Q, '01, 5; 3Q, '02, 5

○ Ⓝ **C1730** Catheter, electrophysiology, diagnostic, other than 3D mapping (19 or fewer electrodes)
AHA: 1Q, '01, 5; 3Q, '01, 4, 5; 3Q, '02, 5

○ Ⓝ **C1731** Catheter, electrophysiology, diagnostic, other than 3D mapping (20 or more electrodes)
AHA: 1Q, '01, 5; 3Q, '02, 5

○ Ⓝ **C1732** Catheter, electrophysiology, diagnostic/ablation, 3D or vector mapping
AHA: 1Q, '01, 5; 3Q, '01, 53Q, '02, 5

○ Ⓝ **C1733** Catheter, electrophysiology, diagnostic/ablation, other than 3D or vector mapping, other than cool-tip
AHA: 3Q, '01, 4, 5; 1Q, '01, 5; 3Q, '02, 5

○ Ⓝ **C1750** Catheter, hemodialysis, long-term
AHA: 1Q, '01, 5; 3Q, '02, 5; 4Q, '03, 8

○ Ⓝ **C1751** Catheter, infusion, inserted peripherally, centrally or midline (other than hemodialysis)
AHA: 1Q, '01, 4, 5; 3Q, '01, 5; 3Q, '02, 5; 4Q, '03, 8

○ Ⓝ **C1752** Catheter, hemodialysis, short-term
AHA: 1Q, '01, 5; 3Q, '02, 5; 4Q, '03, 8

○ Ⓝ **C1753** Catheter, intravascular ultrasound
AHA: 1Q, '01, 5; 3Q, '02, 5; 4Q, '03, 8

○ Ⓝ **C1754** Catheter, intradiscal
AHA: 1Q, '01, 5; 3Q, '02, 5; 4Q, '03, 8

○ Ⓝ **C1755** Catheter, intraspinal
AHA: 1Q, '01, 5; 3Q, '02, 5; 4Q, '03, 8

○ Ⓝ **C1756** Catheter, pacing, transesophageal
AHA: 1Q, '01, 5; 3Q, '02, 5; 4Q, '03, 8

○ Ⓝ **C1757** Catheter, thrombectomy/embolectomy
AHA: 1Q, '01, 5; 3Q, '02, 5; 4Q, '03, 8

○ Ⓝ **C1758** Catheter, ureteral
AHA: 1Q, '01, 6; 3Q, '02, 5; 4Q, '03, 8

○ Ⓝ **C1759** Catheter, intracardiac echocardiography
AHA: 1Q, '01, 5; 3Q, '01, 4; 3Q, '02, 5; 4Q, '03, 8

○ Ⓝ **C1760** Closure device, vascular (implantable/insertable)
AHA: 1Q, '01, 6; 3Q, '02, 5; 4Q, '03, 8

○ Ⓝ **C1762** Connective tissue, human (includes fascia lata)
AHA: 1Q, '01, 6; 3Q, '02, 5; 3Q, '03, 12; 4Q, '03, 8

○ Ⓝ **C1763** Connective tissue, non-human (includes synthetic)
AHA: 1Q, '01, 6; 3Q, '02, 5; 3Q, '03, 12; 4Q, '03, 8

○ Ⓝ **C1764** Event recorder, cardiac (implantable)
AHA: 1Q, '01, 6; 3Q, '02, 5; 4Q, '03, 8

Ⓝ **C1765** Adhesion barrier   ⊘

○ Ⓝ **C1766** Introducer/sheath, guiding, intracardiac electrophysiological, steerable, other than peel-away
AHA: 3Q, '01, 5; 3Q, '02, 5

○ Ⓝ **C1767** Generator, neurostimulator (implantable)
AHA: 1Q, '01, 4, 6; 1Q, '02, 9; 3Q, '02, 5; 4Q, '03, 8

○ Ⓝ **C1768** Graft, vascular
AHA: 1Q, '01, 6; 3Q, '02, 5; 4Q, '03, 8

○ Ⓝ **C1769** Guide wire
AHA: 1Q, '01, 6; 3Q, '01, 4; 3Q, '02, 5; 4Q, '03, 8

○ Ⓝ **C1770** Imaging coil, magnetic resonance (insertable)
AHA: 1Q, '01, 6; 3Q, '02, 5; 4Q, '03, 8

○ Ⓝ **C1771** Repair device, urinary, incontinence, with sling graft
AHA: 1Q, '01, 6; 3Q, '01, 4, 5; 3Q, '02, 5; 4Q, '03, 8

○ Ⓝ **C1772** Infusion pump, programmable (implantable)
AHA: 1Q, '01, 6; 3Q, '02, 5

○ Ⓝ **C1773** Retrieval device, insertable (used to retrieve fractured medical devices)
AHA: 1Q, '01, 6; 3Q, '02, 5; 4Q, '03, 8

Ⓚ ☑ **C1775** Supply of radiopharmaceutical diagnostic imaging agent, fluorodeoxyglucose f18 (2-deoxy-2-[18f] fluoro-d-glucose), per dose (4-40 mci/ml)   ⊘

○ Ⓝ **C1776** Joint device (implantable)
AHA: 1Q, '01, 6; 3Q, '01, 5; 3Q, '02, 5

○ Ⓝ **C1777** Lead, cardioverter-defibrillator, endocardial single coil (implantable)
AHA: 1Q, '01, 6; 3Q, '02, 5

○ Ⓝ **C1778** Lead, neurostimulator (implantable)
AHA: 1Q, '01, 4, 6; 3Q, '02, 5; 1Q, '02, 9

○ Ⓝ **C1779** Lead, pacemaker, transvenous VDD single pass
AHA: 1Q, '01, 6; 3Q, '02, 5

○ Ⓝ **C1780** Lens, intraocular (new technology)
AHA: 1Q, '01, 6; 3Q, '02, 5

○ Ⓝ **C1781** Mesh (implantable)
AHA: 1Q, '01, 6; 3Q, '02, 5

○ Ⓝ **C1782** Morcellator
AHA: 1Q, '01, 6; 3Q, '02, 5

Ⓗ **C1783** Ocular implant, aqueous drainage assist device   ⊘

○ Ⓝ **C1784** Ocular device, intraoperative, detached retina
AHA: 1Q, '01, 6; 3Q, '02, 5

○ Ⓝ **C1785** Pacemaker, dual chamber, rate-responsive (implantable)
AHA: 1Q, '01, 6; 3Q, '02, 5; 4Q, '03, 8

○ Ⓝ **C1786** Pacemaker, single chamber, rate-responsive (implantable)
AHA: 1Q, '01, 6; 3Q, '02, 5; 4Q, '03, 8

○ Ⓝ **C1787** Patient programmer, neurostimulator
AHA: 1Q, '01, 6; 3Q, '02, 5; 4Q, '03, 8

○ Ⓝ **C1788** Port, indwelling (implantable)
AHA: 1Q, '01, 6; 3Q, '01, 4; 3Q, '02, 5; 4Q, '03, 8

○ Ⓝ **C1789** Prosthesis, breast (implantable)
AHA: 1Q, '01, 6; 3Q, '02, 5; 4Q, '03, 8

○ Ⓝ **C1813** Prosthesis, penile, inflatable
AHA: 1Q, '01, 6; 3Q, '02, 5; 4Q, '03, 8

Ⓗ **C1814** Retinal tamponade device, silicone oil   ⊘

○ Ⓝ **C1815** Prosthesis, urinary sphincter (implantable)
AHA: 1Q, '01, 6; 3Q, '02, 5; 4Q, '03, 8

○ Ⓝ **C1816** Receiver and/or transmitter, neurostimulator (implantable)
AHA: 1Q, '01, 6; 3Q, '02, 5; 4Q, '03, 8

○ Ⓝ **C1817** Septal defect implant system, intracardiac
AHA: 1Q, '01, 6; 3Q, '02, 5; 4Q, '03, 8

Ⓗ **C1818** Integrated keratoprosthesis   ⊘
AHA: 4Q, '03, 4

Special Coverage Instructions   Noncovered by Medicare   Carrier Discretion   ☑ Quantity Alert   ● New Code   ○ Reinstated Code   ▲ Revised Code

24 — C Codes   Ⓐ Adult   Ⓜ Maternity   Ⓟ Pediatrics   Ⓘ Infant   Ⓐ-Ⓨ APC Status Indicator   *2005 HCPCS*

○ [H]   **C1819** Surgical tissue localization and excision device (implantable)
This code has been added, effective January 1, 2004.

○ [N]   **C1874** Stent, coated/covered, with delivery system
AHA: 1Q, '01, 6; 3Q, '01, 4, 5; 3Q, '02, 5, 9; 4Q, '03, 8

○ [N]   **C1875** Stent, coated/covered, without delivery system
AHA: 1Q, '01, 6; 3Q, '02, 5, 9; 4Q, '03, 8

○ [N]   **C1876** Stent, non-coated/non-covered, with delivery system
AHA: 1Q, '01, 6; 3Q, '01, 4, 5; 3Q, '01, 4; 3Q, '02, 5; 4Q, '03, 8

○ [N]   **C1877** Stent, non-coated/non-covered, without delivery system
AHA: 1Q, '01, 6; 3Q, '01, 4; 3Q, '02, 5; 4Q, '03, 8

○ [N]   **C1878** Material for vocal cord medialization, synthetic (implantable)
AHA: 1Q, '01, 6; 3Q, '02, 5

○ [N]   **C1879** Tissue marker (implantable)
AHA: 1Q, '01, 6; 3Q, '02, 5; 4Q, '03, 8

○ [N]   **C1880** Vena cava filter
AHA: 1Q, '01, 6; 3Q, '02, 5; 4Q, '03, 8

○ [N]   **C1881** Dialysis access system (implantable)
AHA: 1Q, '01, 6; 3Q, '02, 5; 4Q, '03, 8

○ [N]   **C1882** Cardioverter-defibrillator, other than single or dual chamber (implantable)
AHA: 1Q, '01, 5; 3Q, '02, 5

○ [N]   **C1883** Adaptor/extension, pacing lead or neurostimulator lead (implantable)
AHA: 1Q, '01, 5; 1Q, '02, 9; 3Q, '02, 5

[H]   **C1884** Embolization protective system   ⊘

○ [N]   **C1885** Catheter, transluminal angioplasty, laser
AHA: 1Q, '01, 5; 3Q, '02, 5; 4Q, '03, 8

○ [N]   **C1887** Catheter, guiding (may include infusion/perfusion capability)
AHA: 1Q, '01, 5; 3Q, '01, 4, 5; 3Q, '02, 5

[H]   **C1888** Catheter, ablation, non-cardiac, endovascular (implantable)   ⊘

○ [N]   **C1891** Infusion pump, non-programmable, permanent (implantable)
AHA: 1Q, '01, 6; 3Q, '02, 5; 4Q, '03, 8

○ [N]   **C1892** Introducer/sheath, guiding, intracardiac electrophysiological, fixed-curve, peel-away
AHA: 1Q, '01, 6; 3Q, '02, 5

○ [N]   **C1893** Introducer/sheath, guiding, intracardiac electrophysiological, fixed-curve, other than peel-away
AHA: 1Q, '01, 6; 3Q, '01, 4; 3Q, '02, 5

○ [N]   **C1894** Introducer/sheath, othe than guiding, intracardiac electrophysiological, non-laser
AHA: 1Q, '01, 4, 6; 3Q, '02, 5

○ [N]   **C1895** Lead, cardioverter-defibrillator, endocardial dual coil (implantable)
AHA: 1Q, '01, 6; 3Q, '02, 5

○ [N]   **C1896** Lead, cardioverter-defibrillator, other than endocardial single or dual coil (implantable)
AHA: 1Q, '01, 6; 3Q, '02, 5

○ [N]   **C1897** Lead, neurostimulator test kit (implantable)
AHA: 1Q, '01, 6; 1Q, '02, 9; 3Q, '02, 5

○ [N]   **C1898** Lead, pacemaker, other than transvenous VDD single pass
AHA: 1Q, '01, 6; 3Q, '01, 4; 3Q, '02, 5, 8

○ [N]   **C1899** Lead, pacemaker/cardioverter-defibrillator combination (implantable)
AHA: 1Q, '01, 6; 3Q, '02, 5

[H]   **C1900** Lead, left ventricular coronary venous system   ⊘

[H]   **C2614** Probe, percutaneous lumbar discectomy   ⊘

○ [N]   **C2615** Sealant, pulmonary, liquid
AHA: 1Q, '01, 6; 3Q, '02, 5

▲ [H]   **C2616** Brachytherapy source, yttrium 90, per source   ⊘
AHA: 3Q, '02, 5; 3Q, '03, 11

○ [N]   **C2617** Stent, non-coronary, temporary, without delivery system
AHA: 1Q, '01, 6; 3Q, '02, 5; 4Q, '03, 8

[N]   **C2618** Probe, cryoablation   ⊘
AHA: 1Q, '01, 6; 3Q, '02, 5; 4Q, '03, 8

○ [N]   **C2619** Pacemaker, dual chamber, non-rate-responsive (implantable)
AHA: 1Q, '01, 6; 3Q, '01, 4; 3Q, '02, 5

○ [N]   **C2620** Pacemaker, single chamber, non-rate-responsive (implantabe)
AHA: 1Q, '01, 6; 3Q, '02, 5; 4Q, '03, 8

○ [N]   **C2621** Pacemaker, other than single or dual chamber (implantable)
AHA: 1Q, '01, 6; 3Q, '02, 5, 8; 4Q, '03, 8

○ [N]   **C2622** Prosthesis, penile, non-inflatable
AHA: 1Q, '01, 6; 3Q, '02, 5; 4Q, '03, 8

○ [N]   **C2625** Stent, non-coronary, temporary, with delivery system
AHA: 1Q, '01, 6; 3Q, '02, 5; 4Q, '03, 8

○ [N]   **C2626** Infusion pump, non-programmable, temporary (implantable)
AHA: 1Q, '01, 6; 3Q, '02, 5

○ [N]   **C2627** Catheter, suprapubic/cystoscopic
AHA: 1Q, '01, 5; 3Q, '02, 5; 4Q, '03, 8

○ [N]   **C2628** Catheter, occlusion
AHA: 1Q, '01, 5; 3Q, '02, 5; 4Q, '03, 8

○ [N]   **C2629** Introducer/sheath, other than guiding, intracardiac electrophysiological, laser
AHA: 1Q, '01, 6; 3Q, '02, 5

○ [N]   **C2630** Catheter, electrophysiology, diagnostic/ablation, other than 3D or vector mapping, cool-tip
AHA: 1Q, '01, 5; 3Q, '02, 5

○ [N]   **C2631** Repair device, urinary, incontinence, without sling graft
AHA: 1Q, '01, 6; 3Q, '02, 5; 4Q, '03, 8

[H] ☑   **C2632** Brachytherapy solution, iodine 125, per mci   ⊘

▲ [H]   **C2633** Brachytherapy source, cesium 131, per source

● ☑   **C2634** Brachytherapy source, high activity, iodine 125, per source

● ☑   **C2635** Brachytherapy source, high activity, palladium 103, per source

●   **C2636** Brachytherapy linear source, palladium 103, per 1 mm

[S]   **C8900** Magnetic resonance angiography with contrast, abdomen

---

S	**C8901**	Magnetic resonance angiography without contrast, abdomen
S	**C8902**	Magnetic resonance angiography without contrast followed by with contrast, abdomen
S	**C8903**	Magnetic resonance imaging with contrast, breast; unilateral
S	**C8904**	Magnetic resonance imaging without contrast, breast; unilateral
S	**C8905**	Magnetic resonance imaging without contrast followed by with contrast, breast; unilateral
S	**C8906**	Magnetic resonance imaging with contrast, breast; bilateral
S	**C8907**	Magnetic resonance imaging without contrast, breast; bilateral
S	**C8908**	Magnetic resonance imaging without contrast followed by with contrast, breast; bilateral
S	**C8909**	Magnetic resonance angiography with contrast, chest (excluding myocardium)
S	**C8910**	Magnetic resonance angiography without contrast, chest (excluding myocardium)
S	**C8911**	Magnetic resonance angiography without contrast followed by with contrast, chest (excluding myocardium)
S	**C8912**	Magnetic resonance angiography with contrast, lower extremity
S	**C8913**	Magnetic resonance angiography without contrast, lower extremity
S	**C8914**	Magnetic resonance angiography without contrast followed by with contrast, lower extremity
S	**C8918**	Magnetic resonance angiography with contrast, pelvis AHA: 4Q, '03, 4
S	**C8919**	Magnetic resonance angiography without contrast, pelvis AHA: 4Q, '03, 4
S	**C8920**	Magnetic resonance angiography without contrast followed by with contrast, pelvis AHA: 4Q, '03, 4
N	**C9000**	Injection, sodium chromate Cr-51, per 0.25 millicurie ⊘ See Radiology CPT code 73225. AHA: 2Q, '02, 9
K	**C9003**	Palivizumab-RSV-igM, per 50 mg ⊘ Use this code for Synagis.
N	**C9007**	Baclofen intrathecal screening kit (1 amp) ⊘ Use this code for Lioresal Intrathecal.
K	**C9008**	Baclofen intrathecal refill kit, per 500 mcg ⊘
K	**C9009**	Baclofen intrathecal refill kit, per 2000 mcg ⊘ Use this code for Lioresal.
K	**C9013**	Supply of Co-57 cobaltous chloride, radiopharmaceutical diagnostic imaging agent ⊘ AHA: 2Q, '02, 9
N ☑	**C9102**	Supply of radiopharmaceutical diagnostic imaging agent, 51 sodium chromate, per 50 millicurie ⊘ AHA: 2Q, '02, 9
N ☑	**C9103**	Supply of radiopharmaceutical diagnostic imaging agent, sodium iothalamate I-125 injection, per 10 uci ⊘

K ☑	**C9105**	Injection, hepatitis B immune globulin, per 1 ml ⊘ Use this code for Bayhep B, H-BIG.	
	~~C9100~~	~~Injection, tirofiban HCl, 6.25 mg~~ See code(s): J3246	
G	**C9112**	Injection, perflutren lipid microsphere, per 2 ml vial ⊘ Use this code for Definity.	
G	**C9113**	Injection, pantoprazole sodium, per vial ⊘ Use this code for Profonix.	
G	**C9121**	Injection, argatroban, per 5 mg ⊘ Use this code for Acova.	
▲ G ☑	**C9123**	Human fibroblast derived temporary skin substitute, per 247 sq. cm ⊘ AHA: 4Q, '03, 4	
	~~C9124~~	~~Injection, daptomycin, per 1 mg~~ See code(s): J0878	
	~~C9125~~	~~Injection, risperidone, per 12.5 mg~~ See code(s): J2794	
▲ G	**C9200**	Bilayered cellular matrix, per 36 sq. cm ⊘	
▲ G ☑	**C9201**	Human fibroblast-derived dermal substitute, per 37.5 sq. cm ⊘ Use this code for Dermal tissue of human origin. See also J7340, J7342, J7350.	
K ☑	**C9202**	Injection, suspension of microspheres of human serum albumin with octafluoropropane, per 3 ml ⊘ AHA: 2Q, '03, 7	
G ☑	**C9203**	Injection, perflexane lipid microspheres, per 10 ml vial ⊘ AHA: 2Q, '03, 7	
○ G ☑	**C9205**	Injection, oxaliplatin, per 5 mg ⊘ Use this code for Eloxafin. AHA: 4Q, '03, 4	
● ☑	C9206	Collagen-glycosaminoglycan bilayer matrix, per cm^2	
	~~C9207~~	~~Injection, bortezomib, per 3.5 mg~~ See code(s): J9041	
	~~C9208~~	~~Injection, agalsidase beta, per 1 mg~~ See code(s): J0180	
	~~C9209~~	~~Injection, laronidase, per 2.9 mg~~ See code(s): J1931	
	~~C9210~~	~~Injection, palonosetron hydrochloride, per 250 mcg~~ See code(s): J2469	
● G ☑	**C9211**	Injection, alefacept, for intravenous use, per 7.5 mg Use this code for Amevive.	
● G ☑	**C9212**	Injection, alefacept, for intramuscular use, per 7.5 mg Use this code for Amevive.	
	~~C9213~~	~~Injection, pemetrexed, per 10 mg~~ See code(s): J9305	
	~~C9214~~	~~Injection, bevacizumab, per 10 mg~~ See code(s): J9035	
	~~C9215~~	~~Injection, cetuximab, per 10 mg~~ See code(s): J9055	
	~~C9216~~	~~Injection, abarelix for injectable suspension, per 10 mg~~ See code(s): J0128	

Special Coverage Instructions	Noncovered by Medicare	Carrier Discretion	☑ Quantity Alert	● New Code	○ Reinstated Code	▲ Revised Code

C9217 ~~Injection, omalizumab, per 5 mg~~
See code(s): J2357

● K ☑ **C9218** Injection, azacitidine, per 1 mg
Use this code for Vidaza.

C9219 ~~Mycophenolic acid, oral, per 180 mg~~
See code(s): J7518

● **C9220** Sodium hyaluronate per 30 mg dose, for intra-articular injection

● **C9221** Acellular dermal tissue matrix, per 16 cm²

● **C9222** Decellularized soft tissue scaffold, per 1 cc

● A **C9399** Unclassified drugs or biologicals

● K ☑ **C9400** Supply of radiopharmaceutical diagnostic imaging agent, thallous chloride TL-201, per mci, brand name
See code(s): A9505

● K ☑ **C9401** Supply of therapeutic radiopharmaceutical, strontium 89 chloride, brand name, per mci

● K ☑ **C9402** Supply of radiopharmaceutical therapeutic imaging agent, I-131 sodium iodide capsule, per mci, brand name
See code(s): A9517

● K ☑ **C9403** Supply of radiopharmaceutical diagnostic agent, I-131 sodium iodide capsule, per millicurie
See code(s): A9528

● K ☑ **C9404** Supply of radiopharmaceutical diagnostic agent, I-131 sodium iodide solution, per millicurie, brand name
See code(s): A9529

● K ☑ **C9405** Supply of radiopharmaceutical therapeutic agent, I-131 sodium iodide solution, per millicurie, brand name
See code(s): A9530

C9408 ~~Supply of radiopharmaceutical diagnostic imaging agent, fluorodeoxyglucose f18 (2-deoxy-2-[18f]fluoro-d-glucose), per dose (4-40 mci/ml), brand name~~

● K ☑ **C9410** Injection, dexrazoxane hydrochloride, per 250 mg, brand name
See code(s): J1190

Use this code for Zinecard.

● K ☑ **C9411** Injection, pamidronate disodium, per 30 mg, brand name
See code(s): J2430

Use this code for Aredia.

C9412 ~~Ganciclovir, 4.5 mg, long-acting implant, brand name~~
See code(s): J7310

● K ☑ **C9413** Sodium hyaluronate, per 20 to 25 mg dose for intra-articular injection, brand name
See code(s): J7317

● K ☑ **C9414** Etoposide; oral, 50 mg, brand name
See code(s): J8560

● K ☑ **C9415** Doxorubicin HCl, 10 mg, brand name
See code(s): J9000

C9416 ~~BCG (intravesical) per instillation, brand name~~

● K ☑ **C9417** Bleomycin sulfate, 15 units, brand name
See code(s): J9040

● K ☑ **C9418** Cisplatin, powder or solution, per 10 mg, brand name
See code(s): J9060

● K ☑ **C9419** Injection, cladribine, per 1 mg, brand name
See code(s): J9065

Use this code for Leustat.

● K ☑ **C9420** Cyclophosphamide, 100 mg, brand name
See code(s): J9070

● K ☑ **C9421** Cyclophosphamide, lyophilized, 100 mg, brand name
See code(s): J9093

● K ☑ **C9422** Cytarabine, 100 mg, brand name
See code(s): J9100

Use this code for Ara-C, Cytosar-U, Tarabine CFS.

● K ☑ **C9423** Dacarbazine, 100 mg, brand name
See code(s): J9130

Use this code for DTIC-Dome.

● K ☑ **C9424** Daunorubicin, 10 mg
See code(s): J9150

● K ☑ **C9425** Etoposide, 10 mg, brand name
See code(s): J9181

● K ☑ **C9426** Floxuridine, 500 mg, brand name
See code(s): J9200

● K ☑ **C9427** Ifosfamide, 1 gm, brand name
See code(s): J9208

Use this code for Mitoxana.

● K ☑ **C9428** Mesna, 200 mg, brand name
See code(s): J9209

Use this code for Mesnex.

● K ☑ **C9429** Idarubicin hydrochloride, 5 mg, brand name
See code(s): J9211

● K ☑ **C9430** Leuprolide acetate, per 1 mg, brand name
See code(s): J9218

● K ☑ **C9431** Paclitaxel, 30 mg, brand name
See code(s): J9265

Use this code for Taxol.

● K ☑ **C9432** Mitomycin, 5 mg, brand name
See code(s): J9280

● K ☑ **C9433** Thiotepa, 15 mg, brand name
See code(s): J9340

C9434 ~~Supply of radiopharmaceutical diagnostic imaging agent, Gallium Ga 67, per mci, brand name~~

● **C9435** Injection, gonadorelin hydrochloride, brand name, per 100 mcg

● **C9436** Azathioprine, parenteral, brand name, per 100 mg

● **C9437** Carmustine, brand name, 100 mg

● K **C9438** Cyclosporine, oral, 100 mg, brand name
See code(s): J7502

● **C9439** Diethylstilbestrol diphosphate, brand name, 250 mg

C9701 ~~Stretta system~~

C9703 ~~Bard endoscopic suturing system~~

● T **C9704** Injection or insertion of inert substance for submucosal/intramuscular injection(s) into the upper gastrointestinal tract, under fluoroscopic guidance

Special Coverage Instructions | Noncovered by Medicare | Carrier Discretion | ☑ Quantity Alert | ● New Code | ○ Reinstated Code | ▲ Revised Code

2005 HCPCS | ♀ Female Only | ♂ Male Only | **1**-**9** ASC Groups | **MED:** Pub 100/NCD Reference | ᕑ DMEPOS Paid | Ⓝ SNF Excluded | **C Codes — 27**

~~C9712~~ ~~Insertion of a pH capsule for measurement and monitoring of gastroesophageal reflux disease, includes data collection and interpretation~~
See code(s): 91035

● Ⓢ **C9713** Non-contact laser vaporization of prostate, including coagulation control of intraoperative and postoperative bleeding
See code(s): 52647

~~C9714~~ ~~Placement of balloon catheter into the breast for interstitial radiation therapy following a partial mastectomy; concurrent/immediate (add on)~~
See code(s): 19297

~~C9715~~ ~~Placement of balloon catheter into the breast for interstitial radiation therapy following a partial mastectomy; delayed~~
See code(s): 19296

● Ⓢ **C9716** Creations of thermal anal lesions by radiofrequency energy

~~C9717~~ ~~Hemorrhoidopexy, complex or extensive, by a circular stapler~~
See code(s): 46947

● **C9718** Kyphoplasty, one vertebral body, unilateral or bilateral injection

● **C9719** Kyphoplasty, one vertebral body, unilateral or bilateral injection; each additional vertebral body (list separately in addition to code for primary procedure)

● **C9720** High-energy (greater than 0.22 mj/mm²) extracorporeal shock wave (ESW) treatment for chronic lateral epicondylitis (tennis elbow)

● **C9721** High-energy (greater than 0.22 mj/mm²) extracorporeal shock wave (ESW) treatment for chronic plantar fasciitis

● **C9722** Stereoscopic kilovolt x-ray imaging with infrared tracking for localization of target volume (Do not report C9722 in conjunction with G0173, G0243, G0251, G0339, or G0340)

Special Coverage Instructions   Noncovered by Medicare   Carrier Discretion   ☑ Quantity Alert   ● New Code   ○ Reinstated Code   ▲ Revised Code

28 — C Codes   Ⓐ Adult   Ⓜ Maternity   Ⓟ Pediatrics   Ⓘ Infant   Ⓐ-Ⓨ APC Status Indicator   **2005 HCPCS**

DENTAL PROCEDURES *D0000–D9999*

The D, or dental, codes are a separate category of national codes. The Current Dental Terminology (CDT 2005) code set is copyrighted by the American Dental Association (ADA). CDT 2005 is included in HCPCS Level II. Decisions regarding the modification, deletion, or addition of CDT 2005 codes are made by the ADA and not the national panel responsible for the administration of HCPCS.

The Department of Health and Human Services has an agreement with the AMA pertaining to the use of the CPT codes for physician services; it also has an agreement with the ADA to include CDT 2005 as a set of HCPCS Level II codes for use in billing for dental services.

DIAGNOSTIC D0100–D0999

CLINICAL ORAL EVALUATION
All dental codes fall under the jurisdiction of the Medicare local carrier.

E　　**D0120** Periodic oral examination
This procedure is covered if its purpose is to identify a patient's existing infections prior to kidney transplantation.

E　　**D0140** Limited oral evaluation — problem focused

S　　**D0150** Comprehensive oral evaluation — new or established patient
This procedure is covered if its purpose is to identify a patient's existing infections prior to kidney transplantation.
MED: 100-2, 15, 150; 100-2, 16, 140; 100-3, 260.6

E　　**D0160** Detailed and extensive oral evaluation — problem focused, by report
Pertinent documentation to evaluate medical appropriateness should be included when this code is reported.

E　　**D0170** Re-evaluation — limited, problem focused (established patient; not postoperative visit)

E　　**D0180** Comprehensive periodontal evaluation — new or established patient
See also equivalent CPT E&M codes.

RADIOGRAPHS

E　　**D0210** Intraoral — complete series (including bitewings)
See code(s): 70320

E ☑　**D0220** Intraoral — periapical, first film
See code(s): 70300

E ☑　**D0230** Intraoral — periapical, each additional film
See code(s): 70310

S　　**D0240** Intraoral — occlusal film
MED: 100-2, 15, 150; 100-2, 16, 140

S ☑　**D0250** Extraoral — first film
MED: 100-2, 15, 150; 100-2, 16, 140

S ☑　**D0260** Extraoral — each additional film
MED: 100-2, 15, 150; 100-2, 16, 140

S ☑　**D0270** Bitewing — single film
MED: 100-2, 15, 150; 100-2, 16, 140

S ☑　**D0272** Bitewings — two films
MED: 100-2, 15, 150; 100-2, 16, 140

S ☑　**D0274** Bitewings — four films
MED: 100-2, 15, 150; 100-2, 16, 140

S ☑　**D0277** Vertical bitewings — 7 to 8 films
MED: 100-2, 15, 150; 100-2, 16, 140

E　　**D0290** Posterior-anterior or lateral skull and facial bone survey film
See code(s): 70150

E　　**D0310** Sialography
See code(s): 70390

E　　**D0320** Temporomandibular joint arthrogram, including injection
See code(s): 70332

E　　**D0321** Other temporomandibular joint films, by report
See code(s): 76499

E　　**D0322** Tomographic survey
MED: 100-3, 260.6

E　　**D0330** Panoramic film
See code(s): 70320

E　　**D0340** Cephalometric film
See code(s): 70350

▲ E　**D0350** Oral/facial photographic images
This code excludes conventional radiographs.

TEST AND LABORATORY EXAMINATIONS

▲ E　**D0415** Collection of microorganisms for culture and sensitivity
This procedure is covered if its purpose is to identify a patient's existing infections prior to kidney transplantation.
See code(s): D0410

●　　**D0416** Viral culture

●　　**D0421** Genetic test for susceptibility to oral diseases

E　　**D0425** Caries susceptibility tests
This procedure is covered by Medicare if its purpose is to identify a patient's existing infections prior to kidney transplantation.
See code(s): D0420

●　　**D0431** Adjunctive pre-diagnostic test that aids in detection of mucosal abnormalities including premalignant and malignant lesions, not to include cytology or biopsy procedures

S　　**D0460** Pulp vitality tests
This procedure is covered by Medicare if its purpose is to identify a patient's existing infections prior to kidney transplantation.
MED: 100-2, 15, 150; 100-2, 16, 140; 100-3, 260.6

E　　**D0470** Diagnostic casts

S　　**D0472** Accession of tissue, gross examination, preparation and transmission of written report
MED: 100-2, 15, 150; 100-2, 16, 140; 100-3, 260.6

S　　**D0473** Accession of tissue, gross and microscopic examination, preparation and transmission of written report
MED: 100-2, 15, 150; 100-2, 16, 140; 100-3, 260.6

S　　**D0474** Accession of tissue, gross and microscopic examination, including assessment of surgical margins for presence of disease, preparation and transmission of written report
MED: 100-2, 15, 150; 100-2, 16, 140; 100-3, 260.6

●　　**D0475** Decalcification procedure

●　　**D0476** Special stains for microorganisms

●　　**D0477** Special stains, not for microorganisms

●　　**D0478** Immunohistochemical stains

●　　**D0479** Tissue in-situ hybridization, including interpretation

Special Coverage Instructions　　Noncovered by Medicare　　Carrier Discretion　　☑ Quantity Alert　● New Code　○ Reinstated Code　▲ Revised Code

2005 HCPCS　♀ Female Only　♂ Male Only　**1-9** ASC Groups　MED: Pub 100/NCD Reference　⅃ DMEPOS Paid　⊘ SNF Excluded　**D Codes — 29**

Dental Procedures

D0480 — D2722

▲ Ⓢ **D0480** Processing and interpretation of exfoliative cytologic smears, including the preparation and transmission of written report
MED: 100-2, 15, 150; 100-2, 16, 140; 100-3, 260.6

● **D0481** Electron microscopy — diagnostic

● **D0482** Direct immunofluorescence

● **D0483** Indirect immunofluorescence

● **D0484** Consultation on slides prepared elsewhere

● **D0485** Consultation, including preparation of slides from biopsy material supplied by referring source

Ⓢ **D0502** Other oral pathology procedures, by report
Pertinent documentation to evaluate medical appropriateness should be included when this code is reported. This procedure is covered by Medicare if its purpose is to identify a patient's existing infections prior to kidney transplantation.
MED: 100-2, 15, 150; 100-2, 16, 140; 100-3, 260.6

Ⓢ **D0999** Unspecified diagnostic procedure, by report
Determine if an alternative HCPCS Level II or a CPT code better describes the service being reported. This code should be used only if a more specific code is unavailable.
MED: 100-2, 15, 150; 100-2, 16, 140; 100-3, 260.6

PREVENTIVE D1000–D1999

DENTAL PROPHYLAXIS

Ⓔ **D1110** Prophylaxis — adult   Ⓐ

Ⓔ **D1120** Prophylaxis — child   Ⓟ

TOPICAL FLUORIDE TREATMENT (OFFICE PROCEDURE)

Ⓔ **D1201** Topical application of fluoride (including prophylaxis) — child   Ⓟ

Ⓔ **D1203** Topical application of fluoride (prophylaxis not included) — child   Ⓟ

Ⓔ **D1204** Topical application of fluoride (prophylaxis not included) — adult   Ⓐ

Ⓔ **D1205** Topical application of fluoride (including prophylaxis) — adult   Ⓐ
See code(s): D1202

OTHER PREVENTIVE SERVICES

Ⓔ **D1310** Nutritional counseling for control of dental disease
MED: 100-2, 16, 10

Ⓔ **D1320** Tobacco counseling for the control and prevention of oral disease
MED: 100-2, 16, 10

Ⓔ **D1330** Oral hygiene instructions
MED: 100-2, 16, 10

Ⓔ ☑ **D1351** Sealant — per tooth

SPACE MAINTENANCE (PASSIVE APPLIANCES)

Ⓢ **D1510** Space maintainer — fixed-unilateral
MED: 100-2, 16, 140

Ⓢ **D1515** Space maintainer — fixed-bilateral
MED: 100-2, 15, 150; 100-2, 16, 140

Ⓢ **D1520** Space maintainer — removable-unilateral
MED: 100-2, 15, 150; 100-2, 16, 140

Ⓢ **D1525** Space maintainer — removable-bilateral
MED: 100-2, 15, 150; 100-2, 16, 140

Ⓢ **D1550** Recementation of space maintainer
MED: 100-2, 15, 150; 100-2, 16, 140

Ⓔ ☑ **D2140** Amalgam — one surface, primary or permanent

Ⓔ ☑ **D2150** Amalgam — two surfaces, primary or permanent

Ⓔ ☑ **D2160** Amalgam — three surfaces, primary or permanent

Ⓔ ☑ **D2161** Amalgam — four or more surfaces, primary or permanent

RESIN RESTORATIONS

Ⓔ ☑ **D2330** Resin-based composite — one surface, anterior

Ⓔ ☑ **D2331** Resin-based composite — two surfaces, anterior

Ⓔ ☑ **D2332** Resin-based composite — three surfaces, anterior

Ⓔ ☑ **D2335** Resin-based composite — four or more surfaces or involving incisal angle (anterior)

Ⓔ **D2390** Resin-based composite crown, anterior

Ⓔ **D2391** Resin-based composite — one surface, posterior

Ⓔ **D2392** Resin-based composite — two surfaces, posterior

Ⓔ **D2393** Resin-based composite — three surfaces, posterior

Ⓔ **D2394** Resin-based composite — four or more surfaces, posterior

GOLD FOIL RESTORATIONS

Ⓔ ☑ **D2410** Gold foil — one surface

Ⓔ ☑ **D2420** Gold foil — two surfaces

Ⓔ ☑ **D2430** Gold foil — three surfaces

INLAY/ONLAY RESTORATIONS

Ⓔ ☑ **D2510** Inlay — metallic — one surface

Ⓔ ☑ **D2520** Inlay — metallic — two surfaces

Ⓔ ☑ **D2530** Inlay — metallic — three or more surfaces

Ⓔ ☑ **D2542** Onlay — metallic — two surfaces

Ⓔ ☑ **D2543** Onlay — metallic — three surfaces

Ⓔ ☑ **D2544** Onlay — metallic — four or more surfaces

Ⓔ ☑ **D2610** Inlay — porcelain/ceramic — one surface

Ⓔ ☑ **D2620** Inlay — porcelain/ceramic — two surfaces

Ⓔ ☑ **D2630** Inlay — porcelain/ceramic — three or more surfaces

Ⓔ ☑ **D2642** Onlay — porcelain/ceramic — two surfaces

Ⓔ ☑ **D2643** Onlay — porcelain/ceramic — three surfaces

Ⓔ ☑ **D2644** Onlay — porcelain/ceramic — four or more surfaces

Ⓔ ☑ **D2650** Inlay — resin-based composite composite/resin — one surface

Ⓔ ☑ **D2651** Inlay — resin-based composite composite/resin — two surfaces

Ⓔ ☑ **D2652** Inlay — resin-based composite composite/resin — three or more surfaces

Ⓔ ☑ **D2662** Onlay — resin-based composite composite/resin — two surfaces

Ⓔ ☑ **D2663** Onlay — resin-based composite composite/resin — three surfaces

Ⓔ ☑ **D2664** Onlay — resin-based composite composite/resin — four or more surfaces

CROWNS — SINGLE RESTORATION ONLY

▲ Ⓔ **D2710** Crown — resin-based composite (indirect)

● **D2712** Crown — 3/4 resin-based composite (indirect)

Ⓔ **D2720** Crown — resin with high noble metal

Ⓔ **D2721** Crown — resin with predominantly base metal

Ⓔ **D2722** Crown — resin with noble metal

E   **D2740** Crown — porcelain/ceramic substrate

E   **D2750** Crown — porcelain fused to high noble metal

E   **D2751** Crown — porcelain fused to predominantly base metal

E   **D2752** Crown — porcelain fused to noble metal

E   **D2780** Crown — 3/4 cast high noble metal

E   **D2781** Crown — 3/4 cast predominately base metal

E   **D2782** Crown — 3/4 cast noble metal

E   **D2783** Crown — 3/4 porcelain/ceramic

E   **D2790** Crown — full cast high noble metal

E   **D2791** Crown — full cast predominantly base metal

E   **D2792** Crown — full cast noble metal

●   **D2794** Crown — titanium

E   **D2799** Provisional crown
Do not use this code to report a temporary crown for routine prosthetic restoration.

OTHER RESTORATIVE SERVICES

▲ E   **D2910** Recement inlay, onlay or partial coverage restoration

●   **D2915** Recement cast or prefabricated post and core

E   **D2920** Recement crown

E   **D2930** Prefabricated stainless steel crown — primary tooth

E   **D2931** Prefabricated stainless steel crown — permanent tooth

E   **D2932** Prefabricated resin crown

E   **D2933** Prefabricated stainless steel crown with resin window

●   **D2934** Prefabricated esthetic coated stainless steel crown — primary tooth

E   **D2940** Sedative filling

E   **D2950** Core buildup, including any pins

E   **D2951** Pin retention — per tooth, in addition to restoration

E   **D2952** Cast post and core in addition to crown

E   **D2953** Each additional cast post — same tooth
Report in addition to code D2952.

E   **D2954** Prefabricated post and core in addition to crown

E   **D2955** Post removal (not in conjunction with endodontic therapy)

E   **D2957** Each additional prefabricated post — same tooth
Report in addition to code D2954.

E   **D2960** Labial veneer (resin laminate) — chairside

E   **D2961** Labial veneer (resin laminate) — laboratory

E   **D2962** Labial veneer (porcelain laminate) — laboratory

~~**D2970** Temporary crown (fractured tooth)~~

●   **D2971** Additional procedures to construct new crown under existing partial denture framework

●   **D2975** Coping

E   **D2980** Crown repair, by report
Pertinent documentation to evaluate medical appropriateness should be included when this code is reported.

S   **D2999** Unspecified restorative procedure, by report
Determine if an alternative HCPCS Level II or a CPT code better describes the service being reported. This code should be used only if a more specific code is unavailable.

MED: 100-2, 15, 150; 100-2, 16, 140

ENDODONTICS D3000–D3999

PULP CAPPING

E   **D3110** Pulp cap — direct (excluding final restoration)

E   **D3120** Pulp cap — indirect (excluding final restoration)

PULPOTOMY

E   **D3220** Therapeutic pulpotomy (excluding final restoration) — removal of pulp coronal to the dentinocemental junction and application of medicament
Do not use this code to report the first stage of root canal therapy.

E   **D3221** Pulpal debridement, primary and permanent teeth

PULPAL THERAPY ON PRIMARY TEETH (INCLUDES PRIMARY TEETH WITH SUCCEDANEOUS TEETH AND PLACEMENT OF RESORBABLE FILLING)

E   **D3230** Pulpal therapy (resorbable filling) — anterior, primary tooth (excluding final restoration)

E   **D3240** Pulpal therapy (resorbable filling) — posterior, primary tooth (excluding final restoration)

ROOT CANAL THERAPY (INCLUDING TREATMENT PLAN, CLINICAL PROCEDURES, AND FOLLOW-UP CARE, INCLUDES PRIMARY TEETH WITHOUT SUCCEDANEOUS TEETH AND PERMANENT TEETH)

E   **D3310** Anterior (excluding final restoration)

E   **D3320** Bicuspid (excluding final restoration)

E   **D3330** Molar (excluding final restoration)

E   **D3331** Treatment of root canal obstruction; non-surgical access

▲ E   **D3332** Incomplete endodontic therapy; inoperable, unrestorable or fractured tooth

E   **D3333** Internal root repair of perforation defects

E   **D3346** Retreatment of previous root canal therapy — anterior

E   **D3347** Retreatment of previous root canal therapy — bicuspid

E   **D3348** Retreatment of previous root canal therapy — molar

E   **D3351** Apexification/recalcification — initial visit (apical closure/calcific repair of perforations, root resorption, etc.)

E   **D3352** Apexification/recalcification — interim medication replacement (apical closure/calcific repair of perforations, root resorption, etc.)

E   **D3353** Apexification/recalcification — final visit (includes completed root canal therapy — apical closure/calcific repair of perforations, root resorption, etc.)

APICOECTOMY/PERIRADICULAR SERVICES

E   **D3410** Apicoectomy/periradicular surgery — anterior

E   **D3421** Apicoectomy/periradicular surgery — bicuspid (first root)

E   **D3425** Apicoectomy/periradicular surgery — molar (first root)

E ☑   **D3426** Apicoectomy/periradicular surgery (each additional root)

E ☑   **D3430** Retrograde filling — per root

E ☑   **D3450** Root amputation — per root

Special Coverage Instructions   Noncovered by Medicare   Carrier Discretion   ☑ Quantity Alert   ● New Code   ○ Reinstated Code   ▲ Revised Code

2005 HCPCS   ♀ Female Only   ♂ Male Only   **1**-**9** ASC Groups   MED: Pub 100/NCD Reference   DMEPOS Paid   ○ SNF Excluded   **D Codes — 31**

Dental Procedures

D3460 — D5211

D3460   Endodontic endosseous implant
MED: 100-2, 15, 150; 100-2, 16, 140

D3470   Intentional reimplantation (including necessary splinting)

OTHER ENDODONTIC PROCEDURES

D3910   Surgical procedure for isolation of tooth with rubber dam

D3920   Hemisection (including any root removal), not including root canal therapy

D3950   Canal preparation and fitting of preformed dowel or post

[S]   D3999   Unspecified endodontic procedure, by report
Determine if an alternative HCPCS Level II or a CPT code better describes the service being reported. This code should be used only if a more specific code is unavailable.
MED: 100-2, 15, 150; 100-2, 16, 140

PERIODONTICS D4000–D4999

SURGICAL SERVICES (INCLUDING USUAL POSTOPERATIVE SERVICES)

▲ [E] ☑   D4210   Gingivectomy or gingivoplasty — four or more contiguous teeth or bounded teeth spaces per quadrant
See code(s): 41820

▲ [E] ☑   D4211   Gingivectomy or gingivoplasty — one to three contiguous teeth or bounded teeth spaces per quadrant
See also CPT code (64400-64530).

▲ [E] ☑   D4240   Gingival flap procedure, including root planing — four or more contiguous teeth or bounded teeth spaces per quadrant

▲ [E]   D4241   Gingival flap procedure, including root planing — one to three contiguous teeth or bounded teeth spaces per quadrant
See also D4240.

[E]   D4245   Apically positioned flap

[E]   D4249   Clinical crown lengthening — hard tissue

▲ [S] ☑   D4260   Osseous surgery (including flap entry and closure) — four or more contiguous teeth or bounded teeth spaces per quadrant
MED: 100-2, 15, 150; 100-2, 16, 140

▲ [E]   D4261   Osseous surgery (including flap entry and closure) — one to three contiguous teeth or bounded teeth spaces per quadrant
See CPT code 41823.

[S] ☑   D4263   Bone replacement graft — first site in quadrant
MED: 100-2, 15, 150; 100-2, 16, 140; 100-3, 260.6

[S] ☑   D4264   Bone replacement graft — each additional site in quadrant (use if performed on same date of service as D4263)
MED: 100-2, 15, 150; 100-2, 16, 140; 100-3, 260.6

[E]   D4265   Biologic materials to aid in soft and osseous tissue regeneration

[E] ☑   D4266   Guided tissue regeneration — resorbable barrier, per site

[E] ☑   D4267   Guided tissue regeneration — nonresorbable barrier, per site (includes membrane removal)

[S] ☑   D4268   Surgical revision procedure, per tooth
MED: 100-2, 15, 150; 100-2, 16, 140

[S]   D4270   Pedicle soft tissue graft procedure
MED: 100-2, 15, 150; 100-2, 16, 140

[S]   D4271   Free soft tissue graft procedure (including donor site surgery)
MED: 100-2, 15, 150; 100-2, 16, 140

▲ [S]   D4273   Subepithelial connective tissue graft procedures, per tooth
For tissue grafts, see CPT 15000 and related codes.
MED: 100-2, 15, 150; 100-2, 16, 140; 100-3, 260.6

[E]   D4274   Distal or proximal wedge procedure (when not performed in conjunction with surgical procedures in the same anatomical area)

[E]   D4275   Soft tissue allograft
For tissue grafts, see CPT 15000 and related codes.

▲ [E]   D4276   Combined connective tissue and double pedicle graft, per tooth
For tissue/pedicle grafts see CPT 15000 and related codes.

ADJUNCTIVE PERIODONTAL SERVICES

[E]   D4320   Provisional splinting — intracoronal

[E]   D4321   Provisional splinting — extracoronal

▲ [E] ☑   D4341   Periodontal scaling and root planing — four or more teeth per quadrant

[E]   D4342   Periodontal scaling and root planing — one to three teeth, per quadrant

[S]   D4355   Full mouth debridement to enable comprehensive evaluation and diagnosis
This procedure is covered by Medicare if its purpose is to identify a patient's existing infections prior to kidney transplantation. For debridement see CPT 11000 and related codes.
MED: 100-2, 15, 150; 100-2, 16, 140; 100-3, 260.6

▲ [S]   D4381   Localized delivery of antimicrobial agents via a controlled release vehicle into diseased crevicular tissue, per tooth, by report
Pertinent documentation to evaluate medical appropriateness should be included when this code is reported.
MED: 100-2, 15, 150; 100-2, 16, 140; 100-3, 260.6

OTHER PERIODONTAL SERVICES

[E]   D4910   Periodontal maintenance

[E]   D4920   Unscheduled dressing change (by someone other than treating dentist)

[E]   D4999   Unspecified periodontal procedure, by report
Determine if an alternative HCPCS Level II or a CPT code better describes the service being reported. This code should be used only if a more specific code is unavailable.

PROSTHODONTICS (REMOVABLE) D5000–D5899

COMPLETE DENTURES (INCLUDING ROUTINE POST DELIVERY CARE)

[E]   D5110   Complete denture — maxillary

[E]   D5120   Complete denture — mandibular

[E]   D5130   Immediate denture — maxillary

[E]   D5140   Immediate denture — mandibular

PARTIAL DENTURES (INCLUDING ROUTINE POST DELIVERY CARE)

[E]   D5211   Maxillary partial denture — resin base (including any conventional clasps, rests and teeth)

Special Coverage Instructions   Noncovered by Medicare   Carrier Discretion   ☑ Quantity Alert   ● New Code   ○ Reinstated Code   ▲ Revised Code

32 — D Codes   [A] Adult   [M] Maternity   [P] Pediatrics   [I] Infant   [A-Y] APC Status Indicator   **2005 HCPCS**

E	D5212	Mandibular partial denture — resin base (including any conventional clasps, rests and teeth)	

| E | D5213 | Maxillary partial denture — cast metal framework with resin denture bases (including any conventional clasps, rests and teeth) |

| E | D5214 | Mandibular partial denture — cast metal framework with resin denture bases (including any conventional clasps, rests and teeth) |

● D5225   Maxillary partial denture — flexible base (including any clasps, rests and teeth)

● D5226   Mandibular partial denture — flexible base (including any clasps, rests and teeth)

E   D5281   Removable unilateral partial denture — one piece cast metal (including clasps and teeth)

ADJUSTMENTS TO REMOVABLE PROSTHESES

E   D5410   Adjust complete denture — maxillary

E   D5411   Adjust complete denture — mandibular

E   D5421   Adjust partial denture — maxillary

E   D5422   Adjust partial denture — mandibular

REPAIRS TO COMPLETE DENTURES

E   D5510   Repair broken complete denture base

E   D5520   Replace missing or broken teeth — complete denture (each tooth)

REPAIRS TO PARTIAL DENTURES

E   D5610   Repair resin denture base

E   D5620   Repair cast framework

E   D5630   Repair or replace broken clasp

E   ☑   D5640   Replace broken teeth — per tooth

E   D5650   Add tooth to existing partial denture

E   D5660   Add clasp to existing partial denture

E   D5670   Replace all teeth and acrylic on cast metal framework (maxillary)

E   D5671   Replace all teeth and acrylic on cast metal framework (mandibular)

DENTURE REBASE PROCEDURES

E   D5710   Rebase complete maxillary denture

E   D5711   Rebase complete mandibular denture

E   D5720   Rebase maxillary partial denture

E   D5721   Rebase mandibular partial denture

DENTURE RELINE PROCEDURES

E   D5730   Reline complete maxillary denture (chairside)

E   D5731   Reline complete mandibular denture (chairside)

E   D5740   Reline maxillary partial denture (chairside)

E   D5741   Reline mandibular partial denture (chairside)

E   D5750   Reline complete maxillary denture (laboratory)

E   D5751   Reline complete mandibular denture (laboratory)

E   D5760   Reline maxillary partial denture (laboratory)

E   D5761   Reline mandibular partial denture (laboratory)

OTHER REMOVABLE PROSTHETIC SERVICES

E   D5810   Interim complete denture (maxillary)

E   D5811   Interim complete denture (mandibular)

E   D5820   Interim partial denture (maxillary)

E   D5821   Interim partial denture (mandibular)

E   D5850   Tissue conditioning, maxillary

E   D5851   Tissue conditioning, mandibular

E   D5860   Overdenture — complete, by report
Pertinent documentation to evaluate medical appropriateness should be included when this code is reported.

E   D5861   Overdenture — partial, by report
Pertinent documentation to evaluate medical appropriateness should be included when this code is reported.

E   D5862   Precision attachment, by report
Pertinent documentation to evaluate medical appropriateness should be included when this code is reported.

E   D5867   Replacement of replaceable part of semi-precision or precision attachment (male or female component)

E   D5875   Modification of removable prosthesis following implant surgery

E   D5899   Unspecified removable prosthodontic procedure, by report
Determine if an alternative HCPCS Level II or a CPT code better describes the service being reported. This code should be used only if a more specific code is unavailable.

MAXILLOFACIAL PROSTHETICS D5900–D5999

S   D5911   Facial moulage (sectional)
MED: 100-2, 15, 120; 100-2, 15, 150

S   D5912   Facial moulage (complete)
MED: 100-2, 15, 120

E   D5913   Nasal prosthesis
See code(s): 21087

E   D5914   Auricular prosthesis
See code(s): 21086

E   D5915   Orbital prosthesis
See code(s): L8611

E   D5916   Ocular prosthesis
See also CPT code (21077, 65770, 66982-66985, 92330-92335, 92358, 92393).
See code(s): V2623, V2629

E   D5919   Facial prosthesis
See code(s): 21088

E   D5922   Nasal septal prosthesis
See code(s): 30220

E   D5923   Ocular prosthesis, interim
See code(s): 92330

E   D5924   Cranial prosthesis
See code(s): 62143

E   D5925   Facial augmentation implant prosthesis
See code(s): 21208

E   D5926   Nasal prosthesis, replacement
See code(s): 21087

E   D5927   Auricular prosthesis, replacement
See code(s): 21086

E   D5928   Orbital prosthesis, replacement
See code(s): 67550

E   D5929   Facial prosthesis, replacement
See code(s): 21088

Special Coverage Instructions   Noncovered by Medicare   Carrier Discretion   ☑ Quantity Alert   ● New Code   ○ Reinstated Code   ▲ Revised Code

2005 HCPCS   ♀ Female Only   ♂ Male Only   1-9 ASC Groups   MED: Pub 100/NCD Reference   ᕆ DMEPOS Paid   ⊘ SNF Excluded   **D Codes — 33**

Dental Procedures

D5931 — D6071

[E] **D5931** Obturator prosthesis, surgical
See code(s): 21079

[E] **D5932** Obturator prosthesis, definitive
See code(s): 21080

[E] **D5933** Obturator prosthesis, modification
See code(s): 21080

[E] **D5934** Mandibular resection prosthesis with guide flange
See code(s): 21081

[E] **D5935** Mandibular resection prosthesis without guide flange
See code(s): 21081

[E] **D5936** Obturator/prosthesis, interim
See code(s): 21079

[E] **D5937** Trismus appliance (not for TMD treatment)
MED: 100-2, 15, 120

[E] **D5951** Feeding aid
MED: 100-2, 15, 120; 100-2, 16, 140

[E] **D5952** Speech aid prosthesis, pediatric
See code(s): 21084

[E] **D5953** Speech aid prosthesis, adult
See code(s): 21084

[E] **D5954** Palatal augmentation prosthesis
See code(s): 21082

[E] **D5955** Palatal lift prosthesis, definitive
See code(s): 21083

[E] **D5958** Palatal lift prosthesis, interim
See code(s): 21083

[E] **D5959** Palatal lift prosthesis, modification
See code(s): 21083

[E] **D5960** Speech aid prosthesis, modification
See code(s): 21084

[E] **D5982** Surgical stent
For oral surgical stent see CPT code. Surgical stent. Periodontal stent, skin graft stent, columellar stent.
See code(s): 21085

[S] **D5983** Radiation carrier
MED: 100-2, 15, 150; 100-2, 16, 140

[S] **D5984** Radiation shield
MED: 100-2, 15, 150; 100-2, 16, 140

[S] **D5985** Radiation cone locator
MED: 100-2, 15, 150; 100-2, 16, 140

[E] **D5986** Fluoride gel carrier

[S] **D5987** Commissure splint
MED: 100-2, 15, 150; 100-2, 16, 140

[E] **D5988** Surgical splint. See also CPT.
See also CPT code (21085)

[E] **D5999** Unspecified maxillofacial prosthesis, by report
Determine if an alternative HCPCS Level II or a CPT code better describes the service being reported. This code should be used only if a more specific code is unavailable.

IMPLANT SERVICES D6000–D6199

[E] **D6010** Surgical placement of implant body: endosteal implant
See code(s): 21248

~~D6020~~ ~~Abutment placement or substitution: endosteal implant~~
See code(s): 21248

[E] **D6040** Surgical placement: eposteal implant
See code(s): 21245

[E] **D6050** Surgical placement: transosteal implant
See code(s): 21244

[E] **D6053** Implant/abutment supported removable denture for completely edentulous arch
MED: 100-2, 15, 150

[E] **D6054** Implant/abutment supported removable denture for partially edentulous arch
MED: 100-2, 15, 150

[E] **D6055** Dental implant supported connecting bar
MED: 100-2, 15, 150

▲ [E] **D6056** Prefabricated abutment — includes placement
MED: 100-2, 15, 150

▲ [E] **D6057** Custom abutment — includes placement
MED: 100-2, 15, 150

[E] **D6058** Abutment supported porcelain/ceramic crown
MED: 100-2, 15, 150

[E] **D6059** Abutment supported porcelain fused to metal crown (high noble metal)
MED: 100-2, 15, 150

[E] **D6060** Abutment supported porcelain fused to metal crown (predominantly base metal)
MED: 100-2, 15, 150

[E] **D6061** Abutment supported porcelain fused to metal crown (noble metal)
MED: 100-2, 15, 150

[E] **D6062** Abutment supported cast metal crown (high noble metal)
MED: 100-2, 15, 150

[E] **D6063** Abutment supported cast metal crown (predominantly base metal)
MED: 100-2, 15, 150

[E] **D6064** Abutment supported cast metal crown (noble metal)
MED: 100-2, 15, 150

[E] **D6065** Implant supported porcelain/ceramic crown
MED: 100-2, 15, 150

[E] **D6066** Implant supported porcelain fused to metal crown (titanium, titanium alloy, high noble metal)
MED: 100-2, 15, 150

[E] **D6067** Implant supported metal crown (titanium, titanium alloy, high noble metal)
MED: 100-2, 15, 150

[E] **D6068** Abutment supported retainer for porcelain/ceramic FPD
MED: 100-2, 15, 150

[E] **D6069** Abutment supported retainer for porcelain fused to metal FPD (high noble metal)
MED: 100-2, 15, 150

[E] **D6070** Abutment supported retainer for porcelain fused to metal FPD (predominately base metal)
MED: 100-2, 15, 150

[E] **D6071** Abutment supported retainer for porcelain fused to metal FPD (noble metal)
MED: 100-2, 15, 150

Special Coverage Instructions   Noncovered by Medicare   Carrier Discretion   ☑ Quantity Alert   ● New Code   ○ Reinstated Code   ▲ Revised Code

34 — D Codes   [A] Adult   [M] Maternity   [P] Pediatrics   [I] Infant   [A]-[Y] APC Status Indicator   *2005 HCPCS*

E D6072 Abutment supported retainer for cast metal FPD (high noble metal)
MED: 100-2, 15, 150

E D6073 Abutment supported retainer for cast metal FPD (predominately base metal)
MED: 100-2, 15, 150

E D6074 Abutment supported retainer for cast metal FPD (noble metal)
MED: 100-2, 15, 150

E D6075 Implant supported retainer for ceramic FPD
MED: 100-2, 15, 150

E D6076 Implant supported retainer for porcelain fused to metal FPD (titanium, titanium alloy, or high noble metal)
MED: 100-2, 15, 150

E D6077 Implant supported retainer for cast metal FPD (titanium, titanium alloy, or high noble metal)
MED: 100-2, 15, 150

E D6078 Implant/abutment supported fixed denture for completely edentulous arch
MED: 100-2, 15, 150

E D6079 Implant/abutment supported fixed denture for partially edentulous arch
MED: 100-2, 15, 150

E D6080 Implant maintenance procedures, including removal of prosthesis, cleansing of prosthesis and abutments, reinsertion of prosthesis
MED: 100-2, 15, 150

E D6090 Repair implant supported prosthesis, by report
Pertinent documentation to evaluate medical appropriateness should be included when this code is reported.

See code(s): 21299

● D6094 Abutment supported crown — (titanium)

E D6095 Repair implant abutment, by report
Pertinent documentation to evaluate medical appropriateness should be included when this code is reported.

See code(s): 21299

E D6100 Implant removal, by report
Pertinent documentation to evaluate medical appropriateness should be included when this code is reported.

See code(s): 21299

● D6190 Radiographic/surgical implant index, by report

● D6194 Abutment supported retainer crown for FPD — (titanium)

E D6199 Unspecified implant procedure, by report
See code(s): 21299

● D6205 Pontic — indirect resin based composite

PROSTHODONTICS (FIXED) D6200–D6999

FIXED PARTIAL DENTURE PONTICS

E D6210 Pontic — cast high noble metal
Each abutment and each pontic constitute a unit in a prosthesis. An alloy of at least 60 percent gold (Au), palladium (Pd), or platinum (Pt) is considered a high noble metal.

E D6211 Pontic — cast predominantly base metal
Each abutment and each pontic constitute a unit in a prosthesis. An alloy of less than 25 percent gold (Au), palladium (Pd), or platinum (Pt) is considered a high noble metal.

E D6212 Pontic — cast noble metal
Each abutment and each pontic constitute a unit in a prosthesis. An alloy of at least 25 percent gold (Au), palladium (Pd), or platinum (Pt) is considered a high noble metal.

● D6214 Pontic — titanium

E D6240 Pontic — porcelain fused to high noble metal
Each abutment and each pontic constitute a unit in a prosthesis. An alloy of at least 60 percent gold (Au), palladium (Pd), or platinum (Pt) is considered a high noble metal.

E D6241 Pontic — porcelain fused to predominantly base metal
Each abutment and each pontic constitute a unit in a prosthesis. An alloy of less than 25 percent gold (Au), palladium (Pd), or platinum (Pt) is considered a high noble metal.

E D6242 Pontic — porcelain fused to noble metal
Each abutment and each pontic constitute a unit in a prosthesis. An alloy of at least 60 percent gold (Au), palladium (Pd), or platinum (Pt) is considered a high noble metal.

E D6245 Pontic — porcelain/ceramic
MED: 100-2, 15, 150

E D6250 Pontic — resin with high noble metal
Each abutment and each pontic constitute a unit in a prosthesis. An alloy of at least 60 percent gold (Au), palladium (Pd), or platinum (Pt) is considered a high noble metal.

E D6251 Pontic — resin with predominantly base metal
Each abutment and each pontic constitute a unit in a prosthesis. An alloy of less than 25 percent gold (Au), palladium (Pd), or platinum (Pt) is considered a high noble metal.

E D6252 Pontic — resin with noble metal
Each abutment and each pontic constitute a unit in a prosthesis. An alloy of at least 25 percent gold (Au), palladium (Pd), or platinum (Pt) is considered a high noble metal.

E D6253 Provisional pontic

E D6545 Retainer — cast metal for resin bonded fixed prosthesis

E D6548 Retainer — porcelain/ceramic for resin bonded fixed prosthesis
MED: 100-2, 15, 150

E D6600 Inlay — porcelain/ceramic, two surfaces
MED: 100-2, 15, 150

E D6601 Inlay — porcelain/ceramic, three or more surfaces
MED: 100-2, 15, 150

E D6602 Inlay — cast high noble metal, two surfaces
MED: 100-2, 15, 150

E D6603 Inlay — cast high noble metal, three or more surfaces
MED: 100-2, 15, 150

E D6604 Inlay — cast predominantly base metal, two surfaces
MED: 100-2, 15, 150

E D6605 Inlay — cast predominantly base metal, three or more surfaces
MED: 100-2, 15, 150

E D6606 Inlay — cast noble metal, two surfaces
MED: 100-2, 15, 150

E D6607 Inlay — cast noble metal, three or more surfaces
MED: 100-2, 15, 150

Special Coverage Instructions   Noncovered by Medicare   Carrier Discretion   ☑ Quantity Alert   ● New Code   ○ Reinstated Code   ▲ Revised Code

2005 HCPCS   ♀ Female Only   ♂ Male Only   1-9 ASC Groups   MED: Pub 100/NCD Reference   ৬ DMEPOS Paid   ⊘ SNF Excluded   D Codes — 35

Dental Procedures

D6608 — D7240

E **D6608** Onlay — porcelain/ceramic, two surfaces
MED: 100-2, 15, 150

E **D6609** Onlay — porcelain/ceramic, three or more surfaces
MED: 100-2, 15, 150

E **D6610** Onlay — cast high noble metal, two surfaces
MED: 100-2, 15, 150

E **D6611** Onlay — cast high noble metal, three or more surfaces
MED: 100-2, 15, 150

E **D6612** Onlay — cast predominantly base metal, two surfaces
MED: 100-2, 15, 150

E **D6613** Onlay — cast predominantly base metal, three or more surfaces
MED: 100-2, 15, 150

E **D6614** Onlay — cast noble metal, two surfaces
MED: 100-2, 15, 150

E **D6615** Onlay — cast noble metal, three or more surfaces
MED: 100-2, 15, 150

● **D6624** Inlay — titanium

● **D6634** Onlay — titanium

● **D6710** Crown — indirect resin based composite

FIXED PARTIAL DENTURE RETAINERS — CROWNS

E **D6720** Crown — resin with high noble metal
An alloy of at least 60 percent gold (Au), palladium (Pd), or platinum (Pt) is considered a high noble metal.

E **D6721** Crown — resin with predominantly base metal
An alloy of less than 25 percent gold (Au), palladium (Pd), or platinum (Pt) is considered a base metal.

E **D6722** Crown — resin with noble metal
An alloy of at least 25 percent gold (Au), palladium (Pd), or platinum (Pt) is considered a noble metal.

E **D6740** Crown — porcelain/ceramic
MED: 100-2, 15, 150

E **D6750** Crown — porcelain fused to high noble metal
An alloy of at least 60 percent gold (Au), palladium (Pd), or platinum (Pt) is considered a high noble metal.

E **D6751** Crown — porcelain fused to predominantly base metal
An alloy of less than 25 percent gold (Au), palladium (Pd), or platinum (Pt) is considered a base metal.

E **D6752** Crown — porcelain fused to noble metal
An alloy of at least 25 percent gold (Au), palladium (Pd), or platinum (Pt) is considered a noble metal.

E **D6780** Crown — 3/4 cast high noble metal
An alloy of at least 60 percent gold (Au), palladium (Pd), or platinum (Pt) is considered a high noble metal.

E **D6781** Crown — 3/4 cast predominately base metal
An alloy of less than 25 percent gold (Au), palladium (Pd), or platinum (Pt) is considered a base metal.
MED: 100-2, 15, 150

E **D6782** Crown — 3/4 cast noble metal
An alloy of at least 25 percent gold (Au), palladium (Pd), or platinum (Pt) is considered a noble metal.
MED: 100-2, 15, 150

E **D6783** Crown — 3/4 porcelain/ceramic
MED: 100-2, 15, 150

E **D6790** Crown — full cast high noble metal
An alloy of at least 60 percent gold (Au), palladium (Pd), or platinum (Pt) is considered a high noble metal.

E **D6791** Crown — full cast predominantly base metal
An alloy of less than 25 percent gold (Au), palladium (Pd), or platinum (Pt) is considered a base metal.

E **D6792** Crown — full cast noble metal
An alloy of at least 25 percent gold (Au), palladium (Pd), or platinum (Pt) is considered a noble metal.

E **D6793** Provisional retainer crown

● **D6794** Crown — titanium

OTHER FIXED PARTIAL DENTURE SERVICES

S **D6920** Connector bar
MED: 100-2, 15, 150; 100-2, 16, 140; 100-3, 260.6

E **D6930** Recement fixed partial denture

E **D6940** Stress breaker

E **D6950** Precision attachment

E **D6970** Cast post and core in addition to fixed partial denture retainer

E **D6971** Cast post as part of fixed partial denture retainer

E **D6972** Prefabricated post and core in addition to fixed partial denture retainer

E **D6973** Core build up for retainer, including any pins

E **D6975** Coping — metal

E **D6976** Each additional cast post — same tooth
Report this code in addition to codes D6970 or D6971.
MED: 100-2, 15, 150

E **D6977** Each additional prefabricated post — same tooth
Report this code in addition to code D6972.
MED: 100-2, 15, 150

E **D6980** Fixed partial denture repair, by report
Pertinent documentation to evaluate medical appropriateness should be included when this code is reported.

E **D6985** Pediatric partial denture, fixed P

E **D6999** Unspecified, fixed prosthodontic procedure, by report
Determine if an alternative HCPCS Level II or a CPT code better describes the service being reported. This code should be used only if a more specific code is unavailable.

▲ S **D7111** Extraction, coronal remnants — deciduous tooth
MED: 100-2, 16, 140

S **D7140** Extraction, erupted tooth or exposed root (elevation and/or forceps removal)
MED: 100-2, 16, 140

SURGICAL EXTRACTIONS (INCLUDES LOCAL ANESTHESIA AND ROUTINE POSTOPERATIVE CARE)

S **D7210** Surgical removal of erupted tooth requiring elevation of mucoperiosteal flap and removal of bone and/or section of tooth
MED: 100-2, 15, 150; 100-2, 16, 140

S **D7220** Removal of impacted tooth — soft tissue
MED: 100-2, 15, 150; 100-2, 16, 140

S **D7230** Removal of impacted tooth — partially bony
MED: 100-2, 15, 150; 100-2, 16, 140

S **D7240** Removal of impacted tooth — completely bony
MED: 100-2, 15, 150; 100-2, 16, 140

Special Coverage Instructions   Noncovered by Medicare   Carrier Discretion   ☑ Quantity Alert   ● New Code   ○ Reinstated Code   ▲ Revised Code

36 — D Codes   A Adult   M Maternity   P Pediatrics   I Infant   A-Y APC Status Indicator   *2005 HCPCS*

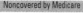
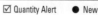
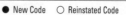

S		D7241	Removal of impacted tooth — completely bony, with unusual surgical complications MED: 100-2, 15, 150; 100-2, 16, 140
S		D7250	Surgical removal of residual tooth roots (cutting procedure) MED: 100-2, 15, 150; 100-2, 16, 140

OTHER SURGICAL PROCEDURES

S	D7260	Orolantral fistula closure MED: 100-2, 15, 150; 100-2, 16, 140
S	D7261	Primary closure of a sinus perforation See equivalent CPT code for repair of mucous membranes. MED: 100-2, 16, 140
E	D7270	Tooth reimplantation and/or stabilization of accidentally evulsed or displaced tooth
E	D7272	Tooth transplantation (includes reimplantation from one site to another and splinting and/or stabilization)
E	D7280	Surgical access of an unerupted tooth
	D7281	~~Surgical exposure of impacted or unerupted tooth to aid eruption~~
E	D7282	Mobilization of erupted or malpositioned tooth to aid eruption
●	D7283	Placement of device to facilitate eruption of impacted tooth
E	D7285	Biopsy of oral tissue — hard (bone, tooth) See code(s): 20220, 20225, 20240, 20245
▲ E	D7286	Biopsy of oral tissue — soft See code(s): 40808
▲ E	D7287	Exfoliative cytological sample collection
●	D7288	Brush biopsy — transepithelial sample collection
E	D7290	Surgical repositioning of teeth
S	D7291	Transseptal fiberotomy/supra crestal fiberotomy, by report Pertinent documentation to evaluate medical appropriateness should be included when this code is reported. MED: 100-2, 15, 150; 100-2, 16, 140

ALVEOLOPLASTY — SURGICAL PREPARATION OF RIDGE FOR DENTURES

E	☑	D7310	Alveoloplasty in conjunction with extractions — per quadrant See code(s): 41874
●	☑	D7311	Alveoloplasty in conjunction with extractions — one to three teeth or tooth spaces, per quadrant
E	☑	D7320	Alveoloplasty not in conjunction with extractions — per quadrant See code(s): 41870
●	☑	D7321	Alveoloplasty not in conjunction with extractions — one to three teeth or tooth spaces, per quadrant

VESTIBULOPLASTY

E	D7340	Vestibuloplasty — ridge extension (second epithelialization) See code(s): 40840, 40842, 40843, 40844
E	D7350	Vestibuloplasty — ridge extension (including soft tissue grafts, muscle reattachments, revision of soft tissue attachment and management of hypertrophied and hyperplastic tissue) See code(s): 40845

SURGICAL EXCISION OF REACTIVE INFLAMMATORY LESIONS (SCAR TISSUE OR LOCALIZED CONGENITAL LESIONS)

E	☑	D7410	Excision of benign lesion up to 1.25 cm
E		D7411	Excision of benign lesion greater than 1.25 cm See CPT codes in the surgical section (11440 & 40520)
E		D7412	Excision of benign lesion, complicated See CPT code in the surgical section (10000 & 40000)
E		D7413	Excision of malignant lesion up to 1.25 cm See CPT code in the surgical section (11442)
E		D7414	Excision of malignant lesion greater than 1.25 cm See CPT codes in the surgical section (11442-11446)
E		D7415	Excision of malignant lesion, complicated See CPT codes in the surgical section (11440-11446 with modifier 22 for complicated)
E	☑	D7440	Excision of malignant tumor — lesion diameter up to 1.25 cm
E	☑	D7441	Excision of malignant tumor — lesion diameter greater than 1.25 cm
E	☑	D7450	Removal of benign odontogenic cyst or tumor — lesion diameter up to 1.25 cm
E	☑	D7451	Removal of benign odontogenic cyst or tumor — lesion diameter greater than 1.25 cm
E	☑	D7460	Removal of benign nonodontogenic cyst or tumor — lesion diameter up to 1.25 cm
E	☑	D7461	Removal of benign nonodontogenic cyst or tumor — lesion diameter greater than 1.25 cm
E		D7465	Destruction of lesion(s) by physical or chemical method, by report Pertinent documentation to evaluate medical appropriateness should be included when this code is reported. See code(s): 41850
E	☑	D7471	Removal of lateral exostosis (maxilla or mandible) See code(s): 21031, 21032
E		D7472	Removal of torus palatinus See CPT code in the surgical section (21029, 21030, 21031)
E		D7473	Removal of torus mandibularis
E		D7485	Surgical reduction of osseous tuberosity
▲ E		D7490	Radical resection of maxilla or mandible See code(s): 21095

SURGICAL INCISION

E	D7510	Incision and drainage of abscess — intraoral soft tissue See code(s): 41800
●	D7511	Incision and drainage of abscess — intraoral soft tissue — complicated (includes drainage of multiple fascial spaces)
E	D7520	Incision and drainage of abscess — extraoral soft tissue See code(s): 40800
●	D7521	Incision and drainage of abscess — extraoral soft tissue — complicated (includes drainage of multiple fascial spaces)
E	D7530	Removal of foreign body from mucosa, skin, or subcutaneous alveolar tissue See code(s): 41805, 41828
E	D7540	Removal of reaction-producing foreign bodies, musculoskeletal system See code(s): 20520, 41800, 41806

Dental Procedures

D7550 — D7941

E   **D7550** Partial ostectomy/sequestrectomy for removal of non-vital bone
See code(s): 20999

E   **D7560** Maxillary sinusotomy for removal of tooth fragment or foreign body
See code(s): 31020

TREATMENT OF FRACTURES — SIMPLE

E   **D7610** Maxilla — open reduction (teeth immobilized, if present

E   **D7620** Maxilla — closed reduction (teeth immobilized, if present)

E   **D7630** Mandible — open reduction (teeth immobilized, if present)

E   **D7640** Mandible — closed reduction (teeth immobilized, if present)

E   **D7650** Malar and/or zygomatic arch — open reduction

E   **D7660** Malar and/or zygomatic arch — closed reduction

E   **D7670** Alveolus — closed reduction, may include stabilization of teeth

E   **D7671** Alveolus — open reduction, may include stabilization of teeth

E   **D7680** Facial bones — complicated reduction with fixation and multiple surgical approaches

TREATMENT OF FRACTURES — COMPOUND

E   **D7710** Maxilla — open reduction
See code(s): 21346

E   **D7720** Maxilla — closed reduction
See code(s): 21345

E   **D7730** Mandible — open reduction
See code(s): 21461, 21462

E   **D7740** Mandible — closed reduction
See code(s): 21455

E   **D7750** Malar and/or zygomatic arch — open reduction
See code(s): 21360, 21365

E   **D7760** Malar and/or zygomatic arch — closed reduction
See code(s): 21355

E   **D7770** Alveolus — open reduction stabilization of teeth
See code(s): 21422

E   **D7771** Alveolus, closed reduction stabilization of teeth
See CPT code in the surgical section (21421)

E   **D7780** Facial bones — complicated reduction with fixation and multiple surgical approaches
See code(s): 21433, 21435

REDUCTION OF DISLOCATION AND MANAGEMENT OF OTHER TEMPOROMANDIBULAR JOINT DYSFUNCTIONS

Procedures which are an integral part of a primary procedure should not be reported separately.

E   **D7810** Open reduction of dislocation
See code(s): 21490

E   **D7820** Closed reduction of dislocation
See code(s): 21480

E   **D7830** Manipulation under anesthesia

E   **D7840** Condylectomy
See code(s): 21050

E   **D7850** Surgical discectomy, with/without implant
See code(s): 21060

E   **D7852** Disc repair
See code(s): 21299

E   **D7854** Synovectomy
See code(s): 21299

E   **D7856** Myotomy
See code(s): 21299

E   **D7858** Joint reconstruction
See code(s): 21242, 21243

E   **D7860** Arthrotomy
MED: 100-2, 15, 150; 100-2, 16, 140

E   **D7865** Arthroplasty
See code(s): 21240

E   **D7870** Arthrocentesis
See code(s): 21060

E   **D7871** Non-arthroscopic lysis and lavage

E   **D7872** Arthroscopy — diagnosis, with or without biopsy
See code(s): 29800

E   **D7873** Arthroscopy — surgical: lavage and lysis of adhesions
See code(s): 29804

E   **D7874** Arthroscopy — surgical: disc repositioning and stabilization
See code(s): 29804

E   **D7875** Arthroscopy — surgical: synovectomy
See code(s): 29804

E   **D7876** Arthroscopy — surgical: discectomy
See code(s): 29804

E   **D7877** Arthroscopy — surgical: debridement
See code(s): 29804

E   **D7880** Occlusal orthotic device, by report
See code(s): 21499

E   **D7899** Unspecified TMD therapy, by report
Determine if an alternative HCPCS Level II or a CPT code better describes the service being reported. This code should be used only if a more specific code is unavailable.
See code(s): 21499

REPAIR OF TRAUMATIC WOUNDS

E   ☑   **D7910** Suture of recent small wounds up to 5 cm
See code(s): 12011, 12013

COMPLICATED SUTURING (RECONSTRUCTION REQUIRING DELICATE HANDLING OF TISSUES AND WIDE UNDERMINING FOR METICULOUS CLOSURE)

E   **D7911** Complicated suture — up to 5 cm
See code(s): 12051, 12052

E   **D7912** Complicated suture — greater than 5 cm
See code(s): 13132

OTHER REPAIR PROCEDURES

E   **D7920** Skin graft (identify defect covered, location and type of graft)

S   **D7940** Osteoplasty — for orthognathic deformities
MED: 100-2, 15, 150; 100-2, 16, 140

E   **D7941** Osteotomy — mandibular rami
See code(s): 21193, 21195, 21196

Special Coverage Instructions   Noncovered by Medicare   Carrier Discretion   ☑ Quantity Alert   ● New Code   ○ Reinstated Code   ▲ Revised Code

38 — D Codes   A Adult   M Maternity   P Pediatrics   I Infant   A-Y APC Status Indicator   *2005 HCPCS*

E		**D7943**	Osteotomy — mandibular rami with bone graft; includes obtaining the graft See code(s): 21194

☑ | E | **D7944** | Osteotomy — segmented or subapical — per sextant or quadrant
See code(s): 21198, 21206

E | **D7945** | Osteotomy — body of mandible
See code(s): 21193, 21194, 21195, 21196

E | **D7946** | LeFort I (maxilla — total)
See code(s): 21147

E | **D7947** | LeFort I (maxilla — segmented)
See code(s): 21145, 21146

E | **D7948** | LeFort II or LeFort III (osteoplasty of facial bones for midface hypoplasia or retrusion) — without bone graft
See code(s): 21150

E | **D7949** | LeFort II or LeFort III — with bone graft

E | **D7950** | Osseous, osteoperiosteal, or cartilage graft of the mandible or facial bones — autogenous or nonautogenous, by report
Pertinent documentation to evaluate medical appropriateness should be included when this code is reported.
See code(s): 21247

● ☑ | **D7953** | Bone replacement graft for ridge preservation — per site

▲ E | **D7955** | Repair of maxillofacial soft and/or hard tissue defect
See code(s): 21299

E | **D7960** | Frenulectomy (frenectomy or frenotomy) — separate procedure
See code(s): 40819, 41010, 41115

● | **D7963** | Frenuloplasty

E ☑ | **D7970** | Excision of hyperplastic tissue — per arch

E | **D7971** | Excision of pericoronal gingiva
See code(s): 41821

E | **D7972** | Surgical reduction of fibrous tuberosity

E | **D7980** | Sialolithotomy
See code(s): 42330, 42335, 42340

E | **D7981** | Excision of salivary gland, by report
Pertinent documentation to evaluate medical appropriateness should be included when this code is reported.
See code(s): 42408

E | **D7982** | Sialodochoplasty
See code(s): 42500

E | **D7983** | Closure of salivary fistula
See code(s): 42600

E | **D7990** | Emergency tracheotomy
See code(s): 31605

E | **D7991** | Coronoidectomy
See code(s): 21070

E | **D7995** | Synthetic graft — mandible or facial bones, by report
Pertinent documentation to evaluate medical appropriateness should be included when this code is reported.
See code(s): 21299

E | **D7996** | Implant — mandible for augmentation purposes (excluding alveolar ridge), by report
Pertinent documentation to evaluate medical appropriateness should be included when this code is reported.
See code(s): 21299

E | **D7997** | Appliance removal (not by dentist who placed appliance), includes removal of archbar

E | **D7999** | Unspecified oral surgery procedure, by report
Determine if an alternative HCPCS Level II or a CPT code better describes the service being reported. This code should be used only if a more specific code is unavailable.
See code(s): 21299

ORTHODONTICS D8000–D8999

E | **D8010** | Limited orthodontic treatment of the primary dentition P

E | **D8020** | Limited orthodontic treatment of the transitional dentition

E | **D8030** | Limited orthodontic treatment of the adolescent dentition P

E | **D8040** | Limited orthodontic treatment of the adult dentition A

E | **D8050** | Interceptive orthodontic treatment of the primary dentition P

E | **D8060** | Interceptive orthodontic treatment of the transitional dentition

E | **D8070** | Comprehensive orthodontic treatment of the transitional dentition

E | **D8080** | Comprehensive orthodontic treatment of the adolescent dentition P

E | **D8090** | Comprehensive orthodontic treatment of the adult dentition A

MINOR TREATMENT TO CONTROL HARMFUL HABITS

E | **D8210** | Removable appliance therapy

E | **D8220** | Fixed appliance therapy

OTHER ORTHODONTIC SERVICES

E | **D8660** | Pre-orthodontic treatment visit

E | **D8670** | Periodic orthodontic treatment visit (as part of contract)

E | **D8680** | Orthodontic retention (removal of appliances, construction and placement of retainer(s))

E | **D8690** | Orthodontic treatment (alternative billing to a contract fee)

E | **D8691** | Repair of orthodontic appliance

E | **D8692** | Replacement of lost or broken retainer

E | **D8999** | Unspecified orthodontic procedure, by report
Determine if an alternative HCPCS Level II or a CPT code better describes the service being reported. This code should be used only if a more specific code is unavailable.

ADJUNCTIVE GENERAL SERVICES D9110–D9999

UNCLASSIFIED TREATMENT

N | **D9110** | Palliative (emergency) treatment of dental pain — minor procedure
MED: 100-2, 15, 150; 100-2, 16, 140

Special Coverage Instructions Noncovered by Medicare Carrier Discretion ☑ Quantity Alert ● New Code ○ Reinstated Code ▲ Revised Code

2005 HCPCS ♀ Female Only ♂ Male Only **1-9** ASC Groups MED: Pub 100/NCD Reference ᧖ DMEPOS Paid ⊘ SNF Excluded **D Codes — 39**

Dental Procedures

D9210 — D9999

ANESTHESIA

E   **D9210**   Local anesthesia not in conjunction with operative or surgical procedures
See code(s): 90784

E   **D9211**   Regional block anesthesia

E   **D9212**   Trigeminal division block anesthesia
See code(s): 64400

E   **D9215**   Local anesthesia
See code(s): 90784

E ☑   **D9220**   Deep sedation/general anesthesia — first 30 minutes
See also CPT code 00172-00176.

E ☑   **D9221**   Deep sedation/general anesthesia — each additional 15 minutes
MED: 100-2, 15, 150; 100-2, 16, 140

N   **D9230**   Analgesia, anxiolysis, inhalation of nitrous oxide
MED: 100-2, 15, 150; 100-2, 16, 140

E ☑   **D9241**   Intravenous conscious sedation/analgesia — first 30 minutes
See also CPT code 90784, 99141.

See code(s): 90784

E ☑   **D9242**   Intravenous conscious sedation/analgesia — each additional 15 minutes
See also CPT code 90784, 99141.

See code(s): 90784

N   **D9248**   Non-intravenous conscious sedation

PROFESSIONAL CONSULTATION

E   **D9310**   Consultation (diagnostic service provided by dentist or physician other than practitioner providing treatment)

PROFESSIONAL VISITS

E   **D9410**   House/extended care facility call

E   **D9420**   Hospital call
See also CPT E & M codes

E   **D9430**   Office visit for observation (during regularly scheduled hours) — no other services performed
See also CPT E & M codes

E   **D9440**   Office visit — after regularly scheduled hours
See code(s): 99050

E   **D9450**   Case presentation, detailed and extensive treatment planning

DRUGS

E   **D9610**   Therapeutic drug injection, by report
Pertinent documentation to evaluate medical appropriateness should be included when this code is reported.

See code(s): 90788, 90784

S   **D9630**   Other drugs and/or medicaments, by report
Determine if an alternative HCPCS Level II or a CPT code better describes the service being reported. This code should be used only if a more specific code is unavailable.

MED: 100-2, 15, 150; 100-2, 16, 140

MISCELLANEOUS SERVICES

E   **D9910**   Application of desensitizing medicament

E ☑   **D9911**   Application of desensitizing resin for cervical and/or root surface, per tooth

E   **D9920**   Behavior management, by report
Pertinent documentation to evaluate medical appropriateness should be included when this code is reported.

S   **D9930**   Treatment of complications (postsurgical) — unusual circumstances, by report
MED: 100-2, 15, 150; 100-2, 16, 140

S   **D9940**   Occlusal guard, by report
Pertinent documentation to evaluate medical appropriateness should be included when this code is reported.

MED: 100-2, 15, 150; 100-2, 16, 140

E   **D9941**   Fabrication of athletic mouthguard
See code(s): 21089

●   **D9942**   Repair and/or reline of occlusal guard

S   **D9950**   Occlusion analysis — mounted case
MED: 100-2, 15, 150; 100-2, 16, 140

S   **D9951**   Occlusal adjustment — limited
MED: 100-2, 15, 150; 100-2, 16, 140

S   **D9952**   Occlusal adjustment — complete
MED: 100-2, 15, 150; 100-2, 16, 140

E   **D9970**   Enamel microabrasion

E ☑   **D9971**   Odontoplasty 1-2 teeth; includes removal of enamel projections

E ☑   **D9972**   External bleaching — per arch

E ☑   **D9973**   External bleaching — per tooth

E ☑   **D9974**   Internal bleaching — per tooth

E   **D9999**   Unspecified adjunctive procedure, by report
Determine if an alternative HCPCS Level II or a CPT code better describes the service being reported. This code should be used only if a more specific code is unavailable.

See code(s): 21499

Special Coverage Instructions   Noncovered by Medicare   Carrier Discretion   ☑ Quantity Alert   ● New Code   ○ Reinstated Code   ▲ Revised Code

40 — D Codes   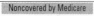 A Adult   M Maternity   P Pediatrics   I Infant   A-Y APC Status Indicator   *2005 HCPCS*

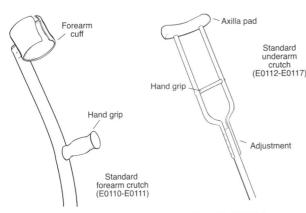

Forearm cuff

Axilla pad

Standard underarm crutch (E0112-E0117)

Hand grip

Hand grip

Adjustment

Standard forearm crutch (E0110-E0111)

DURABLE MEDICAL EQUIPMENT *E0100–E9999*

E codes include durable medical equipment such as canes, crutches, walkers, commodes, decubitus care, bath and toilet aids, hospital beds, oxygen and related respiratory equipment, monitoring equipment, pacemakers, patient lifts, safety equipment, restraints, traction equipment, fracture frames, wheelchairs, and artificial kidney machines.

CANES

E0100 Cane, includes canes of all materials, adjustable or fixed, with tip
White canes for the blind are not covered under Medicare.
MED: 100-2, 15, 110.1; 100-3, 280.1; 100-3, 280.2

E0105 Cane, quad or three-prong, includes canes of all materials, adjustable or fixed, with tips
MED: 100-2, 15, 110.1; 100-3, 280.1; 100-3, 280.5

CRUTCHES

E0110 Crutches, forearm, includes crutches of various materials, adjustable or fixed, pair, complete with tips and handgrips
MED: 100-2, 15, 110.1; 100-3, 280.1

E0111 Crutch, forearm, includes crutches of various materials, adjustable or fixed, each, with tip and handgrip
MED: 100-2, 15, 110.1; 100-3, 280.1

E0112 Crutches, underarm, wood, adjustable or fixed, pair, with pads, tips and handgrips
MED: 100-2, 15, 110.1; 100-3, 280.1

E0113 Crutch, underarm, wood, adjustable or fixed, each, with pad, tip and handgrip
MED: 100-2, 15, 110.1; 100-3, 280.1

E0114 Crutches, underarm, other than wood, adjustable or fixed, pair, with pads, tips and handgrips
MED: 100-2, 15, 110.1; 100-3, 280.1

E0116 Crutch, underarm, other than wood, adjustable or fixed, each, with pad, tip and handgrip
MED: 100-2, 15, 110.1; 100-3, 280.1

E0117 Crutch, underarm, articulating, spring assisted, each
MED: 100-2, 15, 110.1

E0118 Crutch substitute, lower leg platform, with or without wheels, each

WALKERS

E0130 Walker, rigid (pickup), adjustable or fixed height
Medicare covers walkers if patient's ambulation is impaired.
MED: 100-2, 15, 110.1; 100-3, 280.1

E0135 Walker, folding (pickup), adjustable or fixed height
Medicare covers walkers if patient's ambulation is impaired.
MED: 100-2, 15, 110.1; 100-3, 280.1

E0140 Walker, with trunk support, adjustable or fixed height, any type
MED: 100-2, 15, 110.1; 100-3, 280.1

E0141 Walker, rigid, wheeled, adjustable or fixed height
Medicare covers walkers if patient's ambulation is impaired.
MED: 100-2, 15, 110.1; 100-3, 280.1

E0143 Walker, folding, wheeled, adjustable or fixed height
Medicare covers walkers if patient's ambulation is impaired.
MED: 100-2, 15, 110.1; 100-3, 280.1

E0144 Walker, enclosed, four sided framed, rigid or folding, wheeled with posterior seat
MED: 100-2, 15, 110.1; 100-3, 280.1

E0147 Walker, heavy duty, multiple braking system, variable wheel resistance
Medicare covers safety roller walkers only in patients with severe neurological disorders or restricted use of one hand. In some cases, coverage will be extended to patients with a weight exceeding the limits of a standard wheeled walker.
MED: 100-2, 15, 110.1; 100-3, 280.5

E0148 Walker, heavy duty, without wheels, rigid or folding, any type, each

E0149 Walker, heavy duty, wheeled, rigid or folding, any type

E0153 Platform attachment, forearm crutch, each

E0154 Platform attachment, walker, each

E0155 Wheel attachment, rigid pick-up walker, per pair seat attachment, walker

ATTACHMENTS

E0156 Seat attachment, walker

E0157 Crutch attachment, walker, each

E0158 Leg extensions for walker, per set of four (4)

E0159 Brake attachment for wheeled walker, replacement, each

COMMODES

E0160 Sitz type bath or equipment, portable, used with or without commode
Medicare covers sitz baths if medical record indicates that the patient has an infection or injury of the perineal area and the sitz bath is prescribed by the physician.
MED: 100-3, 280.1

E0161 Sitz type bath or equipment, portable, used with or without commode, with faucet attachment(s)
Medicare covers sitz baths if medical record indicates that the patient has an infection or injury of the perineal area and the sitz bath is prescribed by the physician.
MED: 100-3, 280.1

E0162   Sitz bath chair
Medicare covers sitz baths if medical record indicates that the patient has an infection or injury of the perineal area and the sitz bath is prescribed by the physician.

MED: 100-3, 280.1

E0163   Commode chair, stationary, with fixed arms
Medicare covers commodes for patients confined to their beds or rooms, for patients without indoor bathroom facilities, and to patients who cannot climb or descend the stairs necessary to reach the bathrooms in their homes.

MED: 100-2, 15, 110.1; 100-3, 280.1

E0164   Commode chair, mobile, with fixed arms
Medicare covers commodes for patients confined to their beds or rooms, for patients without indoor bathroom facilities, and to patients who cannot climb or descend the stairs necessary to reach the bathrooms in their homes.

MED: 100-2, 15, 110.1; 100-3, 280.1

E0165   Commode chair, stationary, with detachable arms
Medicare covers commodes for patients confined to their beds or rooms, for patients without indoor bathroom facilities, and to patients who cannot climb or descend the stairs necessary to reach the bathrooms in their homes.

MED: 100-2, 15, 110.1; 100-3, 280.1

E0166   Commode chair, mobile, with detachable arms
Medicare covers commodes for patients confined to their beds or rooms, for patients without indoor bathroom facilities, and to patients who cannot climb or descend the stairs necessary to reach the bathrooms in their homes.

MED: 100-2, 15, 110.1; 100-3, 280.1

E0167   Pail or pan for use with commode chair
Medicare covers commodes for patients confined to their beds or rooms, for patients without indoor bathroom facilities, and to patients who cannot climb or descend the stairs necessary to reach the bathrooms in their homes.

MED: 100-3, 280.1

E0168   Commode chair, extra wide and/or heavy duty, stationary or mobile, with or without arms, any type, each

E0169   Commode chair with seat lift mechanism

E0175   Foot rest, for use with commode chair, each

DECUBITUS CARE EQUIPMENT

~~**E0176**   Air pressure pad or cushion, nonpositioning~~

~~**E0177**   Water pressure pad or cushion, nonpositioning~~

~~**E0178**   Gel or gel like pressure pad or cushion, nonpositioning~~

~~**E0179**   Dry pressure pad or cushion, nonpositioning~~

E0180   Pressure pad, alternating with pump
Medicare covers pads if physicians supervise their use in patients who have decubitus ulcers or susceptibility to them. Prior authorization is required by Medicare for this item.

MED: 100-3, 280.1; 100-8, 5, 5.1.1.2.1

E0181   Pressure pad, alternating with pump, heavy duty
Medicare covers pads if physicians supervise their use in patients who have decubitus ulcers or susceptibility to them. Prior authorization is required by Medicare for this item.

MED: 100-3, 280.1; 100-8, 5, 5.1.1.2.1

E0182   Pump for alternating pressure pad
Medicare covers pads if physicians supervise their use in patients who have decubitus ulcers or susceptibility to them. Prior authorization is required by Medicare for this item.

MED: 100-3, 280.1; 100-8, 5, 5.1.1.2.1

E0184   Dry pressure mattress
Medicare covers pads if physicians supervise their use in patients who have decubitus ulcers or susceptibility to them. Prior authorization is required by Medicare for this item.

MED: 100-3, 280.1; 100-8, 5, 5.1.1.2.1

E0185   Gel or gel-like pressure pad for mattress, standard mattress length and width
Medicare covers pads if physicians supervise their use in patients who have decubitus ulcers or susceptibility to them. Prior authorization is required by Medicare for this item.

MED: 100-3, 280.1; 100-8, 5, 5.1.1.2.1

E0186   Air pressure mattress
Medicare covers pads if physicians supervise their use in patients who have decubitus ulcers or susceptibility to them.

MED: 100-3, 280.1

E0187   Water pressure mattress
Medicare covers pads if physicians supervise their use in patients who have decubitus ulcers or susceptibility to them.

MED: 100-3, 280.1

E0188   Synthetic sheepskin pad
Medicare covers pads if physicians supervise their use in patients who have decubitus ulcers or susceptibility to them. Prior authorization is required by Medicare for this item.

MED: 100-3, 280.1; 100-8, 5, 5.1.1.2.1

E0189   Lambswool sheepskin pad, any size
Medicare covers pads if physicians supervise their use in patients who have decubitus ulcers or susceptibility to them. Prior authorization is required by Medicare for this item.

MED: 100-3, 280.1; 100-8, 5, 5.1.1.2.1

●   **E0190**   Positioning cushion/pillow/wedge, any shape or size

MED: 100-2, 15, 110.1

E0191   Heel or elbow protector, each

~~**E0192**   Low pressure and positioning equalization pad, for wheelchair~~

E0193   Powered air flotation bed (low air loss therapy)

E0194   Air fluidized bed
An air fluidized bed is covered by Medicare if the patient has a stage 3 or stage 4 pressure sore and, without the bed, would require institutionalization. A physician's prescription is required.

MED: 100-3, 280.8

E0196   Gel pressure mattress
Medicare covers pads if physicians supervise their use in patients who have decubitus ulcers or susceptibility to them.

MED: 100-3, 280.1

E0197   Air pressure pad for mattress, standard mattress length and width
Medicare covers pads if physicians supervise their use in patients who have decubitus ulcers or susceptibility to them.

MED: 100-3, 280.1

E0198   Water pressure pad for mattress, standard mattress length and width
Medicare covers pads if physicians supervise their use in patients who have decubitus ulcers or susceptibility to them.

MED: 100-3, 280.1

E0199   Dry pressure pad for mattress, standard mattress length and width
Medicare covers pads if physicians supervise their use in patients who have decubitus ulcers or susceptibility to them.

MED: 100-3, 280.1

Special Coverage Instructions   Noncovered by Medicare   Carrier Discretion   ☑ Quantity Alert   ● New Code   ○ Reinstated Code   ▲ Revised Code

42 — E Codes   Ⓐ Adult   Ⓜ Maternity   Ⓟ Pediatrics   Ⓘ Infant   Ⓐ-Ⓨ APC Status Indicator   **2005 HCPCS**

HEAT/COLD APPLICATION

Y	E0200	Heat lamp, without stand (table model), includes bulb, or infrared element MED: 100-2, 15, 110.1; 100-3, 280.1	&. ⊘
Y	E0202	Phototherapy (bilirubin) light with photometer	&. ⊘
A	E0203	Therapeutic lightbox, minimum 10,000 lux, table top model	
Y	E0205	Heat lamp, with stand, includes bulb, or infrared element MED: 100-2, 15, 110.1; 100-3, 280.1	&. ⊘
Y	E0210	Electric heat pad, standard MED: 100-3, 280.1	&. ⊘
Y	E0215	Electric heat pad, moist MED: 100-3, 280.1	&. ⊘
Y	E0217	Water circulating heat pad with pump MED: 100-3, 280.1	&. ⊘
Y	E0218	Water circulating cold pad with pump MED: 100-3, 280.1	⊘
Y	E0220	Hot water bottle	&. ⊘
Y ☑	E0221	Infrared heating pad system MED: 100-3, 270.2	&. ⊘
Y	E0225	Hydrocollator unit, includes pads MED: 100-2, 15, 230; 100-3, 280.1	&. ⊘
Y	E0230	Ice cap or collar	&. ⊘
E	E0231	Non-contact wound warming device (temperature control unit, AC adapter and power cord) for use with warming card and wound cover MED: 100-2, 16, 20	⊘
E	E0232	Warming card for use with the non-contact wound warming device and non-contact wound warming wound cover MED: 100-2, 16, 20	⊘
Y	E0235	Paraffin bath unit, portable (see medical supply code A4265 for paraffin) MED: 100-2, 15, 230; 100-3, 280.1	&. ⊘
Y	E0236	Pump for water circulating pad MED: 100-3, 280.1	&. ⊘
Y	E0238	Nonelectric heat pad, moist MED: 100-3, 280.1	&. ⊘
Y	E0239	Hydrocollator unit, portable MED: 100-2, 15, 230; 100-3, 280.1	&. ⊘
● E	E0240	Bath/shower chair, with or without wheels, any size MED: 100-3, 280.1	⊘

BATH AND TOILET AIDS

E ☑	E0241	Bathtub wall rail, each MED: 100-2, 15, 110.1; 100-3, 280.1	⊘
E	E0242	Bathtub rail, floor base MED: 100-2, 15, 110.1; 100-3, 280.1	⊘
E ☑	E0243	Toilet rail, each MED: 100-2, 15, 110.1; 100-3, 280.1	⊘
E	E0244	Raised toilet seat MED: 100-3, 280.1	⊘
E	E0245	Tub stool or bench MED: 100-3, 280.1	⊘
E	E0246	Transfer tub rail attachment	⊘
● E	E0247	Transfer bench for tub or toilet with or without commode opening MED: 100-3, 280.1	⊘
● E	E0248	Transfer bench, heavy duty, for tub or toilet with or without commode opening MED: 100-3, 280.1	⊘
Y	E0249	Pad for water circulating heat unit MED: 100-3, 280.1	&. ⊘

HOSPITAL BEDS AND ACCESSORIES

Y	E0250	Hospital bed, fixed height, with any type side rails, with mattress MED: 100-2, 15, 110.1; 100-3, 280.7	&. ⊘
Y	E0251	Hospital bed, fixed height, with any type side rails, without mattress MED: 100-2, 15, 110.1; 100-3, 280.7	&. ⊘
Y	E0255	Hospital bed, variable height, hi-lo, with any type side rails, with mattress MED: 100-2, 15, 110.1; 100-3, 280.7	&. ⊘
Y	E0256	Hospital bed, variable height, hi-lo, with any type side rails, without mattress MED: 100-2, 15, 110.1; 100-3, 280.7	&. ⊘
Y	E0260	Hospital bed, semi-electric (head and foot adjustment), with any type side rails, with mattress MED: 100-2, 15, 110.1; 100-3, 280.7	&. ⊘
Y	E0261	Hospital bed, semi-electric (head and foot adjustment), with any type side rails, without mattress MED: 100-2, 15, 110.1; 100-3, 280.7	&. ⊘
Y	E0265	Hospital bed, total electric (head, foot, and height adjustments), with any type side rails, with mattress MED: 100-2, 15, 110.1; 100-3, 280.7	&. ⊘
Y	E0266	Hospital bed, total electric (head, foot, and height adjustments), with any type side rails, without mattress MED: 100-2, 15, 110.1; 100-3, 280.7	&. ⊘
E	E0270	Hospital bed, institutional type includes: oscillating, circulating and Stryker frame, with mattress MED: 100-3, 280.1	⊘
Y	E0271	Mattress, inner spring MED: 100-3, 280.1; 100-3, 280.7	&. ⊘
Y	E0272	Mattress, foam rubber MED: 100-3, 280.1; 100-3, 280.7	&. ⊘
E	E0273	Bed board MED: 100-3, 280.1	⊘
E	E0274	Over-bed table MED: 100-3, 280.1	⊘
Y	E0275	Bed pan, standard, metal or plastic Reusable, autoclavable bedpans are covered by Medicare for bed-confined patients. MED: 100-3, 280.1	&. ⊘
Y	E0276	Bed pan, fracture, metal or plastic Reusable, autoclavable bedpans are covered by Medicare for bed-confined patients. MED: 100-3, 280.1	&. ⊘

Special Coverage Instructions | Noncovered by Medicare | Carrier Discretion | ☑ Quantity Alert | ● New Code | ⊘ Reinstated Code | ▲ Revised Code

2005 HCPCS | ♀ Female Only | ♂ Male Only | 1-9 ASC Groups | MED: Pub 100/NCD Reference | &. DMEPOS Paid | ⊘ SNF Excluded | **E Codes — 43**

Durable Medical Equipment

E0277 — E0440

Ⓨ	**E0277**	Powered pressure-reducing air mattress 🖐⃠
		MED: 100-3, 280.1
Ⓨ	**E0280**	Bed cradle, any type 🖐⃠
Ⓨ	**E0290**	Hospital bed, fixed height, without side rails, with mattress 🖐⃠
		MED: 100-2, 15, 110.1; 100-3, 280.7
Ⓨ	**E0291**	Hospital bed, fixed height, without side rails, without mattress 🖐⃠
		MED: 100-2, 15, 110.1; 100-3, 280.7
Ⓨ	**E0292**	Hospital bed, variable height, hi-lo, without side rails, with mattress 🖐⃠
		MED: 100-2, 15, 110.1; 100-3, 280.7
Ⓨ	**E0293**	Hospital bed, variable height, hi-lo, without side rails, without mattress 🖐⃠
		MED: 100-2, 15, 110.1; 100-3, 280.7
Ⓨ	**E0294**	Hospital bed, semi-electric (head and foot adjustment), without side rails, with mattress 🖐⃠
		MED: 100-2, 15, 110.1; 100-3, 280.7
Ⓨ	**E0295**	Hospital bed, semi-electric (head and foot adjustment), without side rails, without mattress 🖐⃠
		MED: 100-2, 15, 110.1; 100-3, 280.7
Ⓨ	**E0296**	Hospital bed, total electric (head, foot, and height adjustments), without side rails, with mattress 🖐⃠
		MED: 100-2, 15, 110.1; 100-3, 280.7
Ⓨ	**E0297**	Hospital bed, total electric (head, foot, and height adjustments), without side rails, without mattress 🖐⃠
		MED: 100-2, 15, 110.1; 100-3, 280.7
Ⓨ	**E0300**	Pediatric crib, hospital grade, fully enclosed 🖐⃠
Ⓨ	**E0301**	Hospital bed, heavy duty, extra wide, with weight capacity greater than 350 pounds, but less than or equal to 600 pounds, with any type side rails, without mattress 🖐⃠
		MED: 100-3, 280.7
Ⓨ	**E0302**	Hospital bed, extra heavy duty, extra wide, with weight capacity greater than 600 pounds, with any type side rails, without mattress 🖐⃠
		MED: 100-3, 280.7
Ⓨ	**E0303**	Hospital bed, heavy duty, extra wide, with weight capacity greater than 350 pounds, but less than or equal to 600 pounds, with any type side rails, with mattress 🖐⃠
		MED: 100-3, 280.7
Ⓨ	**E0304**	Hospital bed, extra heavy duty, extra wide, with weight capacity greater than 600 pounds, with any type side rails, with mattress 🖐⃠
		MED: 100-3, 280.7
Ⓨ	**E0305**	Bedside rails, half-length 🖐⃠
		MED: 100-3, 280.7
Ⓨ	**E0310**	Bedside rails, full-length 🖐⃠
		MED: 100-3, 280.7
Ⓔ	**E0315**	Bed accessory: board, table, or support device, any type ⃠
		MED: 100-3, 280.1
Ⓨ	**E0316**	Safety enclosure frame/canopy for use with hospital bed, any type 🖐⃠
Ⓨ	**E0325**	Urinal; male, jug-type, any material ♂🖐⃠
		MED: 100-3, 280.1

Ⓨ	**E0326**	Urinal; female, jug-type, any material ♀🖐⃠
		MED: 100-3, 280.1
Ⓔ	**E0350**	Control unit for electronic bowel irrigation/evacuation system ⃠
Ⓔ	**E0352**	Disposable pack (water reservoir bag, speculum, valving mechanism and collection bag/box) for use with the electronic bowel irrigation/evacuation system ⃠
Ⓔ	**E0370**	Air pressure elevator for heel ⃠
Ⓨ	**E0371**	Nonpowered advanced pressure reducing overlay for mattress, standard mattress length and width 🖐⃠
Ⓨ	**E0372**	Powered air overlay for mattress, standard mattress length and width 🖐⃠
Ⓨ	**E0373**	Nonpowered advanced pressure reducing mattress 🖐⃠

OXYGEN AND RELATED RESPIRATORY EQUIPMENT

Ⓨ	**E0424**	Stationary compressed gaseous oxygen system, rental; includes container, contents, regulator, flowmeter, humidifier, nebulizer, cannula or mask, and tubing 🖐⃠
		For the first claim filed for home oxygen equipment or therapy, submit a certificate of medical necessity that includes the oxygen flow rate, anticipated frequency and duration of oxygen therapy, and physician signature. Medicare accepts oxygen therapy as medically necessary in cases documenting any of the following: erythocythemia with a hematocrit greater than 56 percent; a P pulmonale on EKG; or dependent edema consistent with congestive heart failure.
		MED: 100-3, 240.2
Ⓔ	**E0425**	Stationary compressed gas system, purchase; includes regulator, flowmeter, humidifier, nebulizer, cannula or mask, and tubing ⃠
		MED: 100-3, 240.2
Ⓔ	**E0430**	Portable gaseous oxygen system, purchase; includes regulator, flowmeter, humidifier, cannula or mask, and tubing ⃠
		MED: 100-3, 240.2
Ⓨ	**E0431**	Portable gaseous oxygen system, rental; includes portable container, regulator, flowmeter, humidifier, cannula or mask, and tubing 🖐⃠
		MED: 100-3, 240.2
Ⓨ	**E0434**	Portable liquid oxygen system, rental; includes portable container, supply reservoir, humidifier, flowmeter, refill adaptor, contents gauge, cannula or mask, and tubing 🖐⃠
		MED: 100-3, 240.2
Ⓔ	**E0435**	Portable liquid oxygen system, purchase; includes portable container, supply reservoir, flowmeter, humidifier, contents gauge, cannula or mask, tubing, and refill adapter ⃠
		MED: 100-3, 240.2
Ⓨ	**E0439**	Stationary liquid oxygen system, rental; includes container, contents, regulator, flowmeter, humidifier, nebulizer, cannula or mask, and tubing 🖐⃠
		MED: 100-3, 240.2
Ⓔ	**E0440**	Stationary liquid oxygen system, purchase; includes use of reservoir, contents indicator, regulator, flowmeter, humidifier, nebulizer, cannula or mask, and tubing ⃠
		MED: 100-3, 240.2

Special Coverage Instructions   Noncovered by Medicare   Carrier Discretion   ☑ Quantity Alert   ● New Code   ○ Reinstated Code   ▲ Revised Code

44 — E Codes   Ⓐ Adult   Ⓜ Maternity   Ⓟ Pediatrics   Ⓘ Infant   Ⓐ-Ⓨ APC Status Indicator   *2005 HCPCS*

Y ☑ **E0441** Oxygen contents, gaseous (for use with owned gaseous stationary systems or when both a stationary and portable gaseous system are owned), one month's supply = 1 unit ♿⃠
MED: 100-3, 240.2

Y ☑ **E0442** Oxygen contents, liquid (for use with owned liquid stationary systems or when both a stationary and portable liquid system are owned), one month's supply = 1 unit ♿⃠
MED: 100-3, 240.2

Y ☑ **E0443** Portable oxygen contents, gaseous (for use only with portable gaseous systems when no stationary gas or liquid system is used), one month's supply = 1 unit ♿⃠
MED: 100-3, 240.2

Y ☑ **E0444** Portable oxygen contents, liquid (for use only with portable liquid systems when no stationary gas or liquid system is used), one month's supply = 1 unit ♿⃠
MED: 100-3, 240.2

A **E0445** Oximeter device for measuring blood oxygen levels non-invasively

▲ Y **E0450** Volume control ventilator, without pressure support mode, may include pressure control mode, used with invasive interface (e.g., tracheostomy tube) ♿⃠
MED: 100-3, 280.1

~~E0454~~ ~~Pressure ventilator with pressure control, pressure support and flow triggering features~~

Y **E0455** Oxygen tent, excluding croup or pediatric tents ⃠
MED: 100-3, 240.2

Y **E0457** Chest shell (cuirass) ♿⃠

Y **E0459** Chest wrap ♿⃠

Y **E0460** Negative pressure ventilator; portable or stationary ♿⃠
MED: 100-3, 280.1

▲ Y **E0461** Volume control ventilator, without pressure support mode, may include pressure control mode, used with non-invasive interface (e.g., mask) ♿
MED: 100-3, 280.1

Y **E0462** Rocking bed, with or without side rails ♿⃠

● **E0463** Pressure support ventilator with volume control mode, may include pressure control mode, used with invasive interface (e.g., tracheostomy tube)

● **E0464** Pressure support ventilator with volume control mode, may include pressure control mode, used with non-invasive interface (e.g., mask)

Y **E0470** Respiratory assist device, bi-level pressure capability, without backup rate feature, used with noninvasive interface, e.g., nasal or facial mask (intermittent assist device with continuous positive airway pressure device) ♿⃠
MED: 100-3, 280.1

Y **E0471** Respiratory assist device, bi-level pressure capability, with back-up rate feature, used with noninvasive interface, e.g., nasal or facial mask (intermittent assist device with continuous positive airway pressure device) ♿⃠
MED: 100-3, 280.1

Y **E0472** Respiratory assist device, bi-level pressure capability, with backup rate feature, used with invasive interface, e.g., tracheostomy tube (intermittent assist device with continuous positive airway pressure device) ♿⃠
MED: 100-3, 280.1

Y **E0480** Percussor, electric or pneumatic, home model ♿⃠
MED: 100-3, 280.1

E **E0481** Intrapulmonary percussive ventilation system and related accessories ⃠
MED: 100-3, 240.5

Y **E0482** Cough stimulating device, alternating positive and negative airway pressure ♿⃠

Y **E0483** High frequency chest wall oscillation air-pulse generator system, (includes hoses and vest), each ♿

Y **E0484** Oscillatory positive expiratory pressure device, non-electric, any type, each ♿

IPPB MACHINES

Y **E0500** IPPB machine, all types, with built-in nebulization; manual or automatic valves; internal or external power source ♿⃠
MED: 100-3, 280.1

HUMIDIFIERS/COMPRESSORS/NEBULIZERS FOR USE WITH OXYGEN IPPB EQUIPMENT

Y **E0550** Humidifier, durable for extensive supplemental humidification during IPPB treatments or oxygen delivery ♿⃠
MED: 100-3, 280.1

Y **E0555** Humidifier, durable, glass or autoclavable plastic bottle type, for use with regulator or flowmeter ⃠
MED: 100-3, 280.1

Y **E0560** Humidifier, durable for supplemental humidification during IPPB treatment or oxygen delivery ♿⃠
MED: 100-3, 280.1

Y **E0561** Humidifier, non-heated, used with positive airway pressure device ♿⃠

Y **E0562** Humidifier, heated, used with positive airway pressure device ♿⃠

Y **E0565** Compressor, air power source for equipment which is not self-contained or cylinder driven ♿⃠

Y **E0570** Nebulizer, with compressor ♿⃠
MED: 100-3, 280.1

Y **E0571** Aerosol compressor, battery powered, for use with small volume nebulizer ♿⃠
MED: 100-3, 280.1

Intermittent Positive Pressure Breathing (IPPB) devices

Special Coverage Instructions | Noncovered by Medicare | Carrier Discretion | ☑ Quantity Alert ● New Code ○ Reinstated Code ▲ Revised Code

2005 HCPCS | ♀ Female Only | ♂ Male Only | 1-9 ASC Groups | MED: Pub 100/NCD Reference | ♿ DMEPOS Paid | ⃠ SNF Excluded | **E Codes — 45**

Ⓨ **E0572** Aerosol compressor, adjustable pressure, light duty for intermittent use   ♿⊘

Ⓨ **E0574** Ultrasonic/electronic aerosol generator with small volume nebulizer   ♿⊘

Ⓨ **E0575** Nebulizer, ultrasonic, large volume   ♿⊘
MED: 100-3, 280.1

Ⓨ **E0580** Nebulizer, durable, glass or autoclavable plastic, bottle type, for use with regulator or flowmeter ♿⊘
MED: 100-3, 280.1

Ⓨ **E0585** Nebulizer, with compressor and heater   ♿⊘
MED: 100-3, 280.1

Ⓨ **E0590** Dispensing fee covered drug administered through DME nebulizer suction pump, home model, portable   ⊘

SUCTION PUMP/ROOM VAPORIZERS

Ⓨ **E0600** Respiratory suction pump, home model, portable or stationary, electric   ♿⊘
MED: 100-3, 280.1

Ⓨ **E0601** Continuous airway pressure (CPAP) device   ♿⊘
MED: 100-3, 240.4

Ⓨ **E0602** Breast pump, manual, any type   Ⓜ♀♿⊘

Ⓐ **E0603** Breast pump, electric (AC and/or DC), any type   Ⓜ♀⊘

Ⓐ **E0604** Breast pump, heavy duty, hospital grade, piston operated, pulsatile vacuum suction/release cycles, vacuum regulator, supplies, transformer, electric (AC and/or DC)   Ⓜ♀⊘

Ⓨ **E0605** Vaporizer, room type   ♿⊘
MED: 100-3, 280.1

Ⓨ **E0606** Postural drainage board   ♿⊘
MED: 100-3, 280.1

MONITORING EQUIPMENT

Ⓨ **E0607** Home blood glucose monitor   ♿⊘
Medicare covers home blood testing devices for diabetic patients when the devices are prescribed by the patients' physicians. Many commercial payers provide this coverage to non-insulin dependent diabetics as well.
MED: 100-3, 230.16

PACEMAKER MONITOR

Ⓨ **E0610** Pacemaker monitor, self-contained, checks battery depletion, includes audible and visible check systems   ♿⊘
MED: 100-3, 20.8; 100-3, 20.8; 100-3, 20.8.1; 100-3, 20.8.1; 100-3, 20.8.2

Ⓨ **E0615** Pacemaker monitor, self-contained, checks battery depletion and other pacemaker components, includes digital/visible check systems   ♿⊘
MED: 100-3, 20.8; 100-3, 20.8; 100-3, 20.8.1; 100-3, 20.8.1; 100-3, 20.8.2

Ⓝ **E0616** Implantable cardiac event recorder with memory, activator and programmer   ⊘

Ⓨ **E0617** External defibrillator with integrated electrocardiogram analysis   ♿⊘

Ⓐ **E0618** Apnea monitor, without recording feature   ♿

Ⓐ **E0619** Apnea monitor, with recording feature   ♿

Ⓨ **E0620** Skin piercing device for collection of capillary blood, laser, each   ♿⊘

PATIENT LIFTS

Ⓨ **E0621** Sling or seat, patient lift, canvas or nylon   ♿⊘
MED: 100-3, 280.1

▲ Ⓔ **E0625** Patient lift, bathroom or toilet, not otherwise classified   ⊘
MED: 100-3, 280.1

Ⓨ **E0627** Seat lift mechanism incorporated into a combination lift-chair mechanism   ♿⊘
MED: 100-3, 280.4; 100-4, 20, 100; 100-4, 20, 130.2; 100-4, 20, 130.3; 100-4, 20, 130.4; 100-4, 20, 130.5
See code(s): Q0080

Ⓨ **E0628** Separate seat lift mechanism for use with patient owned furniture — electric   ♿⊘
MED: 100-3, 280.4; 100-4, 20, 100; 100-4, 20, 130.2; 100-4, 20, 130.3; 100-4, 20, 130.4; 100-4, 20, 130.5
See code(s): Q0078

Ⓨ **E0629** Separate seat lift mechanism for use with patient owned furniture — nonelectric   ♿⊘
MED: 100-4, 20, 100; 100-4, 20, 130.2; 100-4, 20, 130.3; 100-4, 20, 130.4; 100-4, 20, 130.5
See code(s): Q0079

Ⓨ **E0630** Patient lift, hydraulic, with seat or sling   ♿⊘
MED: 100-3, 280.1

Ⓨ **E0635** Patient lift, electric, with seat or sling   ♿⊘
MED: 100-3, 280.1

Ⓨ **E0636** Multipositional patient support system, with integrated lift, patient accessible controls   ♿

● Ⓨ **E0637** Combination sit to stand system, any size, with seat lift feature, with or without wheels   ♿⊘
MED: 100-3, 280.1

Ⓨ **E0638** Standing frame system, any size, with or without wheels   ♿⊘
MED: 100-3, 280.1

● **E0639** Patient lift, moveable from room to room with disassembly and reassembly, includes all components/accessories

● **E0640** Patient lift, fixed system, includes all components/accessories

PNEUMATIC COMPRESSOR AND APPLIANCES

Ⓨ **E0650** Pneumatic compressor, nonsegmental home model   ♿⊘
MED: 100-3, 280.6

Ⓨ **E0651** Pneumatic compressor, segmental home model without calibrated gradient pressure   ♿⊘
MED: 100-3, 280.6

Ⓨ **E0652** Pneumatic compressor, segmental home model with calibrated gradient pressure   ♿⊘
MED: 100-3, 280.6

Ⓨ **E0655** Nonsegmental pneumatic appliance for use with pneumatic compressor, half arm   ♿⊘
MED: 100-3, 280.6

Ⓨ **E0660** Nonsegmental pneumatic appliance for use with pneumatic compressor, full leg   ♿⊘
MED: 100-3, 280.6

Ⓨ **E0665** Nonsegmental pneumatic appliance for use with pneumatic compressor, full arm   ♿⊘
MED: 100-3, 280.6

Ⓨ **E0666** Nonsegmental pneumatic appliance for use with pneumatic compressor, half leg   ♿⊘
MED: 100-3, 280.6

Special Coverage Instructions   Noncovered by Medicare   Carrier Discretion   ☑ Quantity Alert   ● New Code   ○ Reinstated Code   ▲ Revised Code

46 — E Codes   Ⓐ Adult   Ⓜ Maternity   Ⓟ Pediatrics   Ⓘ Infant   Ⓐ-Ⓨ APC Status Indicator   **2005 HCPCS**

☑ **E0667** Segmental pneumatic appliance for use with pneumatic compressor, full leg   ♿⊘
MED: 100-3, 280.6

☑ **E0668** Segmental pneumatic appliance for use with pneumatic compressor, full arm   ♿⊘
MED: 100-3, 280.6

☑ **E0669** Segmental pneumatic appliance for use with pneumatic compressor, half leg   ♿⊘
MED: 100-3, 280.6

☑ **E0671** Segmental gradient pressure pneumatic appliance, full leg   ♿⊘
MED: 100-3, 280.6

☑ **E0672** Segmental gradient pressure pneumatic appliance, full arm   ♿⊘
MED: 100-3, 280.6

☑ **E0673** Segmental gradient pressure pneumatic appliance, half leg   ♿⊘
MED: 100-3, 280.6

☑ **E0675** Pneumatic compression device, high pressure, rapid inflation/deflation cycle, for arterial insufficiency (unilateral or bilateral system)   ♿⊘

☑ **E0691** Ultraviolet light therapy system panel, includes bulbs/lamps, timer and eye protection; treatment area two sq. feet or less   ♿

☑ **E0692** Ultraviolet light therapy system panel, includes bulbs/lamps, timer and eye protection, four foot panel   ♿

☑ **E0693** Ultraviolet light therapy system panel, includes bulbs/lamps, timer and eye protection, six foot panel   ♿

☑ **E0694** Ultraviolet multidirectional light therapy system in six foot cabinet, includes bulbs/lamps, timer and eye protection   ♿

SAFETY EQUIPMENT

Ⓔ **E0700** Safety equipment (e.g., belt, harness or vest)   ⊘

☑ **E0701** Helmet with face guard and soft interface material, prefabricated   ♿

RESTRAINTS

Ⓔ **E0710** Restraint, any type (body, chest, wrist or ankle)   ⊘

Fabric wrist restraint

Padded leather restraints may feature a locking device

Restraints (E0710)

Body restraint

Fabric gait belt for assistance in walking (E0700)

TRANSCUTANEOUS AND/OR NEUROMUSCULAR ELECTRICAL NERVE STIMULATORS — TENS

☑ **E0720** TENS, two lead, localized stimulation   ♿⊘
While TENS is covered when employed to control chronic pain, it is not covered for experimental treatment, as in motor function disorders like MS. Prior authorization is required by Medicare for this item.

MED: 100-3, 130.5; 100-3, 130.5; 100-3, 130.6; 100-3, 130.6; 100-3, 160.2; 100-3, 160.2; 100-3, 160.2; 100-3, 160.7.1; 100-3, 230.1; 100-3, 230.1; 100-3, 40.5; 100-3, 40.5; 100-3, 40.5; 100-3, 40.5; 100-3, 40.5; 100-3, 40.5; 100-3, 40.5; 100-3, 40.5; 100-3, 40.5; 100-3, 40.5; 100-3, 40.5; 100-3, 40.5; 100-3, 40.5; 100-3, 40.5; 100-8, 5, 5.1.1.2.1

☑ **E0730** TENS, four or more leads, for multiple nerve stimulation   ♿⊘
While TENS is covered when employed to control chronic pain, it is not covered for experimental treatment, as in motor function disorders like MS. Prior authorization is required by Medicare for this item.

MED: 100-3, 130.5; 100-3, 130.5; 100-3, 130.6; 100-3, 130.6; 100-3, 160.2; 100-3, 160.2; 100-3, 160.2; 100-3, 160.2; 100-3, 160.7.1; 100-3, 230.1; 100-3, 230.1; 100-3, 40.5; 100-3, 40.5; 100-3, 40.5; 100-3, 40.5; 100-3, 40.5; 100-3, 40.5; 100-3, 40.5; 100-3, 40.5; 100-3, 40.5; 100-3, 40.5; 100-3, 40.5; 100-3, 40.5; 100-3, 40.5; 100-3, 40.5; 100-8, 5, 5.1.1.2.1

☑ **E0731** Form-fitting conductive garment for delivery of TENS or NMES (with conductive fibers separated from the patient's skin by layers of fabric)   ♿⊘
MED: 100-3, 160.13

☑ **E0740** Incontinence treatment system, pelvic floor stimulator, monitor, sensor and/or trainer   ♿⊘
MED: 100-3, 230.8

☑ **E0744** Neuromuscular stimulator for scoliosis   ♿⊘

☑ **E0745** Neuromuscular stimulator, electronic shock unit   ♿⊘
MED: 100-3, 160.12

Ⓔ **E0746** Electromyography (EMG), biofeedback device   ⊘
Biofeedback therapy is covered by Medicare only for re-education of specific muscles or for treatment of incapacitating muscle spasm or weakness. Medicare jurisdiction: local carrier.

MED: 100-3, 30.1; 100-3, 30.1.1

☑ **E0747** Osteogenesis stimulator, electrical, noninvasive, other than spinal applications   ♿⊘
Medicare covers noninvasive osteogenic stimulation for nonunion of long bone fractures, failed fusion, or congenital pseudoarthroses.

MED: 100-3, 150.2

☑ **E0748** Osteogenesis stimulator, electrical, noninvasive, spinal applications   ♿⊘
Medicare covers noninvasive osteogenic stimulation as an adjunct to spinal fusion surgery for patients at high risk of pseudoarthroses due to previously failed spinal fusion, or for those undergoing fusion of three or more vertebrae.

MED: 100-3, 150.2

Ⓝ **E0749** Osteogenesis stimulator, electrical, surgically implanted   ♿⊘
Medicare covers invasive osteogenic stimulation for nonunion of long bone fractures or as an adjunct to spinal fusion surgery for patients at high risk of pseudoarthroses due to previously failed spinal fusion, or for those undergoing fusion of three or more vertebrae.

MED: 100-3, 150.2

Ⓑ **E0752** Implantable neurostimulator electrode, each   ♿⊘
MED: 100-3, 160.7

AHA: 1Q, '02, 9

Special Coverage Instructions   Noncovered by Medicare   Carrier Discretion   ☑ Quantity Alert   ● New Code   ○ Reinstated Code   ▲ Revised Code

2005 HCPCS   ♀ Female Only   ♂ Male Only   **1**-**9** ASC Groups   MED: Pub 100/NCD Reference   ♿ DMEPOS Paid   ⊘ SNF Excluded   **E Codes — 47**

Durable Medical Equipment

E0754 — E0920

[A] **E0754** Patient programmer (external) for use with implantable programmable neurostimulator pulse generator   ⅄⊘
MED: 100-3, 160.7

[E] **E0755** Electronic salivary reflex stimulator (intraoral/noninvasive)   ⊘

[B] **E0756** Implantable neurostimulator pulse generator   ⅄
Medicare jurisdiction: local carrier.
MED: 100-3, 160.7
AHA: 1Q, '02, 9

[N] **E0757** Implantable neurostimulator radiofrequency receiver   ⅄
Medicare jurisdiction: local carrier.
MED: 100-3, 160.7

[A] **E0758** Radiofrequency transmitter (external) for use with implantable neurostimulator radiofrequency receiver   ⅄
Medicare jurisdiction: local carrier.
MED: 100-3, 160.7

[A] **E0759** Radiofrequency transmitter (external) for use with implantable sacral root neurostimulator receiver for bowel and bladder management, replacement   ⅄⊘

[Y] **E0760** Osteogenesis stimulator, low intensity ultrasound, non-invasive   ⅄⊘
MED: 100-3, 150.2

[E] **E0761** Non-thermal pulsed high frequency radiowaves, high peak power electromagnetic energy treatment device

[Y] **E0765** FDA approved nerve stimulator, with replaceable batteries, for treatment of nausea and vomiting ⅄⊘

● **E0769** Electrical stimulation or electromagnetic wound treatment device, not otherwise classified
MED: 100-4, 32, 11.1

INFUSION SUPPLIES

[Y] **E0776** IV pole   ⅄⊘

[Y] **E0779** Ambulatory infusion pump, mechanical, reusable, for infusion 8 hours or greater   ⅄⊘

[Y] **E0780** Ambulatory infusion pump, mechanical, reusable, for infusion less than 8 hours   ⅄⊘

[Y] **E0781** Ambulatory infusion pump, single or multiple channels, electric or battery operated, with administrative equipment, worn by patient   ⅄⊘
Medicare jurisdiction: DME local or regional carrier. Bill Medicare claims for regional carrier when the infusion is initiated in the physician's office but the patient does not return during the same day of business.
MED: 100-3, 280.14

[N] **E0782** Infusion pump, implantable, non-programmable (includes all components, e.g., pump, catheter, connectors, etc.)   ⅄⊘
Medicare jurisdiction: local carrier.
MED: 100-3, 280.14

[N] **E0783** Infusion pump system, implantable, programmable (includes all components, e.g., pump, catheter, connectors, etc.)   ⅄⊘
Medicare jurisdiction: local carrier.
MED: 100-3, 280.14

[Y] **E0784** External ambulatory infusion pump, insulin ⅄⊘
Covered by some commercial payers with preauthorization.
MED: 100-3, 280.14

[N] **E0785** Implantable intraspinal (epidural/intrathecal) catheter used with implantable infusion pump, replacement   ⅄⊘
Medicare jurisdiction: local carrier.
MED: 100-3, 280.14

[N] **E0786** Implantable programmable infusion pump, replacement (excludes implantable intraspinal catheter)   ⅄⊘
Medicare jurisdiction: local carrier.
MED: 100-3, 280.14

[Y] **E0791** Parenteral infusion pump, stationary, single or multichannel   ⅄⊘
MED: 100-2, 15, 120; 100-3, 180.2; 100-4, 20, 100.2.2; 100-4, 20, 100.2.2.3

TRACTION — ALL TYPES

[N] **E0830** Ambulatory traction device, all types, each   ⊘
MED: 100-3, 280.1

TRACTION — CERVICAL

[Y] **E0840** Traction frame, attached to headboard, cervical traction   ⅄⊘
MED: 100-3, 280.1

● **E0849** Traction equipment, cervical, free-standing stand/frame, pneumatic, applying traction force to other than mandible

[Y] **E0850** Traction stand, freestanding, cervical traction   ⅄⊘
MED: 100-3, 280.1

[Y] **E0855** Cervical traction equipment not requiring additional stand or frame   ⅄⊘

TRACTION — OVERDOOR

[Y] **E0860** Traction equipment, overdoor, cervical   ⅄⊘
MED: 100-3, 280.1

TRACTION — EXTREMITY

[Y] **E0870** Traction frame, attached to footboard, extremity traction (e.g., Buck's)   ⅄⊘
MED: 100-3, 280.1

[Y] **E0880** Traction stand, freestanding, extremity traction (e.g., Buck's)   ⅄⊘
MED: 100-3, 280.1

TRACTION — PELVIC

[Y] **E0890** Traction frame, attached to footboard, pelvic traction   ⅄⊘
MED: 100-3, 280.1

[Y] **E0900** Traction stand, freestanding, pelvic traction (e.g., Buck's)   ⅄⊘
MED: 100-3, 280.1

TRAPEZE EQUIPMENT, FRACTURE FRAME, AND OTHER ORTHOPEDIC DEVICES

[Y] **E0910** Trapeze bars, also known as Patient Helper, attached to bed, with grab bar   ⅄⊘
MED: 100-3, 280.1

[Y] **E0920** Fracture frame, attached to bed, includes weights   ⅄⊘
MED: 100-3, 280.1

Special Coverage Instructions   Noncovered by Medicare   Carrier Discretion   ☑ Quantity Alert   ● New Code   ○ Reinstated Code   ▲ Revised Code

48 — E Codes   [A] Adult   [M] Maternity   [P] Pediatrics   [I] Infant   [A]-[Y] APC Status Indicator   **2005 HCPCS**

Y	**E0930**	Fracture frame, freestanding, includes weights MED: 100-3, 280.1	ᵫ⊘
Y	**E0935**	Passive motion exercise device MED: 100-3, 280.1	ᵫ⊘
Y	**E0940**	Trapeze bar, freestanding, complete with grab bar MED: 100-3, 280.1	ᵫ⊘
Y	**E0941**	Gravity assisted traction device, any type MED: 100-3, 280.1	ᵫ⊘
Y	**E0942**	Cervical head harness/halter	ᵫ⊘
Y	**E0944**	Pelvic belt/harness/boot	ᵫ⊘
Y	**E0945**	Extremity belt/harness	ᵫ⊘
Y	**E0946**	Fracture frame, dual with cross bars, attached to bed (e.g., Balken, Four Poster) MED: 100-3, 280.1	ᵫ⊘
Y	**E0947**	Fracture frame, attachments for complex pelvic traction MED: 100-3, 280.1	ᵫ⊘
Y	**E0948**	Fracture frame, attachments for complex cervical traction MED: 100-3, 280.1	ᵫ⊘
E	**E0950**	Wheelchair accessory, tray, each MED: 100-3, 280.1	ᵫ⊘
▲ E	**E0951**	Heel loop/holder, any type, with or without ankle strap, each	ᵫ⊘
▲ E	**E0952**	Toe loop/holder, any type, each MED: 100-3, 280.1	ᵫ⊘
E ☑	**E0953**	Pneumatic tire, each MED: 100-3, 280.1 See code(s): K0067	⊘
E ☑	**E0954**	Semi-pneumatic caster, each MED: 100-3, 280.1 See code(s): K0075	⊘
▲ Y ☑	**E0955**	Wheelchair accessory, headrest, cushioned, any type, including fixed mounting hardware, each	ᵫ⊘
▲ Y ☑	**E0956**	Wheelchair accessory, lateral trunk or hip support, any type, including fixed mounting hardware, each	ᵫ⊘
▲ Y ☑	**E0957**	Wheelchair accessory, medial thigh support, any type, including fixed mounting hardware, each	ᵫ⊘
▲ A	**E0958**	Manual wheelchair accessory, one-arm drive attachment, each MED: 100-3, 280.1	ᵫ⊘
▲ B	**E0959**	Manual wheelchair accessory, adapter for amputee, each	ᵫ⊘
Y	**E0960**	Wheelchair accessory, shoulder harness/straps or chest strap, including any type mounting hardware	ᵫ⊘
▲ B	**E0961**	Manual wheelchair accessory, wheel lock brake extension (handle), each MED: 100-3, 280.1	ᵫ⊘
	~~**E0962**~~	~~One inch cushion, for wheelchair~~	
	~~**E0963**~~	~~Two inch cushion, for wheelchair~~	
	~~**E0964**~~	~~Three inch cushion, for wheelchair~~	
	~~**E0965**~~	~~Four inch cushion, for wheelchair~~	
▲ B	**E0966**	Manual wheelchair accessory, headrest extension, each MED: 100-3, 280.1	
▲ Y ☑	**E0967**	Manual wheelchair accessory, hand rim with projections, any type, replacement only, each MED: 100-3, 280.1	ᵫ⊘
Y	**E0968**	Commode seat, wheelchair MED: 100-3, 280.1	ᵫ⊘
Y	**E0969**	Narrowing device, wheelchair MED: 100-3, 280.1	ᵫ⊘
B	**E0970**	No. 2 footplates, except for elevating legrest MED: 100-3, 280.1 See code(s): K0037, K0042	⊘
B	**E0971**	Anti-tipping device, wheelchair MED: 100-3, 280.1 See code(s): K0021	ᵫ⊘
▲ B	**E0972**	Wheelchair accessory, transfer board or device, each	ᵫ⊘
▲ B	**E0973**	Wheelchair accessory, adjustable height, detachable armrest, complete assembly, each MED: 100-3, 280.1	ᵫ⊘
▲ B	**E0974**	Manual wheelchair accessory, anti-rollback device, each MED: 100-3, 280.1	ᵫ⊘
Y	**E0977**	Wedge cushion, wheelchair	ᵫ⊘
▲ B	**E0978**	Wheelchair accessory, positioning belt/safety belt/pelvic strap, each	ᵫ⊘
Y	**E0980**	Safety vest, wheelchair	ᵫ⊘
Y ☑	**E0981**	Wheelchair accessory, seat upholstery, replacement only, each	ᵫ⊘
Y ☑	**E0982**	Wheelchair accessory, back upholstery, replacement only, each	ᵫ⊘
Y	**E0983**	Manual wheelchair accessory, power add-on to convert manual wheelchair to motorized wheelchair, joystick control	ᵫ⊘
Y	**E0984**	Manual wheelchair accessory, power add-on to convert manual wheelchair to motorized wheelchair, tiller control	ᵫ⊘
Y	**E0985**	Wheelchair accessory, seat lift mechanism	ᵫ⊘
▲ Y ☑	**E0986**	Manual wheelchair accessory, push activated power assist, each	ᵫ⊘
▲ B	**E0990**	Wheelchair accessory, elevating leg rest, complete assembly, each MED: 100-3, 280.1	ᵫ⊘
▲ B	**E0992**	Manual wheelchair accessory, solid seat insert	ᵫ⊘
Y ☑	**E0994**	Armrest, each MED: 100-3, 280.1	ᵫ⊘
▲ B	**E0995**	Wheelchair accessory, calf rest/pad, each MED: 100-3, 280.1	ᵫ⊘
B ☑	**E0996**	Tire, solid, each MED: 100-3, 280.1 See code(s): K0066	⊘
Y	**E0997**	Caster with fork MED: 100-3, 280.1	ᵫ⊘
Y	**E0998**	Caster without fork MED: 100-3, 280.1	ᵫ⊘

Special Coverage Instructions   Noncovered by Medicare   Carrier Discretion   ☑ Quantity Alert   ● New Code   ○ Reinstated Code   ▲ Revised Code

2005 HCPCS   ♀ Female Only   ♂ Male Only   **1**-**9** ASC Groups   MED: Pub 100/NCD Reference   ᵫ DMEPOS Paid   ⊘ SNF Excluded   **E Codes — 49**

☑   **E0999** Pneumatic tire with wheel   ↱○
MED: 100-3, 280.1

Ⓑ   **E1000** Tire, pneumatic caster   ○
MED: 100-3, 280.1
See code(s): K0074

☑ ☑   **E1001** Wheel, single   ↱○
MED: 100-3, 280.1

☑   **E1002** Wheelchair accessory, power seating system, tilt only   ↱○

☑   **E1003** Wheelchair accessory, power seating system, recline only, without shear reduction   ↱○

☑   **E1004** Wheelchair accessory, power seating system, recline only, with mechanical shear reduction   ↱○

☑   **E1005** Wheelchair accessory, power seating system, recline only, with power shear reduction   ↱○

☑   **E1006** Wheelchair accessory, power seating system, combination tilt and recline, without shear reduction   ↱○

☑   **E1007** Wheelchair accessory, power seating system, combination tilt and recline, with mechanical shear reduction   ↱○

☑   **E1008** Wheelchair accessory, power seating system, combination tilt and recline, with power shear reduction   ↱○

☑ ☑   **E1009** Wheelchair accessory, addition to power seating system, mechanically linked leg elevation system, including pushrod and leg rest, each   ↱○

▲ ☑ ☑   **E1010** Wheelchair accessory, addition to power seating system, power leg elevation system, including leg rest, pair   ↱○

▲ ☑   **E1011** Modification to pediatric size wheelchair, width adjustment package (not to be dispensed with initial chair)   ↱
MED: 100-3, 280.1

   ~~**E1012** Integrated seating system, planar, for pediatric wheelchair~~

   ~~**E1013** Integrated seating system, contoured, for pediatric wheelchair~~

▲ ☑   **E1014** Reclining back, addition to pediatric size wheelchair   ↱
MED: 100-3, 280.1

☑   **E1015** Shock absorber for manual wheelchair, each   ↱
MED: 100-3, 280.1

☑   **E1016** Shock absorber for power wheelchair, each   ↱
MED: 100-3, 280.1

☑   **E1017** Heavy duty shock absorber for heavy duty or extra heavy duty manual wheelchair, each   ↱
MED: 100-3, 280.1

☑   **E1018** Heavy duty shock absorber for heavy duty or extra heavy duty power wheelchair, each   ↱
MED: 100-3, 280.1

▲ ☑   **E1019** Wheelchair accessory, power seating system, heavy duty feature, patient weight capacity greater than 250 pounds and less than or equal to 400 pounds   ○

☑   **E1020** Residual limb support system for wheelchair   ↱
MED: 100-3, 280.3

▲ ☑   **E1021** Wheelchair accessory, power seating system, extra heavy duty feature, weight capacity greater than 400 pounds   ○

☑   **E1025** Lateral thoracic support, non-contoured, for pediatric wheelchair, each (includes hardware)   ↱

☑   **E1026** Lateral thoracic support, contoured, for pediatric wheelchair, each (includes hardware)   ↱

☑   **E1027** Lateral/anterior support, for pediatric wheelchair, each (includes hardware)   ↱

☑   **E1028** Wheelchair accessory, manual swingaway, retractable or removable mounting hardware for joystick, other control interface or positioning accessory   ↱○

☑   **E1029** Wheelchair accessory, ventilator tray, fixed   ↱○

☑   **E1030** Wheelchair accessory, ventilator tray, gimbaled   ↱○

ROLLABOUT CHAIR

☑   **E1031** Rollabout chair, any and all types with casters five in. or greater   ↱○
MED: 100-3, 280.1

☑   **E1035** Multi-positional patient transfer system, with integrated seat, operated by care giver   ↱○
MED: 100-2, 15, 110

☑   **E1037** Transport chair, pediatric size   ↱
MED: 100-3, 280.1

▲ ☑   **E1038** Transport chair, adult size, patient weight capacity less than 250 pounds   ↱
MED: 100-3, 280.1

●   **E1039** Transport chair, adult size, heavy duty, patient weight capacity 250 pounds or greater

WHEELCHAIRS — FULLY RECLINING

Ⓐ   **E1050** Fully reclining wheelchair; fixed full-length arms, swing-away, detachable, elevating legrests   ↱○
MED: 100-3, 280.1

Ⓐ   **E1060** Fully reclining wheelchair; detachable arms, desk or full-length, swing-away, detachable, elevating legrests   ↱○
MED: 100-3, 280.1

Ⓐ   **E1070** Fully reclining wheelchair; detachable arms, desk or full-length, swing-away, detachable footrests   ↱○
MED: 100-3, 280.1

Ⓐ   **E1083** Hemi-wheelchair; fixed full-length arms, swing-away, detachable, elevating legrests   ↱○
MED: 100-3, 280.1

Ⓐ   **E1084** Hemi-wheelchair; detachable arms, desk or full-length, swing-away, detachable, elevating legrests   ↱○
MED: 100-3, 280.1

Ⓐ   **E1085** Hemi-wheelchair; fixed full-length arms, swing-away, detachable footrests   ○
MED: 100-3, 280.1
See code(s): K0002

Ⓐ   **E1086** Hemi-wheelchair; detachable arms, desk or full-length, swing-away, detachable footrests   ○
MED: 100-3, 280.1
See code(s): K0002

Ⓐ   **E1087** High-strength lightweight wheelchair; fixed full-length arms, swing-away, detachable, elevating legrests   ↱○
MED: 100-3, 280.1

| Special Coverage Instructions | Noncovered by Medicare | Carrier Discretion | ☑ Quantity Alert | ● New Code | ○ Reinstated Code | ▲ Revised Code |

50 — E Codes   Ⓐ Adult   Ⓜ Maternity   Ⓟ Pediatrics   Ⓘ Infant   Ⓐ-Ⓨ APC Status Indicator   **2005 HCPCS**

Ⓐ **E1088** High-strength lightweight wheelchair; detachable arms, desk or full-length, swing-away, detachable, elevating legrests   🦽⊘
MED: 100-3, 280.1

Ⓐ **E1089** High-strength lightweight wheelchair; fixed-length arms, swing-away, detachable footrests   ⊘
MED: 100-3, 280.1
See code(s): K0004

Ⓐ **E1090** High-strength lightweight wheelchair; detachable arms, desk or full-length, swing-away, detachable footrests   ⊘
MED: 100-3, 280.1
See code(s): K0004

Ⓐ **E1092** Wide, heavy-duty wheelchair; detachable arms, desk or full-length, swing-away, detachable, elevating legrests   🦽⊘
MED: 100-3, 280.1

Ⓐ **E1093** Wide, heavy-duty wheelchair; detachable arms, desk or full-length arms, swing-away, detachable footrests   🦽⊘
MED: 100-3, 280.1

WHEELCHAIR — SEMI-RECLINING

Ⓐ **E1100** Semi-reclining wheelchair; fixed full-length arms, swing-away, detachable, elevating legrests   🦽⊘
MED: 100-3, 280.1

Ⓐ **E1110** Semi-reclining wheelchair; detachable arms, desk or full-length, elevating legrest   🦽⊘
MED: 100-3, 280.1

WHEELCHAIR — STANDARD

Ⓐ **E1130** Standard wheelchair; fixed full-length arms, fixed or swing-away, detachable footrests   ⊘
MED: 100-3, 280.1
See code(s): K0001

Ⓐ **E1140** Wheelchair; detachable arms, desk or full-length, swing-away, detachable footrests   ⊘
MED: 100-3, 280.1
See code(s): K0001

Ⓨ **E1150** Wheelchair; detachable arms, desk or full-length, swing-away, detachable, elevating legrests   🦽⊘
MED: 100-3, 280.1

Ⓐ **E1160** Wheelchair; fixed full-length arms, swing-away, detachable, elevating legrests   🦽⊘
MED: 100-3, 280.1

Ⓐ **E1161** Manual adult size wheelchair, includes tilt in space   🦽

WHEELCHAIR — AMPUTEE

Ⓐ **E1170** Amputee wheelchair; fixed full-length arms, swing-away, detachable, elevating legrests   🦽⊘
MED: 100-3, 280.1

Ⓐ **E1171** Amputee wheelchair; fixed full-length arms, without footrests or legrests   🦽⊘
MED: 100-3, 280.1

Ⓐ **E1172** Amputee wheelchair; detachable arms, desk or full-length, without footrests or legrests   🦽⊘
MED: 100-3, 280.1

Ⓐ **E1180** Amputee wheelchair; detachable arms, desk or full-length, swing-away, detachable footrests   🦽⊘
MED: 100-3, 280.1

Ⓐ **E1190** Amputee wheelchair; detachable arms, desk or full-length, swing-away, detachable, elevating legrests   🦽⊘
MED: 100-3, 280.1

Ⓐ **E1195** Heavy duty wheelchair; fixed full-length arms, swing-away, detachable, elevating legrests   🦽⊘
MED: 100-3, 280.1

Ⓐ **E1200** Amputee wheelchair; fixed full-length arms, swing-away, detachable footrests   🦽⊘
MED: 100-3, 280.1

WHEELCHAIR — POWER

Ⓨ **E1210** Motorized wheelchair; fixed full-length arms, swing-away, detachable, elevating legrests   🦽⊘
MED: 100-3, 280.1; 100-3, 280.9

Ⓨ **E1211** Motorized wheelchair; detachable arms, desk or full-length, swing-away, detachable, elevating legrests   🦽⊘
MED: 100-3, 280.1; 100-3, 280.9

Ⓐ **E1212** Motorized wheelchair; fixed full-length arms, swing-away, detachable footrests   ⊘
MED: 100-3, 280.1; 100-3, 280.9
See code(s): K0010

Ⓐ **E1213** Motorized wheelchair; detachable arms, desk or full-length, swing-away, detachable footrests   ⊘
MED: 100-3, 280.1; 100-3, 280.9
See code(s): K0010

WHEELCHAIR — SPECIAL SIZE

Ⓐ **E1220** Wheelchair; specially sized or constructed (indicate brand name, model number, if any, and justification)   ⊘
MED: 100-3, 280.3

Ⓐ **E1221** Wheelchair with fixed arm, footrests   🦽⊘
MED: 100-3, 280.3

Ⓐ **E1222** Wheelchair with fixed arm, elevating legrests   🦽⊘
MED: 100-3, 280.3

Ⓐ **E1223** Wheelchair with detachable arms, footrests   🦽⊘
MED: 100-3, 280.3

Ⓐ **E1224** Wheelchair with detachable arms, elevating legrests   🦽⊘
MED: 100-3, 280.3

▲ Ⓨ **E1225** Wheelchair accessory, manual semi-reclining back, (recline greater than 15 degrees, but less than 80 degrees), each   🦽⊘
MED: 100-3, 280.3

▲ Ⓑ **E1226** Wheelchair accessory, manual fully reclining back, (recline greater than 80 degrees), each   🦽⊘
See also K0028
MED: 100-3, 280.1

Ⓨ **E1227** Special height arms for wheelchair   🦽⊘
MED: 100-3, 280.3

Ⓨ **E1228** Special back height for wheelchair   🦽⊘
MED: 100-3, 280.3

● **E1229** Wheelchair, pediatric size, not otherwise specified

Ⓨ **E1230** Power operated vehicle (three- or four-wheel nonhighway), specify brand name and model number   🦽⊘
Prior authorization is required by Medicare for this item.
MED: 100-3, 280.9; 100-8, 5, 5.1.1.2.1

| Special Coverage Instructions | Noncovered by Medicare | Carrier Discretion | ☑ Quantity Alert ● New Code ○ Reinstated Code ▲ Revised Code |

2005 HCPCS   ♀ Female Only   ♂ Male Only   1-9 ASC Groups   MED: Pub 100/NCD Reference   🦽 DMEPOS Paid   ⊘ SNF Excluded   **E Codes — 51**

Durable Medical Equipment

E1231 — E1520

☒   **E1231** Wheelchair, pediatric size, tilt-in-space, rigid, adjustable, with seating system   ♿
MED: 100-3, 280.1

☒   **E1232** Wheelchair, pediatric size, tilt-in-space, folding, adjustable, with seating system   ♿
MED: 100-3, 280.1

☒   **E1233** Wheelchair, pediatric size, tilt-in-space, rigid, adjustable, without seating system   ♿
MED: 100-3, 280.1

☒   **E1234** Wheelchair, pediatric size, tilt-in-space, folding, adjustable, without seating system   ♿
MED: 100-3, 280.1

☒   **E1235** Wheelchair, pediatric size, rigid, adjustable, with seating system   ♿
MED: 100-3, 280.1

☒   **E1236** Wheelchair, pediatric size, folding, adjustable, with seating system   ♿
MED: 100-3, 280.1

☒   **E1237** Wheelchair, pediatric size, rigid, adjustable, without seating system   ♿
MED: 100-3, 280.1

☒   **E1238** Wheelchair, pediatric size, folding, adjustable, without seating system   ♿
MED: 100-3, 280.1

●   **E1239** Power wheelchair, pediatric size, not otherwise specified

WHEELCHAIR — LIGHTWEIGHT

Ⓐ   **E1240** Lightweight wheelchair; detachable arms, desk or full-length, swing-away, detachable, elevating legrest   ♿⊘
MED: 100-3, 280.1

Ⓐ   **E1250** Lightweight wheelchair; fixed full-length arms, swing-away, detachable footrests   ⊘
MED: 100-3, 280.1
See code(s): K0003

Ⓐ   **E1260** Lightweight wheelchair; detachable arms, desk or full-length, swing-away, detachable footrests   ⊘
MED: 100-3, 280.1
See code(s): K0003

Ⓐ   **E1270** Lightweight wheelchair; fixed full-length arms, swing-away, detachable elevating legrests   ♿⊘
MED: 100-3, 280.1

WHEELCHAIR — HEAVY-DUTY

Ⓐ   **E1280** Heavy-duty wheelchair; detachable arms, desk or full-length, elevating legrests   ♿⊘
MED: 100-3, 280.1

Ⓐ   **E1285** Heavy-duty wheelchair; fixed full-length arms, swing-away, detachable footrests   ⊘
MED: 100-3, 280.1
See code(s): K0006

Ⓐ   **E1290** Heavy-duty wheelchair; detachable arms, desk or full-length, swing-away, detachable footrests   ⊘
MED: 100-3, 280.1
See code(s): K0006

Ⓐ   **E1295** Heavy-duty wheelchair; fixed full-length arms, elevating legrests   ♿⊘
MED: 100-3, 280.1

☒   **E1296** Special wheelchair seat height from floor   ♿⊘
MED: 100-3, 280.3

☒   **E1297** Special wheelchair seat depth, by upholstery   ♿⊘
MED: 100-3, 280.3

☒   **E1298** Special wheelchair seat depth and/or width, by construction   ♿⊘
MED: 100-3, 280.3

WHIRLPOOL — EQUIPMENT

Ⓔ   **E1300** Whirlpool, portable (overtub type)   ⊘
MED: 100-3, 280.1

☒   **E1310** Whirlpool, nonportable (built-in type)   ♿⊘
MED: 100-3, 280.1

REPAIRS AND REPLACEMENT SUPPLIES

☒   ☑   **E1340** Repair or nonroutine service for durable medical equipment requiring the skill of a technician, labor component, per 15 minutes
Medicare jurisdiction: local carrier if repair or implanted DME.

MED: 100-2, 15, 110.2

ADDITIONAL OXYGEN RELATED EQUIPMENT

☒   **E1353** Regulator   ⊘
MED: 100-3, 240.2

☒   **E1355** Stand/rack   ⊘
MED: 100-3, 240.2

☒   **E1372** Immersion external heater for nebulizer   ♿⊘
MED: 100-3, 240.2

☒   **E1390** Oxygen concentrator, single delivery port, capable of delivering 85 percent or greater oxygen concentration at the prescribed flow rate   ♿⊘
MED: 100-3, 240.2

☒   ☑   **E1391** Oxygen concentrator, dual delivery port, capable of delivering 85 percent or greater oxygen concentration at the prescribed flow rate, each   ♿⊘
MED: 100-3, 240.2

Ⓝ   **E1399** Durable medical equipment, miscellaneous   ⊘
Determine if an alternative HCPCS Level II or a CPT code better describes the service being reported. This code should be used only if a more specific code is unavailable. Medicare jurisdiction: local carrier if repair or implanted DME.

☒   **E1405** Oxygen and water vapor enriching system with heated delivery   ♿⊘
MED: 100-3, 240.2; 100-4, 20, 20; 100-4, 20, 20.4

☒   **E1406** Oxygen and water vapor enriching system without heated delivery   ♿⊘
MED: 100-3, 240.2; 100-4, 20, 20; 100-4, 20, 20.4

ARTIFICIAL KIDNEY MACHINES AND ACCESSORIES

For glucose monitors, see A4253–A4256. For supplies for ESRD, see procedure codes A4651–A4929.

Ⓐ   **E1500** Centrifuge, for dialysis   ⊘

Ⓐ   **E1510** Kidney, dialysate delivery system kidney machine, pump recirculating, air removal system, flowrate meter, power off, heater and temp control with alarm, IV poles, pressure gauge, concentrate container   ⊘

Ⓐ   **E1520** Heparin infusion pump for hemodialysis   ⊘

Special Coverage Instructions   Noncovered by Medicare   Carrier Discretion   ☑ Quantity Alert   ● New Code   ○ Reinstated Code   ▲ Revised Code

52 — E Codes   Ⓐ Adult   Ⓜ Maternity   Ⓟ Pediatrics   Ⓘ Infant   Ⓐ-☒ APC Status Indicator   ***2005 HCPCS***

Ⓐ		E1530	Air bubble detector for hemodialysis, each, replacement	⊘
Ⓐ		E1540	Pressure alarm for hemodialysis, each, replacement	⊘
Ⓐ		E1550	Bath conductivity meter for hemodialysis, each	⊘
Ⓐ		E1560	Blood leak detector for hemodialysis, each, replacement	⊘
Ⓐ		E1570	Adjustable chair, for ESRD patients	⊘
Ⓐ	☑	E1575	Transducer protectors/fluid barriers, for hemodialysis, any size, per 10	⊘
Ⓐ		E1580	Unipuncture control system for hemodialysis	⊘
Ⓐ		E1590	Hemodialysis machine	⊘
Ⓐ		E1592	Automatic intermittent peritoneal dialysis system	⊘
Ⓐ		E1594	Cycler dialysis machine for peritoneal dialysis	⊘
Ⓐ		E1600	Delivery and/or installation charges for hemodialysis equipment	⊘
Ⓐ		E1610	Reverse osmosis water purification system, for hemodialysis MED: 100-3, 230.7	⊘
Ⓐ		E1615	Deionizer water purification system, for hemodialysis MED: 100-3, 230.7	⊘
Ⓐ		E1620	Blood pump for hemodialysis, replacement	⊘
Ⓐ		E1625	Water softening system, for hemodialysis MED: 100-3, 230.7	⊘
Ⓐ		E1630	Reciprocating peritoneal dialysis system	⊘
Ⓐ		E1632	Wearable artificial kidney, each	⊘
Ⓑ	☑	E1634	Peritoneal dialysis clamps, each MED: 100-4, 8, 130; 100-4, 8, 70; 100-4, 8, 80; 100-4, 8, 90; 100-4, 8, 90.1; 100-4, 8, 90.3.2	⊘
Ⓐ		E1635	Compact (portable) travel hemodialyzer system	⊘
Ⓐ	☑	E1636	Sorbent cartridges, for hemodialysis, per 10	⊘
Ⓐ	☑	E1637	Hemostats, each	⊘
Ⓐ	☑	E1639	Scale, each	⊘
Ⓐ		E1699	Dialysis equipment, not otherwise specified Determine if an alternative HCPCS Level II or a CPT code better describes the service being reported. This code should be used only if a more specific code is unavailable. Pertinent documentation to evaluate medical appropriateness should be included when this code is reported.	⊘

JAW MOTION REHABILITATION SYSTEM AND ACCESSORIES

Ⓨ		E1700	Jaw motion rehabilitation system Medicare jurisdiction: local carrier.	⅄⊘
Ⓨ	☑	E1701	Replacement cushions for jaw motion rehabilitation system, package of six Medicare jurisdiction: local carrier.	⅄⊘
Ⓨ	☑	E1702	Replacement measuring scales for jaw motion rehabilitation system, package of 200 Medicare jurisdiction: local carrier.	⅄⊘

OTHER ORTHOPEDIC DEVICES

Ⓨ		E1800	Dynamic adjustable elbow extension/flexion device, includes soft interface material	⅄⊘
Ⓨ		E1801	Bi-directional static progressive stretch elbow device with range of motion adjustment, includes cuffs	⅄⊘
Ⓨ		E1802	Dynamic adjustable forearm pronation/supination device, includes soft interface material	⅄
Ⓨ		E1805	Dynamic adjustable wrist extension/flexion device, includes soft interface material	⅄⊘
Ⓨ		E1806	Bi-directional static progressive stretch wrist device with range of motion adjustment, includes cuffs	⅄⊘
Ⓨ		E1810	Dynamic adjustable knee extension/flexion device, includes soft interface material	⅄⊘
Ⓨ		E1811	Bi-directional progressive stretch knee device with range of motion adjustment, includes cuffs	⅄⊘
Ⓨ		E1815	Dynamic adjustable ankle extension/flexion, includes soft interface material	⅄⊘
Ⓨ		E1816	Bi-directional static progressive stretch ankle device with range of motion adjustment, includes cuffs	⅄⊘
Ⓨ		E1818	Bi-directional static progressive stretch forearm pronation/supination device with range of motion adjustment, includes cuffs	⅄
Ⓨ		E1820	Replacement soft interface material, dynamic adjustable extension/flexion device	⅄⊘
Ⓨ		E1821	Replacement soft interface material/cuffs for bi-directional static progressive stretch device	⅄⊘
Ⓨ		E1825	Dynamic adjustable finger extension/flexion device, includes soft interface material	⅄⊘
Ⓨ		E1830	Dynamic adjustable toe extension/flexion device, includes soft interface material	⅄⊘
Ⓨ		E1840	Dynamic adjustable shoulder flexion/abduction/rotation device, includes soft interface material	⅄⊘
●		E1841	Multi-directional static progressive stretch shoulder device, with range of motion adjustability, includes cuffs	
Ⓐ		E1902	Communication board, non-electronic augmentative or alternative communication device	⊘
		E2000	Gastric suction pump, home model, portable or stationary, electric	⅄⊘
		E2100	Blood glucose monitor with integrated voice synthesizer MED: 100-3, 230.16	⅄
		E2101	Blood glucose monitor with integrated lancing/blood sample MED: 100-3, 230.16	⅄⊘
Ⓨ		E2120	Pulse generator system for tympanic treatment of inner ear endolymphatic fluid	⅄⊘
Ⓨ	☑	E2201	Manual wheelchair accessory, nonstandard seat frame, width greater than or equal to 20 in. and less than 24 in.	⅄⊘
Ⓨ	☑	E2202	Manual wheelchair accessory, nonstandard seat frame width, 24-27 in.	⅄⊘
Ⓨ	☑	E2203	Manual wheelchair accessory, nonstandard seat frame depth, 20 to less than 22 in.	⅄⊘
Ⓨ	☑	E2204	Manual wheelchair accessory, nonstandard seat frame depth, 22 to 25 in.	⅄⊘
●		E2205	Manual wheelchair accessory, handrim without projections, any type, replacement only, each	
●		E2206	Manual wheelchair accessory, wheel lock assembly, complete, each	
●		E2291	Back, planar, for pediatric size wheelchair including fixed attaching hardware	

Special Coverage Instructions   Noncovered by Medicare   Carrier Discretion   ☑ Quantity Alert   ● New Code   ○ Reinstated Code   ▲ Revised Code

Durable Medical Equipment

E1530 — E2291

Durable Medical Equipment

E2292 — E2506

●   **E2292** Seat, planar, for pediatric size wheelchair including fixed attaching hardware

●   **E2293** Back, contoured, for pediatric size wheelchair including fixed attaching hardware

●   **E2294** Seat, contoured, for pediatric size wheelchair including fixed attaching hardware

Ⓨ   **E2300** Power wheelchair accessory, power seat elevation system ⊘

Ⓨ   **E2301** Power wheelchair accessory, power standing system ⊘

Ⓨ   **E2310** Power wheelchair accessory, electronic connection between wheelchair controller and one power seating system motor, including all related electronics, indicator feature, mechanical function selection switch, and fixed mounting hardware ♿⊘

Ⓨ   **E2311** Power wheelchair accessory, electronic connection between wheelchair controller and two or more power seating system motors, including all related electronics, indicator feature, mechanical function selection switch, and fixed mounting hardware ♿⊘

Ⓨ   **E2320** Power wheelchair accessory, hand or chin control interface, remote joystick or touchpad, proportional, including all related electronics, and fixed mounting hardware ♿⊘

Ⓨ   **E2321** Power wheelchair accessory, hand control interface, remote joystick, nonproportional, including all related electronics, mechanical stop switch, and fixed mounting hardware ♿⊘

Ⓨ   **E2322** Power wheelchair accessory, hand control interface, multiple mechanical switches, nonproportional, including all related electronics, mechanical stop switch, and fixed mounting hardware ♿⊘

Ⓨ   **E2323** Power wheelchair accessory, specialty joystick handle for hand control interface, prefabricated ♿⊘

Ⓨ   **E2324** Power wheelchair accessory, chin cup for chin control interface ♿⊘

Ⓨ   **E2325** Power wheelchair accessory, sip and puff interface, nonproportional, including all related electronics, mechanical stop switch, and manual swingaway mounting hardware ♿⊘

Ⓨ   **E2326** Power wheelchair accessory, breath tube kit for sip and puff interface ♿⊘

Ⓨ   **E2327** Power wheelchair accessory, head control interface, mechanical, proportional, including all related electronics, mechanical direction change switch, and fixed mounting hardware ♿⊘

Ⓨ   **E2328** Power wheelchair accessory, head control or extremity control interface, electronic, proportional, including all related electronics and fixed mounting hardware ♿⊘

Ⓨ   **E2329** Power wheelchair accessory, head control interface, contact switch mechanism, nonproportional, including all related electronics, mechanical stop switch, mechanical direction change switch, head array, and fixed mounting hardware ♿⊘

Ⓨ   **E2330** Power wheelchair accessory, head control interface, proximity switch mechanism, nonproportional, including all related electronics, mechanical stop switch, mechanical direction change switch, head array, and fixed mounting hardware ♿⊘

Ⓨ   **E2331** Power wheelchair accessory, attendant control, proportional, including all related electronics and fixed mounting hardware ⊘

Ⓨ ☑   **E2340** Power wheelchair accessory, nonstandard seat frame width, 20-23 in. ♿⊘

Ⓨ ☑   **E2341** Power wheelchair accessory, nonstandard seat frame width, 24-27 in. ♿⊘

Ⓨ ☑   **E2342** Power wheelchair accessory, nonstandard seat frame depth, 20 or 21 in. ♿⊘

Ⓨ ☑   **E2343** Power wheelchair accessory, nonstandard seat frame depth, 22-25 in. ♿⊘

Ⓨ   **E2351** Power wheelchair accessory, electronic interface to operate speech generating device using power wheelchair control interface ♿⊘

Ⓨ ☑   **E2360** Power wheelchair accessory, 22 NF non-sealed lead acid battery, each ♿⊘

Ⓨ   **E2361** Power wheelchair accessory, 22 NF sealed lead acid battery, each, (e.g., gel cell, absorbed glassmat) ♿⊘

Ⓨ ☑   **E2362** Power wheelchair accessory, group 24 non-sealed lead acid battery, each ♿⊘

Ⓨ ☑   **E2363** Power wheelchair accessory, group 24 sealed lead acid battery, each (e.g., gel cell, absorbed glassmat) ♿⊘

Ⓨ ☑   **E2364** Power wheelchair accessory, U-1 non-sealed lead acid battery, each ♿⊘

Ⓨ ☑   **E2365** Power wheelchair accessory, U-1 sealed lead acid battery, each (e.g., gel cell, absorbed glassmat) ♿⊘

Ⓨ ☑   **E2366** Power wheelchair accessory, battery charger, single mode, for use with only one battery type, sealed or non-sealed, each ♿⊘

Ⓨ ☑   **E2367** Power wheelchair accessory, battery charger, dual mode, for use with either battery type, sealed or non-sealed, each ♿⊘

●   **E2368** Power wheelchair component, motor, replacement only

●   **E2369** Power wheelchair component, gear box, replacement only

●   **E2370** Power wheelchair component, motor and gear box combination, replacement only

Ⓨ   **E2399** Power wheelchair accessory, not otherwise classified interface, including all related electronics and any type mounting hardware ⊘

Ⓨ   **E2402** Negative pressure wound therapy electrical pump, stationary or portable ♿⊘

Ⓨ ☑   **E2500** Speech generating device, digitized speech, using pre-recorded messages, less than or equal to 8 minutes recording time ♿⊘
MED: 100-3, 50.1

Ⓨ ☑   **E2502** Speech generating device, digitized speech, using pre-recorded messages, greater than 8 minutes but less than or equal to 20 minutes recording time ♿⊘
MED: 100-3, 50.1

Ⓨ ☑   **E2504** Speech generating device, digitized speech, using pre-recorded messages, greater than 20 minutes but less than or equal to 40 minutes recording time ♿⊘
MED: 100-3, 50.1

Ⓨ ☑   **E2506** Speech generating device, digitized speech, using pre-recorded messages, greater than 40 minutes recording time ♿⊘
MED: 100-3, 50.1

■ Special Coverage Instructions   ■ Noncovered by Medicare   ■ Carrier Discretion   ☑ Quantity Alert   ● New Code   ○ Reinstated Code   ▲ Revised Code

☑ **E2508** Speech generating device, synthesized speech, requiring message formulation by spelling and access by physical contact with the device   ⅄⊘
MED: 100-3, 50.1

☑ **E2510** Speech generating device, synthesized speech, permitting multiple methods of message formulation and multiple methods of device access   ⅄⊘
MED: 100-3, 50.1

☑ **E2511** Speech generating software program, for personal computer or personal digital assistant   ⅄⊘
MED: 100-3, 50.1

☑ **E2512** Accessory for speech generating device, mounting system   ⅄⊘
MED: 100-3, 50.1

☑ **E2599** Accessory for speech generating device, not otherwise classified   ⊘
MED: 100-3, 50.1

● **E2601** General use wheelchair seat cushion, width less than 22 in., any depth

● **E2602** General use wheelchair seat cushion, width 22 in. or greater, any depth

● **E2603** Skin protection wheelchair seat cushion, width less than 22 in., any depth

● **E2604** Skin protection wheelchair seat cushion, width 22 in. or greater, any depth

● **E2605** Positioning wheelchair seat cushion, width less than 22 in., any depth

● **E2606** Positioning wheelchair seat cushion, width 22 in. or greater, any depth

● **E2607** Skin protection and positioning wheelchair seat cushion, width less than 22 in., any depth

● **E2608** Skin protection and positioning wheelchair seat cushion, width 22 in. or greater, any depth

● **E2609** Custom fabricated wheelchair seat cushion, any size

● **E2610** Wheelchair seat cushion, powered

● **E2611** General use wheelchair back cushion, width less than 22 in., any height, including any type mounting hardware

● **E2612** General use wheelchair back cushion, width 22 in. or greater, any height, including any type mounting hardware

● **E2613** Positioning wheelchair back cushion, posterior, width less than 22 in., any height, including any type mounting hardware

● **E2614** Positioning wheelchair back cushion, posterior, width 22 in. or greater, any height, including any type mounting hardware

● **E2615** Positioning wheelchair back cushion, posterior-lateral, width less than 22 in., any height, including any type mounting hardware

● **E2616** Positioning wheelchair back cushion, posterior-lateral, width 22 in. or greater, any height, including any type mounting hardware

● **E2617** Custom fabricated wheelchair back cushion, any size, including any type mounting hardware

● **E2618** Wheelchair accessory, solid seat support base (replaces sling seat), for use with manual wheelchair or lightweight power wheelchair, includes any type mounting hardware

● **E2619** Replacement cover for wheelchair seat cushion or back cushion, each

● **E2620** Positioning wheelchair back cushion, planar back with lateral supports, width less than 22 in., any height, including any type mounting hardware

● **E2621** Positioning wheelchair back cushion, planar back with lateral supports, width 22 in. or greater, any height, including any type mounting hardware

● **E8000** Gait trainer, pediatric size, posterior support, includes all accessories and components

● **E8001** Gait trainer, pediatric size, upright support, includes all accessories and components

● **E8002** Gait trainer, pediatric size, anterior support, includes all accessories and components

Special Coverage Instructions   Noncovered by Medicare   Carrier Discretion   ☑ Quantity Alert   ● New Code   ○ Reinstated Code   ▲ Revised Code

2005 HCPCS   ♀ Female Only   ♂ Male Only   **1**-**9** ASC Groups   **MED:** Pub 100/NCD Reference   ⅄ DMEPOS Paid   ⊘ SNF Excluded   **E Codes — 55**

PROCEDURES/PROFESSIONAL SERVICES (TEMPORARY) *G0000–G9999*

The G codes are used to identify professional health care procedures and services that would otherwise be coded in CPT but for which there are no CPT codes.

PET SCAN MODIFIERS

CMS will no longer require the designation of the four PET scan modifiers (N, E, P, S) and has made the determination that no paper documentation needs to be submitted up front with PET scan claims. Documentation requirements such as physician referral and medical necessity determination are to be maintained by the provider as part of the beneficiary's medical record. Review the expanded coverage of PET scans and revised billing instructions. (PM AB-02-115 Aug. 2002)

G codes fall under the jurisdiction of the local carrier.

G0001 ~~Routine venipuncture for collection of specimen(s)~~

▲ Ⓛ **G0008** Administration of influenza virus vaccine when no physician fee schedule service on the same day

▲ Ⓛ **G0009** Administration of pneumococcal vaccine when no physician fee schedule service on the same day

▲ Ⓚ **G0010** Administration of hepatitis B vaccine when no physician fee schedule service on the same day

○ Ⓐ **G0027** Semen analysis; presence and/or motility of sperm excluding Huhner   ⊘

Ⓢ **G0030** PET myocardial perfusion imaging, (following previous PET, G0030-G0047); single study, rest or stress (exercise and/or pharmacologic)
MED: 100-3, 220.6

Ⓢ **G0031** PET myocardial perfusion imaging, (following previous PET, G0030-G0047); multiple studies, rest or stress (exercise and/or pharmacologic)
MED: 100-3, 220.6

Ⓢ **G0032** PET myocardial perfusion imaging, (following rest SPECT, 78464); single study, rest or stress (exercise and/or pharmacologic)
MED: 100-3, 220.6

Ⓢ **G0033** PET myocardial perfusion imaging, (following rest SPECT, 78464); multiple studies, rest or stress (exercise and/or pharmacologic)
MED: 100-3, 220.6

Ⓢ **G0034** PET myocardial perfusion imaging, (following stress SPECT, 78465); single study, rest or stress (exercise and/or pharmacologic)
MED: 100-3, 220.6

Ⓢ **G0035** PET myocardial perfusion imaging, (following stress SPECT, 78465); multiple studies, rest or stress (exercise and/or pharmacologic)
MED: 100-3, 220.6

Ⓢ **G0036** PET myocardial perfusion imaging, (following coronary angiography, 93510-93529); single study, rest or stress (exercise and/or pharmacologic)
MED: 100-3, 220.6

Ⓢ **G0037** PET myocardial perfusion imaging, (following coronary angiography, 93510-93529); multiple studies, rest or stress (exercise and/or pharmacologic)
MED: 100-3, 220.6

Ⓢ **G0038** PET myocardial perfusion imaging, (following stress planar myocardial perfusion, 78460); single study, rest or stress (exercise and/or pharmacologic)
MED: 100-3, 220.6

Ⓢ **G0039** PET myocardial perfusion imaging, (following stress planar myocardial perfusion, 78460); multiple studies, rest or stress (exercise and/or pharmacologic)
MED: 100-3, 220.6

Ⓢ **G0040** PET myocardial perfusion imaging, (following stress echocardiogram, 93350); single study, rest or stress (exercise and/or pharmacologic)
MED: 100-3, 220.6

Ⓢ **G0041** PET myocardial perfusion imaging, (following stress echocardiogram, 93350); multiple studies, rest or stress (exercise and/or pharmacologic)
MED: 100-3, 220.6

Ⓢ **G0042** PET myocardial perfusion imaging, (following stress nuclear ventriculogram, 78481 or 78483); single study, rest or stress (exercise and/or pharmacologic)
MED: 100-3, 220.6

Ⓢ **G0043** PET myocardial perfusion imaging, (following stress nuclear ventriculogram, 78481 or 78483); multiple studies, rest or stress (exercise and/or pharmacologic)
MED: 100-3, 220.6

Ⓢ **G0044** PET myocardial perfusion imaging, (following rest ECG, 93000); single study, rest or stress (exercise and/or pharmacologic)
MED: 100-3, 220.6

Ⓢ **G0045** PET myocardial perfusion imaging, (following rest ECG, 93000); multiple studies, rest or stress (exercise and/or pharmacologic)
MED: 100-3, 220.6

Ⓢ **G0046** PET myocardial perfusion imaging, (following stress ECG, 93015); single study, rest or stress (exercise and/or pharmacologic)
MED: 100-3, 220.6

Ⓢ **G0047** PET myocardial perfusion imaging, (following stress ECG, 93015); multiple studies, rest or stress (exercise and/or pharmacologic)
MED: 100-3, 220.6

Ⓥ **G0101** Cervical or vaginal cancer screening; pelvic and clinical breast examination   ♀
G0101 can be reported with an E/M code when a separately identifiable E/M service was provided.
AHA: 3Q, '01, 6; 4Q, '02, 8

Ⓝ **G0102** Prostate cancer screening; digital rectal examination   ♂
MED: 100-3, 210.1; 100-4, 18, 50

Ⓐ **G0103** Prostate cancer screening; prostate specific antigen test (PSA), total   ♂
MED: 100-3, 210.1; 100-4, 18, 50

Ⓢ **G0104** Colorectal cancer screening; flexible sigmoidoscopy   ⊘
Medicare covers colorectal screening for cancer via flexible sigmoidoscopy once every four years for patients 50 years or older.

Ⓣ **G0105** Colorectal cancer screening; colonoscopy on individual at high risk   ❷⊘
An individual with ulcerative enteritis or a history of a malignant neoplasm of the lower gastrointestinal tract is considered at high-risk for colorectal cancer, as defined by CMS.
AHA: 3Q, '01, 6

Special Coverage Instructions	Noncovered by Medicare	Carrier Discretion	☑ Quantity Alert	● New Code	○ Reinstated Code	▲ Revised Code

2005 HCPCS   ♀ Female Only   ♂ Male Only   ❶-❾ ASC Groups   MED: Pub 100/NCD Reference   ᕑ DMEPOS Paid   ⊘ SNF Excluded   **G Codes — 57**

Procedures/Professional Services (Temporary)

G0106 — G0175

[S] **G0106** Colorectal cancer screening; alternative to G0104, screening sigmoidoscopy, barium enema
Medicare covers colorectal screening for cancer via barium enema once every four years for patients 50 years or older.

[A] **G0107** Colorectal cancer screening; fecal-occult blood test, 1-3 simultaneous determinations
Medicare covers colorectal screening for cancer via fecal-occult blood test once every year for patients 50 years or older.

[A] **G0108** Diabetes outpatient self-management training services, individual, per 30 minutes ⊘

[A] **G0109** Diabetes self-management training services, group session (2 or more), per 30 minutes ⊘

● [A] **G0110** NETT pulmonary rehabilitation; education/skills training, individual ⊘
MED: 100-3, 240.1

● [A] **G0111** NETT pulmonary rehabilitation; education/skills, group ⊘
MED: 100-3, 240.1

● [A] **G0112** NETT pulmonary rehabilitation; nutritional guidance, initial ⊘
MED: 100-3, 240.1

● [A] **G0113** NETT pulmonary rehabilitation; nutritional guidance, subsequent ⊘
MED: 100-3, 240.1

● [A] **G0114** NETT pulmonary rehabilitation; psychosocial consultation ⊘
MED: 100-3, 240.1

● [A] **G0115** NETT pulmonary rehabilitation; psychological testing ⊘
MED: 100-3, 240.1

● [A] **G0116** NETT pulmonary rehabilitation; psychosocial counselling ⊘
MED: 100-3, 240.1

[S] **G0117** Glaucoma screening for high risk patients furnished by an optometrist or ophthalmologist
AHA: 3Q, '01, 12; 1Q, '02, 4

[S] **G0118** Glaucoma screening for high risk patient furnished under the direct supervision of an optometrist or ophthalmologist
AHA: 3Q, '01, 12; 1Q, '02, 4

[S] **G0120** Colorectal cancer screening; alternative to G0105, screening colonoscopy, barium enema

[T] **G0121** Colorectal cancer screening; colonoscopy on individual not meeting criteria for high risk ☑⊘
AHA: 3Q, '01, 12; 1Q, '02, 4

[E] **G0122** Colorectal cancer screening; barium enema ⊘

[A] **G0123** Screening cytopathology, cervical or vaginal (any reporting system), collected in preservative fluid, automated thin layer preparation, screening by cytotechnologist under physician supervision ♀
See also P3000-P3001.
MED: 100-3, 190.2

[A] **G0124** Screening cytopathology, cervical or vaginal (any reporting system), collected in preservative fluid, automated thin layer preparation, requiring interpretation by physician ♀
See also P3000-P3001.
MED: 100-3, 190.2

[S] **G0125** PET imaging regional or whole body; single pulmonary nodule
MED: 100-3, 220.6; 100-4, 13, 60

[T] **G0127** Trimming of dystrophic nails, any number ⊘
MED: 100-2, 15, 290; 100-2, 15, 290

[B] **G0128** Direct (face-to-face with patient) skilled nursing services of a registered nurse provided in a comprehensive outpatient rehabilitation facility, each 10 minutes beyond the first 5 minutes ⊘

[P] **G0129** Occupational therapy requiring the skills of a qualified occupational therapist, furnished as a component of a partial hospitalization treatment program, per day ⊘

[X] **G0130** Single energy x-ray absorptiometry (SEXA) bone density study, one or more sites; appendicular skeleton (peripheral) (e.g., radius, wrist, heel)
MED: 100-3, 150.3

[E] **G0141** Screening cytopathology smears, cervical or vaginal, performed by automated system, with manual rescreening, requiring interpretation by physician ♀ ⊘

[A] **G0143** Screening cytopathology, cervical or vaginal (any reporting system), collected in preservative fluid, automated thin layer preparation, with manual screening and rescreening by cytotechnologist under physician supervision ♀

[A] **G0144** Screening cytopathology, cervical or vaginal (any reporting system), collected in preservative fluid, automated thin layer preparation, with screening by automated system, under physician supervision ♀

[A] **G0145** Screening cytopathology, cervical or vaginal (any reporting system), collected in preservative fluid, automated thin layer preparation, with screening by automated system and manual rescreening under physician supervision ♀

[A] **G0147** Screening cytopathology smears, cervical or vaginal, performed by automated system under physician supervision ♀

[A] **G0148** Screening cytopathology smears, cervical or vaginal, performed by automated system with manual rescreening ♀

[B] **G0151** Services of physical therapist in home health setting, each 15 minutes ⊘

[B] **G0152** Services of occupational therapist in home health setting, each 15 minutes ⊘

[B] **G0153** Services of speech and language pathologist in home health setting, each 15 minutes ⊘

[B] **G0154** Services of skilled nurse in home health setting, each 15 minutes ⊘

[B] **G0155** Services of clinical social worker in home health setting, each 15 minutes ⊘

[B] **G0156** Services of home health aide in home health setting, each 15 minutes ⊘

[T] **G0166** External counterpulsation, per treatment session ⊘
MED: 100-3, 20.20

[X] **G0168** Wound closure utilizing tissue adhesive(s) only ⊘
AHA: 3Q, '01, 13; 4Q, '01, 12

▲ [S] **G0173** Linear accelerator based stereotactic radiosurgery, complete course of therapy in one session

[V] **G0175** Scheduled interdisciplinary team conference (minimum of three exclusive of patient care nursing staff) with patient present ⊘

Special Coverage Instructions   Noncovered by Medicare   Carrier Discretion   ☑ Quantity Alert   ● New Code   ○ Reinstated Code   ▲ Revised Code

58 — G Codes   [A] Adult   [M] Maternity   [P] Pediatrics   [I] Infant   [A]-[Y] APC Status Indicator   **2005 HCPCS**

P	**G0176**	Activity therapy, such as music, dance, art or play therapies not for recreation, related to the care and treatment of patient's disabling mental health problems, per session (45 minutes or more) ⊘
P	**G0177**	Training and educational services related to the care and treatment of patient's disabling mental health problems per session (45 minutes or more) ⊘
E	**G0179**	Physician re-certification for Medicare-covered home health services under a home health plan of care (patient not present), including contacts with home health agency and review of reports of patient status required by physicians to affirm the initial implementation of the plan of care that meets patient's needs, per re-certification period ⊘
E	**G0180**	Physician certification for Medicare-covered home health services under a home health plan of care (patient not present), including contacts with home health agency and review of reports of patient status required by physicians to affirm the initial implementation of the plan of care that meets patient's needs, per certification period ⊘
E	**G0181**	Physician supervision of a patient receiving Medicare-covered services provided by a participating home health agency (patient not present) requiring complex and multidisciplinary care modalities involving regular physician development and/or revision of care plans, review of subsequent reports of patient status, review of laboratory and other studies, communication (including telephone calls) with other health care professionals involved in the patient's care, integration of new information into the medical treatment plan and/or adjustment of medical therapy, within a calendar month, 30 minutes or more ⊘
E	**G0182**	Physician supervision of a patient under a Medicare-approved hospice (patient not present) requiring complex and multidisciplinary care modalities involving regular physician development and/or revision of care plans, review of subsequent reports of patient status, review of laboratory and other studies, communication (including telephone calls) with other health care professionals involved in the patient's care, integration of new information into the medical treatment plan and/or adjustment of medical therapy, within a calendar month, 30 minutes or more ⊘
T	**G0186**	Destruction of localized lesion of choroid (for example, choroidal neovascularization); photocoagulation, feeder vessel technique (one or more sessions) ⊘
A	**G0202**	Screening mammography, producing direct digital image, bilateral, all views AHA: 1Q, '02, 3; 1Q, '03, 7, 10
S	**G0204**	Diagnostic mammography, producing direct digital image, bilateral, all views AHA: 1Q, '03, 7
S	**G0206**	Diagnostic mammography, producing direct digital image, unilateral, all views AHA: 1Q, '03, 7
S	**G0210**	PET imaging whole body; diagnosis; lung cancer, non-small cell MED: 100-3, 220.6; 100-4, 13, 60 AHA: 1Q, '02, 10
S	**G0211**	PET imaging whole body; initial staging; lung cancer; non-small cell MED: 100-3, 220.6; 100-4, 13, 60 AHA: 1Q, '02, 10
S	**G0212**	PET imaging whole body; restaging; lung cancer; non-small MED: 100-3, 220.6; 100-4, 13, 60 AHA: 1Q, '02, 10
S	**G0213**	PET imaging whole body; diagnosis; colorectal MED: 100-3, 220.6; 100-4, 13, 60 AHA: 1Q, '02, 10
S	**G0214**	PET imaging whole body; initial staging; colorectal MED: 100-3, 220.6; 100-4, 13, 60 AHA: 1Q, '02, 10
S	**G0215**	PET imaging whole body; restaging; colorectal cancer MED: 100-3, 220.6; 100-4, 13, 60 AHA: 1Q, '02, 10
S	**G0216**	PET imaging whole body; diagnosis; melanoma MED: 100-3, 220.6; 100-4, 13, 60 AHA: 1Q, '02, 10
S	**G0217**	PET imaging whole body; initial staging; melanoma MED: 100-3, 220.6; 100-4, 13, 60 AHA: 1Q, '02, 10
S	**G0218**	PET imaging whole body; restaging; melanoma MED: 100-3, 220.6; 100-4, 13, 60 AHA: 1Q, '02, 10
E	**G0219**	PET imaging whole body; melanoma for non-covered indications MED: 100-3, 220.6; 100-4, 13, 60 AHA: 1Q, '02, 10
S	**G0220**	PET imaging whole body; diagnosis; lymphoma MED: 100-3, 220.6; 100-4, 13, 60 AHA: 1Q, '02, 10
S	**G0221**	PET imaging whole body; initial staging; lymphoma MED: 100-3, 220.6; 100-4, 13, 60 AHA: 1Q, '02, 10
S	**G0222**	PET imaging whole body; restaging; lymphoma MED: 100-3, 220.6; 100-4, 13, 60 AHA: 1Q, '02, 10
S	**G0223**	PET imaging whole body or regional; diagnosis; head and neck cancer; excluding thyroid and CNS cancers MED: 100-3, 220.6; 100-4, 13, 60 AHA: 1Q, '02, 10
S	**G0224**	PET imaging whole body or regional; initial staging; head and neck cancer; excluding thyroid and CNS cancers MED: 100-3, 220.6; 100-4, 13, 60 AHA: 1Q, '02, 10
S	**G0225**	PET imaging whole body or regional; restaging; head and neck cancer, excluding thyroid and CNS cancers MED: 100-3, 220.6; 100-4, 13, 60 AHA: 1Q, '02, 10
S	**G0226**	PET imaging whole body; diagnosis; esophageal cancer MED: 100-3, 220.6; 100-4, 13, 60 AHA: 1Q, '02, 10

Procedures/Professional Services (Temporary)

G0227 — G0248

⑤ **G0227** PET imaging whole body; initial staging; esophageal cancer
MED: 100-3, 220.6; 100-4, 13, 60

AHA: 1Q, '02, 12

⑤ **G0228** PET imaging whole body; restaging; esophageal cancer
MED: 100-3, 220.6; 100-4, 13, 60

AHA: 1Q, '02, 12

⑤ **G0229** PET imaging; metabolic brain imaging for pre-surgical evaluation of refractory seizures
MED: 100-3, 220.6; 100-4, 13, 60

AHA: 1Q, '02, 12

⑤ **G0230** PET imaging; metabolic assessment for myocardial viability following inconclusive SPECT study
MED: 100-3, 220.6; 100-4, 13, 60

AHA: 1Q, '02, 12

⑤ **G0231** PET, whole body, for recurrence of colorectal or colorectal metastatic cancer; gamma cameras only
MED: 100-3, 220.6

AHA: 1Q, '02, 12

⑤ **G0232** PET, whole body, for recurrence of lymphoma; gamma cameras only
MED: 100-3, 220.6

AHA: 1Q, '02, 12

⑤ **G0233** PET, whole body, for recurrence of melanoma; gamma cameras only
MED: 100-3, 220.6

AHA: 1Q, '02, 12

⑤ **G0234** PET, regional or whole body, for solitary pulmonary nodule following CT or for initial staging of pathologically diagnosed nonsmall cell lung cancer; gamma cameras only
MED: 100-3, 220.6

AHA: 1Q, '02, 12

⑤ **G0237** Therapeutic procedures to increase strength or endurance of respiratory muscles, face-to-face, one-on-one, each 15 minutes (includes monitoring) ⊘

⑤ **G0238** Therapeutic procedures to improve respiratory function, other than described by G0237, one-on-one, face-to-face, per 15 minutes (includes monitoring) ⊘

⑤ **G0239** Therapeutic procedures to improve respiratory function or increase strength or endurance of respiratory muscles, two or more individuals (includes monitoring) ⊘

⑤ **G0242** Multi-source photon stereotactic radiosurgery (cobalt 60 multi-source converging beams) plan, including dose volume histograms for target and critical structure tolerances, plan optimization performed for highly conformal distributions, plan positional accuracy and dose verification, all lesions treated, per course of treatment
AHA: 1Q, '03, 6

⑤ **G0243** Multi-source photon stereotactic radiosurgery, delivery including collimator changes and custom plugging, complete course of treatment, all lesions

▲ ⑤ **G0244** Observation care provided by a facility to a patient with CHF, chest pain, or asthma, minimum eight hours ⊘
AHA: 4Q, '01, 2; 4Q, '02, 6, 7; 4Q, '03, 7

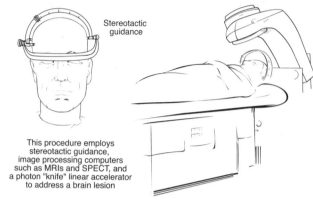

Stereotactic guidance

This procedure employs stereotactic guidance, image processing computers such as MRIs and SPECT, and a photon "knife" linear accelerator to address a brain lesion

Ⓥ **G0245** Initial physician evaluation and management of a diabetic patient with diabetic sensory neuropathy resulting in a loss of protective sensation (LOPS) which must include: (1) the diagnosis of LOPS, (2) a patient history, (3) a physical examination that consists of at least the following elements: (a) visual inspection of the forefoot, hindfoot and toe web spaces, (b) evaluation of a protective sensation, (c) evaluation of foot structure and biomechanics, (d) evaluation of vascular status and skin integrity, and (e) evaluation and recommendation of footwear and (4) patient education
MED: 100-3, 70.2.1

AHA: 4Q, '02, 9

Ⓥ **G0246** Follow-up physician evaluation and management of a diabetic patient with diabetic sensory neuropathy resulting in a loss of protective sensation (LOPS) to include at least the following: (1) a patient history, (2) a physical examination that includes: (a) visual inspection of the forefoot, hindfoot and toe web spaces, (b) evaluation of protective sensation, (c) evaluation of foot structure and biomechanics, (d) evaluation of vascular status and skin integrity, and (e) evaluation and recommendation of footwear, and (3) patient education
MED: 100-3, 70.2.1

AHA: 4Q, '02, 9

Ⓣ **G0247** Routine foot care by a physician of a diabetic patient with diabetic sensory neuropathy resulting in a loss of protective sensation (LOPS) to include, the local care of superficial wounds (i.e., superficial to muscle and fascia) and at least the following if present: (1) local care of superficial wounds, (2) debridement of corns and calluses, and (3) trimming and debridement of nails ⊘
MED: 100-3, 70.2.1

AHA: 4Q, '02, 9

⑤ **G0248** Demonstration, at initial use, of home INR monitoring for patient with mechanical heart valve(s) who meets Medicare coverage criteria, under the direction of a physician; includes: demonstrating use and care of the INR monitor, obtaining at least one blood sample, provision of instructions for reporting home INR test results, and documentation of patient ability to perform testing ⊘
MED: 100-3, 210.1

AHA: 4Q, '02, 9

| Special Coverage Instructions | Noncovered by Medicare | Carrier Discretion | ☑ Quantity Alert | ● New Code | ○ Reinstated Code | ▲ Revised Code |

60 — G Codes   Ⓐ Adult   Ⓜ Maternity   Ⓟ Pediatrics   Ⓘ Infant   Ⓐ-Ⓨ APC Status Indicator   **2005 HCPCS**

Ⓢ   G0249   Provision of test materials and equipment for home INR monitoring to patient with mechanical heart valve(s) who meets Medicare coverage criteria; includes provision of materials for use in the home and reporting of test results to physician; per four tests ⊘
MED: 100-3, 210.1
AHA: 4Q, '02, 9

Ⓔ   G0250   Physician review, interpretation and patient management of home INR testing for a patient with mechanical heart valve(s) who meets other coverage criteria; per four tests (does not require face-to-face service) ⊘
MED: 100-3, 210.1
AHA: 4Q, '02, 9

Ⓢ   G0251   Linear accelerator based stereotactic radiosurgery, delivery including collimator changes and custom plugging, fractionated treatment, all lesions, per session, maximum five sessions per course of treatment ⊘

Ⓔ   G0252   PET imaging, full and partial-ring PET scanners only, for initial diagnosis of breast cancer and/or surgical planning for breast cancer (e.g., initial staging of axillary lymph nodes) ⊘
MED: 100-3, 220.6
AHA: 4Q, '02, 9

Ⓢ   G0253   PET imaging for breast cancer, full and partial-ring PET scanners only, staging/restaging of local regional recurrence or distant metastases (i.e., staging/restaging after or prior to course of treatment) ⊘
MED: 100-3, 220.6
AHA: 4Q, '02, 9

Ⓢ   G0254   PET imaging for breast cancer, full and partial ring PET scanners only, evaluation of response to treatment, performed during course of treatment ⊘
MED: 100-3, 220.6
AHA: 4Q, '02, 9

Ⓔ   G0255   Current perception threshold/sensory nerve conduction test, (SNCT) per limb, any nerve ⊘
MED: 100-3, 160.23
AHA: 4Q, '02, 9

Ⓢ   G0257   Unscheduled or emergency dialysis treatment for an ESRD patient in a hospital outpatient department that is not certified as an ESRD facility ⊘
AHA: 4Q, '02, 9; 1Q, '03, 9

G0258   Intravenous infusion during separately payable observation stay, per observation stay (must be reported with G0244) ⊘
AHA: 4Q, '02, 9

Ⓝ   G0259   Injection procedure for sacroiliac joint; arthrography ⊘
AHA: 4Q, '02, 9

● Ⓣ   G0260   Injection procedure for sacroiliac joint; provision of anesthetic, steroid and/or other therapeutic agent, with or without arthrography ❶⊘
AHA: 4Q, '02, 9

Ⓝ   G0263   Direct admission of patient with diagnosis of congestive heart failure, chest pain or asthma for observation services that meet all criteria for G0244
AHA: 4Q, '02, 6, 7, 9; 1Q, '03, 11; 4Q, '03, 7

Ⓥ   G0264   Initial nursing assessment of patient directly admitted to observation with diagnosis other than CHF, chest pain or asthma or patient directly admitted to observation with diagnosis of CHF, chest pain or asthma when the observation stay does not qualify for G0244
AHA: 4Q, '02, 6, 7, 9; 1Q, '03, 11

Ⓐ   G0265   Cryopreservation, freezing and storage of cells for therapeutic use, each cell line

Ⓐ   G0266   Thawing and expansion of frozen cells for therapeutic use, each aliquot

Ⓢ   G0267   Bone marrow or peripheral stem cell harvest, modification or treatment to eliminate cell type(s) (e.g., T-cells, metastatic carcinoma)

Ⓧ   G0268   Removal of impacted cerumen (one or both ears) by physician on same date of service as audiologic function testing
AHA: 1Q, '03, 12

Ⓝ   G0269   Placement of occlusive device into either a venous or arterial access site, post surgical or interventional procedure (e.g., angioseal plug, vascular plug)

Ⓐ   G0270   Medical nutrition therapy; reassessment and subsequent intervention(s) following second referral in same year for change in diagnosis, medical condition or treatment regimen (including additional hours needed for renal disease), individual, face to face with the patient, each 15 minutes ⊘

Ⓐ   G0271   Medical nutrition therapy, reassessment and subsequent intervention(s) following second referral in same year for change in diagnosis, medical condition, or treatment regimen (including additional hours needed for renal disease), group (2 or more individuals), each 30 minutes ⊘

▲ Ⓝ   G0275   Renal artery angiography (unilateral or bilateral) performed at the time of cardiac catheterization, includes catheter placement, injection of dye, flush aortogram and radiologic supervision and interpretation and production of images (list separately in addition to primary procedure)

▲ Ⓝ   G0278   Iliac artery angiography performed at the same time of cardiac catheterization, includes catheter placement, injection of dye, radiologic supervision and interpretation and production of images (list separately in addition to primary procedure) ⊘

Ⓐ   G0279   Extracorporeal shock wave therapy; involving elbow epicondylitis

Ⓐ   G0280   Extracorporeal shock wave therapy; involving other than elbow epicondylitis or plantar fascitis

Ⓐ   G0281   Electrical stimulation, (unattended), to one or more areas, for chronic Stage III and Stage IV pressure ulcers, arterial ulcers, diabetic ulcers, and venous stasis ulcers not demonstrating measurable signs of healing after 30 days of conventional care, as part of a therapy plan of care
AHA: 1Q, '03, 7; 2Q, '03, 7

Ⓔ   G0282   Electrical stimulation, (unattended), to one or more areas, for wound care other than described in G0281 ⊘
MED: 100-3, 270.1; 100-3, 270.1; 100-3, 270.1; 100-3, 270.1
AHA: 1Q, '03, 7; 2Q, '03, 7

| Special Coverage Instructions | Noncovered by Medicare | Carrier Discretion | ☑ Quantity Alert   ● New Code   ○ Reinstated Code   ▲ Revised Code |

2005 HCPCS   ♀ Female Only   ♂ Male Only   ❶-❾ ASC Groups   MED: Pub 100/NCD Reference   ᗷ DMEPOS Paid   ⊘ SNF Excluded   **G Codes — 61**

Procedures/Professional Services (Temporary)

G0283 — G0314

[A] **G0283** Electrical stimulation (unattended), to one or more areas for indication(s) other than wound care, as part of a therapy plan of care
AHA: 1Q, '03, 7; 2Q, '03, 7

[T] **G0288** Reconstruction, computed tomographic angiography of aorta for surgical planning for vascular surgery

[N] **G0289** Arthroscopy, knee, surgical, for removal of loose body, foreign body, debridement/shaving of articular cartilage (chondroplasty) at the time of other surgical knee arthroscopy in a different compartment of the same knee ⊘

[T] **G0290** Transcatheter placement of a drug eluting intracoronary stent(s), percutaneous, with or without other therapeutic intervention, any method; single vessel ⊘
AHA: 4Q, '02, 9; 3Q, '03, 11; 4Q, '03, 7

[T] **G0291** Transcatheter placement of a drug eluting intracoronary stent(s), percutaneous, with or without other therapeutic intervention, any method; each additional vessel ⊘
AHA: 4Q, '02, 9; 3Q, '03, 11; 4Q, '03, 7

~~G0292~~ ~~Administration(s) of experimental drug(s) only in a Medicare qualifying clinical trial (includes administration for chemotherapy and other types of therapy via infusion and/or other than infusion), per day~~

[S] **G0293** Noncovered surgical procedure(s) using conscious sedation, regional, general or spinal anesthesia in a Medicare qualifying clinical trial, per day ⊘
AHA: 4Q, '02, 9

[S] **G0294** Noncovered procedure(s) using either no anesthesia or local anesthesia only, in a Medicare qualifying clinical trial, per day ⊘
AHA: 4Q, '02, 9

▲ [E] **G0295** Electromagnetic therapy, to one or more areas, for wound care other than described in G0329 or for other uses
MED: 100-3, 270.1; 100-3, 270.1; 100-3, 270.1; 100-3, 270.1
AHA: 1Q, '03, 7

[S] **G0296** PET imaging, full and partial ring PET scanner only, for restaging of previously treated thyroid cancer of follicular cell origin following negative I-131 whole body scan
AHA: 4Q, '03, 4

[T] **G0297** Insertion of single chamber pacing cardioverter defibrillator pulse generator ⊘
AHA: 4Q, '03, 4, 7

[T] **G0298** Insertion of dual chamber pacing cardioverter defibrillator pulse generator ⊘
AHA: 4Q, '03, 4, 7

[T] **G0299** Insertion or repositioning of electrode lead for single chamber pacing cardioverter defibrillator and insertion of pulse generator ⊘
AHA: 4Q, '03, 4, 7

[T] **G0300** Insertion or repositioning of electrode lead(s) for dual chamber pacing cardioverter defibrillator and insertion of pulse generator ⊘
AHA: 4Q, '03, 4, 7

[S] ☑ **G0302** Preoperative pulmonary surgery services for preparation for LVRS, complete course of services, to include a minimum of 16 days of services ⊘

[S] ☑ **G0303** Preoperative pulmonary surgery services for preparation for LVRS, 10 to 15 days of services ⊘

[S] ☑ **G0304** Preoperative pulmonary surgery services for preparation for LVRS, 1 to 9 days of services ⊘

[S] ☑ **G0305** Postdischarge pulmonary surgery services after LVRS, minimum of 6 days of services ⊘

[A] **G0306** Complete CBC, automated (HgB, HCT, RBC, WBC, without platelet count) and automated WBC differential count

[A] **G0307** Complete CBC, automated (HgB, HCT, RBC, WBC; without platelet count)

● [A] **G0308** ESRD related services during the course of treatment, for patients under 2 years of age to include monitoring for the adequacy of nutrition, assessment of growth and development, and counseling of parents; with 4 or more face-to-face physician visits per month [P]⊘
MED: 100-2, 11, 130.1

● [A] **G0309** ESRD related services during the course of treatment, for patients under 2 years of age to include monitoring for the adequacy of nutrition, assessment of growth and development, and counseling of parents; with 2 or 3 face-to-face physician visits per month [P]⊘
MED: 100-2, 11, 130.1

● [A] **G0310** ESRD related services during the course of treatment, for patients under 2 years of age to include monitoring for the adequacy of nutrition, assessment of growth and development, and counseling of parents; with 1 face-to-face physician visit per month [P]⊘
MED: 100-2, 11, 130.1

● [A] **G0311** ESRD related services during the course of treatment, for patients between 2 and 11 years of age to include monitoring for the adequacy of nutrition, assessment of growth and development, and counseling of parents; with 4 or more face-to-face physician visits per month [P]⊘
MED: 100-2, 11, 130.1

● [A] **G0312** ESRD related services during the course of treatment, for patients between 2 and 11 years of age to include monitoring for the adequacy of nutrition, assessment of growth and development, and counseling of parents; with 2 or 3 face-to-face physician visits per month [P]⊘
MED: 100-2, 11, 130.1

● [A] **G0313** ESRD related services during the course of treatment, for patients between 2 and 11 years of age to include monitoring for the adequacy of nutrition, assessment of growth and development, and counseling of parents; with 1 face-to-face physician visit per month [P]⊘
MED: 100-2, 11, 130.1

● [A] **G0314** ESRD related services during the course of treatment, for patients between 12 and 19 years of age to include monitoring for the adequacy of nutrition, assessment of growth and development, and counseling of parents; with 4 or more face-to-face physician visits per month [P]⊘
MED: 100-2, 11, 130.1

| Special Coverage Instructions | Noncovered by Medicare | Carrier Discretion | ☑ Quantity Alert | ● New Code | ○ Reinstated Code | ▲ Revised Code |

● Ⓐ **G0315** ESRD related services during the course of treatment, for patients between 12 and 19 years of age to include monitoring for the adequacy of nutrition, assessment of growth and development, and counseling of parents; with 2 or 3 face-to-face physician visits per month Ⓟ ⊘
MED: 100-2, 11, 130.1

● Ⓐ **G0316** ESRD related services during the course of treatment, for patients between 12 and 19 years of age to include monitoring for the adequacy of nutrition, assessment of growth and development, and counseling of parents; with 1 face-to-face physician visit per month Ⓟ ⊘
MED: 100-2, 11, 130.1

● Ⓐ **G0317** ESRD related services during the course of treatment, for patients 20 years of age and over; with 4 or more face-to-face physician visits per month Ⓐ ⊘
MED: 100-2, 11, 130.1

● Ⓐ **G0318** ESRD related services during the course of treatment, for patients 20 years of age and over; with 2 or 3 face-to-face physician visits per month Ⓐ ⊘
MED: 100-2, 11, 130.1

● Ⓐ **G0319** ESRD related services during the course of treatment, for patients 20 years of age and over; with 1 face-to-face physician visit per month Ⓐ ⊘
MED: 100-2, 11, 130.1

● Ⓐ **G0320** ESRD related services for home dialysis patients per full month; for patients under 2 years of age to include monitoring for adequacy of nutrition, assessment of growth and development, and counseling of parents Ⓟ ⊘
MED: 100-2, 11, 130.1

● Ⓐ **G0321** ESRD related services for home dialysis patients per full month; for patients 2 to 11 years of age to include monitoring for adequacy of nutrition, assessment of growth and development, and counseling of parents Ⓟ ⊘
MED: 100-2, 11, 130.1

● Ⓐ **G0322** ESRD related services for home dialysis patients per full month; for patients 12 to 19 years of age to include monitoring for adequacy of nutrition, assessment of growth and development, and counseling of parents Ⓟ ⊘
MED: 100-2, 11, 130.1

● Ⓐ **G0323** ESRD related services for home dialysis patients per full month; for patients 20 years of age and older Ⓐ ⊘
MED: 100-2, 11, 130.1

● Ⓐ **G0324** ESRD related services for home dialysis (less than full month), per day; for patients under 2 years of age Ⓟ ⊘
MED: 100-2, 11, 130.1

● Ⓐ **G0325** ESRD related services for home dialysis (less than full month), per day; for patients between 2 and 11 years of age Ⓟ ⊘
MED: 100-2, 11, 130.1

● Ⓐ **G0326** ESRD related services for home dialysis (less than full month), per day; for patients between 12 and 19 years of age Ⓟ ⊘
MED: 100-2, 11, 130.1

● Ⓐ **G0327** ESRD related services for home dialysis (less than full month), per day; for patients 20 years of age and over Ⓐ ⊘
MED: 100-2, 11, 130.1

● Ⓐ **G0328** Colorectalcancer screening; fecal-occult blood test, immunoassay, 1-3 simultaneous determinations

● Ⓐ **G0329** Electromagnetic therapy, to one or more areas for chronic Stage III and Stage IV pressure ulcers, arterial ulcers, diabetic ulcers and venous stasis ulcers not demonstrating measurable signs of healing after 30 days of conventional care as part of a therapy plan of care

● Ⓔ G0330 PET imaging initial diagnosis cervical
Short description only available from CMS.

● Ⓔ G0331 PET imaging restaging ovarian
Short description only available from CMS.

● Ⓢ **G0336** PET imaging, brain imaging for the differential diagnosis of Alzheimer's disease with aberrant features vs. fronto-temporal dementia
MED: 100-3, 260.3

● **G0337** Hospice evaluation and counseling services, pre-election

● Ⓢ **G0338** Linear accelerator based stereotactic radiosurgery plan, including does volume histograms for target and critical structure tolerances, plan optimization performed for highly conformal distributions, plan postitional accuracy and does verification, all lesions treated, per course of treatment

● Ⓢ **G0339** Image guided robotic linear accelerator base stereotactic radiosurgery, complete course of therapy in one session, or first session of fractionated treatment

● Ⓢ **G0340** Image guided robotic linear accelerator based stereotactic radiosurgery, delivery including collimator changes and custom plugging, fractionated treatment, all lesions, per session, second through fifth sessions, maximum five sessions per course of treatment

● Ⓒ **G0341** Percutaneous islet cell transplant, includes portal vein catheterization and infusion
MED: 100-3, 260.3

● Ⓒ **G0342** Laparoscopy for islet cell transplant, includes portal vein catheterization and infusion
MED: 100-3, 260.3

● Ⓒ **G0343** Laparotomy for islet cell transplant, includes portal vein catheterization and infusion
MED: 100-3, 260.3

● **G0344** Initial preventive physical examination; face-to-face visit, services limited to new beneficiary during the first six months of Medicare enrollment

● ☑ **G0345** Intravenous infusion, hydration; initial, up to one hour

● ☑ **G0346** Each additional hour, up to eight (8) hours (list separately in addition to code for primary procedure)

● ☑ **G0347** Intravenous infusion, for therapeutic/diagnostic (specify substance or drug); initial, up to one hour

● ☑ **G0348** Each additional hour, up to eight (8) hours (list separately in addition to code for primary procedure and report in conjunction with G0347)

● ☑ **G0349** Additional sequential infusion, up to one hour (list separately in addition to code for primary procedure)

Special Coverage Instructions   Noncovered by Medicare   Carrier Discretion   ☑ Quantity Alert   ● New Code   ○ Reinstated Code   ▲ Revised Code

2005 HCPCS   ♀ Female Only   ♂ Male Only   🔟-�«9» ASC Groups   **MED:** Pub 100/NCD Reference   ♿ DMEPOS Paid   ⊘ SNF Excluded   **G Codes — 63**

Procedures/Professional Services (Temporary)

G0350 — G9027

●   **G0350** Concurrent infusion (list separately in addition to code for primary procedure) report only once per substance/drug regardless of duration, report G0350 in conjunction with G0345

● ☑ **G0351** Therapeutic or diagnostic injection (specify substance or drug); subcutaneous or intramuscular

● ☑ **G0353** Intravenous push, single or initial substance/drug

● ☑ **G0354** Each additional sequential intravenous push (list separately in addition to code for primary procedure)

●   **G0355** Chemotherapy administration, subcutaneous or intramuscular non-hormonal antineoplastic

●   **G0356** Hormonal antineoplastic

●   **G0357** Intravenous, push technique, single or initial substance/drug

● ☑ **G0358** Intravenous, push technique, each additional substance/drug (list separately in addition to code for primary procedure)

●   **G0359** Chemotherapy administration, intravenous infusion technique; up to one hour, single or initial substance/drug

● ☑ **G0360** Each additional hour, one to eight (8) hours (list separately in addition to code for primary procedure) use G0360 in conjunction with G0359

● ☑ **G0361** Initiation of prolonged chemotherapy infusion (more than eight hours), requiring use of a portable or implantable pump

● ☑ **G0362** Each additional sequential infusion (different substance/drug), up to one hour (use with G0359)

●   **G0363** Irrigation of implanted venous access device for drug delivery systems (do not report G0363 if an injection or infusion is provided on the same day)

●   **G0364** Bone marrow aspiration performed with bone marrow biopsy through the same incision on the same date of service

●   **G0365** Vessel mapping of vessels for hemodialysis access (services for preoperative vessel mapping prior to creation of hemodialysis access using an autogenous hemodialysis conduit, including arterial inflow and venous outflow)

●   **G0366** Electrocardiogram, routine ECG with at least 12 leads; with interpretation and report, performed as a component of the initial preventive physical examination

●   **G0367** Tracing only, without interpretation and report, performed as a component of the initial preventive physical examination

●   **G0368** Interpretation and report only, performed as a component of the initial preventive physical examination

Ⓢ ☑ **G3001** Administration and supply of tositumomab, 450 mg
Use this code for Bexxar.

Ⓑ   **G9001** Coordinated care fee, initial rate ⊘

Ⓑ   **G9002** Coordinated care fee, maintenance rate ⊘

Ⓑ   **G9003** Coordinated care fee, risk adjusted high, initial ⊘

Ⓑ   **G9004** Coordinated care fee, risk adjusted low, initial ⊘

Ⓑ   **G9005** Coordinated care fee, risk adjusted maintenance ⊘

Ⓑ   **G9006** Coordinated care fee, home monitoring ⊘

Ⓑ   **G9007** Coordinated care fee, schedule team conference ⊘

Ⓑ   **G9008** Coordinated care fee, physician coordinated care oversight services ⊘

Ⓔ   **G9009** Coordinated care fee, risk adjusted maintenance, Level 3

Ⓔ   **G9010** Coordinated care fee, risk adjusted maintenance, Level 4 ⊘

Ⓔ   **G9011** Coordinated care fee, risk adjusted maintenance, Level 5 ⊘

Ⓔ   **G9012** Coordinated care fee, risk adjusted maintenance, other specified care management ⊘

●   **G9013** ESRD demo basic bundle Level 1

●   **G9014** ESRD demo expanded bundle including venous access and related services

Ⓔ   **G9016** Smoking cessation counseling, individual, in the absence of or in addition to any other evaluation and management service, per session (6-10 minutes) [demonstration project code only] ⊘

● ☑ **G9017** Amantadine hydrochloride, oral, per 100 mg (for use as a Medicare-approved demonstration project)

● ☑ **G9018** Zanamivir, inhalation powder administered through inhaler, per 10 mg (for use as a Medicare-approved demonstration project)

● ☑ **G9019** Oseltamivir phosphate, oral, per 75 mg (for use as a Medicare-approved demonstration project)

● ☑ **G9020** Rimantadine hydrochloride, oral, per 100 mg (for use as a Medicare-approved demonstration project)

     G9021 Chemotherapy assessment for nausea and/or vomiting, patient reported, performed at the time of chemotherapy administration; assessment Level 1: not at all (for use in a Medicare-approved demonstration project)

●   **G9022** Chemotherapy assessment for nausea and/or vomiting, patient reported, performed at the time of chemotherapy administration; assessment Level 2: a little (for use in a Medicare-approved demonstration project)

●   **G9023** Chemotherapy assessment for nausea and/or vomiting, patient reported, performed at the time of chemotherapy administration; assessment Level 3: quite a bit (for use in a Medicare-approved demonstration project)

●   **G9024** Chemotherapy assessment for nausea and/or vomiting, patient reported, performed at the time of chemotherapy administration; assessment Level 4: very much (for use in a Medicare-approved demonstration project)

●   **G9025** Chemotherapy assessment for pain, patient reported, performed at the time of chemotherapy administration, assessment Level 1: not at all (for use in a Medicare-approved demonstration project)

●   **G9026** Chemotherapy assessment for pain, patient reported, performed at the time of chemotherapy administration, assessment Level 2: a little (for use in a Medicare-approved demonstration project)

●   **G9027** Chemotherapy assessment for pain, patient reported, performed at the time of chemotherapy administration assessment Level 3: quite a bit (for use in a Medicare-approved demonstration project)

Special Coverage Instructions   Noncovered by Medicare   Carrier Discretion   ☑ Quantity Alert   ● New Code   ○ Reinstated Code   ▲ Revised Code

64 — G Codes   Ⓐ Adult   Ⓜ Maternity   Ⓟ Pediatrics   Ⓘ Infant   Ⓐ-Ⓨ APC Status Indicator   *2005 HCPCS*

●   **G9028**   Chemotherapy assessment for pain, patient reported, performed at the time of chemotherapy administration, assessment Level 4: very much (for use in a Medicare-approved demonstration project)

●   **G9029**   Chemotherapy assessment for lack of energy (fatigue), patient reported, performed at the time of chemotherapy administration, assessment Level 1: not at all (for use in a Medicare-approved demonstration project)

●   **G9030**   Chemotherapy assessment for lack of energy (fatigue), patient reported, performed at the time of chemotherapy administration, assessment Level 2: a little (for use in a Medicare-approved demonstration project)

●   **G9031**   Chemotherapy assessment for lack of energy (fatigue), patient reported, performed at the time of chemotherapy administration, assessment Level 3: quite a bit (for use in a Medicare-approved demonstration project)

●   **G9032**   Chemotherapy assessment for lack of energy (fatigue), patient reported, performed at the time of chemotherapy administration, assessment Level 4: very much (for use in a Medicare-approved demonstration project)

●   **G9034**   Services provided by occupational therapist (demonstration project)

●   **G9035**   Services provided by orientation and mobility specialist (demonstration project)

●   **G9036**   Services provided by low vision therapist (demonstration project)

●   **G9037**   Services provided by rehabilitation teacher (demonstration project)

Special Coverage Instructions   Noncovered by Medicare   Carrier Discretion   ☑ Quantity Alert   ● New Code   ○ Reinstated Code   ▲ Revised Code

2005 HCPCS   ♀ Female Only   ♂ Male Only   **1**-**9** ASC Groups   MED: Pub 100/NCD Reference   ♿ DMEPOS Paid   ⊘ SNF Excluded   **G Codes — 65**

ALCOHOL AND DRUG ABUSE TREATMENT SERVICES
H0001–H2037

The H codes are used by those state Medicaid agencies that are mandated by state law to establish separate codes for identifying mental health services that include alcohol and drug treatment services.

E H0001 Alcohol and/or drug assessment

E H0002 Behavioral health screening to determine eligibility for admission to treatment program

E H0003 Alcohol and/or drug screening; laboratory analysis of specimens for presence of alcohol and/or drugs

E H0004 Behavioral health counseling and therapy, per 15 minutes

E H0005 Alcohol and/or drug services; group counseling by a clinician

E H0006 Alcohol and/or drug services; case management

E H0007 Alcohol and/or drug services; crisis intervention (outpatient)

E H0008 Alcohol and/or drug services; sub-acute detoxification (hospital inpatient)

E H0009 Alcohol and/or drug services; acute detoxification (hospital inpatient)

E H0010 Alcohol and/or drug services; sub-acute detoxification (residential addiction program inpatient)

E H0011 Alcohol and/or drug services; acute detoxification (residential addiction program inpatient)

E H0012 Alcohol and/or drug services; sub-acute detoxification (residential addiction program outpatient)

E H0013 Alcohol and/or drug services; acute detoxification (residential addiction program outpatient)

E H0014 Alcohol and/or drug services; ambulatory detoxification

E H0015 Alcohol and/or drug services; intensive outpatient (treatment program that operates at least 3 hours/day and at least 3 days/week and is based on an individualized treatment plan), including assessment, counseling; crisis intervention, and activity therapies or education

E H0016 Alcohol and/or drug services; medical/somatic (medical intervention in ambulatory setting)

E H0017 Behavioral health; residential (hospital residential treatment program), without room and board, per diem

E H0018 Behavioral health; short-term residential (non-hospital residential treatment program), without room and board, per diem

E H0019 Behavioral health; long-term residential (non-medial, non-acute care in a residential treatment program where stay is typically longer than 30 days), without room and board, per diem

E H0020 Alcohol and/or drug services; methadone administration and/or service (provision of the drug by a licensed program)

E H0021 Alcohol and/or drug training service (for staff and personnel not employed by providers)

E H0022 Alcohol and/or drug intervention service (planned facilitation)

E H0023 Behavioral health outreach service (planned approach to reach a targeted population)

E H0024 Behavioral health prevention information dissemination service (one-way direct or non-direct contact with service audiences to affect knowledge and attitude)

E H0025 Behavioral health prevention education service (delivery of services with target population to affect knowledge, attitude and/or behavior)

E H0026 Alcohol and/or drug prevention process service, community-based (delivery of services to develop skills of impactors)

E H0027 Alcohol and/or drug prevention environmental service (broad range of external activities geared toward modifying systems in order to mainstream prevention through policy and law)

E H0028 Alcohol and/or drug prevention problem identification and referral service (e.g., student assistance and employee assistance programs), does not include assessment

E H0029 Alcohol and/or drug prevention alternatives service (services for populations that exclude alcohol and other drug use e.g., alcohol free social events)

E H0030 Behavioral health hotline service

E H0031 Mental health assessment, by nonphysician

E H0032 Mental health service plan development by nonphysician

E H0033 Oral medication administration, direct observation

E H0034 Medication training and support, per 15 minutes

E H0035 Mental health partial hospitalization, treatment, less than 24 hours

E H0036 Community psychiatric supportive treatment, face-to-face, per 15 minutes

E H0037 Community psychiatric supportive treatment program, per diem

E H0038 Self-help/peer services, per 15 minutes

E H0039 Assertive community treatment, face-to-face, per 15 minutes

E H0040 Assertive community treatment program, per diem

E H0041 Foster care, child, non-therapeutic, per diem P

E H0042 Foster care, child, non-therapeutic, per month P

E H0043 Supported housing, per diem

E H0044 Supported housing, per month

E H0045 Respite care services, not in the home, per diem

E H0046 Mental health services, not otherwise specified

E H0047 Alcohol and/or other drug abuse services, not otherwise specified

E H0048 Alcohol and/or other drug testing: collection and handling only, specimens other than blood

A H1000 Prenatal care, at-risk assessment M ♀

A H1001 Prenatal care, at-risk enhanced service; antepartum management M ♀

A H1002 Prenatal care, at risk enhanced service; care coordination M ♀

A H1003 Prenatal care, at-risk enhanced service; education M ♀

A H1004 Prenatal care, at-risk enhanced service; follow-up home visit M ♀

A H1005 Prenatal care, at-risk enhanced service package (includes H1001-H1004) M ♀

| Special Coverage Instructions | Noncovered by Medicare | Carrier Discretion | ☑ Quantity Alert | ● New Code | ○ Reinstated Code | ▲ Revised Code |

2005 HCPCS   ♀ Female Only   ♂ Male Only   **1**-**9** ASC Groups   **MED**: Pub 100/NCD Reference   ♿ DMEPOS Paid   ⊘ SNF Excluded   **H Codes — 67**

E	H1010	Non-medical family planning education, per session
E	H1011	Family assessment by licensed behavioral health professional for state defined purposes
E	H2000	Comprehensive multidisciplinary evaluation
E	H2001	Rehabilitation program, per 1/2 day
E	H2010	Comprehensive medication services, per 15 minutes
E	H2011	Crisis intervention service, per 15 minutes
E	H2012	Behavioral health day treatment, per hour
E	H2013	Psychiatric health facility service, per diem
E	H2014	Skills training and development, per 15 minutes
E	H2015	Comprehensive community support services, per 15 minutes
E	H2016	Comprehensive community support services, per diem
E	H2017	Psychosocial rehabilitation services, per 15 minutes
E	H2018	Psychosocial rehabilitation services, per diem
	H2019	Therapeutic behavioral services, per 15 minutes
E	H2020	Therapeutic behavioral services, per diem
E	H2021	Community-based wrap-around services, per 15 minutes
E	H2022	Community-based wrap-around services, per diem
E	H2023	Supported employment, per 15 minutes
E	H2024	Supported employment, per diem
E	H2025	Ongoing support to maintain employment, per 15 minutes
E	H2026	Ongoing support to maintain employment, per diem
E	H2027	Psychoeducational service, per 15 minutes
E	H2028	Sexual offender treatment service, per 15 minutes
E	H2029	Sexual offender treatment service, per diem
E	H2030	Mental health clubhouse services, per 15 minutes
E	H2031	Mental health clubhouse services, per diem
E	H2032	Activity therapy, per 15 minutes
E	H2033	Multisystemic therapy for juveniles, per 15 minutes
E	H2034	Alcohol and/or drug abuse halfway house services, per diem
E	H2035	Alcohol and/or other drug treatment program, per hour
E	H2036	Alcohol and/or other drug treatment program, per diem
E	H2037	Developmental delay prevention activities, dependent child of client, per 15 minutes ▣P

Special Coverage Instructions   Noncovered by Medicare   Carrier Discretion   ☑ Quantity Alert   ● New Code   ○ Reinstated Code   ▲ Revised Code

68 — H Codes   Ⓐ Adult   Ⓜ Maternity   ▣P Pediatrics   ▣I Infant   Ⓐ-Ⓨ APC Status Indicator   *2005 HCPCS*

DRUGS ADMINISTERED OTHER THAN ORAL METHOD
J0000–J9999

J codes include drugs that ordinarily cannot be self-administered, chemotherapy drugs, immunosuppressive drugs, inhalation solutions, and other miscellaneous drugs and solutions.

EXCEPTION: ORAL IMMUNOSUPPRESSIVE DRUGS

J codes fall under the jurisdiction of the DME Regional office for Medicare, unless incidental or otherwise noted.

J0120 Injection, tetracycline, up to 250 mg
Use this code for Achromycin, Panmycin, Sumycin.
MED: 100-2, 15, 50

J0128 Injection, abarelix, 10 mg
Use this code for Plenaxis.

J0130 Injection abciximab, 10 mg
Use this code for ReoPro.
MED: 100-2, 15, 50

J0135 Injection, adalimumab, 20 mg
Use this code for Humira.

J0150 Injection, adenosine for therapeutic use, 6 mg (not to be used to report any adenosine phosphate compounds, instead use A9270)
Use this code for Adenocard.
MED: 100-2, 15, 50
AHA: 2Q, '02, 10

J0152 Injection, adenosine for diagnostic use, 30 mg (not to be used to report any adenosine phosphate compounds; instead use A9270)

J0170 Injection, adrenalin, epinephrine, up to 1 ml ampule
Use this code for Adrenalin Chloride, Sus-Phrine.
MED: 100-2, 15, 50

J0180 Injection, agalsidase beta, 1 mg
Use this code for Fabrazyme.

J0190 Injection, biperiden lactate, per 5 mg
Use this code for Akineton.
MED: 100-2, 15, 50

J0200 Injection, alatrofloxacin mesylate, 100 mg
Use this code for Trovan.
MED: 100-2, 15, 50.5

J0205 Injection, alglucerase, per 10 units
Use this code for Ceredase.
MED: 100-2, 15, 50

J0207 Injection, amifostine, 500 mg
Use this code for Ethyol.
MED: 100-2, 15, 50

J0210 Injection, methyldopa HCl, up to 250 mg
Use this code for Aldomet.
MED: 100-2, 15, 50

J0215 Injection, alefacept, 0.5 mg

J0256 Injection, alpha 1-proteinase inhibitor — human, 10 mg
Use this code for Prolastin.
MED: 100-2, 15, 50

J0270 Injection, alprostadil, 1.25 mcg (code may be used for Medicare when drug administered under direct supervision of a physician, not for use when drug is self-administered)
Use this code for Prostin VR Pediatric.
MED: 100-2, 15, 50

J0275 Alprostadil urethral suppository (code may be used for Medicare when drug administered under direct supervision of a physician, not for use when drug is self-administered)
Use this code for Muse.
MED: 100-2, 15, 50

J0280 Injection, aminophyllin, up to 250 mg
Use this code for Phyllocontin.
MED: 100-2, 15, 50

J0282 Injection, amiodarone HCl, 30 mg
Use this code for Cordarone IV.
MED: 100-2, 15, 50

J0285 Injection, amphotericin B, 50 mg
MED: 100-2, 15, 50

J0287 Injection, amphotericin B lipid complex, 10 mg
Use this code for Albecet.
MED: 100-2, 15, 50

J0288 Injection, amphotericin B cholesteryl sulfate complex, 10 mg
Use this code for Amphotec.
MED: 100-2, 15, 50

J0289 Injection, amphotericin B liposome, 10 mg
Use this code for Ambisome.
MED: 100-2, 15, 50

J0290 Injection, ampicillin sodium, 500 mg
Use this code for Omnipen-N, Totacillin-N.
MED: 100-2, 15, 50

J0295 Injection, ampicillin sodium/sulbactam sodium, per 1.5 g
Use this code for Unasyn.
MED: 100-2, 15, 50

J0300 Injection, amobarbital, up to 125 mg
Use this code for Amytal.
MED: 100-2, 15, 50

J0330 Injection, succinylcholine chloride, up to 20 mg
Use this code for Anectine, Quelicin, Sucostrin.
MED: 100-2, 15, 50

J0350 Injection, anistreplase, per 30 units
Use this code for Eminase.
MED: 100-2, 15, 50

J0360 Injection, hydralazine HCl, up to 20 mg
Use this code for Apresoline.
MED: 100-2, 15, 50

J0380 Injection, metaraminol bitartrate, per 10 mg
Use this code for Aramine.
MED: 100-2, 15, 50

J0390 Injection, chloroquine HCl, up to 250 mg
Use this code for Aralen.
MED: 100-2, 15, 50

Drugs Administered Other Than Oral Method

J0395 — J0702

N ☑ **J0395** Injection, arbutamine HCl, 1 mg ⊘
Use this code for GenESA.
MED: 100-2, 15, 50

N ☑ **J0456** Injection, azithromycin, 500 mg ⊘
Use this code for Zithromax.
MED: 100-2, 15, 50.5

N ☑ **J0460** Injection, atropine sulfate, up to 0.3 mg ⊘
MED: 100-2, 15, 50

N ☑ **J0470** Injection, dimercaprol, per 100 mg ⊘
Use this code for BAL in oil.
MED: 100-2, 15, 50

N ☑ **J0475** Injection, baclofen, 10 mg ⊘
Use this code for Lioresal.
MED: 100-2, 15, 50

B ☑ **J0476** Injection, baclofen, 50 mcg for intrathecal trial ⊘
Use this code for Lioresal for intrathecal trial.
MED: 100-2, 15, 50

N ☑ **J0500** Injection, dicyclomine HCl, up to 20 mg ⊘
Use this code for Bentyl, Dilomine, Antispas, Dibent, Di-Spaz, Neoquess, Or-Tyl, Spasmoject.
MED: 100-2, 15, 50

N ☑ **J0515** Injection, benztropine mesylate, per 1 mg ⊘
Use this code for Cogentin.
MED: 100-2, 15, 50

N ☑ **J0520** Injection, bethanechol chloride, Mytonachol or Urecholine, up to 5 mg ⊘
Use this code for Urecholine.
MED: 100-2, 15, 50

N ☑ **J0530** Injection, penicillin G benzathine and penicillin G procaine, up to 600,000 units ⊘
Use this code for Bicillin C-R.
MED: 100-2, 15, 50

N ☑ **J0540** Injection, penicillin G benzathine and penicillin G procaine, up to 1,200,000 units ⊘
Use this code for Bicillin C-R, Bicillin C-R 900/300.
MED: 100-2, 15, 50

N ☑ **J0550** Injection, penicillin G benzathine and penicillin G procaine, up to 2,400,000 units ⊘
Use this code for Bicillin C-R.
MED: 100-2, 15, 50

N ☑ **J0560** Injection, penicillin G benzathine, up to 600,000 units ⊘
Use this code for Bicillin L-A, Permapen.
MED: 100-2, 15, 50

N ☑ **J0570** Injection, penicillin G benzathine, up to 1,200,000 units ⊘
Use this code for Bicillin L-A, Permapen.
MED: 100-2, 15, 50

N ☑ **J0580** Injection, penicillin G benzathine, up to 2,400,000 units ⊘
Use this code for Bicillin L-A, Permapen.
MED: 100-2, 15, 50

G ☑ **J0583** Injection, bivalirudin, 1 mg ⊘

K ☑ **J0585** Botulinum toxin type A, per unit ⊘
Use this code for Botox.
MED: 100-2, 15, 50

K ☑ **J0587** Botulinum toxin type B, per 100 units ⊘
Use this code for Myobloc.
MED: 100-2, 15, 50
AHA: 2Q, '02, 8

N **J0592** Injection, buprenorphine hydrochloride, 0.1 mg
Use this code for Buprenix.
MED: 100-2, 15, 50

N ☑ **J0595** Injection, butorphanol tartrate, 1 mg ⊘

N ☑ **J0600** Injection, edetate calcium disodium, up to 1000 mg ⊘
Use this code for Calcium Disodium Versenate, Calcium EDTA.
MED: 100-2, 15, 50

N ☑ **J0610** Injection, calcium gluconate, per 10 ml ⊘
Use this code for Kaleinate.
MED: 100-2, 15, 50

N ☑ **J0620** Injection, calcium glycerophosphate and calcium lactate, per 10 ml ⊘
Use this code for Calphosan.
MED: 100-2, 15, 50

N ☑ **J0630** Injection, calcitonin-salmon, up to 400 units ⊘
Use this code for Calcimar, Miacalcin.
MED: 100-2, 15, 50

N **J0636** Injection, calcitriol, 0.1 mcg
Use this code for Calcijex.
MED: 100-2, 15, 50

K **J0637** Injection, caspofungin acetate, 5 mg
Use this code for Cancidas.

N ☑ **J0640** Injection, leucovorin calcium, per 50 mg ⊘
Use this code for Wellcovorin.
MED: 100-2, 15, 50

N ☑ **J0670** Injection, mepivacaine HCl, per 10 ml ⊘
Use this code for Carbocaine, Polocaine, Isocaine HCl.
MED: 100-2, 15, 50

N ☑ **J0690** Injection, cefazolin sodium, 500 mg ⊘
Use this code for Ancef, Kefzol, Zolicef.
MED: 100-2, 15, 50

N **J0692** Injection, cefepime HCl, 500 mg ⊘
Use this code for Maxipime.

N ☑ **J0694** Injection, cefoxitin sodium, 1 g ⊘
Use this code for Mefoxin.
MED: 100-2, 15, 50
See code(s): Q0090

N ☑ **J0696** Injection, ceftriaxone sodium, per 250 mg ⊘
Use this code for Rocephin.
MED: 100-2, 15, 50

N ☑ **J0697** Injection, sterile cefuroxime sodium, per 750 mg ⊘
Use this code for Kefurox, Zinacef.
MED: 100-2, 15, 50

N ☑ **J0698** Cefotaxime sodium, per g ⊘
Use this code for Claforan.
MED: 100-2, 15, 50

N ☑ **J0702** Injection, betamethasone acetate and betamethasone sodium phosphate, per 3 mg ⊘
MED: 100-2, 15, 50

Special Coverage Instructions   Noncovered by Medicare   Carrier Discretion   ☑ Quantity Alert   ● New Code   ○ Reinstated Code   ▲ Revised Code

N ☑ **J0704** Injection, betamethasone sodium phosphate, per 4 mg ⊘
Use this code for Betameth, Celestone Phosphate, Cel-U-Jec, Selestoject.
MED: 100-2, 15, 50

N **J0706** Injection, caffeine citrate, 5 mg ⊘
Use this code for Cafcet.
AHA: 2Q, '02, 8

N ☑ **J0710** Injection, cephapirin sodium, up to 1 g ⊘
Use this code for Cefadyl.
MED: 100-2, 15, 50

N ☑ **J0713** Injection, ceftazidime, per 500 mg ⊘
Use this code for Fortaz, Tazidime.
MED: 100-2, 15, 50

N ☑ **J0715** Injection, ceftizoxime sodium, per 500 mg ⊘
Use this code for Cefizox.
MED: 100-2, 15, 50

N ☑ **J0720** Injection, chloramphenicol sodium succinate, up to 1 g ⊘
Use this code for Chloromycetin Sodium Succinate.
MED: 100-2, 15, 50

N ☑ **J0725** Injection, chorionic gonadotropin, per 1,000 USP units ⊘
Use this code for Glukor, Follutein, Chorex-5, Corgonject-5, Profasi HP, A.P.L., Pregnyl, Gonic, Choron 10, Chorex-10, Chorignon.
MED: 100-2, 15, 50

N ☑ **J0735** Injection, clonidine HCl, 1 mg ⊘
Use this code for Catapres.
MED: 100-2, 15, 50

N ☑ **J0740** Injection, cidofovir, 375 mg ⊘
Use this code for Vistide.
MED: 100-2, 15, 50

N ☑ **J0743** Injection, cilastatin sodium imipenem, per 250 mg ⊘
Use this code for Primaxin I.M., Primaxin I.V.
MED: 100-2, 15, 50

N **J0744** Injection, ciprofloxacin for intravenous infusion, 200 mg ⊘
Use this code for Cipro.

N ☑ **J0745** Injection, codeine phosphate, per 30 mg ⊘
MED: 100-2, 15, 50

N ☑ **J0760** Injection, colchicine, per 1 mg ⊘
MED: 100-2, 15, 50

N ☑ **J0770** Injection, colistimethate sodium, up to 150 mg ⊘
Use this code for Coly-Mycin M.
MED: 100-2, 15, 50

N ☑ **J0780** Injection, prochlorperazine, up to 10 mg ⊘
Use this code for Compazine, Cotranzine, Compa-Z, Ultrazine-10.
MED: 100-2, 15, 50

N ☑ **J0800** Injection, corticotropin, up to 40 units ⊘
Use this code for Acthar, ACTH.
MED: 100-2, 15, 50

N ☑ **J0835** Injection, cosyntropin, per 0.25 mg ⊘
Use this code for Cortrosyn.
MED: 100-2, 15, 50

K ☑ **J0850** Injection, cytomegalovirus immune globulin intravenous (human), per vial ⊘
MED: 100-2, 15, 50

● ☑ **J0878** Injection, daptomycin, 1 mg
Use this code for Cubicin.

E **J0880** Injection, darbepoetin alfa, 5 mcg ⊘
Use this code for Aranesp.

N ☑ **J0895** Injection, deferoxamine mesylate, 500 mg ⊘
Use this code for Desferal.
MED: 100-2, 15, 50
See code(s): Q0087

N ☑ **J0900** Injection, testosterone enanthate and estradiol valerate, up to 1 cc ⊘
Use this code for Deladumone, Andrest 90-4, Andro-Estro 90-4, Androgyn L.A., Delatestadiol, Dua-Gen L.A., Duoval P.A., Estra-Testrin, TEEV, Testadiate, Testradiol 90/4, Valertest No. 1, Valertest No. 2, Deladumone OB, Ditate-DS.
MED: 100-2, 15, 50

N ☑ **J0945** Injection, brompheniramine maleate, per 10 mg ⊘
Use this code for Histaject, Cophene-B, Dehist, Nasahist B, ND Stat, Oraminic II, Sinusol-B.
MED: 100-2, 15, 50

N ☑ **J0970** Injection, estradiol valerate, up to 40 mg ⊘
Use this code for Delestrogen, Dioval, Dioval XX, Dioval 40, Duragen-10, Duragen-20, Duragen-40, Estradiol L.A., Estradiol L.A. 20, Estradiol L.A. 40, Gynogen L.A. 10, Gynogen L.A. 20, Gynogen L.A. 40, Valergen 10, Valergen 20, Valergen 40, Estra-L 20, Estra-L 40, L.A.E. 20.
MED: 100-2, 15, 50

N ☑ **J1000** Injection, depo-estradiol cypionate, up to 5 mg ⊘
Use this code for Estradiol Cypionate, depGynogen, Depogen, Dura-Estrin, Estra-D, Estro-Cyp, Estroject L.A., Estronol-L.A.
MED: 100-2, 15, 50

N ☑ **J1020** Injection, methylprednisolone acetate, 20 mg ⊘
Use this code for Depo-Medrol.
MED: 100-2, 15, 50

N ☑ **J1030** Injection, methylprednisolone acetate, 40 mg ⊘
Use this code for Depo-Medrol, depMedalone 40, Depoject, Depopred-40, Duralone-40, Medralone 40, M-Prednisol-40, Rep-Pred 40.
MED: 100-2, 15, 50

N ☑ **J1040** Injection, methylprednisolone acetate, 80 mg ⊘
Use this code for Depo-Medrol, depMedalone 80, Depoject, Depopred-80, D-Med 80, Duralone-80, Medralone 80, M-Prednisol-80, Rep-Pred 80.
MED: 100-2, 15, 50

N **J1051** Injection, medroxyprogesterone acetate, 50 mg
Use this code for Depo-Provera.
MED: 100-2, 15, 50

E ☑ **J1055** Injection, medroxyprogesterone acetate for contraceptive use, 150 mg ♀⊘
Use this code for Depo-Provera.

E **J1056** Injection, medroxyprogesterone acetate/estradiol cypionate, 5 mg/25 mg ♀⊘
Use this code for Lunelle monthly contraceptive.

N ☑ **J1060** Injection, testosterone cypionate and estradiol cypionate, up to 1 ml ⊘
Use this code for Depo-Testadial, Andro/Fem, De-Comberol, depAndrogyn, Depotestogen, Duo-Cyp, Duratestrin, Menoject LA, Test-Estro-C, Test-Estro Cypionates.
MED: 100-2, 15, 50

J1070 — J1436   Drugs Administered Other Than Oral Method

N ☑ **J1070** Injection, testosterone cypionate, up to 100 mg ⊘
Use this code for Depo-Testosterone, Duratest-100, Andro-Cyp, Andronaq-LA, Andronate-100, depAndro 100, Depotest, Testoject-LA.
MED: 100-2, 15, 50

N ☑ **J1080** Injection, testosterone cypionate, 1 cc, 200 mg ⊘
Use this code for Depo-Testosterone, Andro-Cyp 200, Andronate 200, depAndro 200, Depotest, Duratest-200, Testa-C, Testadiate-Depo, Testoject-LA.
MED: 100-2, 15, 50

N **J1094** Injection, dexamethasone acetate, 1 mg
Use this code for Dalalone L.A.
MED: 100-2, 15, 50

N ☑ **J1100** Injection, dexamethasone sodium phosphate, 1 mg ⊘
Use this code for Cortastat, Dalalone.
MED: 100-2, 15, 50

N ☑ **J1110** Injection, dihydroergotamine mesylate, per 1 mg ⊘
Use this code for D.H.E. 45.
MED: 100-2, 15, 50

N ☑ **J1120** Injection, acetazolamide sodium, up to 500 mg ⊘
Use this code for Diamox.
MED: 100-2, 15, 50

N ☑ **J1160** Injection, digoxin, up to 0.5 mg ⊘
Use this code for Lanoxin.
MED: 100-2, 15, 50

N ☑ **J1165** Injection, phenytoin sodium, per 50 mg ⊘
Use this code for Dilantin.
MED: 100-2, 15, 50

N ☑ **J1170** Injection, hydromorphone, up to 4 mg ⊘
Use this code for Dilaudid.
MED: 100-2, 15, 50

N ☑ **J1180** Injection, dyphylline, up to 500 mg ⊘
Use this code for Lufyllin, Dilor.
MED: 100-2, 15, 50

K ☑ **J1190** Injection, dexrazoxane HCl, per 250 mg ⊘
Use this code for Zinecard.
MED: 100-2, 15, 50

N ☑ **J1200** Injection, diphenhydramine HCl, up to 50 mg ⊘
Use this code for Benadryl, Benahist 10, Benahist 50, Benoject-10, Benoject-50, Bena-D 10, Bena-D 50, Nordryl, Ben-Allergin-50, Dihydrex, Diphenacen-50, Hyrexin-50, Wehdryl.
MED: 100-2, 15, 50
AHA: 1Q, '02, 2

N ☑ **J1205** Injection, chlorothiazide sodium, per 500 mg ⊘
Use this code for Diuril Sodium.
MED: 100-2, 15, 50

N ☑ **J1212** Injection, DMSO, dimethyl sulfoxide, 50%, 50 ml ⊘
Use this code for Rimso. DMSO is covered only as a treatment of interstitial cystitis.
MED: 100-2, 15, 50; 100-3, 230.12

N ☑ **J1230** Injection, methadone HCl, up to 10 mg ⊘
Use this code for Dolophine HCl.
MED: 100-2, 15, 50

N ☑ **J1240** Injection, dimenhydrinate, up to 50 mg ⊘
Use this code for Dramamine, Dinate, Dommanate, Dramanate, Dramilin, Dramocen, Dramoject, Dymenate, Hydrate, Marmine, Wehamine.
MED: 100-2, 15, 50

K ☑ **J1245** Injection, dipyridamole, per 10 mg
Use this code for Persantine IV.
MED: 100-2, 15, 50

N ☑ **J1250** Injection, dobutamine HCl, per 250 mg ⊘
Use this code for Dobutrex.
MED: 100-2, 15, 50

N ☑ **J1260** Injection, dolasetron mesylate, 10 mg ⊘
Use this code for Anzemet.
MED: 100-2, 15, 50

N **J1270** Injection, doxercalciferol, 1 mcg ⊘
Use this code for Hectorolc.

N ☑ **J1320** Injection, amitriptyline HCl, up to 20 mg ⊘
Use this code for Elavil, Enovil.
MED: 100-2, 15, 50

N ☑ **J1325** Injection, epoprostenol, 0.5 mg ⊘
Use this code for Flolan. See K0455 for infusion pump for epoprosterol.
MED: 100-2, 15, 50

K ☑ **J1327** Injection, eptifibatide, 5 mg ⊘
Use this code for Integrilin.
MED: 100-2, 15, 50

N ☑ **J1330** Injection, ergonovine maleate, up to 0.2 mg ⊘
Medicare jurisdiction: local carrier. Use this code for Ergotrate Maleate.
MED: 100-2, 15, 50

G ☑ **J1335** Injection, ertapenem sodium, 500 mg ⊘

N ☑ **J1364** Injection, erythromycin lactobionate, per 500 mg ⊘
MED: 100-2, 15, 50

N ☑ **J1380** Injection, estradiol valerate, up to 10 mg ⊘
Use this code for Delestrogen, Dioval, Dioval XX, Dioval 40, Duragen-10, Duragen-20, Duragen-40, Estradiol L.A., Estradiol L.A. 20, Estradiol L.A. 40, Gynogen L.A. 10, Gynogen L.A. 20, Gynogen L.A. 40, Valergen 10, Valergen 20, Valergen 40, Estra-L 20, Estra-L 40, L.A.E. 20.
MED: 100-2, 15, 50

N ☑ **J1390** Injection, estradiol valerate, up to 20 mg ⊘
Use this code for Delestrogen, Dioval, Dioval XX, Dioval 40, Duragen-10, Duragen-20, Duragen-40, Estradiol L.A., Estradiol L.A. 20, Estradiol L.A. 40, Gynogen L.A. 10, Gynogen L.A. 20, Gynogen L.A. 40, Valergen 10, Valergen 20, Valergen 40, Estra-L 20, Estra-L 40, L.A.E. 20.
MED: 100-2, 15, 50

N ☑ **J1410** Injection, estrogen conjugated, per 25 mg ⊘
Use this code for Premarin Intravenous.
MED: 100-2, 15, 50

N ☑ **J1435** Injection, estrone, per 1 mg ⊘
Use this code for Estone Aqueous, Estronol, Theelin Aqueous, Estone 5, Kestrone 5.
MED: 100-2, 15, 50

N ☑ **J1436** Injection, etidronate disodium, per 300 mg ⊘
Use this code for Didronel.
MED: 100-2, 15, 50

Special Coverage Instructions   Noncovered by Medicare   Carrier Discretion   ☑ Quantity Alert   ● New Code   ○ Reinstated Code   ▲ Revised Code

72 — J Codes   A Adult   M Maternity   P Pediatrics   I Infant   A-Y APC Status Indicator   *2005 HCPCS*

K ☑ **J1438** Injection, etanercept, 25 mg (code may be used for Medicare when drug administered under the direct supervision of a physician, not for use when drug is self-administered) ⊘
Use this code for Enbrel.
MED: 100-2, 15, 50

K ☑ **J1440** Injection, filgrastim (G-CSF), 300 mcg ⊘
Use this code for Neupogen.
MED: 100-2, 15, 50

K ☑ **J1441** Injection, filgrastim (G-CSF), 480 mcg ⊘
Use this code for Neupogen.
MED: 100-2, 15, 50

N ☑ **J1450** Injection, fluconazole, 200 mg ⊘
Use this code for Diflucan.
MED: 100-2, 15, 50.5

N ☑ **J1452** Injection, fomivirsen sodium, intraocular, 1.65 mg ⊘
Use this code for Vitavene.
MED: 100-2, 15, 50.4; 100-2, 15, 50.4.2

N ☑ **J1455** Injection, foscarnet sodium, per 1,000 mg ⊘
Use this code for Foscavir.
MED: 100-2, 15, 50

● ☑ **J1457** Injection, gallium nitrate, 1 mg

B ☑ **J1460** Injection, gamma globulin, intramuscular, 1 cc ⊘
Use this code for Gammar, Gamastan.
MED: 100-2, 15, 50

B ☑ **J1470** Injection, gamma globulin, intramuscular, 2 cc ⊘
Use this code for Gammar, Gamastan.
MED: 100-2, 15, 50

B ☑ **J1480** Injection, gamma globulin, intramuscular, 3 cc ⊘
Use this code for Gammar, Gamastan.
MED: 100-2, 15, 50

B ☑ **J1490** Injection, gamma globulin, intramuscular, 4 cc ⊘
Use this code for Gammar, Gamastan.
MED: 100-2, 15, 50

B ☑ **J1500** Injection, gamma globulin, intramuscular, 5 cc ⊘
Use this code for Gammar, Gamastan.
MED: 100-2, 15, 50

B ☑ **J1510** Injection, gamma globulin, intramuscular, 6 cc ⊘
Use this code for Gammar, Gamastan.
MED: 100-2, 15, 50

B ☑ **J1520** Injection, gamma globulin, intramuscular, 7 cc ⊘
Use this code for Gammar, Gamastan.
MED: 100-2, 15, 50

B ☑ **J1530** Injection, gamma globulin, intramuscular, 8 cc ⊘
Use this code for Gammar, Gamastan.
MED: 100-2, 15, 50

B ☑ **J1540** Injection, gamma globulin, intramuscular, 9 cc ⊘
Use this code for Gammar, Gamastan.
MED: 100-2, 15, 50

B ☑ **J1550** Injection, gamma globulin, intramuscular, 10 cc ⊘
Use this code for Gammar, Gamastan.
MED: 100-2, 15, 50

B ☑ **J1560** Injection, gamma globulin, intramuscular, over 10 cc ⊘
Use this code for Gammar, Gamastan.
MED: 100-2, 15, 50

K ☑ **J1563** Injection, immune globulin, intravenous, 1 g ⊘
MED: 100-2, 15, 50
AHA: 2Q, '03, 8

▲ K **J1564** Injection, immune globulin, intravenous, 10 mg
MED: 100-2, 15, 50
AHA: 2Q, '03, 8

K ☑ **J1565** Injection, respiratory syncytial virus immune globulin, intravenous, 50 mg ⊘
MED: 100-2, 15, 50

K ☑ **J1570** Injection, ganciclovir sodium, 500 mg ⊘
Use this code for Cytovene.
MED: 100-2, 15, 50

N ☑ **J1580** Injection, garamycin, gentamicin, up to 80 mg ⊘
Use this code for Gentamicin Sulfate, Jenamicin.
MED: 100-2, 15, 50

N ☑ **J1590** Injection, gatifloxacin, 10 mg ⊘
N ☑ **J1595** Injection, glatiramer acetate, 20 mg ⊘
MED: 100-2, 15, 50

N ☑ **J1600** Injection, gold sodium thiomalate, up to 50 mg ⊘
Use this code for Myochrysine.
MED: 100-2, 15, 50

N ☑ **J1610** Injection, glucagon HCl, per 1 mg ⊘
Use this code for glucagon.
MED: 100-2, 15, 50

N ☑ **J1620** Injection, gonadorelin HCl, per 100 mcg ⊘
Use this code for Factrel, Lutrepulse.
MED: 100-2, 15, 50

K ☑ **J1626** Injection, granisetron HCl, 100 mcg ⊘
Use this code for Kytril.
MED: 100-2, 15, 50

N ☑ **J1630** Injection, haloperidol, up to 5 mg ⊘
Use this code for Haldol.
MED: 100-2, 15, 50

N ☑ **J1631** Injection, haloperidol decanoate, per 50 mg ⊘
Use this code for Haldol Decanoate-50.
MED: 100-2, 15, 50

N ☑ **J1642** Injection, heparin sodium, (heparin lock flush), per 10 units ⊘
Use this code for Hep-Lock, Hep-Lock U/P.
MED: 100-2, 15, 50

N ☑ **J1644** Injection, heparin sodium, per 1,000 units ⊘
Use this code for Heparin Sodium, Liquaemin Sodium.
MED: 100-2, 15, 50

N ☑ **J1645** Injection, dalteparin sodium, per 2500 IU ⊘
Use this code for Fragmin.
MED: 100-2, 15, 50

N ☑ **J1650** Injection, enoxaparin sodium, 10 mg ⊘
Use this code for Lovenox.

N **J1652** Injection, fondaparinux sodium, 0.5 mg
Use this code for Atrixtra.
MED: 100-2, 15, 50

N ☑ **J1655** Injection, tinzaparin sodium, 1000 IU ⊘
Use this code for Innohep.

N ☑ **J1670** Injection, tetanus immune globulin, human, up to 250 units ⊘
MED: 100-2, 15, 50

J1700 Injection, hydrocortisone acetate, up to 25 mg ⊘
Use this code for Hydrocortone Acetate.
MED: 100-2, 15, 50

J1710 Injection, hydrocortisone sodium phosphate, up to 50 mg ⊘
Use this code for Hydrocortone Phosphate.
MED: 100-2, 15, 50

J1720 Injection, hydrocortisone sodium succinate, up to 100 mg ⊘
Use this code for Solu-Cortef, A-Hydrocort.
MED: 100-2, 15, 50

J1730 Injection, diazoxide, up to 300 mg ⊘
Use this code for Hyperstat IV.
MED: 100-2, 15, 50

J1742 Injection, ibutilide fumarate, 1 mg ⊘
Use this code for Corvert.
MED: 100-2, 15, 50

J1745 Injection, infliximab, 10 mg ⊘
Use this code for Remicade.
MED: 100-2, 15, 50

J1750 Injection, iron dextran, 50 mg ⊘
Use this code for Infed.
MED: 100-2, 15, 50.5

J1756 Injection, iron sucrose, 1 mg
Use this code for Venofer.

J1785 Injection, imiglucerase, per unit ⊘
Use this code for Cerezyme.
MED: 100-2, 15, 50

J1790 Injection, droperidol, up to 5 mg ⊘
Use this code for Inapsine.
MED: 100-2, 15, 50

J1800 Injection, propranolol HCl, up to 1 mg ⊘
Use this code for Inderal.
MED: 100-2, 15, 50

J1810 Injection, droperidol and fentanyl citrate, up to 2 ml ampule ⊘
Use this code for Innovar.
MED: 100-2, 15, 50
AHA: 2Q, '02, 8

J1815 Injection, insulin, per 5 units
Use this code for Humalog, Humulin, Iletin, Insulin Lispo, Novo Nordisk, NPH, Pork insulin, Regular insulin, Ultralente, Velosulin.
MED: 100-2, 15, 50; 100-3, 280.14

J1817 Insulin for administration through DME (i.e., insulin pump) per 50 units
Use this code for Humalog, Humulin.

J1825 Injection, interferon beta-1a, 33 mcg ⊘
Use this code for Avonex.

J1830 Injection interferon beta-1b, 0.25 mg (code may be used for Medicare when drug administered under direct supervision of a physician, not for use when drug is self-administered) ⊘
MED: 100-2, 15, 50

J1835 Injection, itraconazole, 50 mg ⊘
Use this code for Sporonox IV.

J1840 Injection, kanamycin sulfate, up to 500 mg ⊘
Use this code for Kantrex, Klebcil.
MED: 100-2, 15, 50

J1850 Injection, kanamycin sulfate, up to 75 mg ⊘
Use this code for Kantrex, Klebcil.
MED: 100-2, 15, 50

J1885 Injection, ketorolac tromethamine, per 15 mg ⊘
Use this code for Toradol.
MED: 100-2, 15, 50

J1890 Injection, cephalothin sodium, up to 1 g ⊘
Use this code for Cephalothin Sodium, Keflin.
MED: 100-2, 15, 50

● **J1931** Injection, laronidase, 0.1 mg
Use this code for Aldurazyme.

J1940 Injection, furosemide, up to 20 mg ⊘
Use this code for Lasix, Furomide M.D.
MED: 100-2, 15, 50

J1950 Injection, leuprolide acetate (for depot suspension), per 3.75 mg ⊘
Use this code for Lupron Depot.
MED: 100-2, 15, 50

J1955 Injection, levocarnitine, per 1 g ⊘
Use this code for Carnitor.
MED: 100-2, 15, 50

J1956 Injection, levofloxacin, 250 mg ⊘
Use this code for Levaquin.
MED: 100-2, 15, 50

J1960 Injection, levorphanol tartrate, up to 2 mg ⊘
Use this code for Levo-Dromoran.
MED: 100-2, 15, 50

J1980 Injection, hyoscyamine sulfate, up to 0.25 mg ⊘
Use this code for Levsin.
MED: 100-2, 15, 50

J1990 Injection, chlordiazepoxide HCl, up to 100 mg ⊘
Use this code for Librium.
MED: 100-2, 15, 50

J2001 Injection, lidocaine HCl for intravenous infusion, 10 mg ⊘
MED: 100-2, 15, 50

J2010 Injection, lincomycin HCl, up to 300 mg ⊘
Use this code for Lincocin.
MED: 100-2, 15, 50

J2020 Injection, linezolid, 200 mg ⊘
Use this code for Zyvok.
AHA: 2Q, '02, 8

J2060 Injection, lorazepam, 2 mg ⊘
Use this code for Ativan.
MED: 100-2, 15, 50

J2150 Injection, mannitol, 25% in 50 ml ⊘
MED: 100-2, 15, 50

J2175 Injection, meperidine HCl, per 100 mg ⊘
Use this code for Demerol HCl.
MED: 100-2, 15, 50

J2180 Injection, meperidine and promethazine HCl, up to 50 mg ⊘
Use this code for Mepergan Injection.
MED: 100-2, 15, 50

J2185 Injection, meropenem, 100 mg ⊘

Special Coverage Instructions   Noncovered by Medicare   Carrier Discretion   ☑ Quantity Alert   ● New Code   ○ Reinstated Code   ▲ Revised Code

74 — J Codes   Ⓐ Adult   Ⓜ Maternity   Ⓟ Pediatrics   Ⓘ Infant   Ⓐ-Ⓨ APC Status Indicator   *2005 HCPCS*

N ☑ **J2210** Injection, methylergonovine maleate, up to 0.2 mg ⊘
Use this code for Methergine.
MED: 100-2, 15, 50

N ☑ **J2250** Injection, midazolam HCl, per 1 mg ⊘
Use this code for Versed.
MED: 100-2, 15, 50

K ☑ **J2260** Injection, milrinone lactate, 5 mg ⊘
Use this code for Primacor.
MED: 100-2, 15, 50

N ☑ **J2270** Injection, morphine sulfate, up to 10 mg ⊘
MED: 100-2, 15, 50

N ☑ **J2271** Injection, morphine sulfate, 100 mg ⊘
MED: 100-2, 15, 50; 100-3, 280.14

N ☑ **J2275** Injection, morphine sulfate (preservative-free sterile solution), per 10 mg
Use this code for Astramorph PF, Duramorph.
MED: 100-2, 15, 50; 100-3, 280.14

N ☑ **J2280** Injection, moxifloxacin, 100 mg ⊘

N ☑ **J2300** Injection, nalbuphine HCl, per 10 mg ⊘
Use this code for Nubain.
MED: 100-2, 15, 50

N ☑ **J2310** Injection, naloxone HCl, per 1 mg ⊘
Use this code for Narcan.
MED: 100-2, 15, 50

N ☑ **J2320** Injection, nandrolone decanoate, up to 50 mg ⊘
Use this code for Deca-Durabolin, Hybolin Decanoate, Decolone-50, Neo-Durabolic.
MED: 100-2, 15, 50

N ☑ **J2321** Injection, nandrolone decanoate, up to 100 mg ⊘
Use this code for Deca-Durabolin, Hybolin Decanoate, Decolone-100, Neo-Durabolic, Anabolin LA 100, Androlone-D 100, Nandrobolic L.A.
MED: 100-2, 15, 50

N ☑ **J2322** Injection, nandrolone decanoate, up to 200 mg ⊘
Use this code for Deca-Durabolin, Neo-Durabolic.
MED: 100-2, 15, 50

▲ G **J2324** Injection, nesiritide, 0.25 mg
Use this code for Natrecor.
MED: 100-2, 15, 50

K ☑ **J2353** Injection, octreotide, depot form for intramuscular injection, 1 mg ⊘

K ☑ **J2354** Injection, octreotide, non-depot form for subcutaneous or intravenous injection, 25 mcg ⊘

K ☑ **J2355** Injection, oprelvekin, 5 mg ⊘
Use this code for Neumega.
MED: 100-2, 15, 50

● ☑ **J2357** Injection, omalizumab, 5 mg
Use this code for Xolair.

N ☑ **J2360** Injection, orphenadrine citrate, up to 60 mg ⊘
Use this code for Norflex, Banflex, Flexoject, Flexon, K-Flex, Myolin, Neocyten, O-Flex, Orphenate.
MED: 100-2, 15, 50

N ☑ **J2370** Injection, phenylephrine HCl, up to 1 ml ⊘
Use this code for Neo-Synephrine.
MED: 100-2, 15, 50

N ☑ **J2400** Injection, chloroprocaine HCl, per 30 ml ⊘
Use this code for Nesacaine, Nesacaine-MPF.
MED: 100-2, 15, 50

N ☑ **J2405** Injection, ondansetron HCl, per 1 mg ⊘
Use this code for Zofran.
MED: 100-2, 15, 50

N ☑ **J2410** Injection, oxymorphone HCl, up to 1 mg ⊘
Use this code for Numorphan, Numorphan H.P.
MED: 100-2, 15, 50

K ☑ **J2430** Injection, pamidronate disodium, per 30 mg ⊘
Use this code for Aredia.
MED: 100-2, 15, 50

N ☑ **J2440** Injection, papaverine HCl, up to 60 mg ⊘
MED: 100-2, 15, 50

N ☑ **J2460** Injection, oxytetracycline HCl, up to 50 mg ⊘
Use this code for Terramycin IM.
MED: 100-2, 15, 50

● **J2469** Injection, palonosetron HCl, 25 mcg
Use this code for Aloxi.

N **J2501** Injection, paricalcitol, 1 mcg
Use this code For Zemplar.
MED: 100-2, 15, 50

G ☑ **J2505** Injection, pegfilgrastim, 6 mg ⊘
Use this code for Neulasta.

N ☑ **J2510** Injection, penicillin G procaine, aqueous, up to 600,000 units ⊘
Use this code for Wycillin, Duracillin A.S., Pfizerpen A.S., Crysticillin 300 A.S., Crysticillin 600 A.S.
MED: 100-2, 15, 50

N ☑ **J2515** Injection, pentobarbital sodium, per 50 mg ⊘
Use this code for Nembutal Sodium Solution.
MED: 100-2, 15, 50

N ☑ **J2540** Injection, penicillin G potassium, up to 600,000 units ⊘
Use this code for Pfizerpen.
MED: 100-2, 15, 50

N ☑ **J2543** Injection, piperacillin sodium/tazobactam sodium, 1 g/0.125 g (1.125 g) ⊘
Use this code for Zosyn.
MED: 100-2, 15, 50

Y ☑ **J2545** Pentamidine isethionate, inhalation solution, per 300 mg, administered through a DME ⊘
Use this code for Nebupent, PentacaRinat, Pentam 300.
MED: 100-2, 15, 50
See code(s): Q0077

N ☑ **J2550** Injection, promethazine HCl, up to 50 mg ⊘
Use this code for Phenergan, Anergan 25, Anergan 50, Phenazine 25, Phenazine 50, Prorex-25, Prorex-50, Prothazine, V-Gan 25, V-Gan 50.
MED: 100-2, 15, 50

N ☑ **J2560** Injection, phenobarbital sodium, up to 120 mg ⊘
Use this code for Luminal Sodium.
MED: 100-2, 15, 50

N ☑ **J2590** Injection, oxytocin, up to 10 units ⊘
Use this code for Pitocin, Syntocinon.
MED: 100-2, 15, 50

N ☑ **J2597** Injection, desmopressin acetate, per 1 mcg ⊘
Use this code for DDAVP.
MED: 100-2, 15, 50

N ☑ **J2650** Injection, prednisolone acetate, up to 1 ml ⊘
Use this code for Key-Pred 25, Key-Pred 50, Predcor-25, Predcor-50, Predoject-50, Predalone-50, Predicort-50.
MED: 100-2, 15, 50

N ☑ **J2670** Injection, tolazoline HCl, up to 25 mg ⊘
Use this code for Priscoline HCl.
MED: 100-2, 15, 50

N **J2675** Injection, progesterone, per 50 mg ⊘
MED: 100-2, 15, 50

N ☑ **J2680** Injection, fluphenazine decanoate, up to 25 mg ⊘
Use this code for Prolixin Decanoate.
MED: 100-2, 15, 50

N ☑ **J2690** Injection, procainamide HCl, up to 1 g ⊘
Use this code for Pronestyl.
MED: 100-2, 15, 50

N ☑ **J2700** Injection, oxacillin sodium, up to 250 mg ⊘
Use this code for Bactocill, Prostaphlin.
MED: 100-2, 15, 50

N ☑ **J2710** Injection, neostigmine methylsulfate, up to 0.5 mg ⊘
Use this code for Prostigmin.
MED: 100-2, 15, 50

N ☑ **J2720** Injection, protamine sulfate, per 10 mg ⊘
MED: 100-2, 15, 50

N ☑ **J2725** Injection, protirelin, per 250 mcg ⊘
Use this code for Relefact TRH, Thypinone.
MED: 100-2, 15, 50

N ☑ **J2730** Injection, pralidoxime chloride, up to 1 g ⊘
Use this code for Protopam Chloride.
MED: 100-2, 15, 50

N ☑ **J2760** Injection, phentolamine mesylate, up to 5 mg ⊘
Use this code for Regitine.
MED: 100-2, 15, 50

N ☑ **J2765** Injection, metoclopramide HCl, up to 10 mg ⊘
Use this code for Reglan.
MED: 100-2, 15, 50

N ☑ **J2770** Injection, quinupristin/dalfopristin, 500 mg (150/350) ⊘
Use this code for Synercid.
MED: 100-2, 15, 50

N ☑ **J2780** Injection, ranitidine HCl, 25 mg ⊘
Use this code for Zantac.
MED: 100-2, 15, 50

G ☑ **J2783** Injection, rasburicase, 0.5 mg ⊘

K **J2788** Injection, Rho D immune globulin, human, minidose, 50 mcg
Use this code for RhoGam, BAYRho-D, MICRhoGAM, HYPRho-D.
MED: 100-2, 15, 50

K ☑ **J2790** Injection, Rho D immune globulin, human, full dose, 300 mcg ⊘
Use this code for Gamulin RH, HypRho-D RhoGAM.
MED: 100-2, 15, 50

K ☑ **J2792** Injection, Rho D immune globulin, intravenous, human, solvent detergent, 100 IU
Use this code for BAYRho-D, WINRho SDF.
MED: 100-2, 15, 50

● ☑ **J2794** Injection, risperidone, long acting, 0.5 mg

N ☑ **J2795** Injection, ropivacaine HCl, 1 mg ⊘
Use this code for Naropin.

N ☑ **J2800** Injection, methocarbamol, up to 10 ml ⊘
Use this code for Robaxin.
MED: 100-2, 15, 50

N ☑ **J2810** Injection, theophylline, per 40 mg ⊘
MED: 100-2, 15, 50

K ☑ **J2820** Injection, sargramostim (GM-CSF), 50 mcg ⊘
Use this code for Leukine, Prokine.
MED: 100-2, 15, 50

N ☑ **J2910** Injection, aurothioglucose, up to 50 mg ⊘
Use this code for Solganal.
MED: 100-2, 15, 50

N ☑ **J2912** Injection, sodium chloride, 0.9%, per 2 ml ⊘
MED: 100-2, 15, 50

N **J2916** Injection, sodium ferric gluconate complex in sucrose injection, 12.5 mg
Use this code for Ferrlecit.
MED: 100-2, 15, 50.2; 100-2, 15, 50.2

N ☑ **J2920** Injection, methylprednisolone sodium succinate, up to 40 mg ⊘
Use this code for Solu-Medrol, A-methaPred.
MED: 100-2, 15, 50

N ☑ **J2930** Injection, methylprednisolone sodium succinate, up to 125 mg ⊘
Use this code for Solu-Medrol, A-methaPred.
MED: 100-2, 15, 50

N ☑ **J2940** Injection, somatrem, 1 mg ⊘
Use this code for Protropin.
MED: 100-2, 15, 50
AHA: 2Q, '02, 8

K ☑ **J2941** Injection, somatropin, 1 mg ⊘
Use this code for Humatrope, Genotropin Nutropin.
MED: 100-2, 15, 50
AHA: 2Q, '02, 8

N ☑ **J2950** Injection, promazine HCl, up to 25 mg ⊘
Use this code for Sparine, Prozine-50.
MED: 100-2, 15, 50

K ☑ **J2993** Injection, reteplase, 18.1 mg ⊘
Use this code for Retavase
MED: 100-2, 15, 50

K ☑ **J2995** Injection, streptokinase, per 250,000 IU ⊘
Use this code for Streptase.
MED: 100-2, 15, 50

K ☑ **J2997** Injection, alteplase recombinant, 1 mg ⊘
Use this code for Activase.
MED: 100-2, 15, 50

N ☑ **J3000** Injection, streptomycin, up to 1 g ⊘
Use this code for Streptomycin Sulfate.
MED: 100-2, 15, 50

N ☑	**J3010**	Injection, fentanyl citrate, 0.1 mg	⊘
		Use this code for Sublimaze.	
		MED: 100-2, 15, 50	

N ☑ **J3030** Injection, sumatriptan succinate, 6 mg (code may be used for Medicare when drug administered under the direct supervision of a physician, not for use when drug is self administered) ⊘
Use this code for Imitrex.
MED: 100-2, 15, 50

N ☑ **J3070** Injection, pentazocine, 30 mg ⊘
Use this code for Talwin.
MED: 100-2, 15, 50

K ☑ **J3100** Injection, tenecteplase, 50 mg ⊘
Use this code for TNKase.
AHA: 2Q, '02, 8

N ☑ **J3105** Injection, terbutaline sulfate, up to 1 mg ⊘
Use this code for Brethine, Bricanyl Subcutaneous. For terbutaline in inhalation solution, see K0525 and K0526.
MED: 100-2, 15, 50

● ☑ **J3110** Injection, teriparatide, 10 mcg
Use this code for Forteo.
www.fda.gov/bbs/topics/ANSWERS/2002/ANS01176.htm

N ☑ **J3120** Injection, testosterone enanthate, up to 100 mg ⊘
Use this code for Everone, Delatest, Delatestryl, Andropository 100, Testone LA 100.
MED: 100-2, 15, 50

N ☑ **J3130** Injection, testosterone enanthate, up to 200 mg ⊘
Use this code for Everone, Delatestryl, Andro L.A. 200, Andryl 200, Durathate-200, Testone LA 200, Testrin PA.
MED: 100-2, 15, 50

N ☑ **J3140** Injection, testosterone suspension, up to 50 mg ⊘
Use this code for Andronaq 50, Testosterone Aqueous, Testaqua, Testoject-50, Histerone 50, Histerone 100.
MED: 100-2, 15, 50

N ☑ **J3150** Injection, testosterone propionate, up to 100 mg ⊘
Use this code for Testex.
MED: 100-2, 15, 50

N ☑ **J3230** Injection, chlorpromazine HCl, up to 50 mg ⊘
Use this code for Thorazine.
MED: 100-2, 15, 50

K ☑ **J3240** Injection, thyrotropin alpha, 0.9 mg, provided in 1.1 mg vial ⊘
Use this code for Thyrogen, Thytropar.
MED: 100-2, 15, 50

~~**J3245** Injection, tirofiban HCl, 12.5 mg~~

● ☑ **J3246** Injection, tirofiban HCl, 0.25mg

N ☑ **J3250** Injection, trimethobenzamide HCl, up to 200 mg ⊘
Use this code for Tigan, Ticon, Tiject-20, Arrestin.
MED: 100-2, 15, 50

N ☑ **J3260** Injection, tobramycin sulfate, up to 80 mg ⊘
Use this code for Nebcin.
MED: 100-2, 15, 50

N ☑ **J3265** Injection, torsemide, 10 mg/ml ⊘
Use this code for Demadex.
MED: 100-2, 15, 50

N ☑ **J3280** Injection, thiethylperazine maleate, up to 10 mg ⊘
Use this code for Norzine, Torecan.
MED: 100-2, 15, 50

N ☑ **J3301** Injection, triamcinolone acetonide, per 10 mg ⊘
Use this code for Kenalog-10, Kenalog-40, Tri-Kort, Kenaject-40, Cenacort A-40, Triam-A, Trilog. For triamcinolone in inhalation solution, see K0527 and K0528.
MED: 100-2, 15, 50

N ☑ **J3302** Injection, triamcinolone diacetate, per 5 mg ⊘
Use this code for Aristocort Intralesional, Aristocort Forte, Amcort, Trilone, Cenacort Forte.
MED: 100-2, 15, 50

N ☑ **J3303** Injection, triamcinolone hexacetonide, per 5 mg ⊘
Use this code for Aristospan Intralesional, Aristospan Intra-articular.
MED: 100-2, 15, 50

K ☑ **J3305** Injection, trimetrexate glucoronate, per 25 mg ⊘
Use this code for Neutrexin.
MED: 100-2, 15, 50

N ☑ **J3310** Injection, perphenazine, up to 5 mg ⊘
Use this code for Trilafon.
MED: 100-2, 15, 50

G **J3315** Injection, triptorelin pamoate, 3.75 mg ⊘
Use this code dor Trelstar Depot.
MED: 100-2, 15, 50

N ☑ **J3320** Injection, spectinomycin dihydrochloride, up to 2 g ⊘
Use this code for Trobicin.
MED: 100-2, 15, 50

N ☑ **J3350** Injection, urea, up to 40 g ⊘
Use this code for Ureaphil.
MED: 100-2, 15, 50

N ☑ **J3360** Injection, diazepam, up to 5 mg ⊘
Use this code for Valium, Zetran.
MED: 100-2, 15, 50

N ☑ **J3364** Injection, urokinase, 5,000 IU vial ⊘
Use this code for Abbokinase Open-Cath.

K ☑ **J3365** Injection, IV, urokinase, 250,000 IU vial ⊘
Use this code for Abbokinase.
MED: 100-2, 15, 50
See code(s): Q0089

N ☑ **J3370** Injection, vancomycin HCl, 500 mg ⊘
Use this code for Varocin, Vancoled.
MED: 100-2, 15, 50; 100-3, 280.14

~~**J3395** Injection, verteporfin, 15 mg~~

● ☑ **J3396** Injection, verteporfin, 0.1 mg
MED: 100-3, 80.2; 100-3, 80.2; 100-3, 80.3; 100-3, 80.3; 100-3, 80.3; 100-3, 80.3; 100-3, 80.3; 100-3, 80.3; 100-3, 80.3

N ☑ **J3400** Injection, triflupromazine HCl, up to 20 mg ⊘
Use this code for Vesprin.
MED: 100-2, 15, 50

N ☑ **J3410** Injection, hydroxyzine HCl, up to 25 mg ⊘
Use this code for Vistaril, Vistaject-25, Hyzine-50.
MED: 100-2, 15, 50

N ☑ **J3411** Injection, thiamine HCl, 100 mg ⊘

Special Coverage Instructions   Noncovered by Medicare   Carrier Discretion   ☑ Quantity Alert   ● New Code   ○ Reinstated Code   ▲ Revised Code

2005 HCPCS   ♀ Female Only   ♂ Male Only   1-9 ASC Groups   MED: Pub 100/NCD Reference   ⅄ DMEPOS Paid   ⊘ SNF Excluded   **J Codes — 77**

N ☑ **J3415** Injection, pyridoxine HCl, 100 mg ⊘

N ☑ **J3420** Injection, vitamin B-12 cyanocobalamin, up to 1,000 mcg ⊘
Use this code for Sytobex, Redisol, Rubramin PC, Betalin 12, Berubigen, Cobex.
MED: 100-2, 15, 50; 100-3, 150.6

N ☑ **J3430** Injection, phytonadione (vitamin K), per 1 mg ⊘
Use this code for AquaMephyton, Konakion.
MED: 100-2, 15, 50

N ☑ **J3465** Injection, voriconazole, 10 mg ⊘
MED: 100-2, 15, 50

N ☑ **J3470** Injection, hyaluronidase, up to 150 units ⊘
Use this code for Wydase.
MED: 100-2, 15, 50

N ☑ **J3475** Injection, magnesium sulphate, per 500 mg ⊘
MED: 100-2, 15, 50

N ☑ **J3480** Injection, potassium chloride, per 2 meq ⊘
MED: 100-2, 15, 50

N ☑ **J3485** Injection, zidovudine, 10 mg ⊘
Use this code for Retrovir.
MED: 100-2, 15, 50

G ☑ **J3486** Injection, ziprasidone mesylate, 10 mg ⊘

G **J3487** Injection, zoledronic acid, 1 mg
Use this code for Zometa.

N **J3490** Unclassified drugs ⊘
MED: 100-2, 15, 50

E ☑ **J3520** Edetate disodium, per 150 mg ⊘
Use this code for Endrate, Disotate. This drug is used in chelation therapy, a treatment for atherosclerosis that is not covered by Medicare.
MED: 100-3, 20.21; 100-3, 20.22

E **J3530** Nasal vaccine inhalation ⊘
MED: 100-2, 15, 50

E **J3535** Drug administered through a metered dose inhaler ⊘

E **J3570** Laetrile, amygdalin, vitamin B-17 ⊘
The FDA has found Laetrile to have no safe or effective therapeutic purpose.
MED: 100-3, 30.7

N **J3590** Unclassified biologics

MISCELLANEOUS DRUGS AND SOLUTIONS

N ☑ **J7030** Infusion, normal saline solution, 1,000 cc ⊘
MED: 100-2, 15, 50

N ☑ **J7040** Infusion, normal saline solution, sterile (500 ml = 1 unit) ⊘
MED: 100-2, 15, 50

N ☑ **J7042** 5% dextrose/normal saline (500 ml = 1 unit) ⊘
MED: 100-2, 15, 50

N ☑ **J7050** Infusion, normal saline solution, 250 cc ⊘
MED: 100-2, 15, 50

N ☑ **J7051** Sterile saline or water, up to 5 cc ⊘
MED: 100-2, 15, 50

N ☑ **J7060** 5% dextrose/water (500 ml = 1 unit) ⊘
MED: 100-2, 15, 50

N ☑ **J7070** Infusion, D-5-W, 1,000 cc ⊘
MED: 100-2, 15, 50

N ☑ **J7100** Infusion, dextran 40, 500 ml ⊘
Use this code for Gentran, 10% LMD, Rheomacrodex.
MED: 100-2, 15, 50

N ☑ **J7110** Infusion, dextran 75, 500 ml ⊘
Use this code for Gentran 75.
MED: 100-2, 15, 50

N ☑ **J7120** Ringer's lactate infusion, up to 1,000 cc ⊘
MED: 100-2, 15, 50

N ☑ **J7130** Hypertonic saline solution, 50 or 100 meq, 20 cc vial ⊘
MED: 100-2, 15, 50

K ☑ **J7190** Factor VIII (antihemophilic factor, human) per IU
Use this code for Monarc-M, Koate-HP.
Medicare jurisdiction: local carrier.
MED: 100-2, 15, 50

K ☑ **J7191** Factor VIII (anti-hemophilic factor (porcine), per IU
Use this code for Hyate:C. Medicare jurisdiction: local carrier.
MED: 100-2, 15, 50

K ☑ **J7192** Factor VIII (antihemophilic factor, recombinant) per IU
Use this code for Recombinate, Kogenate, Bioclate, Helixate. Medicare jurisdiction: local carrier.
MED: 100-2, 15, 50

K ☑ **J7193** Factor IX (antihemophilic factor, purified, non-recombinant) per IU
Use this code for AlphaNine SD, mononine.
MED: 100-2, 15, 50
AHA: 2Q, '02, 8

K ☑ **J7194** Factor IX complex, per IU
Use this code for Konyne-80, Profilnine Heat-Treated, Proplex T, Proplex SX-T. Medicare jurisdiction: local carrier.
MED: 100-2, 15, 50

K ☑ **J7195** Factor IX (antihemophilic factor, recombinant) per IU
Use this code for Benefix, Konyne 80, Profilnine SD, Proplex T.
MED: 100-2, 15, 50
AHA: 2Q, '02, 8

N ☑ **J7197** Antithrombin III (human), per IU
Medicare jurisdiction: local carrier. Use this code for Throbate III, ATnativ.
MED: 100-2, 15, 50

K ☑ **J7198** Anti-inhibitor, per IU
Medicare jurisdiction: local carrier. Use this code for Autoplex T, Feiba VH Immuno.
MED: 100-2, 15, 50; 100-3, 110.3; 100-3, 110.3; 100-3, 110.3; 100-3, 110.3; 100-3, 110.3; 100-3, 110.3; 100-3, 110.3; 100-3, 110.3

B **J7199** Hemophilia clotting factor, not otherwise classified
Medicare jurisdiction: local carrier.
MED: 100-2, 15, 50; 100-3, 110.3; 100-3, 110.3; 100-3, 110.3; 100-3, 110.3; 100-3, 110.3; 100-3, 110.3; 100-3, 110.3; 100-3, 110.3

E **J7300** Intrauterine copper contraceptive ⊘
Use this code for Paragard T380A. Medicare jurisdiction: local carrier.

E ☑ **J7302** Levonorgestrel-releasing intrauterine contraceptive system, 52 mg ♀⊘
Use this code for Mirena.

   A Adult   M Maternity   P Pediatrics   I Infant   A-Y APC Status Indicator   *2005 HCPCS*

E	☑	**J7303**	Contraceptive supply, hormone containing vaginal ring, each ♀ ⊘
●	☑	**J7304**	Contraceptive supply, hormone containing patch, each
N	☑	**J7308**	Aminolevulinic acid HCl for topical administration, 20%, single unit dosage form (354 mg) ⊘
K	☑	**J7310**	Ganciclovir, 4.5 mg, long-acting implant ⊘ Use this code for Vitrasert. MED: 100-2, 15, 50
K		**J7317**	Sodium hyaluronate, per 20 to 25 mg dose for intra-articular injection Use this code for Hyalgan (20 mg), Supartz (25 mg).
K	☑	**J7320**	Hylan G-F 20, 16 mg, for intra-articular injection⊘ Use this code for Synvisc.
B	☑	**J7330**	Autologous cultured chondrocytes, implant ⊘ Medicare jurisdiction: local carrier. Use this code for Carticel.
E	☑	**J7340**	Dermal and epidermal tissue of human origin, with or without bioengineered or processed elements, with metabolically active elements, per sq. cm Dermal tissue-not found in the drug table. Use this code for Dermagraft , Dermagraft TC. See also C9201 for Outpatient PPS.
N	☑	**J7342**	Dermal tissue, of human origin, with or without other bioengineered or processed elements, with metabolically active elements, per sq. cm Dermal Tissue, not found in the drug table. Use this code for Dermagraft , Dermagraft TC. See also C9201 for Outpatient PPS.
●	☑	**J7343**	Dermal and epidermal, tissue of non-human origin, with or without other bioengineered or processed elements, without metabolically active elements, per sq. cm
●	☑	**J7344**	Dermal tissue, of human origin, with or without other bioengineered or processed elements, without metabolically active elements, per sq. cm
N	☑	**J7350**	Dermal tissue of human origin, injectable, with or without other bioengineered or processed elements, but without metabolized active elements, per 10 mg Dermal Tissue, not found in the drug table. Use this code for Dermagraft , Dermagraft TC. See also C9201 for Outpatient PPS.
N	☑	**J7500**	Azathioprine, oral, 50 mg Use this code for Imuran. MED: 100-2, 15, 50.5
N	☑	**J7501**	Azathioprine, parenteral, 100 mg MED: 100-2, 15, 50
K	☑	**J7502**	Cyclosporine, oral, 100 mg Use this code for Neoral, Sandimmune. MED: 100-2, 15, 50.5
K	☑	**J7504**	Lymphocyte immune globulin, antithymocyte globulin, equine, parenteral, 250 mg Use this code for Atgam. MED: 100-2, 15, 50; 100-3, 260.7
K	☑	**J7505**	Muromonab-CD3, parenteral, 5 mg Use this code for Orthoclone OKT3. MED: 100-2, 15, 50
N	☑	**J7506**	Prednisone, oral, per 5 mg Use this code for Deltasone meticorten orasone. MED: 100-2, 15, 50.5

K	☑	**J7507**	Tacrolimus, oral, per 1 mg Use this code for Prograf. MED: 100-2, 15, 50.5
N	☑	**J7509**	Methylprednisolone, oral, per 4 mg Use this code for Medrol. MED: 100-2, 15, 50.5
N	☑	**J7510**	Prednisolone, oral, per 5 mg Use this code for Delta-Cortef. MED: 100-2, 15, 50.5
K	☑	**J7511**	Lymphocyte immune globulin, antithymocyte globulin, rabbit, parenteral, 25 mg AHA: 2Q, '02, 8
K	☑	**J7513**	Daclizumab, parenteral, 25 mg Use this code for Zenapax. MED: 100-2, 15, 50.5
N	☑	**J7515**	Cyclosporine, oral, 25 mg ⊘ Use this code for Neoral, Sandimmune.
N	☑	**J7516**	Cyclosporine, parenteral, 250 mg ⊘ Use this code for Neoral, Sandimmune.
G	☑	**J7517**	Mycophenolate mofetil, oral, 250 mg Use this code for CellCept.
●	☑	**J7518**	Mycophenolic acid, oral, 180 mg MED: 100-4, 17, 80.3.1; 100-4, 8, 120.1
K	☑	**J7520**	Sirolimus, oral, 1 mg ⊘ Use this code for Rapamune. MED: 100-2, 15, 50.5
K	☑	**J7525**	Tacrolimus, parenteral, 5 mg Use this code for Prograf. MED: 100-2, 15, 50.5
N		**J7599**	Immunosuppressive drug, NOC ⊘ Determine if an alternative HCPCS Level II or a CPT code better describes the service being reported. This code should be used only if a more specific code is unavailable. MED: 100-2, 15, 50.5

INHALATION SOLUTIONS

Y	☑	**J7608**	Acetylcysteine, inhalation solution administered through DME, unit dose form, per g ⊘ Use this code for Mucomyst, Mucosil. MED: 100-2, 15, 110.3
●	☑	**J7611**	Albuterol, inhalation solution, administered through DME, concentrated form, 1 mg MED: 100-2, 15, 110.3
●	☑	**J7612**	Levalbuterol, inhalation solution, administered through DME, concentrated form, 0.5 mg MED: 100-2, 15, 110.3
●	☑	**J7613**	Albuterol, inhalation solution, administered through DME, unit dose, 1 mg MED: 100-2, 15, 110.3
●	☑	**J7614**	Levalbuterol, inhalation solution, administered through DME, unit dose, 0.5 mg MED: 100-2, 15, 110.3
●	☑	**J7616**	Albuterol, up to 5 mg and ipratropium bromide, up to 1 mg, compounded inhalation solution, administered through DME MED: 100-2, 15, 110.3

Special Coverage Instructions   Noncovered by Medicare   Carrier Discretion   ☑ Quantity Alert   ● New Code   ○ Reinstated Code   ▲ Revised Code

2005 HCPCS   ♀ Female Only   ♂ Male Only   **1-9** ASC Groups   MED: Pub 100/NCD Reference   ⛊ DMEPOS Paid   ⊘ SNF Excluded   **J Codes — 79**

● ☑ **J7617** Levalbuterol, up to 2.5 mg and ipratropium bromide, up to 1 mg, compounded inhalation solution, administered through DME
MED: 100-2, 15, 110.3

~~J7618 Albuterol, all formulations including separated isomers, inhalation solution administered through DME, concentrated form, per 1 mg (albuterol) or per 0.5 mg (levalbuterol)~~

~~J7619 Albuterol, all formulations including separated isomers, inhalation solution administered through DME, unit dose, per 1 mg (albuterol) or per 0.5 mg (levalbuterol)~~

~~J7621 Albuterol, all formulations, including separated isomers, up to 5 mg (albuterol) or 2.5 mg (levoalbuterol), and ipratropium bromide, up to 1 mg, compounded inhalation solution, administered through DME~~

Ⓐ **J7622** Beclomethasone, inhalation solution administered through DME, unit dose form, per mg ⊘

Ⓐ ☑ **J7624** Betamethasone, inhalation solution administered through DME, unit dose form, per mg ⊘

Ⓐ **J7626** Budesonide inhalation solution, administered through DME, unit dose form, 0.25 to 0.50 mg
Use this code for Pulmicort Respules.

Ⓨ ☑ **J7628** Bitolterol mesylate, inhalation solution administered through DME, concentrated form, per mg ⊘
Use this code for Tornalate.
MED: 100-2, 15, 110.3

Ⓨ ☑ **J7629** Bitolterol mesylate, inhalation solution administered through DME, unit dose form, per mg ⊘
Use this code for Tornalate.
MED: 100-2, 15, 110.3

Ⓨ ☑ **J7631** Cromolyn sodium, inhalation solution administered through DME, unit dose form, per 10 mg ⊘
Use this code for Intal, Nasalcrom, Gastrocrom.
MED: 100-2, 15, 110.3

Ⓝ **J7633** Budesonide, inhalation solution administered through DME, concentrated form, per 0.25 milligram
Use this code for Pumocort.

Ⓨ ☑ **J7635** Atropine, inhalation solution administered through DME, concentrated form, per mg ⊘
MED: 100-2, 15, 110.3

Ⓨ ☑ **J7636** Atropine, inhalation solution administered through DME, unit dose form, per mg ⊘
MED: 100-2, 15, 110.3

Ⓨ ☑ **J7637** Dexamethasone, inhalation solution administered through DME, concentrated form, per mg ⊘
MED: 100-2, 15, 110.3

Ⓨ ☑ **J7638** Dexamethasone, inhalation solution administered through DME, unit dose form, per mg ⊘
MED: 100-2, 15, 110.3

Ⓨ ☑ **J7639** Dornase alpha, inhalation solution administered through DME, unit dose form, per mg ⊘
Use this code for Pulmozyme.
MED: 100-2, 15, 110.3

Ⓐ **J7641** Flunisolide, inhalation solution administered through DME, unit dose, per mg ⊘

Ⓨ ☑ **J7642** Glycopyrrolate, inhalation solution administered through DME, concentrated form, per mg ⊘
MED: 100-2, 15, 110.3

Ⓨ ☑ **J7643** Glycopyrrolate, inhalation solution administered through DME, unit dose form, per mg ⊘
MED: 100-2, 15, 110.3

Ⓨ ☑ **J7644** Ipratropium bromide, inhalation solution administered through DME, unit dose form, per mg ⊘
Use this code for Atrovent.
MED: 100-2, 15, 110.3

Ⓨ ☑ **J7648** Isoetharine HCl, inhalation solution administered through DME, concentrated form, per mg ⊘
MED: 100-2, 15, 110.3

Ⓨ ☑ **J7649** Isoetharine HCl, inhalation solution administered through DME, unit dose form, per mg ⊘
MED: 100-2, 15, 110.3

Ⓨ ☑ **J7658** Isoproterenol HCl, inhalation solution administered through DME, concentrated form, per mg ⊘
Use this code for Isuprel HCl, Medihaler-ISO.
MED: 100-2, 15, 110.3

Ⓨ ☑ **J7659** Isoproterenol HCl, inhalation solution administered through DME, unit dose form, per mg ⊘
Use this code for Isuprel HCl, Medihaler-ISO.
MED: 100-2, 15, 110.3

Ⓨ ☑ **J7668** Metaproterenol sulfate, inhalation solution administered through DME, concentrated form, per 10 mg ⊘
Use this code for Alupent.
MED: 100-2, 15, 110.3

Ⓨ ☑ **J7669** Metaproterenol sulfate, inhalation solution administered through DME, unit dose form, per 10 mg ⊘
Use this code for Alupent.
MED: 100-2, 15, 110.3

● ☑ **J7674** Methacholine chloride administered as inhalation solution through a nebulizer, per 1 mg

Ⓨ ☑ **J7680** Terbutaline sulfate, inhalation solution administered through DME, concentrated form, per mg ⊘
Use this code for Brethine, Bricanyl.
MED: 100-2, 15, 110.3

Ⓨ ☑ **J7681** Terbutaline sulfate, inhalation solution administered through DME, unit dose form, per mg ⊘
Use this code for Brethine, Bricanyl.
MED: 100-2, 15, 110.3

Ⓨ ☑ **J7682** Tobramycin, unit dose form, 300 mg, inhalation solution, administered through DME ⊘
Use this code for Tobi.
MED: 100-2, 15, 110.3

Ⓨ ☑ **J7683** Triamcinolone, inhalation solution administered through DME, concentrated form, per mg ⊘
Use this code for Azmacort.
MED: 100-2, 15, 110.3

Ⓨ ☑ **J7684** Triamcinolone, inhalation solution administered through DME, unit dose form, per mg ⊘
Use this code for Azmacort.
MED: 100-2, 15, 110.3

| ▨ Special Coverage Instructions | Noncovered by Medicare | Carrier Discretion | ☑ Quantity Alert | ● New Code | ○ Reinstated Code | ▲ Revised Code |

80 — J Codes　　　Ⓐ Adult　　　Ⓜ Maternity　　　Ⓟ Pediatrics　　　Ⓘ Infant　　　Ⓐ-Ⓨ APC Status Indicator　　　**2005 HCPCS**

Y		**J7699**	NOC drugs, inhalation solution administered through DME MED: 100-2, 15, 110.3	⊘

Y		**J7799** NOC drugs, other than inhalation drugs, administered through DME MED: 100-2, 15, 110.3 ⊘
E		**J8499** Prescription drug, oral, nonchemotherapeutic, NOS MED: 100-2, 15, 50 ⊘
● ☑		**J8501** Aprepitant, oral, 5 mg
K ☑		**J8510** Bulsulfan, oral, 2 mg Use this code for Myleran. MED: 100-2, 15, 50.5
K ☑		**J8520** Capecitabine, oral, 150 mg Use this code for Xeloda. MED: 100-2, 15, 50.5
E ☑		**J8521** Capecitabine, oral, 500 mg Use this code for Xeloda. MED: 100-2, 15, 50.5
N ☑		**J8530** Cyclophosphamide, oral, 25 mg Use this code for Cytoxan. MED: 100-2, 15, 50.5
K ☑		**J8560** Etoposide, oral, 50 mg Use this code for VePesid. MED: 100-2, 15, 50.5
● ☑		**J8565** Gefitinib, oral, 250 mg Use this code for Iressa.
N ☑		**J8600** Melphalan, oral 2 mg Use this code for Alkeran. MED: 100-2, 15, 50.5
N ☑		**J8610** Methotrexate, oral, 2.5 mg Use this code for Rheumatrex Dose Pack. MED: 100-2, 15, 50.5
K ☑		**J8700** Temozolomide, oral, 5 mg Use this code for Temodar. MED: 100-2, 15, 50.5
B		**J8999** Prescription drug, oral, chemotherapeutic, NOS Determine if an alternative HCPCS Level II or a CPT code better describes the service being reported. This code should be used only if a more specific code is unavailable. MED: 100-2, 15, 50.5

CHEMOTHERAPY DRUGS *J9000–J9999*

These codes cover the cost of the chemotherapy drug only, not the administration. See also J8999.

K ☑		**J9000** Doxorubicin HCl, 10 mg Use this code for Adriamycin PFS, Adriamycin RDF, Rubex. MED: 100-2, 15, 50
K ☑		**J9001** Doxorubicin HCl, all lipid formulations, 10 mg Use this code for Doxil. MED: 100-2, 15, 50
K		**J9010** Alemtuzumab, 10 mg Use this code for Campath.
K ☑		**J9015** Aldesleukin, per single use vial Use this code for Proleukin, IL-2, Interleukin. MED: 100-2, 15, 50

K ☑		**J9017** Arsenic trioxide, 1 mg Use this code for Trisenox. AHA: 2Q, '02, 8
K ☑		**J9020** Asparaginase, 10,000 units Use this code for Elspar. MED: 100-2, 15, 50
K ☑		**J9031** BCG live (intravesical), per instillation Use this code for Tice BCG, TheraCys. MED: 100-2, 15, 50
● ☑		**J9035** Injection, bevacizumab, 10 mg Use this code for Avastin, Imuron.
K ☑		**J9040** Bleomycin sulfate, 15 units Use this code for Blenoxane. MED: 100-2, 15, 50
● ☑		**J9041** Injection, bortezomib, 0.1 mg Use this code for Velcade.
K ☑		**J9045** Carboplatin, 50 mg Use this code for Paraplatin. MED: 100-2, 15, 50
N ☑		**J9050** Carmustine, 100 mg Use this code for BiCNU. MED: 100-2, 15, 50
● ☑		**J9055** Injection, cetuximab, 10 mg Use this code for Erbitux.
K ☑		**J9060** Cisplatin, powder or solution, per 10 mg Use this code for Plantinol AQ. MED: 100-2, 15, 50
B ☑		**J9062** Cisplatin, 50 mg Use this code for Plantinol AQ. MED: 100-2, 15, 50
K ☑		**J9065** Injection, cladribine, per 1 mg Use this code for Leustatin. MED: 100-2, 15, 50
K ☑		**J9070** Cyclophosphamide, 100 mg Use this code for Cytoxan, Neosar. MED: 100-2, 15, 50
B ☑		**J9080** Cyclophosphamide, 200 mg Use this code for Cytoxan, Neosar. MED: 100-2, 15, 50
B ☑		**J9090** Cyclophosphamide, 500 mg Use this code for Cytoxan, Neosar. MED: 100-2, 15, 50
B ☑		**J9091** Cyclophosphamide, 1 g Use this code for Cytoxan, Neosar. MED: 100-2, 15, 50
B ☑		**J9092** Cyclophosphamide, 2 g Use this code for Cytoxan, Neosar. MED: 100-2, 15, 50
K ☑		**J9093** Cyclophosphamide, lyophilized, 100 mg Use this code for Cytoxan Lyophilized. MED: 100-2, 15, 50
B ☑		**J9094** Cyclophosphamide, lyophilized, 200 mg Use this code for Cytoxan Lyophilized. MED: 100-2, 15, 50

Chemotherapy Drugs

J9095 — J9260

B ☑ **J9095** Cyclophosphamide, lyophilized, 500 mg
Use this code for Cytoxan Lyophilized.
MED: 100-2, 15, 50

B ☑ **J9096** Cyclophosphamide, lyophilized, 1 g
Use this code for Cytoxan Lyophilized.
MED: 100-2, 15, 50

B ☑ **J9097** Cyclophosphamide, lyophilized, 2 g
Use this code for Cytoxan Lyophilized.
MED: 100-2, 15, 50

K ☑ **J9098** Cytarabine liposome, 10 mg   ⊘

K ☑ **J9100** Cytarabine, 100 mg
Use this code for Cytosar-U.
MED: 100-2, 15, 50

B ☑ **J9110** Cytarabine, 500 mg
Use this code for Cytosar-U.
MED: 100-2, 15, 50

N ☑ **J9120** Dactinomycin, 0.5 mg
Use this code for Cosmegen.
MED: 100-2, 15, 50

K ☑ **J9130** Dacarbazine, 100 mg
Use this code for DTIC-Dome.
MED: 100-2, 15, 50

B ☑ **J9140** Dacarbazine, 200 mg
Use this code for DTIC-Dome.
MED: 100-2, 15, 50

K ☑ **J9150** Daunorubicin HCl, 10 mg
Use this code for Cerubidine.
MED: 100-2, 15, 50

K ☑ **J9151** Daunorubicin citrate, liposomal formulation, 10 mg
Use this code for Daunoxome.
MED: 100-2, 15, 50

K ☑ **J9160** Denileukin diftitox, 300 mcg
Use this code for Ontak.

N ☑ **J9165** Diethylstilbestrol diphosphate, 250 mg
Use this code for Stilphostrol.
MED: 100-2, 15, 50

K ☑ **J9170** Docetaxel, 20 mg
Use this code for Taxotere.
MED: 100-2, 15, 50

K ☑ **J9178** Injection, epirubicin HCl, 2 mg

K ☑ **J9181** Etoposide, 10 mg
Use this code for VesPesid, Toposar.
MED: 100-2, 15, 50

B ☑ **J9182** Etoposide, 100 mg
Use this code for VesPesid, Toposar.
MED: 100-2, 15, 50

K ☑ **J9185** Fludarabine phosphate, 50 mg
Use this code for Fludara.
MED: 100-2, 15, 50

N ☑ **J9190** Fluorouracil, 500 mg
Use this code for Adrucil.
MED: 100-2, 15, 50

K ☑ **J9200** Floxuridine, 500 mg
Use this code for FUDR.
MED: 100-2, 15, 50

K ☑ **J9201** Gemcitabine HCl, 200 mg
Use this code for Gemzar.
MED: 100-2, 15, 50

K ☑ **J9202** Goserelin acetate implant, per 3.6 mg
Use this code for Zoladex.
MED: 100-2, 15, 50

K ☑ **J9206** Irinotecan, 20 mg
Use this code for Camptosar.
MED: 100-2, 15, 50

K ☑ **J9208** Ifosfamide, per 1 g
Use this code for Ifex.
MED: 100-2, 15, 50

K ☑ **J9209** Mesna, 200 mg
Use this code for Mesnex.
MED: 100-2, 15, 50

K ☑ **J9211** Idarubicin HCl, 5 mg
Use this code for Idamycin.
MED: 100-2, 15, 50

N ☑ **J9212** Injection, interferon alfacon-1, recombinant, 1 mcg
Use this code for Infergen.
MED: 100-2, 15, 50

K ☑ **J9213** Interferon alfa-2A, recombinant, 3 million units
Use this code for Roferon-A.
MED: 100-2, 15, 50

K ☑ **J9214** Interferon alfa-2B, recombinant, 1 million units
Use this code for Intron A.
MED: 100-2, 15, 50

K ☑ **J9215** Interferon alfa-N3, (human leukocyte derived), 250,000 IU
Use this code for Alferon N.
MED: 100-2, 15, 50

K ☑ **J9216** Interferon gamma-1B, 3 million units
Use this code for Actimmune.
MED: 100-2, 15, 50

K ☑ **J9217** Leuprolide acetate (for depot suspension), 7.5 mg
Use this code for Lupron Depot, Eligard.
MED: 100-2, 15, 50

K ☑ **J9218** Leuprolide acetate, per 1 mg
Use this code for Lupron.
MED: 100-2, 15, 50

K ☑ **J9219** Leuprolide acetate implant, 65 mg
Use this code for Lupron Implant.
MED: 100-2, 15, 50
AHA: 4Q, '01, 5

N ☑ **J9230** Mechlorethamine HCl, (nitrogen mustard), 10 mg
Use this code for Mustargen.
MED: 100-2, 15, 50

K ☑ **J9245** Injection, melphalan HCl, 50 mg
Use this code for Alkeran, L-phenylalanine mustard.
MED: 100-2, 15, 50

N ☑ **J9250** Methotrexate sodium, 5 mg
Use this code for Folex, Folex PFS, Methotrexate LPF.
MED: 100-2, 15, 50

B ☑ **J9260** Methotrexate sodium, 50 mg
Use this code for Folex, Folex PFS, Methotrexate LPF.
MED: 100-2, 15, 50

Special Coverage Instructions   Noncovered by Medicare   Carrier Discretion   ☑ Quantity Alert   ● New Code   ○ Reinstated Code   ▲ Revised Code

82 — J Codes   **A** Adult   **M** Maternity   **P** Pediatrics   **I** Infant   **A**-**Y** APC Status Indicator   *2005 HCPCS*

B ☑ **J9263** Injection, oxaliplatin, 0.5 mg

K ☑ **J9265** Paclitaxel, 30 mg
Use this code for Taxol.
MED: 100-2, 15, 50

N ☑ **J9266** Pegaspargase, per single dose vial
Use this code for Oncaspar, Peg-L-asparaginase.
MED: 100-2, 15, 50
AHA: 2Q, '02, 8

K ☑ **J9268** Pentostatin, per 10 mg
Use this code for Nipent.
MED: 100-2, 15, 50

K ☑ **J9270** Plicamycin, 2.5 mg
Use this code for Mithacin.
MED: 100-2, 15, 50

K ☑ **J9280** Mitomycin, 5 mg
Use this code for Mitomycin.
MED: 100-2, 15, 50

B ☑ **J9290** Mitomycin, 20 mg
Use this code for Mitomycin.
MED: 100-2, 15, 50

B ☑ **J9291** Mitomycin, 40 mg
Use this code for Mitomycin.
MED: 100-2, 15, 50

K ☑ **J9293** Injection, mitoxantrone HCl, per 5 mg
Use this code for Navantrone.
MED: 100-2, 15, 50

K **J9300** Gemtuzumab ozogamicin, 5 mg
Use this code for Mylotarg.
AHA: 2Q, '02, 8

● ☑ **J9305** Injection, pemetrexed, 10 mg
Use this code for Alimta.

K ☑ **J9310** Rituximab, 100 mg
Use this code for RituXan.
MED: 100-2, 15, 50

K ☑ **J9320** Streptozocin, 1 g
Use this code for Zanosar.
MED: 100-2, 15, 50

K ☑ **J9340** Thiotepa, 15 mg
Use this code for Thioplex.
MED: 100-2, 15, 50

K ☑ **J9350** Topotecan, 4 mg
Use this code for Hycamtin.
MED: 100-2, 15, 50

K ☑ **J9355** Trastuzumab, 10 mg
Use this code for Herceptin.

K ☑ **J9357** Valrubicin, intravesical, 200 mg
Use this code for Valstar.
MED: 100-2, 15, 50

N ☑ **J9360** Vinblastine sulfate, 1 mg
Use this code for Velban.
MED: 100-2, 15, 50

N ☑ **J9370** Vincristine sulfate, 1 mg
Use this code for Oncovin.
MED: 100-2, 15, 50

B ☑ **J9375** Vincristine sulfate, 2 mg
Use this code for Oncovin.
MED: 100-2, 15, 50

B ☑ **J9380** Vincristine sulfate, 5 mg
Use this code for Oncovin.
MED: 100-2, 15, 50

K ☑ **J9390** Vinorelbine tartrate, per 10 mg
Use this code for Navelbine.
MED: 100-2, 15, 50

G ☑ **J9395** Injection, fulvestrant, 25 mg

K ☑ **J9600** Porfimer sodium, 75 mg
Use this code for Photofrin.
MED: 100-2, 15, 50

N **J9999** NOC, antineoplastic drug
Determine if an alternative HCPCS Level II or a CPT code better describes the service being reported. This code should be used only if a more specific code is unavailable.
MED: 100-2, 15, 50; 100-3, 110.2

Special Coverage Instructions   Noncovered by Medicare   Carrier Discretion   ☑ Quantity Alert   ● New Code   ○ Reinstated Code   ▲ Revised Code

2005 HCPCS   ♀ Female Only   ♂ Male Only   1-9 ASC Groups   MED: Pub 100/NCD Reference   ዼ DMEPOS Paid   ⊘ SNF Excluded   **J Codes — 83**

TEMPORARY CODES *K0000–K9999*

The K codes were established for use by the durable medical equipment regional carriers (DMERCs). The K codes are developed when the currently existing permanent national codes for supplies and certain product categories do not include the codes needed to implement a DMERC medical review policy.

K CODES ASSIGNED TO DURABLE MEDICAL EQUIPMENT REGIONAL CARRIERS (DMERC)

WHEELCHAIR AND WHEELCHAIR ACCESSORIES

[Y] **K0001** Standard wheelchair ♿⊘

[Y] **K0002** Standard hemi (low seat) wheelchair ♿⊘

[Y] **K0003** Lightweight wheelchair ♿⊘

[Y] **K0004** High strength, lightweight wheelchair ♿⊘

[Y] **K0005** Ultralightweight wheelchair ♿⊘

[Y] **K0006** Heavy-duty wheelchair ♿⊘

[Y] **K0007** Extra heavy-duty wheelchair ♿⊘

[Y] **K0009** Other manual wheelchair/base ⊘

[Y] **K0010** Standard-weight frame motorized/power wheelchair ♿⊘

[Y] **K0011** Standard-weight frame motorized/power wheelchair with programmable control parameters for speed adjustment, tremor dampening, acceleration control and braking ♿⊘

[Y] **K0012** Lightweight portable motorized/power wheelchair ♿⊘

[Y] **K0014** Other motorized/power wheelchair base ⊘

[Y] ☑ **K0015** Detachable, nonadjustable height armrest, each ♿⊘

[Y] ☑ **K0017** Detachable, adjustable height armrest, base, each ♿⊘

[Y] ☑ **K0018** Detachable, adjustable height armrest, upper portion, each ♿⊘

[Y] ☑ **K0019** Arm pad, each ♿⊘

[Y] ☑ **K0020** Fixed, adjustable height armrest, pair ♿⊘

~~**K0023** Solid back insert, planar back, single density foam, attached with straps~~

~~**K0024** Solid back insert, planar back, single density foam, with adjustable hook on hardware~~

[Y] ☑ **K0037** High mount flip-up footrest, each ♿⊘

[Y] ☑ **K0038** Leg strap, each ♿⊘

[Y] ☑ **K0039** Leg strap, H style, each ♿⊘

[Y] ☑ **K0040** Adjustable angle footplate, each ♿⊘

[Y] ☑ **K0041** Large size footplate, each ♿⊘

[Y] ☑ **K0042** Standard size footplate, each ♿⊘

[Y] ☑ **K0043** Footrest, lower extension tube, each ♿⊘

[Y] ☑ **K0044** Footrest, upper hanger bracket, each ♿⊘

[Y] **K0045** Footrest, complete assembly ♿⊘

[Y] ☑ **K0046** Elevating legrest, lower extension tube, each ♿⊘

[Y] ☑ **K0047** Elevating legrest, upper hanger bracket, each ♿⊘

K0050 Ratchet assembly ♿⊘

[Y] ☑ **K0051** Cam release assembly, footrest or legrest, each ♿⊘

[Y] ☑ **K0052** Swingaway, detachable footrests, each ♿⊘

[Y] ☑ **K0053** Elevating footrests, articulating (telescoping), each ♿⊘

[Y] ☑ **K0056** Seat height less than 17 in. or equal to or greater than 21 in. for a high strength, lightweight, or ultralightweight wheelchair ♿⊘

~~**K0059** Plastic coated handrim, each~~

~~**K0060** Steel handrim, each~~

~~**K0061** Aluminum handrim, each~~

[Y] ☑ **K0064** Zero pressure tube (flat free insert), any size, each ♿⊘

[Y] ☑ **K0065** Spoke protectors, each ♿⊘

[Y] ☑ **K0066** Solid tire, any size, each ♿⊘

[Y] ☑ **K0067** Pneumatic tire, any size, each ♿⊘

[Y] ☑ **K0068** Pneumatic tire tube, each ♿⊘

[Y] ☑ **K0069** Rear wheel assembly, complete, with solid tire, spokes or molded, each ♿⊘

[Y] ☑ **K0070** Rear wheel assembly, complete with pneumatic tire, spokes or molded, each ♿⊘

[Y] ☑ **K0071** Front caster assembly, complete, with pneumatic tire, each ♿⊘

[Y] ☑ **K0072** Front caster assembly, complete, with semipneumatic tire, each ♿⊘

[Y] ☑ **K0073** Caster pin lock, each ♿⊘

[Y] ☑ **K0074** Pneumatic caster tire, any size, each ♿⊘

[Y] ☑ **K0075** Semipneumatic caster tire, any size, each ♿⊘

[Y] ☑ **K0076** Solid caster tire, any size, each ♿⊘

[Y] ☑ **K0077** Front caster assembly, complete, with solid tire, each ♿⊘

[Y] ☑ **K0078** Pneumatic caster tire tube, each ♿⊘

~~**K0081** Wheel lock assembly, complete, each~~
See code(s): E2206

[Y] ☑ **K0090** Rear wheel tire for power wheelchair, any size, each ♿⊘

[Y] ☑ **K0091** Rear wheel tire tube other than zero pressure for power wheelchair, any size, each ♿⊘

[Y] ☑ **K0092** Rear wheel assembly for power wheelchair, complete, each ♿⊘

[Y] ☑ **K0093** Rear wheel zero pressure tire tube (flat free insert) for power wheelchair, any size, each ♿⊘

[Y] ☑ **K0094** Wheel tire for power base, any size, each ♿⊘

[Y] ☑ **K0095** Wheel tire tube other than zero pressure for each base, any size, each ♿⊘

[Y] ☑ **K0096** Wheel assembly for power base, complete, each ♿⊘

[Y] ☑ **K0097** Wheel zero-pressure tire tube (flat free insert) for power base, any size, each ♿⊘

[Y] **K0098** Drive belt for power wheelchair ♿⊘

[Y] **K0099** Front caster for power wheelchair ♿⊘

[Y] ☑ **K0102** Crutch and cane holder, each ♿⊘

[Y] ☑ **K0104** Cylinder tank carrier, each ♿⊘

[Y] ☑ **K0105** IV hanger, each ♿⊘

[Y] ☑ **K0106** Arm trough, each ♿⊘

[Y] **K0108** Other accessories ⊘

~~**K0114** Back support system for use with a wheelchair, with inner frame, prefabricated~~

~~**K0115** Seating system, back module, posterior lateral control, with or without lateral supports, custom fabricated for attachment to wheelchair base~~

Temporary Codes

K0116 — K0633

~~K0116 Seating system, combined back and seat module, custom fabricated for attachment to wheelchair base~~

☒ **K0195** Elevating legrest, pair (for use with capped rental wheelchair base)   🔨⊘
MED: 100-3, 230.10

Ⓑ ☑ **K0415** Prescription antiemetic drug, oral, per 1 mg, for use in conjunction with oral anti-cancer drug, NOS
MED: 100-2, 15, 50.5

Ⓑ ☑ **K0416** Prescription antiemetic drug, rectal, per 1 mg, for use in conjunction with oral anti-cancer drug, NOS
MED: 100-2, 15, 50.5

☒ **K0452** Wheelchair bearings, any type   🔨⊘

☒ **K0455** Infusion pump used for uninterrupted parenteral administration of medication, (e.g., epoprostenol or treprostinol)   🔨⊘
See J1325 for epoprostenol.
MED: 100-3, 280.14

☒ **K0462** Temporary replacement for patient owned equipment being repaired, any type   ⊘
MED: 100-4, 20, 40.2

☒ ☑ **K0552** Supplies for external drug infusion pump, syringe type cartridge, sterile, each   🔨⊘
MED: 100-3, 280.14

☒ **K0600** Functional neuromuscular stimulator, transcutaneous stimulation of muscles of ambulation with computer control, used for walking by spinal cord injured, entire system, after completion of training program   🔨⊘
MED: 100-3, 160.12
AHA: 2Q, '03, 7

☒ ☑ **K0601** Replacement battery for external infusion pump owned by patient, silver oxide, 1.5 volt, each   🔨⊘
AHA: 2Q, '03, 7

☒ ☑ **K0602** Replacement battery for external infusion pump owned by patient, silver oxide, 3 volt, each   🔨⊘
AHA: 2Q, '03, 7

☒ ☑ **K0603** Replacement battery for external infusion pump owned by patient, alkaline, 1.5 volt, each   🔨⊘
AHA: 2Q, '03, 7

☒ ☑ **K0604** Replacement battery for external infusion pump owned by patient, lithium, 3.6 volt, each   🔨⊘
AHA: 2Q, '03, 7

☒ ☑ **K0605** Replacement battery for external infusion pump owned by patient, lithium, 4.5 volt, each   🔨⊘
AHA: 2Q, '03, 7

☒ **K0606** Automatic external defibrillator, with integrated electrocardiogram analysis, garment type   🔨⊘
AHA: 4Q, '03, 4

☒ ☑ **K0607** Replacement battery for automated external defibrillator, garment type only, each   🔨⊘
AHA: 4Q, '03, 4

☒ ☑ **K0608** Replacement garment for use with automated external defibrillator, each   🔨⊘
AHA: 4Q, '03, 4

☒ ☑ **K0609** Replacement electrodes for use with automated external defibrillator, garment type only, each   🔨⊘
AHA: 4Q, '03, 4

Ⓐ **K0618** TLSO, sagittal-coronal control, modular segmented spinal system, two rigid plastic shells, posterior extends from the sacrococcygeal junction and terminates just inferior to the scapular spine, anterior extends from the symphysis pubis to the xiphoid, soft liner, restricts gross trunk motion in the sagittal and coronal planes, lateral strength is provided by overlapping plastic and stabilizing closures, includes straps and closures, prefabricated, includes fitting and adjustment   🔨⊘
AHA: 4Q, '03, 5

Ⓐ **K0619** TLSO, sagittal-coronal control, modular segmented spinal system, three rigid plastic shells, posterior extends from the sacrococcygeal junction and terminates just inferior to the scapular spine, anterior extends from the symphysis pubis to the xiphoid, soft liner, restricts gross trunk motion in the sagittal and coronal planes, lateral strength is provided by overlapping plastic and stabilizing closures, includes straps and closures, prefabricated, includes fitting and adjustment   🔨⊘
AHA: 4Q, '03, 5

Ⓐ ☑ **K0620** Tubular elastic dressing, any width, per linear yard   🔨
AHA: 4Q, '03, 5

~~K0627 Traction equipment, cervical, free standing, pneumatic, applying traction force to other than mandible~~
See code(s): E0849

● ☒ **K0628** For diabetics only, multiple density insert, direct formed, molded to foot after external heat source of 230 degrees fahrenheit or higher, total contact with patient's foot, including arch, base layer minimum of 1/4 inch material of Shore A 35 durometer or 3/16 inch material of Shore A 40 (or higher), prefabricated, each

● ☒ **K0629** For diabetics only, multiple density insert, custom molded from model of patient's foot, total contact with patient's foot, including arch, base layer minimum of 3/16 inch material of Shore A 35 durometer or higher, includes arch filler and other shaping material, custom fabricated, each

● Ⓐ **K0630** SO, flexible, provides pelvic-sacral support, reduces motion about the sacroiliac joint, includes straps, closures, may include pendulous abdomen design, prefabricated, includes fitting and adjustment   🔨

● ☒ **K0631** SO, flexible, provides pelvic-sacral support, reduces motion about the sacroiliac joint, includes straps, closures, may include pendulous abdomen design, custom fabricated   🔨

● Ⓐ **K0632** SO, provides pelvic-sacral support, with rigid or semi-rigid panels over the sacrum and abdomen, reduces motion about the sacroiliac joint, includes straps, closures, may include pendulous abdomen design, prefabricated, includes fitting and adjustment   🔨

● ☒ **K0633** SO, provides pelvic-sacral support, with rigid or semi-rigid panels placed over the sacrum and abdomen, reduces motion about the sacroiliac joint, includes straps, closures, may include pendulous abdomen design, custom fabricated

Special Coverage Instructions   Noncovered by Medicare   Carrier Discretion   ☑ Quantity Alert   ● New Code   ○ Reinstated Code   ▲ Revised Code

86 — K Codes   Ⓐ Adult   Ⓜ Maternity   Ⓟ Pediatrics   Ⓘ Infant   Ⓐ-Ⓨ APC Status Indicator   *2005 HCPCS*

● Ⓐ **K0634** LO, flexible, provides lumbar support, posterior extends from L-1 to below L-5 vertebra, produces intracavitary pressure to reduce load on the intervertebral discs, includes straps, closures, may include pendulous abdomen design, shoulder straps, stays, prefabricated, includes fitting and adjustment   ᕃ

● Ⓐ **K0635** LO, sagittal control, with rigid posterior panel(s), posterior extends from L-1 to below L-5 vertebrae, produces intracavitary pressure to reduce load on the intervertebral discs, includes straps, closures, may include padding, stays, shoulder straps, pendulous abdomen design, prefabricated, includes fitting and adjustment   ᕃ

● Ⓐ **K0636** LO, sagittal control, with rigid anterior and posterior panels, posterior extends from L-1 to below L-5 vertebra, produces intracavitary pressure to reduce load on the intervertebral discs, includes straps, closures, may include padding, shoulder straps, pendulous abdomen design, prefabricated, includes fitting and adjustment   ᕃ

● Ⓐ **K0637** LSO, flexible, provides lumbo-sacral support, posterior extends from sacrococcygeal junction to T-9 vertebra, produces intracavitary pressure to reduce load on the intervertebral discs, includes straps, closures, may include stays, shoulder straps, pendulous abdomen design, prefabricated, includes fitting and adjustment   ᕃ

● Ⓨ **K0638** LSO, flexible, provides lumbo-sacral support, posterior extends from sacrococcygeal junction to T-9 vertebra, produces intracavitary pressure to reduce load on the intervertebral discs, includes straps, closures, may include stays, shoulder straps, pendulous abdomen design, custom fabricated

● Ⓐ **K0639** LSO, sagittal control, with rigid posterior panel(s), posterior extends from sacrococcygeal junction to T-9 vertebra, produces intracavitary pressure to reduce load on the intervertebral discs, includes straps, closures, may include padding, stays, shoulder straps, pendulous abdomen design, prefabricated, includes fitting and adjustment   ᕃ

● Ⓐ **K0640** LSO, sagittal control, with rigid anterior and posterior panels, posterior extends from sacrococcygeal junction to T-9 vertebra, produces intracavitary pressure to reduce load on the intervertebral disks, includes straps, closures, may include padding, shoulder straps, pendulous abdomen design, prefabricated, includes fitting and adjustment   ᕃ

● Ⓨ **K0641** LSO, sagittal control, with rigid anterior and posterior panels, posterior extends from sacrococcygeal junction to T-9 vertebra, produces intracavitary pressure to reduce load on the intervertebral discs, includes straps, closures, may include padding, shoulder straps, pendulous abdomen design, custom fabricated

● Ⓐ **K0642** LSO, sagittal-coronal control, with rigid posterior frame/panel(s), posterior extends from sacrococcygeal junction to T-9 vertebra, lateral strength provided by rigid lateral frame/panels, produces intracavitary pressure to reduce load on intervertebral discs, includes straps, closures, may include padding, stays, shoulder straps, pendulous abdomen design, prefabricated, includes fitting and adjustment   ᕃ

● Ⓨ **K0643** LSO, sagittal-coronal control, with rigid posterior frame/panel(s), posterior extends from sacrococcygeal junction to T-9 vertebra, lateral strength provided by rigid lateral frame/panels, produces intracavitary pressure to reduce load on intervertebral discs, includes straps, closures, may include padding, stays, shoulder straps, pendulous abdomen design, custom fabricated

● Ⓐ **K0644** LSO, sagittal-coronal control, lumbar flexion, rigid posterior frame/panels, lateral articulating design to flex the lumbar spine, posterior extends from sacrococcygeal junction to T-9 vertebra, lateral strength provided by rigid lateral frame/panels, produces intracavitary pressure to reduce load on intervertebral discs, includes straps, closures, may include padding, anterior panel, pendulous abdomen design, prefabricated, includes fitting and adjustment   ᕃ

● Ⓨ **K0645** LSO, sagittal-coronal control, lumbar flexion, rigid posterior frame/panels, lateral articulating design to flex the lumbar spine, posterior extends from sacrococcygeal junction to T-9 vertebra, lateral strength provided by rigid lateral frame/panels, produces intracavitary pressure to reduce load on intervertebral discs, includes straps, closures, may include padding, anterior panel, pendulous abdomen design, custom fabricated   ᕃ

● Ⓐ **K0646** LSO, sagittal-coronal control, with rigid anterior and posterior frame/panels, posterior extends from sacrococcygeal junction to T-9 vertebra, lateral strength provided by rigid lateral frame/panels, produces intracavitary pressure to reduce load on intervertebral discs, includes straps, closures, may include padding, shoulder straps, pendulous abdomen design, prefabricated, includes fitting and adjustment   ᕃ

● Ⓨ **K0647** LSO, sagittal-coronal control, with rigid anterior and posterior frame/panels, posterior extends from sacrococcygeal junction to T-9 vertebra, lateral strength provided by rigid lateral frame/panels, produces intracavitary pressure to reduce load on intervertebral discs, includes straps, closures, may include padding, shoulder straps, pendulous abdomen design, custom fabricated   ᕃ

● Ⓐ **K0648** LSO, sagittal-coronal control, rigid shell(s)/panel(s), posterior extends from sacrococcygeal junction to T-9 vertebra, anterior extends from symphysis pubis to xiphoid, produces intracavitary pressure to reduce load on the intervertebral discs, overall strength is provided by overlapping rigid plastic and stabilizing closures, includes straps, closures, may include soft interface, pendulous abdomen design, prefabricated, includes fitting and adjustment   ᕃ

● Ⓨ **K0649** LSO, sagittal-coronal control, rigid shell(s)/panel(s), posterior extends from sacrococcygeal junction to T-9 vertebra, anterior extends from symphysis pubis to xiphoid, produces intracavitary pressure to reduce load on the intervertebral discs, overall strength is provided by overlapping rigid plastic and stabilizing closures, includes straps, closures, may include soft interface, pendulous abdomen design, custom fabricated   ᕃ

K0650 ~~General use wheelchair seat cushion, width less than 22 in., any depth~~
See code(s): E2601

K0651 ~~General use wheelchair seat cushion width 22 in. or greater, any depth~~
See code(s): E2602

| Special Coverage Instructions | Noncovered by Medicare | Carrier Discretion | ☑ Quantity Alert | ● New Code | ○ Reinstated Code | ▲ Revised Code |

2005 HCPCS   ♀ Female Only   ♂ Male Only   **1**-**9** ASC Groups   **MED:** Pub 100/NCD Reference   ᕃ DMEPOS Paid   ⊘ SNF Excluded   **K Codes — 87**

Temporary Codes

K0652 — K0669

K0652 ~~Skin protection wheelchair seat cushion, width less than 22 in., any depth~~
See code(s): E2603

K0653 ~~Skin protection wheelchair seat cushion, width 22 in. or greater, any depth~~
See code(s): E2604

K0654 ~~Positioning wheelchair seat cushion, width less than 22 in., any depth~~
See code(s): E2605

K0655 ~~Positioning wheelchair seat cushion, width 22 in. or greater, any depth~~
See code(s): E2606

K0656 ~~Skin Protection and positioning wheelchair seat cushion, width less than 22 in., any depth~~
See code(s): E2607

K0657 ~~Skin protection and positioning wheelchair seat cushion, width 22 in. or greater, any depth~~
See code(s): E2608

K0658 ~~Custom fabricated wheelchair seat cushion, any size~~
See code(s): E2609

K0659 ~~Wheelchair seat cushion, powered~~
See code(s): E2610

K0660 ~~General use wheelchair back cushion, width less than 22 in., any height, including any type mounting hardware~~
See code(s): E2611

K0661 ~~General use wheelchair back cushion, width 22 in. or greater, any height, including any type mounting hardware~~
See code(s): E2612

K0662 ~~Positioning wheelchair back cushion, posterior, width less than 22 in., any height, including any type mounting hardware~~
See code(s): E2613

K0663 ~~Positioning wheelchair back cushion, posterior, width 22 in. or greater, any height, including any type mounting hardware~~
See code(s): E2614

K0664 ~~Positioning wheelchair back cushion, posterior-lateral, width less than 22 in., any height, including any type mounting hardware~~
See code(s): E2615

K0665 ~~Positioning wheelchair back cushion, posterior-lateral width 22 in. or greater, any height, including any type mounting hardware~~
See code(s): E2616

K0666 ~~Custom fabricated wheelchair back cushion, any size, including any type mounting hardware~~
See code(s): E2617

K0667 ~~Mounting hardware, any type, for seat cushion or seat support base attached to a manual wheelchair or lightweight power wheelchair, per cushion/base~~

K0668 ~~Replacement cover for wheelchair seat cushion or back cushion, each~~
See code(s): E2619

● ☑ K0669 Wheelchair seat or back cushion, no written coding verification from SADMERC

Special Coverage Instructions   Noncovered by Medicare   Carrier Discretion   ☑ Quantity Alert   ● New Code   ○ Reinstated Code   ▲ Revised Code

88 — K Codes   Ⓐ Adult   Ⓜ Maternity   Ⓟ Pediatrics   Ⓘ Infant   Ⓐ-☑ APC Status Indicator   *2005 HCPCS*

ORTHOTIC PROCEDURES *L0000–L4999*

L codes include orthotic and prosthetic procedures and devices, as well as scoliosis equipment, orthopedic shoes, and prosthetic implants.

ORTHOTIC DEVICES — SPINAL

CERVICAL

Medicare claims for L codes fall under the jurisdiction of the DME regional carrier, unless otherwise noted.

Ⓐ	☑	**L0100**	Cranial orthosis (helmet), with or without soft interface, molded to patient model ⛻
Ⓐ	☑	**L0110**	Cranial orthosis (helmet), with or without soft-interface, non-molded ⛻
Ⓐ		**L0112**	Cranial cervical orthosis, congenital torticollis type, with or without soft interface material, adjustable range of motion joint, custom fabricated ⛻
Ⓐ		**L0120**	Cervical, flexible, nonadjustable (foam collar) ⛻
Ⓐ		**L0130**	Cervical, flexible, thermoplastic collar, molded to patient ⛻
Ⓐ		**L0140**	Cervical, semi-rigid, adjustable (plastic collar) ⛻
Ⓐ		**L0150**	Cervical, semi-rigid, adjustable molded chin cup (plastic collar with mandibular/occipital piece) ⛻
Ⓐ		**L0160**	Cervical, semi-rigid, wire frame occipital/mandibular support ⛻
Ⓐ		**L0170**	Cervical, collar, molded to patient model ⛻
Ⓐ	☑	**L0172**	Cervical, collar, semi-rigid thermoplastic foam, two piece ⛻
Ⓐ	☑	**L0174**	Cervical, collar, semi-rigid, thermoplastic foam, two piece with thoracic extension ⛻

MULTIPLE POST COLLAR

Ⓐ		**L0180**	Cervical, multiple post collar, occipital/mandibular supports, adjustable ⛻
Ⓐ		**L0190**	Cervical, multiple post collar, occipital/mandibular supports, adjustable cervical bars (SOMI, Guilford, Taylor types) ⛻
Ⓐ		**L0200**	Cervical, multiple post collar, occipital/mandibular supports, adjustable cervical bars, and thoracic extension ⛻

THORACIC

Ⓐ		**L0210**	Thoracic, rib belt ⛻
Ⓐ		**L0220**	Thoracic, rib belt, custom fabricated ⛻
▲		**L0430**	Spinal orthosis, anterior-posterior-lateral control, with interface material, custom fitted (dewall posture protector only)
Ⓐ		**L0450**	TLSO, flexible, provides trunk support, upper thoracic region, produces intracavitary pressure to reduce load on the intervertebral disks with rigid stays or panel(s), includes shoulder straps and closures, prefabricated, includes fitting and adjustment ⛻
Ⓐ		**L0452**	TLSO, flexible, provides trunk support, upper thoracic region, produces intracavitary pressure to reduce load on the intervertebral disks with rigid stays or panel(s), includes shoulder straps and closures, custom fabricated ⛻

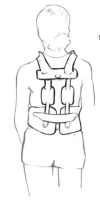
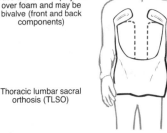

TLSO brace with adjustable straps and pads (L0450). The model at right and similar devices such as the Boston brace are molded polymer over foam and may be bivalve (front and back components)

Thoracic lumbar sacral orthosis (TLSO)

Ⓐ		**L0454**	TLSO flexible, provides trunk support, extends from sacrococcygeal junction to above T-9 vertebra, restricts gross trunk motion in the sagittal plane, produces intracavitary pressure to reduce load on the intervertebral disks with rigid stays or panel(s), includes shoulder straps and closures, prefabricated, includes fitting and adjustment ⛻
Ⓐ		**L0456**	TLSO, flexible, provides trunk support, thoracic region, rigid posterior panel and soft anterior apron, extends from the sacrococcygeal junction and terminates just inferior to the scapular spine, restricts gross trunk motion in the sagittal plane, produces intracavitary pressure to reduce load on the intervertebral disks, includes straps and closures, prefabricated, includes fitting and adjustment ⛻
Ⓐ		**L0458**	TLSO, triplanar control, modular segmented spinal system, two rigid plastic shells, posterior extends from the sacrococcygeal junction and terminates just inferior to the scapular spine, anterior extends from the symphysis pubis to the xiphoid, soft liner, restricts gross trunk motion in the sagittal, coronal, and transverse planes, lateral strength is provided by overlapping plastic and stabilizing closures, includes straps and closures, prefabricated, includes fitting and adjustment ⛻
Ⓐ		**L0460**	TLSO, triplanar control, modular segmented spinal system, two rigid plastic shells, posterior extends from the sacrococcygeal junction and terminates just inferior to the scapular spine, anterior extends from the symphysis pubis to the sternal notch, soft liner, restricts gross trunk motion in the sagittal, coronal, and transverse planes, lateral strength is provided by overlapping plastic and stabilizing closures, includes straps and closures, prefabricated, includes fitting and adjustment ⛻
Ⓐ		**L0462**	TLSO, triplanar control, modular segmented spinal system, three rigid plastic shells, posterior extends from the sacrococcygeal junction and terminates just inferior to the scapular spine, anterior extends from the symphysis pubis to the sternal notch, soft liner, restricts gross trunk motion in the sagittal, coronal, and transverse planes, lateral strength is provided by overlapping plastic and stabilizing closures, includes straps and closures, prefabricated, includes fitting and adjustment ⛻

Special Coverage Instructions   Noncovered by Medicare   Carrier Discretion   ☑ Quantity Alert   ● New Code   ○ Reinstated Code   ▲ Revised Code

2005 HCPCS   ♀ Female Only   ♂ Male Only   **❶-❾** ASC Groups   **MED:**Pub 100/NCD Reference   ⛻ DMEPOS Paid   Ⓢ SNF Excluded   **L Codes — 89**

Orthotic Procedures

L0100 — L0462

Orthotic Procedures

L0464 — L0515

[A] **L0464** TLSO, triplanar control, modular segmented spinal system, four rigid plastic shells, posterior extends from sacrococcygeal junction and terminates just inferior to scapular spine, anterior extends from symphysis pubis to the sternal notch, soft liner, restricts gross trunk motion in sagittal, coronal, and transverse planes, lateral strength is provided by overlapping plastic and stabilizing closures, includes straps and closures, prefabricated, includes fitting and adjustment   ♿

[A] **L0466** TLSO, sagittal control, rigid posterior frame and flexible soft anterior apron with straps, closures and padding, restricts gross trunk motion in sagittal plane, produces intracavity pressure to reduce load on intervertebral disks, includes fitting and shaping the frame, prefabricated, includes fitting and adjustment   ♿

[A] **L0468** TLSO, sagittal-coronal control, rigid posterior frame and flexible soft anterior apron with straps, closures and padding, extends from sacrococcygeal junction over scapulae, lateral strength provided by pelvic, thoracic, and lateral frame pieces, restricts gross trunk motion in sagittal, and coronal planes, produces intracavity pressure to reduce load on intervertebral disks, includes fitting and shaping the frame, prefabricated, includes fitting and adjustment   ♿

[A] **L0470** TLSO, triplanar control, rigid posterior frame and flexible soft anterior apron with straps, closures and padding, extends from sacrococcygeal junction to scapula, lateral strength provided by pelvic, thoracic, and lateral frame pieces, rotational strength provided by subclavicular extensions, restricts gross trunk motion in sagittal, coronal, and transverse planes, produces intracavity pressure to reduce load on the intervertebral disks, includes fitting and shaping the frame, prefabricated, includes fitting and adjustment   ♿

[A] **L0472** TLSO, triplanar control, hyperextension, rigid anterior and lateral frame extends from symphysis pubis to sternal notch with two anterior components (one pubic and one sternal), posterior and lateral pads with straps and closures, limits spinal flexion, restricts gross trunk motion in sagittal, coronal, and transverse planes, includes fitting and shaping the frame, prefabricated, includes fitting and adjustment   ♿

~~**L0476** TLSO, sagittal coronal control, flexion compression jacket, two rigid plastic shells with soft liner, posterior extends from sacrococcygeal junction and terminates at or before the T9 vertebra, anterior extends from symphysis pubis to xiphoid, usually laced together on one side, restricts gross trunk motion in sagittal and coronal planes, allows free flexion and compression of the LS region, includes straps and closures, prefabricated, includes fitting and adjustment~~

~~**L0478** TLSO, sagittal coronal control, flexion compression jacket, two rigid plastic shells with soft liner, posterior extends from sacrococcygeal junction and terminates at or before the T9 vertebra, anterior extends from symphysis pubis to xiphoid, usually laced together on one side, restricts gross trunk motion in sagittal and coronal planes, allows free flexion and compression of LS region, includes straps and closures, custom fabricated~~

[A] **L0480** TLSO, triplanar control, one piece rigid plastic shell without interface liner, with multiple straps and closures, posterior extends from sacrococcygeal junction and terminates just inferior to scapular spine, anterior extends from symphysis pubis to sternal notch, anterior or posterior opening, restricts gross trunk motion in sagittal, coronal, and transverse planes, includes a carved plaster or CAD-CAM model, custom fabricated   ♿

[A] **L0482** TLSO, triplanar control, one piece rigid plastic shell with interface liner, multiple straps and closures, posterior extends from sacrococcygeal junction and terminates just inferior to scapular spine, anterior extends from symphysis pubis to sternal notch, anterior or posterior opening, restricts gross trunk motion in sagittal, coronal, and transverse planes, includes a carved plaster or CAD-CAM model, custom fabricated   ♿

[A] **L0484** TLSO, triplanar control, two piece rigid plastic shell without interface liner, with multiple straps and closures, posterior extends from sacrococcygeal junction and terminates just inferior to scapular spine, anterior extends from symphysis pubis to sternal notch, lateral strength is enhanced by overlapping plastic, restricts gross trunk motion in the sagittal, coronal, and transverse planes, includes a carved plaster or CAD-CAM model, custom fabricated   ♿

[A] **L0486** TLSO, triplanar control, two piece rigid plastic shell with interface liner, multiple straps and closures, posterior extends from sacrococcygeal junction and terminates just inferior to scapular spine, anterior extends from symphysis pubis to sternal notch, lateral strength is enhanced by overlapping plastic, restricts gross trunk motion in the sagittal, coronal, and transverse planes, includes a carved plaster or CAD-CAM model, custom fabricated   ♿

[A] **L0488** TLSO, triplanar control, one piece rigid plastic shell with interface liner, multiple straps and closures, posterior extends from sacrococcygeal junction and terminates just inferior to scapular spine, anterior extends from symphysis pubis to sternal notch, anterior or posterior opening, restricts gross trunk motion in sagittal, coronal, and transverse planes, prefabricated, includes fitting and adjustment   ♿

[A] **L0490** TLSO, sagittal-coronal control, one piece rigid plastic shell, with overlapping reinforced anterior, with multiple straps and closures, posterior extends from sacrococcygeal junction and terminates at or before the T-9 vertebra, anterior extends from symphysis pubis to xiphoid, anterior opening, restricts gross trunk motion in sagittal and coronal planes, prefabricated, includes fitting and adjustment   ♿

LUMBAR-SACRAL ORTHOSIS (LSO)

FLEXIBLE

~~**L0500** Lumbar sacral orthosis (LSO), flexible, (lumbo sacral support)~~

~~**L0510** LSO, flexible (lumbo sacral support), custom fabricated~~

~~**L0515** LSO, anterior posterior control, with rigid or semi-rigid posterior panel, prefabricated~~

Special Coverage Instructions   Noncovered by Medicare   Carrier Discretion   ☑ Quantity Alert   ● New Code   ○ Reinstated Code   ▲ Revised Code

90 — L Codes   [A] Adult   [M] Maternity   [P] Pediatrics   [I] Infant   [A]-[Y] APC Status Indicator   **2005 HCPCS**

ANTERIOR-POSTERIOR-LATERAL CONTROL

~~L0520~~   ~~LSO, anterior posterior lateral control (knight, wilcox types), with apron front~~

ANTERIOR-POSTERIOR CONTROL

~~L0530~~   ~~LSO, anterior posterior control (macausland type), with apron front~~

LUMBAR FLEXION

~~L0540~~   ~~LSO, lumbar flexion (williams flexion type)~~

~~L0550~~   ~~LSO, anterior posterior lateral control, molded to patient model~~

~~L0560~~   ~~LSO, anterior posterior lateral control, molded to patient model, with interface material~~

~~L0561~~   ~~LSO, anterior posterior lateral control, with rigid or semi rigid posterior panel, prefabricated~~

~~L0565~~   ~~LSO, anterior posterior lateral control, custom fitted~~

SACROILIAC

FLEXIBLE

~~L0600~~   ~~Sacroiliac, flexible (sacroiliac surgical support)~~

~~L0610~~   ~~Sacroiliac, flexible (sacroiliac surgical support), custom fabricated~~

SEMI-RIGID

~~L0620~~   ~~Sacroiliac, semi rigid (goldthwaite, osgood types), with apron front~~

CERVICAL-THORACIC-LUMBAR-SACRAL ORTHOSIS (CTLSO)

ANTERIOR-POSTERIOR-LATERAL CONTROL

Ⓐ   L0700   CTLSO, anterior-posterior-lateral control, molded to patient model (Minerva type)   ♿

Ⓐ   L0710   CTLSO, anterior-posterior-lateral control, molded to patient model, with interface material (Minerva type)   ♿

HALO PROCEDURE

Ⓐ   L0810   Halo procedure, cervical halo incorporated into jacket vest   ♿

Ⓐ   L0820   Halo procedure, cervical halo incorporated into plaster body jacket   ♿

Ⓐ   L0830   Halo procedure, cervical halo incorporated into Milwaukee type orthosis   ♿

Ⓐ   L0860   Addition to halo procedure, magnetic resonance image compatible system   ♿

Ⓐ   L0861   Addition to halo procedure, replacement liner/interface material   ♿

Ⓔ   L0960   Torso support, postsurgical support, pads for postsurgical support   ♿

ADDITIONS TO SPINAL ORTHOSIS

Ⓐ   L0970   TLSO, corset front   ♿

Ⓐ   L0972   LSO, corset front   ♿

Ⓐ   L0974   TLSO, full corset   ♿

Ⓐ   L0976   LSO, full corset   ♿

Ⓐ   L0978   Axillary crutch extension   ♿

Ⓐ ☑   L0980   Peroneal straps, pair   ♿

Ⓐ ☑   L0982   Stocking supporter grips, set of four (4)   ♿

Ⓐ ☑   L0984   Protective body sock, each   ♿

Ⓐ   L0999   Addition to spinal orthosis, NOS
Determine if an alternative HCPCS Level II or a CPT code better describes the service being reported. This code should be used only if a more specific code is unavailable.

ORTHOTIC DEVICES — SCOLIOSIS PROCEDURES

The orthotic care of scoliosis differs from other orthotic care in that the treatment is more dynamic in nature and uses continual modification of the orthosis to the patient's changing condition. This coding structure uses the proper names — or eponyms — of the procedures because they have historic and universal acceptance in the profession. It should be recognized that variations to the basic procedures described by the founders/developers are accepted in various medical and orthotic practices throughout the country. All procedures include model of patient when indicated.

CERVICAL-THORACIC-LUMBAR-SACRAL ORTHOSIS (CTLSO) (MILWAUKEE)

Ⓐ   L1000   CTLSO (Milwaukee), inclusive of furnishing initial orthosis, including model   ♿

Ⓐ   L1005   Tension based scoliosis orthosis and accessory pads, includes fitting and adjustment   ♿

Ⓐ   L1010   Addition to CTLSO or scoliosis orthosis, axilla sling   ♿

Ⓐ   L1020   Addition to CTLSO or scoliosis orthosis, kyphosis pad   ♿

Ⓐ   L1025   Addition to CTLSO or scoliosis orthosis, kyphosis pad, floating   ♿

Ⓐ   L1030   Addition to CTLSO or scoliosis orthosis, lumbar bolster pad   ♿

Ⓐ   L1040   Addition to CTLSO or scoliosis orthosis, lumbar or lumbar rib pad   ♿

Ⓐ   L1050   Addition to CTLSO or scoliosis orthosis, sternal pad   ♿

Ⓐ   L1060   Addition to CTLSO or scoliosis orthosis, thoracic pad   ♿

Ⓐ   L1070   Addition to CTLSO or scoliosis orthosis, trapezius sling   ♿

Ⓐ   L1080   Addition to CTLSO or scoliosis orthosis, outrigger   ♿

Ⓐ   L1085   Addition to CTLSO or scoliosis orthosis, outrigger, bilateral with vertical extensions   ♿

Ⓐ   L1090   Addition to CTLSO or scoliosis orthosis, lumbar sling   ♿

Ⓐ   L1100   Addition to CTLSO or scoliosis orthosis, ring flange, plastic or leather   ♿

Ⓐ   L1110   Addition to CTLSO or scoliosis orthosis, ring flange, plastic or leather, molded to patient model   ♿

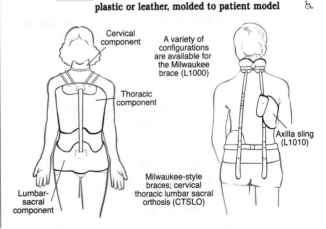

Cervical component

A variety of configurations are available for the Milwaukee brace (L1000)

Thoracic component

Axilla sling (L1010)

Lumbar-sacral component

Milwaukee-style braces; cervical thoracic lumbar sacral orthosis (CTSLO)

Special Coverage Instructions   Noncovered by Medicare   Carrier Discretion   ☑ Quantity Alert   ● New Code   ○ Reinstated Code   ▲ Revised Code

2005 HCPCS   ♀ Female Only   ♂ Male Only   ❶-❾ ASC Groups   MED: Pub 100/NCD Reference   ♿ DMEPOS Paid   Ⓢ SNF Excluded   **L Codes — 91**

Orthotic Procedures

L1120 — L1836

Ⓐ ☑ **L1120** Addition to CTLSO, scoliosis orthosis, cover for upright, each   ♿

THORACIC-LUMBAR-SACRAL ORTHOSIS (TLSO) (LOW PROFILE)

Ⓐ **L1200** TLSO, inclusive of furnishing initial orthosis only   ♿

Ⓐ **L1210** Addition to TLSO, (low profile), lateral thoracic extension   ♿

Ⓐ **L1220** Addition to TLSO, (low profile), anterior thoracic extension   ♿

Ⓐ **L1230** Addition to TLSO, (low profile), Milwaukee type superstructure   ♿

Ⓐ **L1240** Addition to TLSO, (low profile), lumbar derotation pad   ♿

Ⓐ **L1250** Addition to TLSO, (low profile), anterior ASIS pad   ♿

Ⓐ **L1260** Addition to TLSO, (low profile), anterior thoracic derotation pad   ♿

Ⓐ **L1270** Addition to TLSO, (low profile), abdominal pad   ♿

Ⓐ ☑ **L1280** Addition to TLSO, (low profile), rib gusset (elastic), each   ♿

Ⓐ **L1290** Addition to TLSO, (low profile), lateral trochanteric pad   ♿

OTHER SCOLIOSIS PROCEDURES

Ⓐ **L1300** Other scoliosis procedure, body jacket molded to patient model   ♿

Ⓐ **L1310** Other scoliosis procedure, postoperative body jacket   ♿

Ⓐ **L1499** Spinal orthosis, not otherwise specified
Determine if an alternative HCPCS Level II or a CPT code better describes the service being reported. This code should be used only if a more specific code is unavailable.

THORACIC-HIP-KNEE-ANKLE ORTHOSIS (THKAO)

Ⓐ **L1500** THKAO, mobility frame (Newington, Parapodium types)   ♿

Ⓐ **L1510** THKAO, standing frame, with or without tray and accessories   ♿

Ⓐ **L1520** THKAO, swivel walker   ♿

ORTHOTIC DEVICES — LOWER LIMB

The procedures in L1600–L2999 are considered as "base" or "basic procedures" and may be modified by listing procedure from the "additions" sections and adding them to the base procedures.

HIP ORTHOSIS (HO) — FLEXIBLE

Ⓐ **L1600** HO, abduction control of hip joints, flexible, Frejka type with cover, prefabricated, includes fitting and adjustment   ♿

Ⓐ **L1610** HO, abduction control of hip joints, flexible, (Frejka cover only), prefabricated, includes fitting and adjustment   ♿

Ⓐ **L1620** HO, abduction control of hip joints, flexible, (Pavlik harness), prefabricated, includes fitting and adjustment   ♿

Ⓐ **L1630** HO, abduction control of hip joints, semi-flexible (Von Rosen type), custom fabricated   ♿

Ⓐ **L1640** HO, abduction control of hip joints, static, pelvic band or spreader bar, thigh cuffs, custom fabricated   ♿

Ⓐ **L1650** HO, abduction control of hip joints, static, adjustable (Ilfled type), prefabricated, includes fitting and adjustment   ♿

Ⓐ **L1652** HO, bilateral thigh cuffs with adjustable abductor spreader bar, adult size, prefabricated, includes fitting and adjustment, any type   ♿

Ⓐ **L1660** HO, abduction control of hip joints, static, plastic, prefabricated, includes fitting and adjustment   ♿

Ⓐ **L1680** HO, abduction control of hip joints, dynamic, pelvic control, adjustable hip motion control, thigh cuffs (Rancho hip action type), custom fabricated   ♿

Ⓐ **L1685** HO, abduction control of hip joint, postoperative hip abduction type, custom fabricated   ♿

Ⓐ **L1686** HO, abduction control of hip joint, postoperative hip abduction type, prefabricated, includes fitting and adjustments   ♿

Ⓐ **L1690** Combination, bilateral, lumbo-sacral, hip, femur orthosis providing adduction and internal rotation control, prefabricated, includes fitting and adjustment   ♿

LEGG PERTHES

Ⓐ **L1700** Legg Perthes orthosis, (Toronto type), custom fabricated   ♿

Ⓐ **L1710** Legg Perthes orthosis, (Newington type), custom fabricated   ♿

Ⓐ **L1720** Legg Perthes orthosis, trilateral, (Tachdijan type), custom fabricated   ♿

Ⓐ **L1730** Legg Perthes orthosis, (Scottish Rite type), custom fabricated   ♿

Ⓐ **L1750** Legg Perthes orthosis, Legg Perthes sling (Sam Brown type), prefabricated, includes fitting and adjustment   ♿

Ⓐ **L1755** Legg Perthes orthosis, (Patten bottom type), custom fabricated   ♿

KNEE ORTHOSIS (KO)

Ⓐ **L1800** KO, elastic with stays, prefabricated, includes fitting and adjustment   ♿

Ⓐ **L1810** KO, elastic with joints, prefabricated, includes fitting and adjustment   ♿

Ⓐ **L1815** KO, elastic or other elastic type material with condylar pad(s), prefabricated, includes fitting and adjustment   ♿

▲ Ⓐ **L1820** KO, elastic with condylar pads and joints, with or without patellar control, prefabricated, includes fitting and adjustment   ♿

Ⓐ **L1825** KO, elastic knee cap, prefabricated, includes fitting and adjustment   ♿

Ⓐ **L1830** KO, immobilizer, canvas longitudinal, prefabricated, includes fitting and adjustment   ♿

Ⓐ **L1831** KO, locking knee joint(s), positional orthosis, prefabricated, includes fitting and adjustment   ♿

Ⓐ **L1832** KO, adjustable knee joints, positional orthosis, rigid support, prefabricated, includes fitting and adjustment   ♿

Ⓐ **L1834** KO, without knee joint, rigid, custom fabricated   ♿

Ⓐ **L1836** KO, rigid, without joint(s), includes soft interface material, prefabricated, includes fitting and adjustment   ♿

Special Coverage Instructions   Noncovered by Medicare   Carrier Discretion   ☑ Quantity Alert   ● New Code   ○ Reinstated Code   ▲ Revised Code

92 — L Codes   Ⓐ Adult   Ⓜ Maternity   Ⓟ Pediatrics   Ⓘ Infant   Ⓐ-Ⓨ APC Status Indicator   **2005 HCPCS**

Ⓐ **L1840** KO, derotation, medial-lateral, anterior cruciate ligament, custom fabricated 🦽

Ⓐ **L1843** KO, single upright, thigh and calf, with adjustable flexion and extension joint, medial-lateral and rotation control, with or without varus/valgus adjustment, prefabricated, includes fitting and adjustment 🦽

Ⓐ **L1844** KO, single upright, thigh and calf, with adjustable flexion and extension joint, medial-lateral and rotation control, with or without varus/valgus adjustment, custom fabricated 🦽

Ⓐ **L1845** KO, double upright, thigh and calf, with adjustable flexion and extension joint, medial-lateral and rotation control, prefabricated, includes fitting and adjustment 🦽

Ⓐ **L1846** KO, double upright, thigh and calf, with adjustable flexion and extension joint, medial-lateral and rotation control, custom fabricated 🦽

Ⓐ **L1847** KO, double upright with adjustable joint, with inflatable air support chamber(s), prefabricated, includes fitting and adjustment 🦽

Ⓐ **L1850** KO, Swedish type, prefabricated, includes fitting and adjustment 🦽

Ⓐ **L1855** KO, molded plastic, thigh and calf sections, with double upright knee joints, custom fabricated 🦽

Ⓐ **L1858** KO, molded plastic, polycentric knee joints, pneumatic knee pads (CTI), custom fabricated 🦽

Ⓐ **L1860** KO, modification of supracondylar prosthetic socket, custom fabricated (SK) 🦽

Ⓐ **L1870** KO, double upright, thigh and calf lacers, with knee joints, custom fabricated 🦽

Ⓐ **L1880** KO, double upright, nonmolded thigh and calf cuffs/lacers with knee joints, custom fabricated 🦽

ANKLE-FOOT ORTHOSIS (AFO)

Ⓐ **L1900** AFO, spring wire, dorsiflexion assist calf band, custom fabricated 🦽

Ⓐ **L1901** Ankle orthosis, elastic, prefabricated, includes fitting and adjustment (e.g., neoprene, Lycra) 🦽

Ⓐ **L1902** AFO, ankle gauntlet, prefabricated, includes fitting and adjustment 🦽

Ⓐ **L1904** AFO, molded ankle gauntlet, custom fabricated 🦽

Ⓐ **L1906** AFO, multiligamentous ankle support, prefabricated, includes fitting and adjustment 🦽

Ⓐ **L1907** AFO, supramalleolar with straps, with or without interface/pads, custom fabricated 🦽

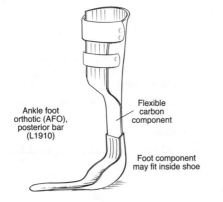

Ankle foot orthotic (AFO), posterior bar (L1910)

Flexible carbon component

Foot component may fit inside shoe

Rigid tibial anterior floor reaction; ankle-foot orthosis (AFO) (L1945)

Spiral; ankle-foot orthosis (AFO) (L1950)

Ⓐ **L1910** AFO, posterior, single bar, clasp attachment to shoe counter, prefabricated, includes fitting and adjustment 🦽

Ⓐ **L1920** AFO, single upright with static or adjustable stop (Phelps or Perlstein type), custom fabricated 🦽

Ⓐ **L1930** AFO, plastic or other material, prefabricated, includes fitting and adjustment 🦽

● **L1932** AFO, rigid anterior tibial section, total Carbon fiber or equal material, prefabricated, includes fitting and adjustment

Ⓐ **L1940** AFO, plastic or other material, custom-fabricated 🦽

Ⓐ **L1945** AFO, molded to patient model, plastic, rigid anterior tibial section (floor reaction), custom fabricated 🦽

Ⓐ **L1950** AFO, spiral, (Institute of Rehabilitative Medicine type), plastic, custom-fabricated 🦽

Ⓐ **L1951** AFO, spiral, (Institute of Rehabilitative Medicine type), plastic or other material, prefabricated, includes fitting and adjustment 🦽

Ⓐ **L1960** AFO, posterior solid ankle, plastic, custom fabricated 🦽

Ⓐ **L1970** AFO, plastic, with ankle joint, custom fabricated 🦽

Ⓐ **L1971** AFO, plastic or other material with ankle joint, prefabricated, includes fitting and adjustment 🦽

Ⓐ **L1980** AFO, single upright free plantar dorsiflexion, solid stirrup, calf band/cuff (single bar BK orthosis), custom fabricated 🦽

Ⓐ **L1990** AFO, double upright free plantar dorsiflexion, solid stirrup, calf band/cuff (double bar BK orthosis), custom fabricated 🦽

KNEE-ANKLE-FOOT ORTHOSIS (KAFO) — OR ANY COMBINATION

L2000, L2020, L2036 are base procedures to be used with any knee joint, L2010 and L2030 are to be used only with no knee joint.

Ⓐ **L2000** KAFO, single upright, free knee, free ankle, solid stirrup, thigh and calf bands/cuffs (single bar AK orthosis), custom fabricated 🦽

● **L2005** KAFO, any material, single or double upright, stance control, automatic lock and swing phase release, mechanical activation, includes ankle joint, any type, custom fabricated

Ⓐ **L2010** KAFO, single upright, free ankle, solid stirrup, thigh and calf bands/cuffs (single bar AK orthosis), without knee joint, custom fabricated 🦽

Ⓐ **L2020** KAFO, double upright, free knee, free ankle, solid stirrup, thigh and calf bands/cuffs (double bar AK orthosis), custom fabricated 🦽

◼ Special Coverage Instructions   ◼ Noncovered by Medicare   ◼ Carrier Discretion   ☑ Quantity Alert   ● New Code   ○ Reinstated Code   ▲ Revised Code

2005 HCPCS   ♀ Female Only   ♂ Male Only   1-9 ASC Groups   MED: Pub 100/NCD Reference   🦽 DMEPOS Paid   ⊘ SNF Excluded   **L Codes — 93**

Orthotic Procedures

L2030 — L2375

[A] **L2030** KAFO, double upright, free ankle, solid stirrup, thigh and calf bands/cuffs, (double bar AK orthosis), without knee joint, custom fabricated

▲ [A] **L2035** KAFO, full plastic, static (pediatric size), without free motion ankle, prefabricated, includes fitting and adjustment

▲ [A] **L2036** KAFO, full plastic, double upright, free knee, with or without free motion ankle, custom fabricated

▲ [A] **L2037** KAFO, full plastic, single upright, free knee, with or without free motion ankle, custom fabricated

▲ [A] **L2038** KAFO, full plastic, without knee joint, multi-axis ankle, custom fabricated

▲ [A] **L2039** KAFO, full plastic, single upright, poly-axial hinge, medial lateral rotation control, with or without free motion ankle, custom fabricated

TORSION CONTROL: HIP-KNEE-ANKLE-FOOT ORTHOSIS (HKAFO)

[A] **L2040** HKAFO, torsion control, bilateral rotation straps, pelvic band/belt, custom fabricated

[A] **L2050** HKAFO, torsion control, bilateral torsion cables, hip joint, pelvic band/belt, custom fabricated

[A] **L2060** HKAFO, torsion control, bilateral torsion cables, ball bearing hip joint, pelvic band/ belt, custom fabricated

[A] **L2070** HKAFO, torsion control, unilateral rotation straps, pelvic band/belt, custom fabricated

[A] **L2080** HKAFO, torsion control, unilateral torsion cable, hip joint, pelvic band/belt, custom fabricated

[A] **L2090** HKAFO, torsion control, unilateral torsion cable, ball bearing hip joint, pelvic band/belt, custom fabricated

[A] **L2106** AFO, fracture orthosis, tibial fracture cast orthosis, thermoplastic type casting material, custom fabricated

[A] **L2108** AFO, fracture orthosis, tibial fracture cast orthosis, custom fabricated

[A] **L2112** AFO, fracture orthosis, tibial fracture orthosis, soft, prefabricated, includes fitting and adjustment

[A] **L2114** AFO, fracture orthosis, tibial fracture orthosis, semi-rigid, prefabricated, includes fitting and adjustment

[A] **L2116** AFO, fracture orthosis, tibial fracture orthosis, rigid, prefabricated, includes fitting and adjustment

[A] **L2126** KAFO, fracture orthosis, femoral fracture cast orthosis, thermoplastic type casting material, custom fabricated

[A] **L2128** KAFO, fracture orthosis, femoral fracture cast orthosis, custom fabricated

[A] **L2132** KAFO, fracture orthosis, femoral fracture cast orthosis, soft, prefabricated, includes fitting and adjustment

[A] **L2134** KAFO, fracture orthosis, femoral fracture cast orthosis, semi-rigid, prefabricated, includes fitting and adjustment

[A] **L2136** KAFO, fracture orthosis, femoral fracture cast orthosis, rigid, prefabricated, includes fitting and adjustment

ADDITIONS TO FRACTURE ORTHOSIS

[A] **L2180** Addition to lower extremity fracture orthosis, plastic shoe insert with ankle joints

[A] **L2182** Addition to lower extremity fracture orthosis, drop lock knee joint

[A] **L2184** Addition to lower extremity fracture orthosis, limited motion knee joint

[A] **L2186** Addition to lower extremity fracture orthosis, adjustable motion knee joint, Lerman type

[A] **L2188** Addition to lower extremity fracture orthosis, quadrilateral brim

[A] **L2190** Addition to lower extremity fracture orthosis, waist belt

[A] **L2192** Addition to lower extremity fracture orthosis, hip joint, pelvic band, thigh flange, and pelvic belt

ADDITIONS TO LOWER EXTREMITY ORTHOSIS: SHOE-ANKLE-SHIN-KNEE

[A] ☑ **L2200** Addition to lower extremity, limited ankle motion, each joint

[A] ☑ **L2210** Addition to lower extremity, dorsiflexion assist (plantar flexion resist), each joint

[A] ☑ **L2220** Addition to lower extremity, dorsiflexion and plantar flexion assist/resist, each joint

[A] **L2230** Addition to lower extremity, split flat caliper stirrups and plate attachment

● **L2232** Addition to lower extremity orthosis, rocker bottom for total contact ankle foot orthosis, for custom fabricated orthosis only

[A] **L2240** Addition to lower extremity, round caliper and plate attachment

[A] **L2250** Addition to lower extremity, foot plate, molded to patient model, stirrup attachment

[A] **L2260** Addition to lower extremity, reinforced solid stirrup (Scott-Craig type)

[A] **L2265** Addition to lower extremity, long tongue stirrup

[A] **L2270** Addition to lower extremity, varus/valgus correction (T) strap, padded/lined or malleolus pad

[A] **L2275** Addition to lower extremity, varus/valgus correction, plastic modification, padded/lined

[A] **L2280** Addition to lower extremity, molded inner boot

[A] **L2300** Addition to lower extremity, abduction bar (bilateral hip involvement), jointed, adjustable

[A] **L2310** Addition to lower extremity, abduction bar, straight

▲ [A] **L2320** Addition to lower extremity, non-molded lacer, for custom fabricated orthosis only

▲ [A] **L2330** Addition to lower extremity, lacer molded to patient model, for custom fabricated orthosis only

[A] **L2335** Addition to lower extremity, anterior swing band

[A] **L2340** Addition to lower extremity, pretibial shell, molded to patient model

[A] **L2350** Addition to lower extremity, prosthetic type, (BK) socket, molded to patient model, (used for PTB, AFO orthoses)

[A] **L2360** Addition to lower extremity, extended steel shank

[A] **L2370** Addition to lower extremity, Patten bottom

[A] **L2375** Addition to lower extremity, torsion control, ankle joint and half solid stirrup

Special Coverage Instructions   Noncovered by Medicare   Carrier Discretion   ☑ Quantity Alert   ● New Code   ○ Reinstated Code   ▲ Revised Code

94 — L Codes   [A] Adult   [M] Maternity   [P] Pediatrics   [I] Infant   [A]-[Y] APC Status Indicator   **2005 HCPCS**

A ☑ **L2380** Addition to lower extremity, torsion control, straight knee joint, each joint ♿

A ☑ **L2385** Addition to lower extremity, straight knee joint, heavy duty, each joint ♿

A ☑ **L2390** Addition to lower extremity, offset knee joint, each joint ♿

A ☑ **L2395** Addition to lower extremity, offset knee joint, heavy duty, each joint ♿

A **L2397** Addition to lower extremity orthosis, suspension sleeve

ADDITIONS TO STRAIGHT KNEE OR OFFSET KNEE JOINTS

A ☑ **L2405** Addition to knee joint, lock; drop, stance or swing phase, each joint ♿

A ☑ **L2415** Addition to knee lock with integrated release mechanism (bail, cable, or equal), any material, each joint ♿

A ☑ **L2425** Addition to knee joint, disc or dial lock for adjustable knee flexion, each joint ♿

A ☑ **L2430** Addition to knee joint, ratchet lock for active and progressive knee extension, each joint ♿

~~L2435 Addition to knee joint, polycentric joint, each joint~~

A **L2492** Addition to knee joint, lift loop for drop lock ring ♿

ADDITIONS: THIGH/WEIGHT BEARING — GLUTEAL/ISCHIAL WEIGHT BEARING

A **L2500** Addition to lower extremity, thigh/weight bearing, gluteal/ischial weight bearing, ring ♿

A **L2510** Addition to lower extremity, thigh/weight bearing, quadri-lateral brim, molded to patient model ♿

A **L2520** Addition to lower extremity, thigh/weight bearing, quadri-lateral brim, custom fitted ♿

A **L2525** Addition to lower extremity, thigh/weight bearing, ischial containment/narrow M-L brim molded to patient model ♿

A **L2526** Addition to lower extremity, thigh/weight bearing, ischial containment/narrow M-L brim, custom fitted ♿

A **L2530** Addition to lower extremity, thigh/weight bearing, lacer, nonmolded ♿

A **L2540** Addition to lower extremity, thigh/weight bearing, lacer, molded to patient model ♿

A **L2550** Addition to lower extremity, thigh/weight bearing, high roll cuff ♿

ADDITIONS: PELVIC AND THORACIC CONTROL

A ☑ **L2570** Addition to lower extremity, pelvic control, hip joint, Clevis type, two position joint, each ♿

A **L2580** Addition to lower extremity, pelvic control, pelvic sling ♿

A ☑ **L2600** Addition to lower extremity, pelvic control, hip joint, Clevis type, or thrust bearing, free, each ♿

A ☑ **L2610** Addition to lower extremity, pelvic control, hip joint, Clevis or thrust bearing, lock, each ♿

A ☑ **L2620** Addition to lower extremity, pelvic control, hip joint, heavy-duty, each ♿

A ☑ **L2622** Addition to lower extremity, pelvic control, hip joint, adjustable flexion, each ♿

A ☑ **L2624** Addition to lower extremity, pelvic control, hip joint, adjustable flexion, extension, abduction control, each ♿

A **L2627** Addition to lower extremity, pelvic control, plastic, molded to patient model, reciprocating hip joint and cables ♿

A **L2628** Addition to lower extremity, pelvic control, metal frame, reciprocating hip joint and cables ♿

A **L2630** Addition to lower extremity, pelvic control, band and belt, unilateral ♿

A **L2640** Addition to lower extremity, pelvic control, band and belt, bilateral ♿

A ☑ **L2650** Addition to lower extremity, pelvic and thoracic control, gluteal pad, each ♿

A **L2660** Addition to lower extremity, thoracic control, thoracic band ♿

A **L2670** Addition to lower extremity, thoracic control, paraspinal uprights ♿

A **L2680** Addition to lower extremity, thoracic control, lateral support uprights ♿

ADDITIONS: GENERAL

A ☑ **L2750** Addition to lower extremity orthosis, plating chrome or nickel, per bar ♿

▲ A **L2755** Addition to lower extremity orthosis, high strength, lightweight material, all hybrid lamination/prepreg composite, per segment, for custom fabricated orthosis only ♿

A ☑ **L2760** Addition to lower extremity orthosis, extension, per extension, per bar (for lineal adjustment for growth) ♿

A ☑ **L2768** Orthotic side bar disconnect device, per bar ♿

A ☑ **L2770** Addition to lower extremity orthosis, any material, per bar or joint ♿

A ☑ **L2780** Addition to lower extremity orthosis, noncorrosive finish, per bar ♿

A ☑ **L2785** Addition to lower extremity orthosis, drop lock retainer, each ♿

A **L2795** Addition to lower extremity orthosis, knee control, full kneecap ♿

▲ A **L2800** Addition to lower extremity orthosis, knee control, knee cap, medial or lateral pull, for use with custom fabricated orthosis only ♿

A **L2810** Addition to lower extremity orthosis, knee control, condylar pad ♿

A **L2820** Addition to lower extremity orthosis, soft interface for molded plastic, below knee section ♿

A **L2830** Addition to lower extremity orthosis, soft interface for molded plastic, above knee section ♿

A ☑ **L2840** Addition to lower extremity orthosis, tibial length sock, fracture or equal, each ♿

A ☑ **L2850** Addition to lower extremity orthosis, femoral length sock, fracture or equal, each ♿

A ☑ **L2860** Addition to lower extremity joint, knee or ankle, concentric adjustable torsion style mechanism, each ♿

A **L2999** Lower extremity orthoses, NOS
Determine if an alternative HCPCS Level II or a CPT code better describes the service being reported. This code should be used only if a more specific code is unavailable.

Special Coverage Instructions   Noncovered by Medicare   Carrier Discretion   ☑ Quantity Alert   ● New Code   ○ Reinstated Code   ▲ Revised Code

2005 HCPCS   ♀ Female Only   ♂ Male Only   ▣-▣ ASC Groups   MED: Pub 100/NCD Reference   ♿ DMEPOS Paid   Ⓢ SNF Excluded   **L Codes — 95**

Orthotic Procedures

L3000 — L3222

ORTHOPEDIC SHOES

INSERTS

B ☑ **L3000** Foot insert, removable, molded to patient model, UCB type, Berkeley shell, each ⊘
MED: 100-2, 15, 290

B ☑ **L3001** Foot insert, removable, molded to patient model, Spenco, each ⊘
MED: 100-2, 15, 290

B ☑ **L3002** Foot insert, removable, molded to patient model, Plastazote or equal, each ⊘
MED: 100-2, 15, 290

B ☑ **L3003** Foot insert, removable, molded to patient model, silicone gel, each ⊘
MED: 100-2, 15, 290

B ☑ **L3010** Foot insert, removable, molded to patient model, longitudinal arch support, each ⊘
MED: 100-2, 15, 290

B ☑ **L3020** Foot insert, removable, molded to patient model, longitudinal/metatarsal support, each ⊘
MED: 100-2, 15, 290

B ☑ **L3030** Foot insert, removable, formed to patient foot, each ⊘
MED: 100-2, 15, 290

E ☑ **L3031** Foot, insert/plate, removable, addition to lower extremity orthosis, high strength, lightweight material, all hybrid lamination/prepreg composite, each ⊘

ARCH SUPPORT, REMOVABLE, PREMOLDED

B ☑ **L3040** Foot, arch support, removable, premolded, longitudinal, each ⊘
MED: 100-2, 15, 290

B ☑ **L3050** Foot, arch support, removable, premolded, metatarsal, each ⊘
MED: 100-2, 15, 290

B ☑ **L3060** Foot, arch support, removable, premolded, longitudinal/metatarsal, each ⊘
MED: 100-2, 15, 290

ARCH SUPPORT, NONREMOVABLE, ATTACHED TO SHOE

B ☑ **L3070** Foot, arch support, nonremovable, attached to shoe, longitudinal, each ⊘
MED: 100-2, 15, 290

B ☑ **L3080** Foot, arch support, nonremovable, attached to shoe, metatarsal, each ⊘
MED: 100-2, 15, 290

B ☑ **L3090** Foot, arch support, nonremovable, attached to shoe, longitudinal/metatarsal, each ⊘
MED: 100-2, 15, 290

B **L3100** Hallus-valgus night dynamic splint ⊘
MED: 100-2, 15, 290

ABDUCTION AND ROTATION BARS

B **L3140** Foot, abduction rotation bar, including shoes ⊘
MED: 100-2, 15, 290

B **L3150** Foot, abduction rotation bar, without shoes ⊘
MED: 100-2, 15, 290

B **L3160** Foot, adjustable shoe-styled positioning device ⊘

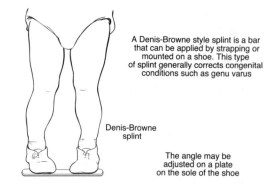

A Denis-Browne style splint is a bar that can be applied by strapping or mounted on a shoe. This type of splint generally corrects congenital conditions such as genu varus

Denis-Browne splint

The angle may be adjusted on a plate on the sole of the shoe

B **L3170** Foot, plastic heel stabilizer ⊘
MED: 100-2, 15, 290

ORTHOPEDIC FOOTWEAR

B **L3201** Orthopedic shoe, Oxford with supinator or pronator, infant ⬛⊘
MED: 100-2, 15, 290

B **L3202** Orthopedic shoe, Oxford with supinator or pronator, child ⬛⊘
MED: 100-2, 15, 290

B **L3203** Orthopedic shoe, Oxford with supinator or pronator, junior ⬛⊘
MED: 100-2, 15, 290

B **L3204** Orthopedic shoe, hightop with supinator or pronator, infant ⬛⊘
MED: 100-2, 15, 290

B **L3206** Orthopedic shoe, hightop with supinator or pronator, child ⬛⊘
MED: 100-2, 15, 290

B **L3207** Orthopedic shoe, hightop with supinator or pronator, junior ⬛⊘
MED: 100-2, 15, 290

B ☑ **L3208** Surgical boot, each, infant ⬛⊘
MED: 100-2, 15, 100

B ☑ **L3209** Surgical boot, each, child ⬛⊘
MED: 100-2, 15, 100

B ☑ **L3211** Surgical boot, each, junior ⬛⊘
MED: 100-2, 15, 100

B ☑ **L3212** Benesch boot, pair, infant ⬛⊘
MED: 100-2, 15, 100

B ☑ **L3213** Benesch boot, pair, child ⬛⊘
MED: 100-2, 15, 100

B ☑ **L3214** Benesch boot, pair, junior ⬛⊘
MED: 100-2, 15, 100

B **L3215** Orthopedic footwear, woman's shoes, Oxford ♀⊘

B **L3216** Orthopedic footwear, woman's shoes, depth inlay ♀⊘

B **L3217** Orthopedic footwear, woman's shoes, hightop, depth inlay ♀⊘

B **L3219** Orthopedic footwear, man's shoes, Oxford ♂⊘

B **L3221** Orthopedic footwear, man's shoes, depth inlay ♂⊘

B **L3222** Orthopedic footwear, man's shoes, hightop, depth inlay ♂⊘

Special Coverage Instructions   Noncovered by Medicare   Carrier Discretion   ☑ Quantity Alert   ● New Code   ○ Reinstated Code   ▲ Revised Code

96 — L Codes   **A** Adult   **M** Maternity   **P** Pediatrics   **I** Infant   **A**-**Y** APC Status Indicator   *2005 HCPCS*

| A | | L3224 | Orthopedic footwear, woman's shoe, Oxford, used as an integral part of a brace (orthosis) ♀ ⅄
MED: 100-2, 15, 290 | |

| A | | L3225 | Orthopedic footwear, man's shoe, Oxford, used as an integral part of a brace (orthosis) ♂ ⅄
MED: 100-2, 15, 290 | |

| B | | L3230 | Orthopedic footwear, custom shoes, depth inlay ⊘
MED: 100-2, 15, 290 | |

| B | ☑ | L3250 | Orthopedic footwear, custom molded shoe, removable inner mold, prosthetic shoe, each
MED: 100-2, 15, 290 | ⊘ |

| B | ☑ | L3251 | Foot, shoe molded to patient model, silicone shoe, each
MED: 100-2, 15, 290 | ⊘ |

| B | ☑ | L3252 | Foot, shoe molded to patient model, Plastazote (or similar), custom fabricated, each
MED: 100-2, 15, 290 | ⊘ |

| B | ☑ | L3253 | Foot, molded shoe Plastazote (or similar), custom fitted, each
MED: 100-2, 15, 290 | ⊘ |

| B | | L3254 | Nonstandard size or width
MED: 100-2, 15, 290 | ⊘ |

| B | | L3255 | Nonstandard size or length
MED: 100-2, 15, 290 | ⊘ |

| B | | L3257 | Orthopedic footwear, additional charge for split size
MED: 100-2, 15, 290 | ⊘ |

| B | ☑ | L3260 | Surgical boot/shoe, each
MED: 100-2, 15, 100 | ⊘ |

| B | ☑ | L3265 | Plastazote sandal, each | ⊘ |

SHOE MODIFICATION — LIFTS

| B | ☑ | L3300 | Lift, elevation, heel, tapered to metatarsals, per inch
MED: 100-2, 15, 290 | ⊘ |

| B | ☑ | L3310 | Lift, elevation, heel and sole, neoprene, per inch
MED: 100-2, 15, 290 | ⊘ |

| B | ☑ | L3320 | Lift, elevation, heel and sole, cork, per inch
MED: 100-2, 15, 290 | ⊘ |

| B | | L3330 | Lift, elevation, metal extension (skate)
MED: 100-2, 15, 290 | ⊘ |

| B | ☑ | L3332 | Lift, elevation, inside shoe, tapered, up to one-half inch
MED: 100-2, 15, 290 | ⊘ |

| B | ☑ | L3334 | Lift, elevation, heel, per inch
MED: 100-2, 15, 290 | ⊘ |

SHOE MODIFICATION — WEDGES

| B | | L3340 | Heel wedge, SACH
MED: 100-2, 15, 290 | ⊘ |

| B | | L3350 | Heel wedge
MED: 100-2, 15, 290 | ⊘ |

| B | | L3360 | Sole wedge, outside sole
MED: 100-2, 15, 290 | ⊘ |

| B | | L3370 | Sole wedge, between sole
MED: 100-2, 15, 290 | ⊘ |

| B | | L3380 | Clubfoot wedge
MED: 100-2, 15, 290 | ⊘ |

| B | | L3390 | Outflare wedge
MED: 100-2, 15, 290 | ⊘ |

| B | | L3400 | Metatarsal bar wedge, rocker
MED: 100-2, 15, 290 | ⊘ |

| B | | L3410 | Metatarsal bar wedge, between sole
MED: 100-2, 15, 290 | ⊘ |

| B | | L3420 | Full sole and heel wedge, between sole
MED: 100-2, 15, 290 | ⊘ |

SHOE MODIFICATIONS — HEELS

| B | | L3430 | Heel, counter, plastic reinforced
MED: 100-2, 15, 290 | ⊘ |

| B | | L3440 | Heel, counter, leather reinforced
MED: 100-2, 15, 290 | ⊘ |

| B | | L3450 | Heel, SACH cushion type
MED: 100-2, 15, 290 | ⊘ |

| B | | L3455 | Heel, new leather, standard
MED: 100-2, 15, 290 | ⊘ |

| B | | L3460 | Heel, new rubber, standard
MED: 100-2, 15, 290 | ⊘ |

| B | | L3465 | Heel, Thomas with wedge
MED: 100-2, 15, 290 | ⊘ |

| B | | L3470 | Heel, Thomas extended to ball
MED: 100-2, 15, 290 | ⊘ |

| B | | L3480 | Heel, pad and depression for spur
MED: 100-2, 15, 290 | ⊘ |

| B | | L3485 | Heel, pad, removable for spur
MED: 100-2, 15, 290 | ⊘ |

MISCELLANEOUS SHOE ADDITIONS

| B | | L3500 | Orthopedic shoe addition, insole, leather
MED: 100-2, 15, 290 | ⊘ |

| B | | L3510 | Orthopedic shoe addition, insole, rubber
MED: 100-2, 15, 290 | ⊘ |

| B | | L3520 | Orthopedic shoe addition, insole, felt covered with leather
MED: 100-2, 15, 290 | ⊘ |

| B | | L3530 | Orthopedic shoe addition, sole, half
MED: 100-2, 15, 290 | ⊘ |

| B | | L3540 | Orthopedic shoe addition, sole, full
MED: 100-2, 15, 290 | ⊘ |

| B | | L3550 | Orthopedic shoe addition, toe tap, standard
MED: 100-2, 15, 290 | ⊘ |

| B | | L3560 | Orthopedic shoe addition, toe tap, horseshoe
MED: 100-2, 15, 290 | ⊘ |

| B | | L3570 | Orthopedic shoe addition, special extension to instep (leather with eyelets)
MED: 100-2, 15, 290 | ⊘ |

| B | | L3580 | Orthopedic shoe addition, convert instep to Velcro closure
MED: 100-2, 15, 290 | ⊘ |

| B | | L3590 | Orthopedic shoe addition, convert firm shoe counter to soft counter
MED: 100-2, 15, 290 | ⊘ |

Special Coverage Instructions   Noncovered by Medicare   Carrier Discretion   ☑ Quantity Alert   ● New Code   ○ Reinstated Code   ▲ Revised Code

2005 HCPCS   ♀ Female Only   ♂ Male Only   **1**-**9** ASC Groups   MED: Pub 100/NCD Reference   ⅄ DMEPOS Paid   ⊘ SNF Excluded   **L Codes — 97**

Orthotic Procedures

L3595 — L3904

B   **L3595**   Orthopedic shoe addition, March bar
MED: 100-2, 15, 290

TRANSFER OR REPLACEMENT

B   **L3600**   Transfer of an orthosis from one shoe to another, caliper plate, existing
MED: 100-2, 15, 290

B   **L3610**   Transfer of an orthosis from one shoe to another, caliper plate, new
MED: 100-2, 15, 290

B   **L3620**   Transfer of an orthosis from one shoe to another, solid stirrup, existing
MED: 100-2, 15, 290

B   **L3630**   Transfer of an orthosis from one shoe to another, solid stirrup, new
MED: 100-2, 15, 290

B   **L3640**   Transfer of an orthosis from one shoe to another, Dennis Browne splint (Riveton), both shoes
MED: 100-2, 15, 290

B   **L3649**   Orthopedic shoe, modification, addition or transfer, NOS
Determine if an alternative HCPCS Level II or a CPT code better describes the service being reported. This code should be used only if a more specific code is unavailable.
MED: 100-2, 15, 290

ORTHOTIC DEVICES — UPPER LIMB

The procedures in this section are considered as "base" or "basic procedures" and may be modified by listing procedures from the "additions" sections and adding them to the base procedure.

SHOULDER ORTHOSIS (SO)

A   **L3650**   SO, figure of eight design abduction restrainer, prefabricated, includes fitting and adjustment

A   **L3651**   SO, single shoulder, elastic, prefabricated, includes fitting and adjustment (e.g., neoprene, Lycra)

A   **L3652**   SO, double shoulder, elastic, prefabricated, includes fitting and adjustment (e.g., neoprene, Lycra)

A   **L3660**   SO, figure of eight design abduction restrainer, canvas and webbing, prefabricated, includes fitting and adjustment

A   **L3670**   SO, acromio/clavicular (canvas and webbing type), prefabricated, includes fitting and adjustment

A   **L3675**   SO, vest type abduction restrainer, canvas webbing type, or equal, prefabricated, includes fitting and adjustment

E   **L3677**   SO, hard plastic, shoulder stabilizer, prefabricated, includes fitting and adjustment
MED: 100-2, 15, 120

ELBOW ORTHOSIS (EO)

A   **L3700**   EO, elastic with stays, prefabricated, includes fitting and adjustment

A   **L3701**   EO, elastic, prefabricated, includes fitting and adjustment (e.g., neoprene, Lycra)

A   **L3710**   EO, elastic with metal joints, prefabricated, includes fitting and adjustment

A   **L3720**   EO, double upright with forearm/arm cuffs, free motion, custom fabricated

A   **L3730**   EO, double upright with forearm/arm cuffs, extension/flexion assist, custom fabricated

A   **L3740**   EO, double upright with forearm/arm cuffs, adjustable position lock with active control, custom fabricated

A   **L3760**   EO, with adjustable position locking joint(s), prefabricated, includes fitting and adjustments, any type

A   **L3762**   EO, rigid, without joints, includes soft interface material, prefabricated, includes fitting and adjustment

WRIST-HAND-FINGER ORTHOSIS (WHFO)

A   **L3800**   WHFO, short opponens, no attachments, custom fabricated

A   **L3805**   WHFO, long opponens, no attachment, custom fabricated

A   **L3807**   WHFO, without joint(s), prefabricated, includes fitting and adjustments, any type

ADDITIONS

A   **L3810**   WHFO, addition to short and long opponens, thumb abduction (C) bar

A   **L3815**   WHFO, addition to short and long opponens, second M.P. abduction assist

A   **L3820**   WHFO, addition to short and long opponens, I.P. extension assist, with M.P. extension stop

A   **L3825**   WHFO, addition to short and long opponens, M.P. extension stop

A   **L3830**   WHFO, addition to short and long opponens, M.P. extension assist

A   **L3835**   WHFO, addition to short and long opponens, M.P. spring extension assist

A   **L3840**   WHFO, addition to short and long opponens, spring swivel thumb

A   **L3845**   WHFO, addition to short and long opponens, thumb I.P. extension assist, with M.P. stop

A   **L3850**   WHFO, addition to short and long opponens, action wrist, with dorsiflexion assist

A   **L3855**   WHFO, addition to short and long opponens, adjustable M.P. flexion control

A   **L3860**   WHFO, addition to short and long opponens, adjustable M.P. flexion control and I.P.

B   **L3890**   Addition to upper extremity joint, wrist or elbow, concentric adjustable torsion style mechanism, each

DYNAMIC FLEXOR HINGE, RECIPROCAL WRIST EXTENSION/FLEXION, FINGER FLEXION/EXTENSION

A   **L3900**   WHFO, dynamic flexor hinge, reciprocal wrist extension/flexion, finger flexion/extension, wrist or finger driven, custom fabricated

A   **L3901**   WHFO, dynamic flexor hinge, reciprocal wrist extension/flexion, finger flexion/extension, cable driven, custom fabricated

EXTERNAL POWER

E   **L3902**   WHFO, external powered, compressed gas, custom fabricated

A   **L3904**   WHFO, external powered, electric, custom fabricated

| Special Coverage Instructions | | Noncovered by Medicare | | Carrier Discretion | | ☑ Quantity Alert | ● New Code | ○ Reinstated Code | ▲ Revised Code |

98 — L Codes   A Adult   M Maternity   P Pediatrics   I Infant   A-Y APC Status Indicator   **2005 HCPCS**

OTHER WHFOS — CUSTOM FITTED

A **L3906** WHO, wrist gauntlet, molded to patient model, custom fabricated

A **L3907** WHFO, wrist gauntlet with thumb spica, molded to patient model, custom fabricated

A **L3908** WHO, wrist extension control cock-up, nonmolded, prefabricated, includes fitting and adjustment

A **L3909** WO, elastic, prefabricated, includes fitting and adjustment (e.g., neoprene, Lycra)

A **L3910** WHFO, Swanson design, prefabricated, includes fitting and adjustment

A **L3911** WHFO, elastic, prefabricated, includes fitting and adjustment (e.g., neoprene, Lycra)

A **L3912** HFO, flexion glove with elastic finger control, prefabricated, includes fitting and adjustment

A **L3914** WHO, wrist extension cock-up, prefabricated, includes fitting and adjustment

A **L3916** WHFO, wrist extension cock-up, with outrigger, prefabricated, includes fitting and adjustment

A **L3917** HO, metacarpal fracture orthosis, prefabricated, includes fitting and adjustment

A **L3918** HFO, knuckle bender, prefabricated, includes fitting and adjustment

A **L3920** HFO, knuckle bender, with outrigger, prefabricated, includes fitting and adjustment

A **L3922** HFO, knuckle bender, two segment to flex joints, prefabricated, includes fitting and adjustment

A **L3923** HFO, without joint(s), prefabricated, includes fitting and adjustments, any type

A **L3924** WHFO, Oppenheimer, prefabricated, includes fitting and adjustment

A **L3926** WHFO, Thomas suspension, prefabricated, includes fitting and adjustment

A **L3928** HFO, finger extension, with clock spring, prefabricated, includes fitting and adjustment

A **L3930** WHFO, finger extension, with wrist support, prefabricated, includes fitting and adjustment

A **L3932** FO, safety pin, spring wire, prefabricated, includes fitting and adjustment

A **L3934** FO, safety pin, modified, prefabricated, includes fitting and adjustment

A **L3936** WHFO, Palmer, prefabricated, includes fitting and adjustment

A **L3938** WHFO, dorsal wrist, prefabricated, includes fitting and adjustment

A **L3940** WHFO, dorsal wrist, with outrigger attachment, prefabricated, includes fitting and adjustment

A **L3942** HFO, reverse knuckle bender, prefabricated, includes fitting and adjustment

A **L3944** HFO, reverse knuckle bender, with outrigger, prefabricated, includes fitting and adjustment

A **L3946** HFO, composite elastic, prefabricated, includes fitting and adjustment

A **L3948** FO, finger knuckle bender, prefabricated, includes fitting and adjustment

A **L3950** WHFO, combination Oppenheimer, with knuckle bender and two attachments, prefabricated, includes fitting and adjustment

A **L3952** WHFO, combination Oppenheimer, with reverse knuckle and two attachments, prefabricated, includes fitting and adjustment

A **L3954** HFO, spreading hand, prefabricated, includes fitting and adjustment

A ☑ **L3956** Addition of joint to upper extremity orthosis, any material; per joint

SHOULDER-ELBOW-WRIST-HAND ORTHOSIS (SEWHO)

ABDUCTION POSITION, CUSTOM FITTED

A **L3960** SEWHO, abduction positioning, airplane design, prefabricated, includes fitting and adjustment

A **L3962** SEWHO, abduction positioning, Erb's palsy design, prefabricated, includes fitting and adjustment

A **L3963** SEWHO, molded shoulder, arm, forearm, and wrist, with articulating elbow joint, custom fabricated

Y **L3964** SEO, mobile arm support attached to wheelchair, balanced, adjustable, prefabricated, includes fitting and adjustment

Y **L3965** SEO, mobile arm support attached to wheelchair, balanced, adjustable Rancho type, prefabricated, includes fitting and adjustment

Y **L3966** SEO, mobile arm support attached to wheelchair, balanced, reclining, prefabricated, includes fitting and adjustment

Y **L3968** SEO, mobile arm support attached to wheelchair, balanced, friction arm support (friction dampening to proximal and distal joints), prefabricated, includes fitting and adjustment

Y **L3969** SEO, mobile arm support, monosuspension arm and hand support, overhead elbow forearm hand sling support, yoke type arm suspension support, prefabricated, includes fitting and adjustment

ADDITIONS TO MOBILE ARM SUPPORTS

Y **L3970** SEO, addition to mobile arm support, elevating proximal arm

Y **L3972** SEO, addition to mobile arm support, offset or lateral rocker arm with elastic balance control

Y **L3974** SEO, addition to mobile arm support, supinator

FRACTURE ORTHOSIS

A **L3980** Upper extremity fracture orthosis, humeral, prefabricated, includes fitting and adjustment

A **L3982** Upper extremity fracture orthosis, radius/ulnar, prefabricated, includes fitting and adjustment

A **L3984** Upper extremity fracture orthosis, wrist, prefabricated, includes fitting and adjustment

A **L3985** Upper extremity fracture orthosis, forearm, hand with wrist hinge, custom fabricated

A **L3986** Upper extremity fracture orthosis, combination of humeral, radius/ulnar, wrist (example: Colles' fracture), custom fabricated

A **L3995** Addition to upper extremity orthosis, sock, fracture or equal, each

A **L3999** Upper limb orthosis, NOS

SPECIFIC REPAIR

A **L4000** Replace girdle for spinal orthosis (CTLSO or SO)

● **L4002** Replacement strap, any orthosis, includes all components, any length, any type

A **L4010** Replace trilateral socket brim

Special Coverage Instructions	Noncovered by Medicare	Carrier Discretion	☑ Quantity Alert	● New Code	○ Reinstated Code	▲ Revised Code

2005 HCPCS ♀ Female Only ♂ Male Only **1-9** ASC Groups **MED:** Pub 100/NCD Reference DMEPOS Paid SNF Excluded **L Codes — 99**

Prosthetic Procedures

L4020 — L5301

[A] **L4020** Replace quadrilateral socket brim, molded to patient model 🔲

[A] **L4030** Replace quadrilateral socket brim, custom fitted 🔲

▲ [A] **L4040** Replace molded thigh lacer, for custom fabricated orthosis only 🔲

▲ [A] **L4045** Replace non-molded thigh lacer, for custom fabricated orthosis only 🔲

▲ [A] **L4050** Replace molded calf lacer, for custom fabricated orthosis only 🔲

▲ [A] **L4055** Replace non-molded calf lacer, for custom fabricated orthosis only 🔲

[A] **L4060** Replace high roll cuff 🔲

[A] **L4070** Replace proximal and distal upright for KAFO 🔲

[A] **L4080** Replace metal bands KAFO, proximal thigh 🔲

[A] **L4090** Replace metal bands KAFO-AFO, calf or distal thigh 🔲

[A] **L4100** Replace leather cuff KAFO, proximal thigh 🔲

[A] **L4110** Replace leather cuff KAFO-AFO, calf or distal thigh 🔲

[A] **L4130** Replace pretibial shell 🔲

REPAIRS

[A] ☑ **L4205** Repair of orthotic device, labor component, per 15 minutes
MED: 100-2, 15, 110.2

[A] **L4210** Repair of orthotic device, repair or replace minor parts
MED: 100-2, 15, 110.2; 100-2, 15, 120; 100-2, 15, 120

[A] **L4350** Ankle control orthosis, stirrup style, rigid, includes any type interface (e.g., pneumatic, gel), prefabricated, includes fitting and adjustment 🔲

[A] **L4360** Walking boot, pneumatic, with or without joints, with or without interface material, prefabricated, includes fitting and adjustment 🔲

[A] **L4370** Pneumatic full leg splint, prefabricated, includes fitting and adjustment 🔲

[A] **L4380** Pneumatic knee splint, prefabricated, includes fitting and adjustment 🔲

[A] **L4386** Walking boot, non-pneumatic, with or without joints, with or without interface material, prefabricated, includes fitting and adjustment 🔲

[A] **L4392** Replacement soft interface material, static AFO 🔲

[A] **L4394** Replace soft interface material, foot drop splint 🔲

[A] **L4396** Static ankle foot orthosis, including soft interface material, adjustable for fit, for positioning, pressure reduction, may be used for minimal ambulation, prefabricated, includes fitting and adjustment 🔲

[A] **L4398** Foot drop splint, recumbent positioning device, prefabricated, includes fitting and adjustment 🔲

PROSTHETIC PROCEDURES *L5000–L9999*

LOWER LIMB

The procedures in this section are considered as "base" or "basic procedures" and may be modified by listing items/procedures or special materials from the "additions" sections and adding them to the base procedure.

PARTIAL FOOT

[A] **L5000** Partial foot, shoe insert with longitudinal arch, toe filler 🔲
MED: 100-2, 15, 290

[A] **L5010** Partial foot, molded socket, ankle height, with toe filler 🔲
MED: 100-2, 15, 290

[A] **L5020** Partial foot, molded socket, tibial tubercle height, with toe filler 🔲
MED: 100-2, 15, 290

ANKLE

[A] **L5050** Ankle, Symes, molded socket, SACH foot 🔲

[A] **L5060** Ankle, Symes, metal frame, molded leather socket, articulated ankle/foot 🔲

BELOW KNEE

[A] **L5100** Below knee, molded socket, shin, SACH foot 🔲

[A] **L5105** Below knee, plastic socket, joints and thigh lacer, SACH foot 🔲

KNEE DISARTICULATION

[A] **L5150** Knee disarticulation (or through knee), molded socket, external knee joints, shin, SACH foot 🔲

[A] **L5160** Knee disarticulation (or through knee), molded socket, bent knee configuration, external knee joints, shin, SACH foot 🔲

ABOVE KNEE

[A] **L5200** Above knee, molded socket, single axis constant friction knee, shin, SACH foot 🔲

[A] ☑ **L5210** Above knee, short prosthesis, no knee joint (stubbies), with foot blocks, no ankle joints, each 🔲

[A] ☑ **L5220** Above knee, short prosthesis, no knee joint (stubbies), with articulated ankle/foot, dynamically aligned, each 🔲

[A] **L5230** Above knee, for proximal femoral focal deficiency, constant friction knee, shin, SACH foot 🔲

HIP DISARTICULATION

[A] **L5250** Hip disarticulation, Canadian type; molded socket, hip joint, single axis constant friction knee, shin, SACH foot 🔲

[A] **L5270** Hip disarticulation, tilt table type; molded socket, locking hip joint, single axis constant friction knee, shin, SACH foot 🔲

HEMIPELVECTOMY

[A] **L5280** Hemipelvectomy, Canadian type; molded socket, hip joint, single axis constant friction knee, shin, SACH foot 🔲

[A] **L5301** Below knee, molded socket, shin, SACH foot, endoskeletal system 🔲

Special Coverage Instructions | Noncovered by Medicare | Carrier Discretion | ☑ Quantity Alert | ● New Code | ○ Reinstated Code | ▲ Revised Code

100 — L Codes | [A] Adult | [M] Maternity | [P] Pediatrics | [I] Infant | [A]-[Y] APC Status Indicator | *2005 HCPCS*

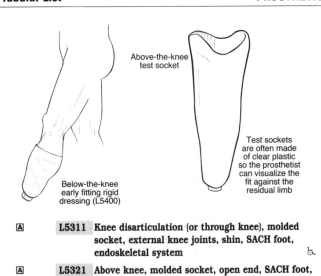

Above-the-knee test socket

Test sockets are often made of clear plastic so the prosthetist can visualize the fit against the residual limb

Below-the-knee early fitting rigid dressing (L5400)

[A] **L5311** Knee disarticulation (or through knee), molded socket, external knee joints, shin, SACH foot, endoskeletal system ⴠ

[A] **L5321** Above knee, molded socket, open end, SACH foot, endoskeletal system, single axis knee ⴠ

[A] **L5331** Hip disarticulation, Canadian type, molded socket, endoskeletal system, hip joint, single axis knee, SACH foot ⴠ

[A] **L5341** Hemipelvectomy, Canadian type, molded socket, endoskeletal system, hip joint, single axis knee, SACH foot ⴠ

IMMEDIATE POSTSURGICAL OR EARLY FITTING PROCEDURES

[A] ☑ **L5400** Immediate postsurgical or early fitting, application of initial rigid dressing, including fitting, alignment, suspension, and one cast change, below knee ⴠ⊘

[A] ☑ **L5410** Immediate postsurgical or early fitting, application of initial rigid dressing, including fitting, alignment and suspension, below knee, each additional cast change and realignment ⴠ⊘

[A] ☑ **L5420** Immediate postsurgical or early fitting, application of initial rigid dressing, including fitting, alignment and suspension and one cast change AK or knee disarticulation ⴠ⊘

[A] ☑ **L5430** Immediate postsurgical or early fitting, application of initial rigid dressing, including fitting, alignment and suspension, AK or knee disarticulation, each additional cast change and realignment ⴠ⊘

[A] **L5450** Immediate postsurgical or early fitting, application of nonweight bearing rigid dressing, below knee ⴠ⊘

[A] **L5460** Immediate postsurgical or early fitting, application of nonweight bearing rigid dressing, above knee ⴠ⊘

INITIAL PROSTHESIS

[A] **L5500** Initial, below knee PTB type socket, non-alignable system, pylon, no cover, SACH foot, plaster socket, direct formed ⴠ

[A] **L5505** Initial, above knee — knee disarticulation, ischial level socket, non-alignable system, pylon, no cover, SACH foot plaster socket, direct formed ⴠ

PREPARATORY PROSTHESIS

[A] **L5510** Preparatory, below knee PTB type socket, non-alignable system, pylon, no cover, SACH foot, plaster socket, molded to model ⴠ

[A] **L5520** Preparatory, below knee PTB type socket, non-alignable system, pylon, no cover, SACH foot, thermoplastic or equal, direct formed ⴠ

[A] **L5530** Preparatory, below knee PTB type socket, non-alignable system, pylon, no cover, SACH foot, thermoplastic or equal, molded to model ⴠ

[A] **L5535** Preparatory, below knee PTB type socket, non-alignable system, pylon, no cover, SACH foot, prefabricated, adjustable open end socket ⴠ

[A] **L5540** Preparatory, below knee PTB type socket, non-alignable system, pylon, no cover, SACH foot, laminated socket, molded to model ⴠ

[A] **L5560** Preparatory, above knee — knee disarticulation, ischial level socket, non-alignable system, pylon, no cover, SACH foot, plaster socket, molded to model ⴠ

[A] **L5570** Preparatory, above knee — knee disarticulation, ischial level socket, non-alignable system, pylon, no cover, SACH foot, thermoplastic or equal, direct formed ⴠ

[A] **L5580** Preparatory, above knee — knee disarticulation, ischial level socket, non-alignable system, pylon, no cover, SACH foot, thermoplastic or equal, molded to model ⴠ

[A] **L5585** Preparatory, above knee — knee disarticulation, ischial level socket, non-alignable system, pylon, no cover, SACH foot, prefabricated adjustable open end socket ⴠ

[A] **L5590** Preparatory, above knee — knee disarticulation, ischial level socket, non-alignable system, pylon, no cover, SACH foot, laminated socket, molded to model ⴠ

[A] **L5595** Preparatory, hip disarticulation — hemipelvectomy, pylon, no cover, SACH foot, thermoplastic or equal, molded to patient model ⴠ

[A] **L5600** Preparatory, hip disarticulation — hemipelvectomy, pylon, no cover, SACH foot, laminated socket, molded to patient model ⴠ

ADDITIONS: LOWER EXTREMITY

[A] **L5610** Addition to lower extremity, endoskeletal system, above knee, hydracadence system ⴠ

[A] **L5611** Addition to lower extremity, endoskeletal system, above knee — knee disarticulation, 4-bar linkage, with friction swing phase control ⴠ

[A] **L5613** Addition to lower extremity, endoskeletal system, above knee — knee disarticulation, 4-bar linkage, with hydraulic swing phase control ⴠ

[A] **L5614** Addition to lower extremity, endoskeletal system, above knee — knee disarticulation, 4-bar linkage, with pneumatic swing phase control ⴠ

[A] **L5616** Addition to lower extremity, endoskeletal system, above knee, universal multiplex system, friction swing phase control ⴠ

[A] ☑ **L5617** Addition to lower extremity, quick change self-aligning unit, above or below knee, each ⴠ

ADDITIONS: TEST SOCKETS

[A] **L5618** Addition to lower extremity, test socket, Symes ⴠ

[A] **L5620** Addition to lower extremity, test socket, below knee ⴠ

[A] **L5622** Addition to lower extremity, test socket, knee disarticulation ⴠ

| Special Coverage Instructions | Noncovered by Medicare | Carrier Discretion | ☑ Quantity Alert | ● New Code | ○ Reinstated Code | ▲ Revised Code |

2005 HCPCS   ♀ Female Only   ♂ Male Only   **1**-**9** ASC Groups   MED: Pub 100/NCD Reference   ⴠ DMEPOS Paid   ⊘ SNF Excluded   **L Codes — 101**

Prosthetic Procedures

L5624 — L5680

Ⓐ **L5624** Addition to lower extremity, test socket, above knee ♿

Ⓐ **L5626** Addition to lower extremity, test socket, hip disarticulation ♿

Ⓐ **L5628** Addition to lower extremity, test socket, hemipelvectomy ♿

Ⓐ **L5629** Addition to lower extremity, below knee, acrylic socket ♿

ADDITIONS: SOCKET VARIATIONS

Ⓐ **L5630** Addition to lower extremity, Symes type, expandable wall socket ♿

Ⓐ **L5631** Addition to lower extremity, above knee or knee disarticulation, acrylic socket ♿

Ⓐ **L5632** Addition to lower extremity, Symes type, PTB brim design socket ♿

Ⓐ **L5634** Addition to lower extremity, Symes type, posterior opening (Canadian) socket ♿

Ⓐ **L5636** Addition to lower extremity, Symes type, medial opening socket ♿

Ⓐ **L5637** Addition to lower extremity, below knee, total contact ♿

Ⓐ **L5638** Addition to lower extremity, below knee, leather socket ♿

Ⓐ **L5639** Addition to lower extremity, below knee, wood socket ♿

Ⓐ **L5640** Addition to lower extremity, knee disarticulation, leather socket ♿

Ⓐ **L5642** Addition to lower extremity, above knee, leather socket ♿

Ⓐ **L5643** Addition to lower extremity, hip disarticulation, flexible inner socket, external frame ♿

Ⓐ **L5644** Addition to lower extremity, above knee, wood socket ♿

Ⓐ **L5645** Addition to lower extremity, below knee, flexible inner socket, external frame ♿

Ⓐ **L5646** Addition to lower extremity, below knee, air, fluid, gel or equal, cushion socket ♿

Ⓐ **L5647** Addition to lower extremity, below knee, suction socket ♿

Ⓐ **L5648** Addition to lower extremity, above knee, air, fluid, gel or equal, cushion socket ♿

Ⓐ **L5649** Addition to lower extremity, ischial containment/narrow M-L socket ♿

Ⓐ **L5650** Addition to lower extremity, total contact, above knee or knee disarticulation socket ♿

Ⓐ **L5651** Addition to lower extremity, above knee, flexible inner socket, external frame ♿

Ⓐ **L5652** Addition to lower extremity, suction suspension, above knee or knee disarticulation socket ♿

Ⓐ **L5653** Addition to lower extremity, knee disarticulation, expandable wall socket ♿

ADDITIONS: SOCKET INSERT AND SUSPENSION

Ⓐ **L5654** Addition to lower extremity, socket insert, Symes (Kemblo, Pelite, Aliplast, Plastazote or equal) ♿

Ⓐ **L5655** Addition to lower extremity, socket insert, below knee (Kemblo, Pelite, Aliplast, Plastazote or equal) ♿

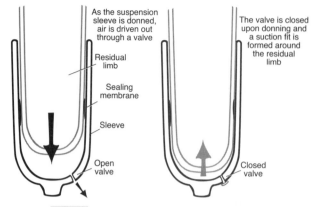

As the suspension sleeve is donned, air is driven out through a valve

Residual limb

Sealing membrane

Sleeve

Open valve

The valve is closed upon donning and a suction fit is formed around the residual limb

Closed valve

Ⓐ **L5656** Addition to lower extremity, socket insert, knee disarticulation (Kemblo, Pelite, Aliplast, Plastazote or equal) ♿

Ⓐ **L5658** Addition to lower extremity, socket insert, above knee (Kemblo, Pelite, Aliplast, Plastazote or equal) ♿

Ⓐ **L5661** Addition to lower extremity, socket insert, multidurometer, Symes ♿

Ⓐ **L5665** Addition to lower extremity, socket insert, multidurometer, below knee ♿

Ⓐ **L5666** Addition to lower extremity, below knee, cuff suspension ♿

Ⓐ **L5668** Addition to lower extremity, below knee, molded distal cushion ♿

Ⓐ **L5670** Addition to lower extremity, below knee, molded supracondylar suspension (PTS or similar) ♿

Ⓐ **L5671** Addition to lower extremity, below knee/above knee suspension locking mechanism (shuttle, lanyard or equal), excludes socket insert ♿

Ⓐ **L5672** Addition to lower extremity, below knee, removable medial brim suspension ♿

Ⓐ **L5673** Addition to lower extremity, below knee/above knee, custom fabricated from existing mold or prefabricated, socket insert, silicone gel, elastomeric or equal, for use with locking mechanism ♿

~~**L5674** Addition to lower extremity, below knee, suspension sleeve, any material, each~~
See code(s): L5685

~~**L5675** Addition to lower extremity, below knee, suspension sleeve, heavy-duty, any material, each~~
See code(s): L5685

Ⓐ ☑ **L5676** Addition to lower extremity, below knee, knee joints, single axis, pair ♿

Ⓐ ☑ **L5677** Addition to lower extremity, below knee, knee joints, polycentric, pair ♿

Ⓐ ☑ **L5678** Addition to lower extremity, below knee joint covers, pair ♿

Ⓐ **L5679** Addition to lower extremity, below knee/above knee, custom fabricated from existing mold or prefabricated, socket insert, silicone gel, elastomeric or equal, not for use with locking mechanism ♿

Ⓐ **L5680** Addition to lower extremity, below knee, thigh lacer, nonmolded ♿

Special Coverage Instructions   Noncovered by Medicare   Carrier Discretion   ☑ Quantity Alert   ● New Code   ○ Reinstated Code   ▲ Revised Code

102 — L Codes   Ⓐ Adult   Ⓜ Maternity   Ⓟ Pediatrics   Ⓘ Infant   Ⓐ-Ⓨ APC Status Indicator   *2005 HCPCS*

A **L5681** Addition to lower extremity, below knee/above knee, custom fabricated socket insert for congenital or atypical traumatic amputee, silicone gel, elastomeric or equal, for use with or without locking mechanism, initial only (for other than initial, use code L5673 or L5679) 🦽

A **L5682** Addition to lower extremity, below knee, thigh lacer, gluteal/ischial, molded 🦽

A **L5683** Addition to lower extremity, below knee/above knee, custom fabricated socket insert for other than congenital or atypical traumatic amputee, silicone gel, elastomeric or equal, for use with or without locking mechanism, initial only (for other than initial, use code L5673 or L5679) 🦽

A **L5684** Addition to lower extremity, below knee, fork strap 🦽

● **L5685** Addition to lower extremity prosthesis, below knee, suspension/sealing sleeve, with or without valve, any material, each

A **L5686** Addition to lower extremity, below knee, back check (extension control) 🦽

A **L5688** Addition to lower extremity, below knee, waist belt, webbing 🦽

A **L5690** Addition to lower extremity, below knee, waist belt, padded and lined 🦽

E **L5692** Addition to lower extremity, above knee, pelvic control belt, light 🦽

A **L5694** Addition to lower extremity, above knee, pelvic control belt, padded and lined 🦽

A ☑ **L5695** Addition to lower extremity, above knee, pelvic control, sleeve suspension, neoprene or equal, each 🦽

A **L5696** Addition to lower extremity, above knee or knee disarticulation, pelvic joint 🦽

A **L5697** Addition to lower extremity, above knee or knee disarticulation, pelvic band 🦽

A **L5698** Addition to lower extremity, above knee or knee disarticulation, Silesian bandage 🦽

A **L5699** All lower extremity prostheses, shoulder harness 🦽

REPLACEMENTS

A **L5700** Replacement, socket, below knee, molded to patient model 🦽

A **L5701** Replacement, socket, above knee/knee disarticulation, including attachment plate, molded to patient model 🦽

A **L5702** Replacement, socket, hip disarticulation, including hip joint, molded to patient model 🦽

A **L5704** Custom shaped protective cover, below knee 🦽

A **L5705** Custom shaped protective cover, above knee 🦽

A **L5706** Custom shaped protective cover, knee disarticulation 🦽

A **L5707** Custom shaped protective cover, hip disarticulation 🦽

ADDITIONS: EXOSKELETAL KNEE-SHIN SYSTEM

A **L5710** Addition, exoskeletal knee-shin system, single axis, manual lock 🦽

A **L5711** Addition, exoskeletal knee-shin system, single axis, manual lock, ultra-light material 🦽

A **L5712** Addition, exoskeletal knee-shin system, single axis, friction swing and stance phase control (safety knee) 🦽

A **L5714** Addition, exoskeletal knee-shin system, single axis, variable friction swing phase control 🦽

A **L5716** Addition, exoskeletal knee-shin system, polycentric, mechanical stance phase lock 🦽

A **L5718** Addition, exoskeletal knee-shin system, polycentric, friction swing and stance phase control 🦽

A **L5722** Addition, exoskeletal knee-shin system, single axis, pneumatic swing, friction stance phase control 🦽

A **L5724** Addition, exoskeletal knee-shin system, single axis, fluid swing phase control 🦽

A **L5726** Addition, exoskeletal knee-shin system, single axis, external joints, fluid swing phase control 🦽

A **L5728** Addition, exoskeletal knee-shin system, single axis, fluid swing and stance phase control 🦽

A **L5780** Addition, exoskeletal knee-shin system, single axis, pneumatic/hydra pneumatic swing phase control 🦽

A **L5781** Addition to lower limb prosthesis, vacuum pump, residual limb volume management and moisture evacuation system 🦽

A **L5782** Addition to lower limb prosthesis, vacuum pump, residual limb volume management and moisture evacuation system, heavy duty 🦽

COMPONENT MODIFICATION

A **L5785** Addition, exoskeletal system, below knee, ultra-light material (titanium, carbon fiber or equal) 🦽

A **L5790** Addition, exoskeletal system, above knee, ultra-light material (titanium, carbon fiber or equal) 🦽

A **L5795** Addition, exoskeletal system, hip disarticulation, ultra-light material (titanium, carbon fiber or equal) 🦽

ADDITIONS: ENDOSKELETAL KNEE-SHIN SYSTEM

A **L5810** Addition, endoskeletal knee-shin system, single axis, manual lock 🦽

A **L5811** Addition, endoskeletal knee-shin system, single axis, manual lock, ultra-light material 🦽

A **L5812** Addition, endoskeletal knee-shin system, single axis, friction swing and stance phase control (safety knee) 🦽

A **L5814** Addition, endoskeletal knee-shin system, polycentric, hydraulic swing phase control, mechanical stance phase lock 🦽

A **L5816** Addition, endoskeletal knee-shin system, polycentric, mechanical stance phase lock 🦽

A **L5818** Addition, endoskeletal knee-shin system, polycentric, friction swing and stance phase control 🦽

A **L5822** Addition, endoskeletal knee-shin system, single axis, pneumatic swing, friction stance phase control 🦽

A **L5824** Addition, endoskeletal knee-shin system, single axis, fluid swing phase control 🦽

A **L5826** Addition, endoskeletal knee-shin system, single axis, hydraulic swing phase control, with miniature high activity frame 🦽

A **L5828** Addition, endoskeletal knee-shin system, single axis, fluid swing and stance phase control 🦽

▨ Special Coverage Instructions   ▨ Noncovered by Medicare   ▨ Carrier Discretion   ☑ Quantity Alert   ● New Code   ○ Reinstated Code   ▲ Revised Code

2005 HCPCS   ♀ Female Only   ♂ Male Only   **1-9** ASC Groups   **MED:** Pub 100/NCD Reference   🦽 DMEPOS Paid   ⊘ SNF Excluded   **L Codes — 103**

Ⓐ   **L5830**   Addition, endoskeletal knee-shin system, single axis, pneumatic/swing phase control   ੬

Ⓐ   **L5840**   Addition, endoskeletal knee-shin system, 4-bar linkage or multiaxial, pneumatic swing phase control   ੬

Ⓐ   **L5845**   Addition, endoskeletal knee-shin system, stance flexion feature, adjustable   ੬

~~**L5846**   Addition, endoskeletal knee-shin system, microprocessor control feature, swing phase only~~

~~**L5847**   Addition, endoskeletal knee-shin system, microprocessor control feature, stance phase~~

Ⓐ   **L5848**   Addition to endoskeletal, knee-shin system, hydraulic stance extension, dampening feature, with or without adjustability   ੬

Ⓐ   **L5850**   Addition, endoskeletal system, above knee or hip disarticulation, knee extension assist   ੬

Ⓐ   **L5855**   Addition, endoskeletal system, hip disarticulation, mechanical hip extension assist   ੬

●   **L5856**   Addition to lower extremity prosthesis, endoskeletal knee-shin system, microprocessor control feature, swing and stance phase, includes electronic sensor(s), any type

●   **L5857**   Addition to lower extremity prosthesis, endoskeletal knee-shin system, microprocessor control feature, swing phase only, includes electronic sensor(s), any type

Ⓐ   **L5910**   Addition, endoskeletal system, below knee, alignable system   ੬

Ⓐ   **L5920**   Addition, endoskeletal system, above knee or hip disarticulation, alignable system   ੬

Ⓐ   **L5925**   Addition, endoskeletal system, above knee, knee disarticulation or hip disarticulation, manual lock   ੬

Ⓐ   **L5930**   Addition, endoskeletal system, high activity knee control frame   ੬

Ⓐ   **L5940**   Addition, endoskeletal system, below knee, ultra-light material (titanium, carbon fiber or equal)   ੬

Ⓐ   **L5950**   Addition, endoskeletal system, above knee, ultra-light material (titanium, carbon fiber or equal)   ੬

Ⓐ   **L5960**   Addition, endoskeletal system, hip disarticulation, ultra-light material (titanium, carbon fiber or equal)   ੬

Ⓐ   **L5962**   Addition, endoskeletal system, below knee, flexible protective outer surface covering system   ੬

Ⓐ   **L5964**   Addition, endoskeletal system, above knee, flexible protective outer surface covering system   ੬

Ⓐ   **L5966**   Addition, endoskeletal system, hip disarticulation, flexible protective outer surface covering system   ੬

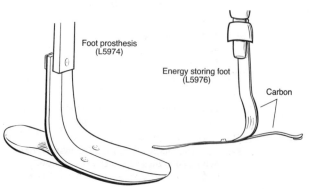

Foot prosthesis
(L5974)

Energy storing foot
(L5976)

Carbon

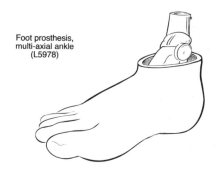

Foot prosthesis,
multi-axial ankle
(L5978)

Ⓐ   **L5968**   Addition to lower limb prosthesis, multiaxial ankle with swing phase active dorsiflexion feature   ੬

Ⓐ   **L5970**   All lower extremity prostheses, foot, external keel, SACH foot   ੬

Ⓐ   **L5972**   All lower extremity prostheses, flexible keel foot (safe, sten, bock dynamic or equal)   ੬

Ⓐ   **L5974**   All lower extremity prostheses, foot, single axis ankle/foot   ੬

Ⓐ   **L5975**   All lower extremity prosthesis, combination single axis ankle and flexible keel foot

Ⓐ   **L5976**   All lower extremity prostheses, energy storing foot (Seattle carbon copy II or equal)   ੬

Ⓐ   **L5978**   All lower extremity prostheses, foot, multi-axial ankle/foot   ੬

Ⓐ   **L5979**   All lower extremity prostheses, multi-axial ankle, dynamic response foot, one piece system   ੬

Ⓐ   **L5980**   All lower extremity prostheses, flex-foot system   ੬

Ⓐ   **L5981**   All lower extremity prostheses, flex-walk system or equal   ੬

Ⓐ   **L5982**   All exoskeletal lower extremity prostheses, axial rotation unit   ੬

Ⓐ   **L5984**   All endoskeletal lower extremity prosthesis, axial rotation unit, with or without adjustability   ੬

Ⓐ   **L5985**   All endoskeletal lower extremity prostheses, dynamic prosthetic pylon   ੬

Ⓐ   **L5986**   All lower extremity prostheses, multi-axial rotation unit (MCP or equal)   ੬

Ⓐ   **L5987**   All lower extremity prosthesis, shank foot system with vertical loading pylon   ੬

Ⓐ   **L5988**   Addition to lower limb prosthesis, vertical shock reducing pylon feature   ੬

~~**L5989**   Addition to lower extremity prosthesis, endoskeletal system, pylon with integrated electronic force sensors~~

Ⓐ   **L5990**   Addition to lower extremity prosthesis, user adjustable heel height   ੬

Ⓐ   **L5995**   Addition to lower extremity prosthesis, heavy duty feature (for patient weight > 300 lbs.)   ੬

Ⓐ   **L5999**   Lower extremity prosthesis, not otherwise specified
Determine if an alternative HCPCS Level II or a CPT code better describes the service being reported. This code should be used only if a more specific code is unavailable.

Special Coverage Instructions   Noncovered by Medicare   Carrier Discretion   ☑ Quantity Alert   ● New Code   ○ Reinstated Code   ▲ Revised Code

104 — L Codes   Ⓐ Adult   Ⓜ Maternity   Ⓟ Pediatrics   Ⓘ Infant   Ⓐ-Ⓨ APC Status Indicator   **2005 HCPCS**

UPPER LIMB

The procedures in L6000–L6590 are considered as "base" or "basic procedures" and may be modified by listing procedures from the "addition" sections. The base procedures include only standard friction wrist and control cable system unless otherwise specified.

PARTIAL HAND

A	**L6000**	Partial hand, Robin-Aids, thumb remaining (or equal)	占
A	**L6010**	Partial hand, Robin-Aids, little and/or ring finger remaining (or equal)	占
A	**L6020**	Partial hand, Robin-Aids, no finger remaining (or equal)	占
A	**L6025**	Transcarpal/metacarpal or partial hand disarticulation prosthesis, external power, self-suspended, inner socket with removable forearm section, electrodes and cables, two batteries, charger, myoelectric control of terminal device	占

WRIST DISARTICULATION

A	**L6050**	Wrist disarticulation, molded socket, flexible elbow hinges, triceps pad	占
A	**L6055**	Wrist disarticulation, molded socket with expandable interface, flexible elbow hinges, triceps pad	占

BELOW ELBOW

A	**L6100**	Below elbow, molded socket, flexible elbow hinge, triceps pad	占
A	**L6110**	Below elbow, molded socket (Muenster or Northwestern suspension types)	占
A	**L6120**	Below elbow, molded double wall split socket, step-up hinges, half cuff	占
A	**L6130**	Below elbow, molded double wall split socket, stump activated locking hinge, half cuff	占

ELBOW DISARTICULATION

A	**L6200**	Elbow disarticulation, molded socket, outside locking hinge, forearm	占
A	**L6205**	Elbow disarticulation, molded socket with expandable interface, outside locking hinges, forearm	占

ABOVE ELBOW

A	**L6250**	Above elbow, molded double wall socket, internal locking elbow, forearm	占

SHOULDER DISARTICULATION

A	**L6300**	Shoulder disarticulation, molded socket, shoulder bulkhead, humeral section, internal locking elbow, forearm	占
A	**L6310**	Shoulder disarticulation, passive restoration (complete prosthesis)	占
A	**L6320**	Shoulder disarticulation, passive restoration (shoulder cap only)	占

INTERSCAPULAR THORACIC

A	**L6350**	Interscapular thoracic, molded socket, shoulder bulkhead, humeral section, internal locking elbow, forearm	占
A	**L6360**	Interscapular thoracic, passive restoration (complete prosthesis)	占
A	**L6370**	Interscapular thoracic, passive restoration (shoulder cap only)	占

IMMEDIATE AND EARLY POSTSURGICAL PROCEDURES

A		**L6380**	Immediate postsurgical or early fitting, application of initial rigid dressing, including fitting alignment and suspension of components, and one cast change, wrist disarticulation or below elbow	占
A	☑	**L6382**	Immediate postsurgical or early fitting, application of initial rigid dressing including fitting alignment and suspension of components, and one cast change, elbow disarticulation or above elbow	占
A	☑	**L6384**	Immediate postsurgical or early fitting, application of initial rigid dressing including fitting alignment and suspension of components, and one cast change, shoulder disarticulation or interscapular thoracic	占
A	☑	**L6386**	Immediate postsurgical or early fitting, each additional cast change and realignment	占
A		**L6388**	Immediate postsurgical or early fitting, application of rigid dressing only	占

ENDOSKELETAL: BELOW ELBOW

A	**L6400**	Below elbow, molded socket, endoskeletal system, including soft prosthetic tissue shaping	占

ENDOSKELETAL: ELBOW DISARTICULATION

A	**L6450**	Elbow disarticulation, molded socket, endoskeletal system, including soft prosthetic tissue shaping	占

ENDOSKELETAL: ABOVE ELBOW

A	**L6500**	Above elbow, molded socket, endoskeletal system, including soft prosthetic tissue shaping	占

ENDOSKELETAL: SHOULDER DISARTICULATION

A	**L6550**	Shoulder disarticulation, molded socket, endoskeletal system, including soft prosthetic tissue shaping	占

ENDOSKELETAL: INTERSCAPULAR THORACIC

A	**L6570**	Interscapular thoracic, molded socket, endoskeletal system, including soft prosthetic tissue shaping	占
A	**L6580**	Preparatory, wrist disarticulation or below elbow, single wall plastic socket, friction wrist, flexible elbow hinges, figure of eight harness, humeral cuff, Bowden cable control, USMC or equal pylon, no cover, molded to patient model	占
A	**L6582**	Preparatory, wrist disarticulation or below elbow, single wall socket, friction wrist, flexible elbow hinges, figure of eight harness, humeral cuff, Bowden cable control, USMC or equal pylon, no cover, direct formed	占
A	**L6584**	Preparatory, elbow disarticulation or above elbow, single wall plastic socket, friction wrist, locking elbow, figure of eight harness, fair lead cable control, USMC or equal pylon, no cover, molded to patient model	占
A	**L6586**	Preparatory, elbow disarticulation or above elbow, single wall socket, friction wrist, locking elbow, figure of eight harness, fair lead cable control, USMC or equal pylon, no cover, direct formed	占

Special Coverage Instructions   Noncovered by Medicare   Carrier Discretion   ☑ Quantity Alert   ● New Code   ○ Reinstated Code   ▲ Revised Code

2005 HCPCS   ♀ Female Only   ♂ Male Only   **1-9** ASC Groups   MED: Pub 100/NCD Reference   占 DMEPOS Paid   Ⓢ SNF Excluded   **L Codes — 105**

Prosthetic Procedures

L6588 — L6697

A   **L6588**   Preparatory, shoulder disarticulation or interscapular thoracic, single wall plastic socket, shoulder joint, locking elbow, friction wrist, chest strap, fair lead cable control, USMC or equal pylon, no cover, molded to patient model   &

A   **L6590**   Preparatory, shoulder disarticulation or interscapular thoracic, single wall socket, shoulder joint, locking elbow, friction wrist, chest strap, fair lead cable control, USMC or equal pylon, no cover, direct formed   &

ADDITIONS: UPPER LIMB
The following procedures/modifications/components may be added to other base procedures. The items in this section should reflect the additional complexity of each modification procedure, in addition to the base procedure, at the time of the original order.

A   ☑   **L6600**   Upper extremity additions, polycentric hinge, pair   &

A   ☑   **L6605**   Upper extremity additions, single pivot hinge, pair   &

A   ☑   **L6610**   Upper extremity additions, flexible metal hinge, pair   &

A   **L6615**   Upper extremity addition, disconnect locking wrist unit   &

A   ☑   **L6616**   Upper extremity addition, additional disconnect insert for locking wrist unit, each   &

A   **L6620**   Upper extremity addition, flexion/extension wrist unit, with or without friction   &

A   **L6623**   Upper extremity addition, spring assisted rotational wrist unit with latch release   &

A   **L6625**   Upper extremity addition, rotation wrist unit with cable lock   &

A   **L6628**   Upper extremity addition, quick disconnect hook adapter, Otto Bock or equal   &

A   **L6629**   Upper extremity addition, quick disconnect lamination collar with coupling piece, Otto Bock or equal   &

A   **L6630**   Upper extremity addition, stainless steel, any wrist   &

A   ☑   **L6632**   Upper extremity addition, latex suspension sleeve, each   &

A   **L6635**   Upper extremity addition, lift assist for elbow   &

A   **L6637**   Upper extremity addition, nudge control elbow lock   &

A   **L6638**   Upper extremity addition to prosthesis, electric locking feature, only for use with manually powered elbow   &

A   ☑   **L6640**   Upper extremity additions, shoulder abduction joint, pair   &

A   **L6641**   Upper extremity addition, excursion amplifier, pulley type   &

A   **L6642**   Upper extremity addition, excursion amplifier, lever type   &

A   ☑   **L6645**   Upper extremity addition, shoulder flexion-abduction joint, each   &

A   **L6646**   Upper extremity addition, shoulder joint, multipositional locking, flexion, adjustable abduction friction control, for use with body powered or external powered system   &

A   **L6647**   Upper extremity addition, shoulder lock mechanism, body powered actuator   &

A   **L6648**   Upper extremity addition, shoulder lock mechanism, external powered actuator   &

A   ☑   **L6650**   Upper extremity addition, shoulder universal joint, each   &

A   **L6655**   Upper extremity addition, standard control cable, extra   &

A   **L6660**   Upper extremity addition, heavy duty control cable   &

A   **L6665**   Upper extremity addition, Teflon, or equal, cable lining   &

A   **L6670**   Upper extremity addition, hook to hand, cable adapter   &

A   **L6672**   Upper extremity addition, harness, chest or shoulder, saddle type   &

A   **L6675**   Upper extremity addition, harness, (e.g., figure of eight type), single cable design   &

A   **L6676**   Upper extremity addition, harness, (e.g., figure of eight type), dual cable design   &

A   **L6680**   Upper extremity addition, test socket, wrist disarticulation or below elbow   &

A   **L6682**   Upper extremity addition, test socket, elbow disarticulation or above elbow   &

A   **L6684**   Upper extremity addition, test socket, shoulder disarticulation or interscapular thoracic   &

A   **L6686**   Upper extremity addition, suction socket   &

A   **L6687**   Upper extremity addition, frame type socket, below elbow or wrist disarticulation   &

A   **L6688**   Upper extremity addition, frame type socket, above elbow or elbow disarticulation   &

A   **L6689**   Upper extremity addition, frame type socket, shoulder disarticulation   &

A   **L6690**   Upper extremity addition, frame type socket, interscapular-thoracic   &

A   ☑   **L6691**   Upper extremity addition, removable insert, each &

A   ☑   **L6692**   Upper extremity addition, silicone gel insert or equal, each   &

A   **L6693**   Upper extremity addition, locking elbow, forearm counterbalance   &

●   **L6694**   Addition to upper extremity prosthesis, below elbow/above elbow, custom fabricated from existing mold or prefabricated, socket insert, silicone gel, elastomeric or equal, for use with locking mechanism

●   **L6695**   Addition to upper extremity prosthesis, below elbow/above elbow, custom fabricated from existing mold or prefabricated, socket insert, silicone gel, elastomeric or equal, not for use with locking mechanism

●   **L6696**   Addition to upper extremity prosthesis, below elbow/above elbow, custom fabricated socket insert for congenital or atypical traumatic amputee, silicone gel, elastomeric or equal, for use with or without locking mechanism, initial only (for other than initial, use code L6694 or L6695)

●   **L6697**   Addition to upper extremity prosthesis, below elbow/above elbow, custom fabricated socket insert for other than congenital or atypical traumatic amputee, silicone gel, elastomeric or equal, for use with or without locking mechanism, initial only (for other than initial, use code L6694 or L6695)

| Special Coverage Instructions | Noncovered by Medicare | Carrier Discretion | ☑ Quantity Alert | ● New Code | ○ Reinstated Code | ▲ Revised Code |

106 — L Codes   A Adult   M Maternity   P Pediatrics   I Infant   A-Y APC Status Indicator   *2005 HCPCS*

●   L6698   Addition to upper extremity prosthesis, below elbow/above elbow, lock mechanism, excludes socket insert

TERMINAL DEVICES

HOOKS

A   L6700   Terminal device, hook, Dorrance or equal, model #3
MED: 100-2, 15, 120

A   L6705   Terminal device, hook, Dorrance or equal, model #5
MED: 100-2, 15, 120

A   L6710   Terminal device, hook, Dorrance or equal, model #5X
MED: 100-2, 15, 120

A   L6715   Terminal device, hook, Dorrance or equal, model #5XA
MED: 100-2, 15, 120

A   L6720   Terminal device, hook, Dorrance or equal, model #6
MED: 100-2, 15, 120

A   L6725   Terminal device, hook, Dorrance or equal, model #7
MED: 100-2, 15, 120

A   L6730   Terminal device, hook, Dorrance or equal, model #7LO
MED: 100-2, 15, 120

A   L6735   Terminal device, hook, Dorrance or equal, model #8
MED: 100-2, 15, 120

A   L6740   Terminal device, hook, Dorrance or equal, model #8X
MED: 100-2, 15, 120

A   L6745   Terminal device, hook, Dorrance or equal, model #88X
MED: 100-2, 15, 120

A   L6750   Terminal device, hook, Dorrance or equal, model #10P
MED: 100-2, 15, 120

A   L6755   Terminal device, hook, Dorrance or equal, model #10X
MED: 100-2, 15, 120

A   L6765   Terminal device, hook, Dorrance or equal, model #12P
MED: 100-2, 15, 120

A   L6770   Terminal device, hook, Dorrance or equal, model #99X
MED: 100-2, 15, 120

A   L6775   Terminal device, hook, Dorrance or equal, model #555
MED: 100-2, 15, 120

A   L6780   Terminal device, hook, Dorrance or equal, model #SS555
MED: 100-2, 15, 120

A   L6790   Terminal device, hook, Accu hook or equal
MED: 100-2, 15, 120

A   L6795   Terminal device, hook, 2 load or equal
MED: 100-2, 15, 120

A   L6800   Terminal device, hook, APRL VC or equal
MED: 100-2, 15, 120

A   L6805   Terminal device, modifier wrist flexion unit
MED: 100-2, 15, 120

A   L6806   Terminal device, hook, TRS Grip, Grip III, VC, or equal
MED: 100-2, 15, 120

A   L6807   Terminal device, hook, Grip I, Grip II, VC, or equal
MED: 100-2, 15, 120

A   L6808   Terminal device, hook, TRS Adept, infant or child, VC, or equal
MED: 100-2, 15, 120

A   L6809   Terminal device, hook, TRS Super Sport, passive
MED: 100-2, 15, 120

A   L6810   Terminal device, Pincher tool, Otto Bock or equal
MED: 100-2, 15, 120

HANDS

A   L6825   Terminal device, hand, Dorrance, VO
MED: 100-2, 15, 120

A   L6830   Terminal device, hand, APRL, VC
MED: 100-2, 15, 120

A   L6835   Terminal device, hand, Sierra, VO
MED: 100-2, 15, 120

A   L6840   Terminal device, hand, Becker Imperial
MED: 100-2, 15, 120

A   L6845   Terminal device, hand, Becker Lock Grip
MED: 100-2, 15, 120

A   L6850   Terminal device, hand, Becker Plylite
MED: 100-2, 15, 120

A   L6855   Terminal device, hand, Robin-Aids, VO
MED: 100-2, 15, 120

A   L6860   Terminal device, hand, Robin-Aids, VO soft
MED: 100-2, 15, 120

A   L6865   Terminal device, hand, passive hand
MED: 100-2, 15, 120

A   L6867   Terminal device, hand, Detroit infant hand (mechanical)
MED: 100-2, 15, 120

A   L6868   Terminal device, hand, passive infant hand, Steeper, Hosmer or equal
MED: 100-2, 15, 120

A   L6870   Terminal device, hand, child mitt
MED: 100-2, 15, 120

A   L6872   Terminal device, hand, NYU child hand
MED: 100-2, 15, 120

A   L6873   Terminal device, hand, mechanical infant hand, steeper or equal
MED: 100-2, 15, 120

A   L6875   Terminal device, hand, Bock, VC
MED: 100-2, 15, 120

A   L6880   Terminal device, hand, Bock, VO
MED: 100-2, 15, 120

Special Coverage Instructions   Noncovered by Medicare   Carrier Discretion   ☑ Quantity Alert   ● New Code   ○ Reinstated Code   ▲ Revised Code

2005 HCPCS   ♀ Female Only   ♂ Male Only   **1-9** ASC Groups   MED: Pub 100/NCD Reference   ᛒ DMEPOS Paid   ⊘ SNF Excluded   **L Codes — 107**

Prosthetic Procedures

L6881 — L7261

Ⓐ **L6881** Automatic grasp feature, addition to upper limb prosthetic terminal device ⅄

Ⓐ **L6882** Microprocessor control feature, addition to upper limb prosthetic terminal device ⅄
MED: 100-2, 15, 120

GLOVES FOR ABOVE HANDS

▲ Ⓐ **L6890** Addition to upper extremity prosthesis, glove for terminal device, any material, prefabricated, includes fitting and adjustment ⅄

▲ Ⓐ **L6895** Addition to upper extremity prosthesis, glove for terminal device, any material, custom fabricated ⅄

HAND RESTORATION

Ⓐ **L6900** Hand restoration (casts, shading and measurements included), partial hand, with glove, thumb or one finger remaining ⅄

Ⓐ **L6905** Hand restoration (casts, shading and measurements included), partial hand, with glove, multiple fingers remaining ⅄

Ⓐ **L6910** Hand restoration (casts, shading and measurements included), partial hand, with glove, no fingers remaining ⅄

Ⓐ **L6915** Hand restoration (shading and measurements included), replacement glove for above ⅄

EXTERNAL POWER

BASE DEVICES

Ⓐ **L6920** Wrist disarticulation, external power, self-suspended inner socket, removable forearm shell, Otto Bock or equal switch, cables, two batteries and one charger, switch control of terminal device ⅄

Ⓐ **L6925** Wrist disarticulation, external power, self-suspended inner socket, removable forearm shell, Otto Bock or equal electrodes, cables, two batteries and one charger, myoelectronic control of terminal device ⅄

Ⓐ **L6930** Below elbow, external power, self-suspended inner socket, removable forearm shell, Otto Bock or equal switch, cables, two batteries and one charger, switch control of terminal device ⅄

Ⓐ **L6935** Below elbow, external power, self-suspended inner socket, removable forearm shell, Otto Bock or equal electrodes, cables, two batteries and one charger, myoelectronic control of terminal device ⅄

Ⓐ **L6940** Elbow disarticulation, external power, molded inner socket, removable humeral shell, outside locking hinges, forearm, Otto Bock or equal switch, cables, two batteries and one charger, switch control of terminal device ⅄

Ⓐ **L6945** Elbow disarticulation, external power, molded inner socket, removable humeral shell, outside locking hinges, forearm, Otto Bock or equal electrodes, cables, two batteries and one charger, myoelectronic control of terminal device ⅄

Ⓐ **L6950** Above elbow, external power, molded inner socket, removable humeral shell, internal locking elbow, forearm, Otto Bock or equal switch, cables, two batteries and one charger, switch control of terminal device ⅄

Ⓐ **L6955** Above elbow, external power, molded inner socket, removable humeral shell, internal locking elbow, forearm, Otto Bock or equal electrodes, cables, two batteries and one charger, myoelectronic control of terminal device ⅄

Ⓐ **L6960** Shoulder disarticulation, external power, molded inner socket, removable shoulder shell, shoulder bulkhead, humeral section, mechanical elbow, forearm, Otto Bock or equal switch, cables, two batteries and one charger, switch control of terminal device ⅄

Ⓐ **L6965** Shoulder disarticulation, external power, molded inner socket, removable shoulder shell, shoulder bulkhead, humeral section, mechanical elbow, forearm, Otto Bock or equal electrodes, cables, two batteries and one charger, myoelectronic control of terminal device ⅄

Ⓐ **L6970** Interscapular-thoracic, external power, molded inner socket, removable shoulder shell, shoulder bulkhead, humeral section, mechanical elbow, forearm, Otto Bock or equal switch, cables, two batteries and one charger, switch control of terminal device ⅄

Ⓐ **L6975** Interscapular-thoracic, external power, molded inner socket, removable shoulder shell, shoulder bulkhead, humeral section, mechanical elbow, forearm, Otto Bock or equal electrodes, cables, two batteries and one charger, myoelectronic control of terminal device ⅄

Ⓐ **L7010** Electronic hand, Otto Bock, Steeper or equal, switch controlled ⅄

Ⓐ **L7015** Electronic hand, System Teknik, Variety Village or equal, switch controlled ⅄

Ⓐ **L7020** Electronic Greifer, Otto Bock or equal, switch controlled ⅄

Ⓐ **L7025** Electronic hand, Otto Bock or equal, myoelectronically controlled ⅄

Ⓐ **L7030** Electronic hand, System Teknik, Variety Village or equal, myoelectronically controlled ⅄

Ⓐ **L7035** Electronic Greifer, Otto Bock or equal, myoelectronically controlled ⅄

Ⓐ **L7040** Prehensile actuator, Hosmer or equal, switch controlled ⅄

Ⓐ **L7045** Electronic hook, child, Michigan or equal, switch controlled ⅄

ELBOW

Ⓐ **L7170** Electronic elbow, Hosmer or equal, switch controlled ⅄

▲ Ⓐ **L7180** Electronic elbow, microprocessor sequential control of elbow and terminal device ⅄

● **L7181** Electronic elbow, microprocessor simultaneous control of elbow and terminal device

Ⓐ **L7185** Electronic elbow, adolescent, Variety Village or equal, switch controlled ⅄

Ⓐ **L7186** Electronic elbow, child, Variety Village or equal, switch controlled ⅄

Ⓐ **L7190** Electronic elbow, adolescent, Variety Village or equal, myoelectronically controlled ⅄

Ⓐ **L7191** Electronic elbow, child, Variety Village or equal, myoelectronically controlled ⅄

Ⓐ **L7260** Electronic wrist rotator, Otto Bock or equal ⅄

Ⓐ **L7261** Electronic wrist rotator, for Utah Arm ⅄

Special Coverage Instructions · Noncovered by Medicare · Carrier Discretion · ☑ Quantity Alert · ● New Code · ○ Reinstated Code · ▲ Revised Code

108 — L Codes · Ⓐ Adult · Ⓜ Maternity · Ⓟ Pediatrics · Ⓘ Infant · Ⓐ-Ⓨ APC Status Indicator · **2005 HCPCS**

A   **L7266** Servo control, Steeper or equal   🦽

A   **L7272** Analogue control, UNB or equal   🦽

A   **L7274** Proportional control, 6-12 volt, Liberty, Utah or equal   🦽

BATTERY COMPONENTS

A   **L7360** Six volt battery, Otto Bock or equal, each   🦽

A   **L7362** Battery charger, six volt, Otto Bock or equal   🦽

A   **L7364** Twelve volt battery, Utah or equal, each   🦽

A   **L7366** Battery charger, twelve volt, Utah or equal   🦽

A   **L7367** Lithium ion battery, replacement   🦽

A   **L7368** Lithium ion battery charger   🦽

A   **L7499** Upper extremity prosthesis, NOS   ⊘

REPAIRS

A   **L7500** Repair of prosthetic device, hourly rate
Medicare jurisdiction: local carrier if repair or implanted prosthetic device.
MED: 100-2, 15, 110.2; 100-2, 15, 120; 100-2, 15, 120

A   **L7510** Repair of prosthetic device, repair or replace minor parts
Medicare jurisdiction: local carrier if repair of implanted prosthetic device.
MED: 100-2, 15, 110.2; 100-2, 15, 120; 100-2, 15, 120

A ☑   **L7520** Repair prosthetic device, labor component, per 15 minutes
Medicare jurisdiction: local carrier if repair of implanted prosthetic device.

GENERAL

A   **L7900** Male vacuum erection system   A ♂ 🦽

PROSTHESIS

A   **L8000** Breast prosthesis, mastectomy bra   A ♀ 🦽
MED: 100-2, 15, 120

A   **L8001** Breast prosthesis, mastectomy bra, with integrated breast prosthesis form, unilateral   A ♀ 🦽
MED: 100-2, 15, 120

A   **L8002** Breast prosthesis, mastectomy bra, with integrated breast prosthesis form, bilateral   A ♀ 🦽
MED: 100-2, 15, 120

A   **L8010** Breast prosthesis, mastectomy sleeve   A ♀
MED: 100-2, 15, 120

A   **L8015** External breast prosthesis garment, with mastectomy form, postmastectomy   A ♀ 🦽
MED: 100-2, 15, 120

A   **L8020** Breast prosthesis, mastectomy form   A ♀ 🦽
MED: 100-2, 15, 120

A   **L8030** Breast prosthesis, silicone or equal   A ♀ 🦽
MED: 100-2, 15, 120

A   **L8035** Custom breast prosthesis, postmastectomy, molded to patient model   A ♀ 🦽
MED: 100-2, 15, 120

A   **L8039** Breast prosthesis, NOS   A ♀

A   **L8040** Nasal prosthesis, provided by a nonphysician   🦽

A   **L8041** Midfacial prosthesis, provided by a nonphysician   🦽

A   **L8042** Orbital prosthesis, provided by a nonphysician   🦽

Orbital and midfacial prosthesis (L8041-L8042)

Nasal prosthesis (L8040)

Frontal bone

Nasal bone

Maxilla

Zygoma

(L8043-L8044)

Facial prosthetics are typically custom manufactured from polymers and carefully matched to the original features. The maxilla, zygoma, frontal, and nasal bones are often involved, either singly or in combination (L8040-L8044)

A   **L8043** Upper facial prosthesis, provided by a nonphysician   🦽

A   **L8044** Hemi-facial prosthesis, provided by a nonphysician   🦽

A   **L8045** Auricular prosthesis, provided by a nonphysician   🦽

A   **L8046** Partial facial prosthesis, provided by a nonphysician   🦽

A   **L8047** Nasal septal prosthesis, provided by a nonphysician   🦽

A   **L8048** Unspecified maxillofacial prosthesis, by report, provided by a nonphysician

A   **L8049** Repair or modification of maxillofacial prosthesis, labor component, 15 minute increments, provided by a nonphysician

ELASTIC SUPPORTS

E ☑   **L8100** Gradient compression stocking, below knee, 18-30 mmHg, each   ⊘
MED: 100-2, 15, 120; 100-3, 280.1

A ☑   **L8110** Gradient compression stocking, below knee, 30-40 mmHg, each   🦽
MED: 100-2, 15, 100
AHA: 4Q, '03, 5

A ☑   **L8120** Gradient compression stocking, below knee, 40-50 mmHg, each   🦽
MED: 100-2, 15, 100
AHA: 4Q, '03, 5

E ☑   **L8130** Gradient compression stocking, thigh length, 18-30 mmHg, each   ⊘
MED: 100-2, 15, 120; 100-3, 280.1

E ☑   **L8140** Gradient compression stocking, thigh length, 30-40 mmHg, each   ⊘
MED: 100-3, 280.1; 100-3, 280.1

E ☑   **L8150** Gradient compression stocking, thigh length, 40-50 mmHg, each   ⊘
MED: 100-2, 15, 120; 100-3, 280.1

E ☑   **L8160** Gradient compression stocking, full length/chap style, 18-30 mmHg, each   ⊘
MED: 100-2, 15, 120; 100-3, 280.1

E ☑   **L8170** Gradient compression stocking, full length/chap style, 30-40 mmHg, each   ⊘
MED: 100-2, 15, 120; 100-3, 280.1

E ☑   **L8180** Gradient compression stocking, full length/chap style, 40-50 mmHg, each   ⊘
MED: 100-2, 15, 120; 100-3, 280.1

Special Coverage Instructions   Noncovered by Medicare   Carrier Discretion   ☑ Quantity Alert   ● New Code   ○ Reinstated Code   ▲ Revised Code

2005 HCPCS   ♀ Female Only   ♂ Male Only   1-9 ASC Groups   MED: Pub 100/NCD Reference   🦽 DMEPOS Paid   ⊘ SNF Excluded   **L Codes — 109**

E ☑ **L8190** Gradient compression stocking, waist length, 18-30 mmHg, each ⊘
MED: 100-2, 15, 120; 100-3, 280.1

E ☑ **L8195** Gradient compression stocking, waist length, 30-40 mmHg, each ⊘
MED: 100-2, 15, 120; 100-3, 280.1

E ☑ **L8200** Gradient compression stocking, waist length, 40-50 mmHg, each ⊘
MED: 100-2, 15, 120; 100-3, 280.1

E **L8210** Gradient compression stocking, custom made ⊘
MED: 100-2, 15, 120; 100-3, 280.1

E **L8220** Gradient compression stocking, lymphedema ⊘
MED: 100-2, 15, 120; 100-3, 280.1

E **L8230** Gradient compression stocking, garter belt ⊘
MED: 100-2, 15, 120; 100-3, 280.1

E **L8239** Gradient compression stocking, NOS

TRUSSES

A **L8300** Truss, single with standard pad ㆓
MED: 100-2, 15, 120; 100-3, 280.11; 100-3, 280.12

A **L8310** Truss, double with standard pads ㆓
MED: 100-2, 15, 120; 100-3, 280.11; 100-3, 280.12

A **L8320** Truss, addition to standard pad, water pad ㆓
MED: 100-2, 15, 120; 100-3, 280.11; 100-3, 280.12

A **L8330** Truss, addition to standard pad, scrotal pad ♂㆓
MED: 100-2, 15, 120; 100-3, 280.11; 100-3, 280.12

PROSTHETIC SOCKS

A ☑ **L8400** Prosthetic sheath, below knee, each ㆓
MED: 100-2, 15, 120

A ☑ **L8410** Prosthetic sheath, above knee, each ㆓
MED: 100-2, 15, 120

A ☑ **L8415** Prosthetic sheath, upper limb, each ㆓
MED: 100-2, 15, 120

A ☑ **L8417** Prosthetic sheath/sock, including a gel cushion layer, below knee or above knee, each ㆓

A ☑ **L8420** Prosthetic sock, multiple ply, below knee, each ㆓
MED: 100-2, 15, 120

A ☑ **L8430** Prosthetic sock, multiple ply, above knee, each ㆓
MED: 100-2, 15, 120

A ☑ **L8435** Prosthetic sock, multiple ply, upper limb, each ㆓
MED: 100-2, 15, 120

A ☑ **L8440** Prosthetic shrinker, below knee, each ㆓
MED: 100-2, 15, 120

A ☑ **L8460** Prosthetic shrinker, above knee, each ㆓
MED: 100-2, 15, 120

A ☑ **L8465** Prosthetic shrinker, upper limb, each ㆓
MED: 100-2, 15, 120

A ☑ **L8470** Prosthetic sock, single ply, fitting, below knee, each ㆓
MED: 100-2, 15, 120

A ☑ **L8480** Prosthetic sock, single ply, fitting, above knee, each ㆓
MED: 100-2, 15, 120

A ☑ **L8485** Prosthetic sock, single ply, fitting, upper limb, each ㆓
MED: 100-2, 15, 120

~~L8400~~ ~~Addition to prosthetic sheath/sock, air seal suction retention system~~

A **L8499** Unlisted procedure for miscellaneous prosthetic services
Determine if an alternative HCPCS Level II or a CPT code better describes the service being reported. This code should be used only if a more specific code is unavailable.

PROSTHETIC IMPLANTS

INTEGUMENTARY SYSTEM

A **L8500** Artificial larynx, any type ㆓
MED: 100-2, 15, 120; 100-3, 50.2

A **L8501** Tracheostomy speaking valve ㆓
MED: 100-3, 50.4

A **L8505** Artificial larynx replacement battery/accessory, any type

A **L8507** Tracheo-esophageal voice prosthesis, patient inserted, any type, each ㆓

A **L8509** Tracheo-esophageal voice prosthesis, inserted by a licensed health care provider, any type ㆓

A **L8510** Voice amplifier ㆓
MED: 100-3, 50.2

A ☑ **L8511** Insert for indwelling tracheoesophageal prosthesis, with or without valve, replacement only, each ㆓

A ☑ **L8512** Gelatin capsules or equivalent, for use with tracheoesophageal voice prosthesis, replacement only, per 10 ㆓

A ☑ **L8513** Cleaning device used with tracheoesophageal voice prosthesis, pipet, brush, or equal, replacement only, each ㆓

A ☑ **L8514** Tracheoesophageal puncture dilator, replacement only, each ㆓

● ☑ **L8515** Gelatin capsule, application device for use with tracheoesophageal voice prosthesis, each

N **L8600** Implantable breast prosthesis, silicone or equal   A ♀㆓
Medicare covers implants inserted in post-mastectomy reconstruction in a breast cancer patient. Always report concurrent to the implant procedure. Medicare jurisdiction: local carrier.

MED: 100-2, 15, 120; 100-3, 140.2

N ☑ **L8603** Injectable bulking agent, collagen implant, urinary tract, 2.5 ml syringe, includes shipping and necessary supplies ㆓
Medicare covers up to five separate collagen implant treatments in patients with intrinsic sphincter deficiency. Who have passed a collagen sensitivity test. Medicare jurisdiction: local carrier.

MED: 100-3, 230.10

N ☑ **L8606** Injectable bulking agent, synthetic implant, urinary tract, 1 ml syringe, includes shipping and necessary supplies ㆓
MED: 100-3, 230.10

HEAD: SKULL, FACIAL BONES, AND TEMPOROMANDIBULAR JOINT

N **L8610** Ocular implant ㆓
Medicare jurisdiction: local carrier.

MED: 100-2, 15, 120

N **L8612** Aqueous shunt ㆓
Medicare jurisdiction: local carrier.

MED: 100-2, 15, 120

See code(s): Q0074

Special Coverage Instructions   Noncovered by Medicare   Carrier Discretion   ☑ Quantity Alert   ● New Code   ○ Reinstated Code   ▲ Revised Code

110 — L Codes   A Adult   M Maternity   P Pediatrics   I Infant   A-Y APC Status Indicator   **2005 HCPCS**

N   **L8613**   Ossicular implant
Medicare jurisdiction: local carrier.
MED: 100-2, 15, 120

N   **L8614**   Cochlear device/system
A cochlear implant is covered by Medicare when the patient has bilateral sensorineural deafness. Medicare jurisdiction: local carrier.
MED: 100-2, 15, 120; 100-3, 50.3
AHA: 3Q, '02, 5; 4Q, '03, 8

●   **L8615**   Headset/headpiece for use with cochlear implant device, replacement
MED: 100-3, 50.3

●   **L8616**   Microphone for use with cochlear implant device, replacement
MED: 100-3, 50.3

●   **L8617**   Transmitting coil for use with cochlear implant device, replacement
MED: 100-3, 50.3

●   **L8618**   Transmitter cable for use with cochlear implant device, replacement
MED: 100-3, 50.3

A   **L8619**   Cochlear implant external speech processor, replacement
Medicare jurisdiction: local carrier.
MED: 100-3, 50.3

● ☑   **L8620**   Lithium ion battery for use with cochlear implant device, replacement, each

   L8621   Zinc air battery for use with cochlear implant device, replacement, each

● ☑   **L8622**   Alkaline battery for use with cochlear implant device, any size, replacement, each

UPPER EXTREMITY

N   **L8630**   Metacarpophalangeal joint implant
Medicare jurisdiction: local carrier.
MED: 100-2, 15, 120

A   **L8631**   Metacarpal phalangeal joint replacement, two or more pieces, metal (e.g., stainless steel or cobalt chrome), ceramic-like material (e.g., pyrocarbon), for surgical implantation (all sizes, includes entire system)
MED: 100-2, 15, 120

LOWER EXTREMITY — JOINT: KNEE, ANKLE, TOE

N   **L8641**   Metatarsal joint implant
Medicare jurisdiction: local carrier.
MED: 100-2, 15, 120

N   **L8642**   Hallux implant
Medicare jurisdiction: local carrier.
MED: 100-2, 15, 120
See code(s): Q0073

MISCELLANEOUS MUSCULAR-SKELETAL

N   **L8658**   Interphalangeal joint spacer, silicone or equal, each
Medicare jurisdiction: local carrier.
MED: 100-2, 15, 120

A   **L8659**   Interphalangeal finger joint replacement, two or more pieces, metal (e.g., stainless steel or cobalt chrome), ceramic-like material (e.g., pyrocarbon) for surgical implantation, any size
MED: 100-2, 15, 120

CARDIOVASCULAR SYSTEM

N   **L8670**   Vascular graft material, synthetic, implant
Medicare jurisdiction: local carrier.
MED: 100-2, 15, 120

GENERAL

N   **L8699**   Prosthetic implant, not otherwise specified
Determine if an alternative HCPCS Level II or a CPT code better describes the service being reported. This code should be used only if a more specific code is unavailable. Medicare jurisdiction: local carrier.

A   **L9900**   Orthotic and prosthetic supply, accessory, and/or service component of another HCPCS L code

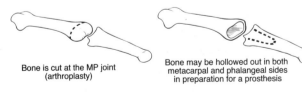

Bone is cut at the MP joint (arthroplasty)

Bone may be hollowed out in both metacarpal and phalangeal sides in preparation for a prosthesis

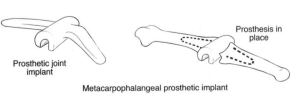

Prosthetic joint implant

Prosthesis in place

Metacarpophalangeal prosthetic implant

Special Coverage Instructions   Noncovered by Medicare   Carrier Discretion   ☑ Quantity Alert   ● New Code   ○ Reinstated Code   ▲ Revised Code

MEDICAL SERVICES *M0000–M0301*

OTHER MEDICAL SERVICES

M codes include office services, cellular therapy, prolotherapy, intragastric hypothermia, IV chelation therapy, and fabric wrapping of an abdominal aneurysm (MNP).

M codes fall under the jurisdiction of the local carrier

☒   **M0064** Brief office visit for the sole purpose of monitoring or changing drug prescriptions used in the treatment of mental psychoneurotic and personality disorders   ⊘
MED: 100-4, 12, 210.1

Ⓔ   **M0075** Cellular therapy   ⊘
The therapeutic efficacy of injecting foreign proteins has not been established.
MED: 100-3, 30.8

Ⓔ   **M0076** Prolotherapy   ⊘
The therapeutic efficacy of prolotherapy and joint sclerotherapy has not been established.
MED: 100-3, 150.7

Ⓔ   **M0100** Intragastric hypothermia using gastric freezing   ⊘
Code with caution: This procedure is considered obsolete.
MED: 100-3, 100.6

CARDIOVASCULAR SERVICES

Ⓔ   **M0300** IV chelation therapy (chemical endarterectomy) ⊘
Chelation therapy is considered experimental in the United States.
MED: 100-3, 20.21

Ⓔ   **M0301** Fabric wrapping of abdominal aneurysm   ⊘
Code with caution: This procedure has largely been replaced with more effective treatment modalities. Submit documentation.
MED: 100-3, 20.23

Special Coverage Instructions	Noncovered by Medicare	Carrier Discretion	☑ Quantity Alert	● New Code	○ Reinstated Code	▲ Revised Code

2005 HCPCS   ♀ Female Only   ♂ Male Only   🔢-🔢 ASC Groups   MED: Pub 100/NCD Reference   ᗱ DMEPOS Paid   ⊘ SNF Excluded   **M Codes — 113**

PATHOLOGY AND LABORATORY SERVICES
P0000–P9999

P codes include chemistry, toxicology, and microbiology tests, screening Papanicolaou procedures, and various blood products.

CHEMISTRY AND TOXICOLOGY TESTS

P codes fall under the jurisdiction of the local carrier.

Ⓐ   **P2028**   Cephalin flocculation, blood   ⊘
Code with caution: This test is considered obsolete. Submit documentation.
MED: 100-3, 300.1

Ⓐ   **P2029**   Congo red, blood   ⊘
Code with caution: This test is considered obsolete. Submit documentation.
MED: 100-3, 300.1

Ⓔ   **P2031**   Hair analysis (excluding arsenic)   ⊘
For hair analysis for arsenic, see CPT codes 83015, 82175.
MED: 100-3, 190.6

Ⓐ   **P2033**   Thymol turbidity, blood   ⊘
Code with caution: This test is considered obsolete. Submit documentation.
MED: 100-3, 300.1

Ⓐ   **P2038**   Mucoprotein, blood (seromucoid) (medical necessity procedure)   ⊘
Code with caution: This test is considered obsolete. Submit documentation.
MED: 100-3, 300.1

PATHOLOGY SCREENING TESTS

Ⓐ   **P3000**   Screening Papanicolaou smear, cervical or vaginal, up to three smears, by technician under physician supervision   Ⓐ ♀
One Pap test is covered by Medicare every three years, unless the physician suspects cervical abnormalities and shortens the interval. See also G0123-G0124.
MED: 100-3, 190.2

Ⓑ   **P3001**   Screening Papanicolaou smear, cervical or vaginal, up to three smears, requiring interpretation by physician   Ⓐ ♀ ⊘
One Pap test is covered by Medicare every three years, unless the physician suspects cervical abnormalities and shortens the interval. See also G0123-G0124.
MED: 100-3, 190.2

MICROBIOLOGY TESTS

Ⓔ   **P7001**   Culture, bacterial, urine; quantitative, sensitivity study   ⊘

MISCELLANEOUS

Ⓚ ☑   **P9010**   Blood (whole), for transfusion, per unit
MED: 100-1, 3, 20.5

Ⓚ ☑   **P9011**   Blood (split unit), specify amount
MED: 100-1, 3, 20.5

Ⓚ ☑   **P9012**   Cryoprecipitate, each unit
MED: 100-1, 3, 20.5

Ⓚ ☑   **P9016**   Red blood cells, leukocytes reduced, each unit
MED: 100-1, 3, 20.5

Ⓚ ☑   **P9017**   Fresh frozen plasma (single donor), frozen within 8 hours of collection, each unit
MED: 100-1, 3, 20.5

Ⓚ ☑   **P9019**   Platelets, each unit
MED: 100-1, 3, 20.5

Ⓚ ☑   **P9020**   Platelet rich plasma, each unit
MED: 100-1, 3, 20.5

Ⓚ ☑   **P9021**   Red blood cells, each unit
MED: 100-1, 3, 20.5

Ⓚ ☑   **P9022**   Red blood cells, washed, each unit
MED: 100-1, 3, 20.5

Ⓚ ☑   **P9023**   Plasma, pooled multiple donor, solvent/detergent treated, frozen, each unit
MED: 100-1, 3, 20.5

Ⓚ ☑   **P9031**   Platelets, leukocytes reduced, each unit
MED: 100-1, 3, 20.5; 100-1, 3, 20.5.2; 100-1, 3, 20.5.3

Ⓚ ☑   **P9032**   Platelets, irradiated, each unit
MED: 100-1, 3, 20.5; 100-1, 3, 20.5.2; 100-1, 3, 20.5.3

Ⓚ ☑   **P9033**   Platelets, leukocytes reduced, irradiated, each unit
MED: 100-1, 3, 20.5; 100-1, 3, 20.5.2; 100-1, 3, 20.5.3

Ⓚ ☑   **P9034**   Platelets, pheresis, each unit
MED: 100-1, 3, 20.5; 100-1, 3, 20.5.2; 100-1, 3, 20.5.3

Ⓚ ☑   **P9035**   Platelets, pheresis, leukocytes reduced, each unit
MED: 100-1, 3, 20.5; 100-1, 3, 20.5.2; 100-1, 3, 20.5.3

Ⓚ ☑   **P9036**   Platelets, pheresis, irradiated, each unit
MED: 100-1, 3, 20.5; 100-1, 3, 20.5.2; 100-1, 3, 20.5.3

Ⓚ ☑   **P9037**   Platelets, pheresis, leukocytes reduced, irradiated, each unit
MED: 100-1, 3, 20.5; 100-1, 3, 20.5.2; 100-1, 3, 20.5.3

Ⓚ ☑   **P9038**   Red blood cells, irradiated, each unit
MED: 100-1, 3, 20.5; 100-1, 3, 20.5.2; 100-1, 3, 20.5.3

Ⓚ ☑   **P9039**   Red blood cells, deglycerolized, each unit
MED: 100-1, 3, 20.5; 100-1, 3, 20.5.2; 100-1, 3, 20.5.3

Ⓚ ☑   **P9040**   Red blood cells, leukocytes reduced, irradiated, each unit
MED: 100-1, 3, 20.5; 100-1, 3, 20.5.2; 100-1, 3, 20.5.3

Ⓚ ☑   **P9041**   Infusion, albumin (human), 5%, 50 ml

Ⓚ ☑   **P9043**   Infusion, plasma protein fraction (human), 5%, 50 ml
MED: 100-1, 3, 20.5

Ⓚ ☑   **P9044**   Plasma, cryoprecipitate reduced, each unit
MED: 100-1, 3, 20.5

Ⓚ ☑   **P9045**   Infusion, albumin (human), 5%, 250 ml

Ⓚ ☑   **P9046**   Infusion, albumin (human), 25%, 20 ml

Ⓚ ☑   **P9047**   Infusion, albumin (human), 25%, 50 ml

Ⓚ ☑   **P9048**   Infusion, plasma protein fraction (human), 5%, 250 ml

Ⓚ ☑   **P9050**   Granulocytes, pheresis, each unit

Ⓚ ☑   **P9051**   Whole blood or red blood cells, leukocytes reduced, CMV-negative, each unit

Ⓚ ☑   **P9052**   Platelets, HLA-matched leukocytes reduced, apheresis/pheresis, each unit

Ⓚ ☑   **P9053**   Platelets, pheresis, leukocytes reduced, CMV-negative, irradiated, each unit

Ⓚ ☑   **P9054**   Whole blood or red blood cells, leukocytes reduced, frozen, deglycerol, washed, each unit

Ⓚ ☑   **P9055**   Platelets, leukocytes reduced, CMV-negative, apheresis/pheresis, each unit

Ⓚ ☑   **P9056**   Whole blood, leukocytes reduced, irradiated, each unit

| Special Coverage Instructions | Noncovered by Medicare | Carrier Discretion | ☑ Quantity Alert | ● New Code | ○ Reinstated Code | ▲ Revised Code |

K ☑ **P9057** Red blood cells, frozen/deglycerolized/washed, leukocytes reduced, irradiated, each unit

K ☑ **P9058** Red blood cells, leukocytes reduced, CMV-negative, irradiated, each unit

K ☑ **P9059** Fresh frozen plasma between 8-24 hours of collection, each unit

K ☑ **P9060** Fresh frozen plasma, donor retested, each unit

A ☑ **P9603** Travel allowance one way in connection with medically necessary laboratory specimen collection drawn from homebound or nursing home bound patient; prorated miles actually traveled
MED: 100-4, 16, 60

A ☑ **P9604** Travel allowance one way in connection with medically necessary laboratory specimen collection drawn from homebound or nursing home bound patient; prorated trip charge
MED: 100-4, 16, 60

N **P9612** Catheterization for collection of specimen, single patient, all places of service ⊘
See also new CPT catheterization codes 51701-51703
MED: 100-4, 16, 60

N **P9615** Catheterization for collection of specimen(s) (multiple patients)
See also new CPT catheterization codes 51701-51703
MED: 100-4, 16, 60

Special Coverage Instructions   Noncovered by Medicare   Carrier Discretion   ☑ Quantity Alert   ● New Code   ○ Reinstated Code   ▲ Revised Code

116 — P Codes   A Adult   M Maternity   P Pediatrics   I Infant   A-Y APC Status Indicator   *2005 HCPCS*

Q CODES (TEMPORARY) *Q0000–Q9999*

New temporary Q codes to pay health care providers for the supplies used in creating casts were established to replace the removal of the practice expense for all HCPCS codes, including the CPT codes for fracture management and for casts and splints. Coders should continue to use the appropriate CPT code to report the work and practice expenses involved with creating the cast or splint; the temporary Q codes replace less specific coding for the casting and splinting supplies.

Q codes fall under the jurisdiction of the local carrier unless they represent an incidental service or are otherwise specified.

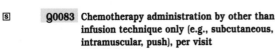

X	**Q0035**	**Cardiokymography**

Covered only in conjunction with electrocardiographic stress testing in male patients with atypical angina or nonischemic chest pain, or female patients with angina.

MED: 100-3, 20.24

T **Q0081** **Infusion therapy, using other than chemotherapeutic drugs, per visit** ⊘

MED: 100-3, 280.14

AHA: 1Q, '02, 7; 2Q, '02, 9, 10; 4Q, '02, 7

S **Q0083** **Chemotherapy administration by other than infusion technique only (e.g., subcutaneous, intramuscular, push), per visit**

AHA: 1Q, '02, 1, 7

S ☑ **Q0084** **Chemotherapy administration by infusion technique only, per visit**

MED: 100-3, 280.14

AHA: 1Q, '02, 1, 7

E ☑ **Q0085** **Chemotherapy administration by both infusion technique and other technique(s) (e.g., subcutaneous, intramuscular, push), per visit**

AHA: 1Q, '02, 1, 7

T **Q0091** **Screening Papanicolaou smear; obtaining, preparing and conveyance of cervical or vaginal smear to laboratory** A ♀

One Pap test is covered by Medicare every three years, unless the physician suspects cervical abnormalities and shortens the interval. Q0091 can be reported with an E/M code when a separately identifiable E/M service is provided.

MED: 100-3, 190.2

AHA: 4Q, '02, 8

N **Q0092** **Set-up portable x-ray equipment**

MED: 100-2, 15, 80.4; 100-4, 13, 90

A **Q0111** **Wet mounts, including preparations of vaginal, cervical or skin specimens**

A **Q0112** **All potassium hydroxide (KOH) preparations**

A **Q0113** **Pinworm examination**

A **Q0114** **Fern test** ♀

A **Q0115** **Post-coital direct, qualitative examinations of vaginal or cervical mucous** A ♀

K ☑ **Q0136** **Injection, epoetin alpha, (for non-ESRD use), per 1,000 units**

This code is for EPO used to treat anemia in patients undergoing chemotherapy for non-myeloid malignancies. Use this code for Epogen, Procrit.

MED: 100-2, 15, 50

K ☑ **Q0137** **Injection, darbepoetin alfa, 1 mcg (non-ESRD use)**

This code is for EPO used to treat anemia in patients undergoing chemotherapy for non-myeloid malignancies. Use this code for Aranesp.

MED: 100-4, 8, 60.4.2; 100-4, 8, 60.4.2.1

E **Q0144** **Azithromycin dihydrate, oral, capsules/powder, 1 gram** ⊘

Use this code for Zithromax, Zithromax Z-PAK.

N **Q0163** **Diphenhydramine HCl, 50 mg, oral, FDA approved prescription anti-emetic, for use as a complete therapeutic substitute for an IV anti-emetic at time of chemotherapy treatment not to exceed a 48-hour dosage regimen**

See also J1200. Medicare covers at the time of chemotherapy if regimen doesn't exceed 48 hours. Submit on the same claim as the chemotherapy.

MED: 100-4, 17, 80.2

AHA: 1Q, '02, 2

N **Q0164** **Prochlorperazine maleate, 5 mg, oral, FDA approved prescription anti-emetic, for use as a complete therapeutic substitute for an IV anti-emetic at the time of chemotherapy treatment, not to exceed a 48-hour dosage regimen**

Medicare covers at the time of chemotherapy if regimen doesn't exceed 48 hours. Submit on the same claim as the chemotherapy. Medicare jurisdiction: DME regional carrier. Use this code for Compazine.

MED: 100-4, 17, 80.2

B **Q0165** **Prochlorperazine maleate, 10 mg, oral, FDA approved prescription anti-emetic, for use as a complete therapeutic substitute for an IV anti-emetic at the time of chemotherapy treatment, not to exceed a 48-hour dosage regimen**

Medicare covers at the time of chemotherapy if regimen doesn't exceed 48 hours. Submit on the same claim as the chemotherapy. Medicare jurisdiction: DME regional carrier. Use this code for Compazine.

MED: 100-4, 17, 80.2

K **Q0166** **Granisetron HCl, 1 mg, oral, FDA approved prescription anti-emetic, for use as a complete therapeutic substitute for an IV anti-emetic at the time of chemotherapy treatment, not to exceed a 24-hour dosage regimen**

Medicare covers at the time of chemotherapy if regimen doesn't exceed 48 hours. Submit on the same claim as the chemotherapy. Medicare jurisdiction: DME regional carrier. Use this code for Kytril.

MED: 100-4, 17, 80.2

N **Q0167** **Dronabinol, 2.5 mg, oral, FDA approved prescription anti-emetic, for use as a complete therapeutic substitute for an IV anti-emetic at the time of chemotherapy treatment, not to exceed a 48-hour dosage regimen**

Medicare covers at the time of chemotherapy if regimen doesn't exceed 48 hours. Submit on the same claim as the chemotherapy. Medicare jurisdiction: DME regional carrier. Use this code for Marinol.

MED: 100-4, 17, 80.2

B **Q0168** **Dronabinol, 5 mg, oral, FDA approved prescription anti-emetic, for use as a complete therapeutic substitute for an IV anti-emetic at the time of chemotherapy treatment, not to exceed a 48-hour dosage regimen**

Medicare jurisdiction: DME regional carrier. Use this code for Marinol.

MED: 100-4, 17, 80.2

N **Q0169** **Promethazine HCl, 12.5 mg, oral, FDA approved prescription anti-emetic, for use as a complete therapeutic substitute for an IV anti-emetic at the time of chemotherapy treatment, not to exceed a 48-hour dosage regimen**

Medicare covers at the time of chemotherapy if regimen doesn't exceed 48 hours. Submit on the same claim as the chemotherapy. Medicare jurisdiction: DME regional carrier. Use this code for Phenergan, Amergan.

MED: 100-4, 17, 80.2

| Special Coverage Instructions | Noncovered by Medicare | Carrier Discretion | ☑ Quantity Alert | ● New Code | ○ Reinstated Code | ▲ Revised Code |

2005 HCPCS   ♀ Female Only   ♂ Male Only   **1-9** ASC Groups   MED: Pub 100/NCD Reference   ℞ DMEPOS Paid   ⊘ SNF Excluded   Q Codes — 117

B **Q0170** Promethazine HCl, 25 mg, oral, FDA approved prescription anti-emetic, for use as a complete therapeutic substitute for an IV anti-emetic at the time of chemotherapy treatment, not to exceed a 48-hour dosage regimen
Medicare covers at the time of chemotherapy if regimen doesn't exceed 48 hours. Submit on the same claim as the chemotherapy. Medicare jurisdiction: DME regional carrier. Use this code for Phenergan, Amergan.

MED: 100-4, 17, 80.2

N **Q0171** Chlorpromazine HCl, 10 mg, oral, FDA approved prescription anti-emetic, for use as a complete therapeutic substitute for an IV anti-emetic at the time of chemotherapy treatment, not to exceed a 48-hour dosage regimen
Medicare covers at the time of chemotherapy if regimen doesn't exceed 48 hours. Submit on the same claim as the chemotherapy. Medicare jurisdiction: DME regional carrier. Use this code for Thorazine.

MED: 100-4, 17, 80.2

B **Q0172** Chlorpromazine HCl, 25 mg, oral, FDA approved prescription anti-emetic, for use as a complete therapeutic substitute for an IV anti-emetic at the time of chemotherapy treatment, not to exceed a 48-hour dosage regimen
Medicare covers at the time of chemotherapy if regimen doesn't exceed 48 hours. Submit on the same claim as the chemotherapy. Medicare jurisdiction: DME regional carrier. Use this code for Thorazine.

MED: 100-4, 17, 80.2

N **Q0173** Trimethobenzamide HCl, 250 mg, oral, FDA approved prescription anti-emetic, for use as a complete therapeutic substitute for an IV anti-emetic at the time of chemotherapy treatment, not to exceed a 48-hour dosage regimen
Medicare covers at the time of chemotherapy if regimen doesn't exceed 48 hours. Submit on the same claim as the chemotherapy. Medicare jurisdiction: DME regional carrier. Use this code for Tebamide, T-Gen, Ticon, Tigan, Triban, Thimazide.

MED: 100-4, 17, 80.2

N **Q0174** Thiethylperazine maleate, 10 mg, oral, FDA approved prescription anti-emetic, for use as a complete therapeutic substitute for an IV anti-emetic at the time of chemotherapy treatment, not to exceed a 48-hour dosage regimen
Medicare covers at the time of chemotherapy if regimen doesn't exceed 48 hours. Submit on the same claim as the chemotherapy. Medicare jurisdiction: DME regional carrier. Use this code for Torecan.

MED: 100-4, 17, 80.2

N **Q0175** Perphenazine, 4 mg, oral, FDA approved prescription anti-emetic, for use as a complete therapeutic substitute for an IV anti-emetic at the time of chemotherapy treatment, not to exceed a 48-hour dosage regimen
Medicare covers at the time of chemotherapy if regimen doesn't exceed 48 hours. Submit on the same claim as the chemotherapy. Medicare jurisdiction: DME regional carrier. Use this code for Trilifon.

MED: 100-4, 17, 80.2

B **Q0176** Perphenazine, 8 mg, oral, FDA approved prescription anti-emetic, for use as a complete therapeutic substitute for an IV anti-emetic at the time of chemotherapy treatment, not to exceed a 48-hour dosage regimen
Medicare covers at the time of chemotherapy if regimen doesn't exceed 48 hours. Submit on the same claim as the chemotherapy. Medicare jurisdiction: DME regional carrier. Use this code for Trilifon.

MED: 100-4, 17, 80.2

N **Q0177** Hydroxyzine pamoate, 25 mg, oral, FDA approved prescription anti-emetic, for use as a complete therapeutic substitute for an IV anti-emetic at the time of chemotherapy treatment, not to exceed a 48-hour dosage regimen
Medicare covers at the time of chemotherapy if regimen doesn't exceed 48 hours. Submit on the same claim as the chemotherapy. Medicare jurisdiction: DME regional carrier. Use this code for Vistaril.

MED: 100-4, 17, 80.2

B **Q0178** Hydroxyzine pamoate, 50 mg, oral, FDA approved prescription anti-emetic, for use as a complete therapeutic substitute for an IV anti-emetic at the time of chemotherapy treatment, not to exceed a 48-hour dosage regimen
Medicare covers at the time of chemotherapy if regimen doesn't exceed 48 hours. Submit on the same claim as the chemotherapy. Medicare jurisdiction: DME regional carrier.

MED: 100-4, 17, 80.2

N **Q0179** Ondansetron HCl 8 mg, oral, FDA approved prescription anti-emetic, for use as a complete therapeutic substitute for an IV anti-emetic at the time of chemotherapy treatment, not to exceed a 48-hour dosage regimen
Medicare covers at the time of chemotherapy if regimen doesn't exceed 48 hours. Submit on the same claim as the chemotherapy. Medicare jurisdiction: DME regional carrier. Use this code for Zofran.

MED: 100-4, 17, 80.2

K **Q0180** Dolasetron mesylate, 100 mg, oral, FDA approved prescription anti-emetic, for use as a complete therapeutic substitute for an IV anti-emetic at the time of chemotherapy treatment, not to exceed a 24-hour dosage regimen
Medicare covers at the time of chemotherapy if regimen doesn't exceed 24 hours. Submit on the same claim as the chemotherapy. Medicare jurisdiction: DME regional carrier. Use this code for Anzemet.

MED: 100-4, 17, 80.2

E **Q0181** Unspecified oral dosage form, FDA approved prescription anti-emetic, for use as a complete therapeutic substitute for an IV anti-emetic at the time of chemotherapy treatment, not to exceed a 48-hour dosage regimen
Medicare covers at the time of chemotherapy if regimen doesn't exceed 48-hours. Submit on the same claim as the chemotherapy. Medicare jurisdiction: DME regional carrier.

MED: 100-4, 17, 80.2

~~Q0182~~ ~~Dermal and epidermal, tissue of non-human origin, with or without other bioengineered or processed elements, without metabolically active elements, per sq. cm~~
See code(s): J7343

~~Q0183~~ ~~Dermal tissue, of human origin, with and without other bioengineered or processed elements, but without metabolically active elements, per sq. cm~~
See code(s): J7344

Special Coverage Instructions   Noncovered by Medicare   Carrier Discretion   ☑ Quantity Alert   ● New Code   ○ Reinstated Code   ▲ Revised Code

118 — Q Codes   A Adult   M Maternity   P Pediatrics   I Infant   A-Y APC Status Indicator   2005 HCPCS

K ☑ **Q0187** Factor VIIa (coagulation factor, recombinant) per 1.2 mg
Use this code for NovoSeven.
MED: 100-2, 15, 50

B **Q1001** New technology intraocular lens category 1 as defined in Federal Register notice, Vol. 65, date May 3, 2000

B **Q1002** New technology intraocular lens category 2 as defined in Federal Register notice, Vol. 65, dated May 3, 2000

B **Q1003** New technology intraocular lens category 3 as defined in Federal Register notice

B **Q1004** New technology intraocular lens category 4 as defined in Federal Register notice

B **Q1005** New technology intraocular lens category 5 as defined in Federal Register notice

E ☑ **Q2001** Oral, cabergoline, 0.5 mg
Use this code for Dostinex.
MED: 100-2, 15, 50.5

N ☑ **Q2002** Injection, Elliott's B solution, per ml
Use this code for Dextrose/electsol, IV.
MED: 100-2, 15, 50

K ☑ **Q2003** Injection, aprotinin, 10,000 kiu
Use this code for Trasylol.
MED: 100-2, 15, 50

N ☑ **Q2004** Irrigation solution for treatment of bladder calculi, for example renacidin, per 500 ml
Use this code for Renacidin.
MED: 100-2, 15, 50

K ☑ **Q2005** Injection, corticorelin ovine triflutate, per dose
Use this code for Acthrel.
MED: 100-2, 15, 50

K ☑ **Q2006** Injection, digoxin immune fab (ovine), per vial
Use this code for Digibind.
MED: 100-2, 15, 50

K ☑ **Q2007** Injection, ethanolamine oleate, 100 mg
Use this code for Ethamolin.
MED: 100-2, 15, 50

K ☑ **Q2008** Injection, fomepizole, 15 mg
Use this code for Antizol.
MED: 100-2, 15, 50
AHA: 2Q, '02, 9

K ☑ **Q2009** Injection, fosphenytoin, 50 mg
Use this code for Cerebryx.
MED: 100-2, 15, 50

K ☑ **Q2011** Injection, hemin, per 1 mg
Use this code for Panhematin.
MED: 100-2, 15, 50

N ☑ **Q2012** Injection, pegademase bovine, 25 IU
Use this code for Adagen.
MED: 100-2, 15, 50

K ☑ **Q2013** Injection, Pentastarch, 10% solution, per 100 ml
Use this code for Pentaspan.
MED: 100-2, 15, 50

N ☑ **Q2014** Injection, sermorelin acetate, 0.5 mg
Use this code for Geref diagnostic.
MED: 100-2, 15, 50

K ☑ **Q2017** Injection, teniposide, 50 mg
Use this code for Vumon.
MED: 100-2, 15, 50

K ☑ **Q2018** Injection, urofollitropin, 75 IU
Use this code for Fertinex.
MED: 100-2, 15, 50

K ☑ **Q2019** Injection, basiliximab, 20 mg
Use this code for Simulect.
MED: 100-2, 15, 50

E ☑ **Q2020** Injection, histrelin acetate, 10 mg
Use this code for Supprelin.
MED: 100-2, 15, 50
AHA: 2Q, '02, 8

N ☑ **Q2021** Injection, lepirudin, 50 mg
Use this code for Refludan.
MED: 100-2, 15, 50

K ☑ **Q2022** Von Willebrand factor complex, human, per IU
MED: 100-2, 15, 50.5; 100-3, 110.8

K ☑ **Q3000** Supply of radiopharmaceutical diagnostic imaging agent, rubidium RB-82, per dose

N ☑ **Q3001** Radioelements for brachytherapy, any type, each
MED: 100-4, 12, 70; 100-4, 13, 20; 100-4, 13, 90

K ☑ **Q3002** Supply of radiopharmaceutical diagnostic imaging agent, gallium Ga-67, per millicurie
MED: 100-4, 12, 70; 100-4, 13, 20; 100-4, 13, 90
AHA: 2Q, '02, 9

K ☑ **Q3003** Supply of radiopharmaceutical diagnostic imaging agent, technetium Tc 99m bicisate, per unit dose
MED: 100-4, 12, 70; 100-4, 13, 20; 100-4, 13, 90

N ☑ **Q3004** Supply of radiopharmaceutical diagnostic imaging agent, xenon Xe-133, per 10 millicurie
MED: 100-4, 12, 70; 100-4, 13, 20; 100-4, 13, 90
AHA: 2Q, '02, 9

K ☑ **Q3005** Supply of radiopharmaceutical diagnostic imaging agent, technetium Tc 99m mertiatide, per millicurie
MED: 100-4, 12, 70; 100-4, 13, 20; 100-4, 13, 90
AHA: 2Q, '02, 9

N ☑ **Q3006** Supply of radiopharmaceutical diagnostic imaging agent, technetium Tc 99m glucepatate, per 5 millicurie
MED: 100-4, 12, 70; 100-4, 13, 20; 100-4, 13, 90
AHA: 2Q, '02, 9

K ☑ **Q3007** Supply of radiopharmaceutical diagnostic imaging agent, sodium phosphate P32, per millicurie
MED: 100-4, 12, 70; 100-4, 13, 20; 100-4, 13, 90
AHA: 2Q, '02, 9

K ☑ **Q3008** Supply of radiopharmaceutical diagnostic imaging agent, indium 111 – in pentetreotide, per 3 millicurie
MED: 100-4, 12, 70; 100-4, 13, 20; 100-4, 13, 90
AHA: 2Q, '02, 9

N ☑ **Q3009** Supply of radiopharmaceutical diagnostic imaging agent, technetium Tc 99m oxidronate, per millicurie
MED: 100-4, 12, 70; 100-4, 13, 20; 100-4, 13, 90
AHA: 2Q, '02, 9

| Special Coverage Instructions | Noncovered by Medicare | Carrier Discretion | ☑ Quantity Alert | ● New Code | ○ Reinstated Code | ▲ Revised Code |

2005 HCPCS   ♀ Female Only   ♂ Male Only   **1-9** ASC Groups   MED: Pub 100/NCD Reference   ১. DMEPOS Paid   ⊘ SNF Excluded   **Q Codes — 119**

Q Codes (Temporary)

Q3010 — Q4045

N ☑	**Q3010**	**Supply of radiopharmaceutical diagnostic imaging agent, technetium Tc 99m — labeled red blood cells, per millicurie** ⊘	
		MED: 100-4, 12, 70; 100-4, 13, 20; 100-4, 13, 90	
		AHA: 2Q, '02, 9	
K ☑	**Q3011**	**Supply of radiopharmaceutical diagnostic imaging agent, chromic phosphate P32 suspension, per millicurie** ⊘	
		MED: 100-4, 12, 70; 100-4, 13, 20; 100-4, 13, 90	
		AHA: 2Q, '02, 9	
K ☑	**Q3012**	**Supply of oral radiopharmaceutical diagnostic imaging agent, cyanocobalamin cobalt Co-57, per 0.5 millicurie** ⊘	
		MED: 100-4, 12, 70; 100-4, 13, 20; 100-4, 13, 90	
		AHA: 2Q, '02, 9	
A	**Q3014**	**Telehealth originating site facility fee** ⊘	
A	**Q3019**	**ALS vehicle used, emergency transport, no ALS level services furnished**	
A	**Q3020**	**ALS vehicle used, non-emergency transport, no ALS level service furnished**	
K	**Q3025**	**Injection, interferon beta-1A, 11 mcg for intramuscular use**	
		Use this code for Avonex. See also J1825.	
		MED: 100-2, 15, 50	
E	**Q3026**	**Injection, interferon beta-1A, 11 mcg for subcutaneous use**	
		Use this code for Avonex. See also J1825.	
N	**Q3031**	**Collagen skin test**	
		MED: 100-3, 230.10	
B	**Q4001**	**Casting supplies, body cast adult, with or without head, plaster**	A
B	**Q4002**	**Cast supplies, body cast adult, with or without head, fiberglass**	A
B	**Q4003**	**Cast supplies, shoulder cast, adult (11 years +), plaster**	A
B	**Q4004**	**Cast supplies, shoulder cast, adult (11 years +), fiberglass**	A
B	**Q4005**	**Cast supplies, long arm cast, adult (11 years +), plaster**	A
B	**Q4006**	**Cast supplies, long arm cast, adult (11 years +), fiberglass**	A
B	**Q4007**	**Cast supplies, long arm cast, pediatric (0-10 years), plaster**	P
B	**Q4008**	**Cast supplies, long arm cast, pediatric (0-10 years), fiberglass**	P
B	**Q4009**	**Cast supplies, short arm cast, adult (11 years +), plaster**	A
B	**Q4010**	**Cast supplies, short arm cast, adult (11 years +), fiberglass**	A
B	**Q4011**	**Cast supplies, short arm cast, pediatric (0-10 years), plaster**	P
B	**Q4012**	**Cast supplies, short arm cast, pediatric (0-10 years), fiberglass**	P
B	**Q4013**	**Cast supplies, gauntlet cast (includes lower forearm and hand), adult (11 years +), plaster**	A
B	**Q4014**	**Cast supplies, gauntlet cast (includes lower forearm and hand), adult (11 years +), fiberglass**	A
B	**Q4015**	**Cast supplies, gauntlet cast (includes lower forearm and hand), pediatric (0-10 years), plaster**	P

B	**Q4016**	**Cast supplies, gauntlet cast (includes lower forearm and hand), pediatric (0-10 years), fiberglass**	P
B	**Q4017**	**Cast supplies, long arm splint, adult (11 years +), plaster**	A
B	**Q4018**	**Cast supplies, long arm splint, adult (11 years +), fiberglass**	A
B	**Q4019**	**Cast supplies, long arm splint, pediatric (0-10 years), plaster**	P
B	**Q4020**	**Cast supplies, long arm splint, pediatric (0-10 years), fiberglass**	P
B	**Q4021**	**Cast supplies, short arm splint, adult (11 years +), plaster**	A
B	**Q4022**	**Cast supplies, short arm splint, adult (11 years +), fiberglass**	A
B	**Q4023**	**Cast supplies, short arm splint, pediatric (0-10 years), plaster**	P
B	**Q4024**	**Cast supplies, short arm splint, pediatric (0-10 years), fiberglass**	P
B	**Q4025**	**Cast supplies, hip spica (one or both legs), adult (11 years +), plaster**	A
B	**Q4026**	**Cast supplies, hip spica (one or both legs), adult (11 years +), fiberglass**	A
B	**Q4027**	**Cast supplies, hip spica (one or both legs), pediatric (0-10 years), plaster**	P
B	**Q4028**	**Cast supplies, hip spica (one or both legs), pediatric (0-10 years), fiberglass**	P
B	**Q4029**	**Cast supplies, long leg cast, adult (11 years +), plaster**	A
B	**Q4030**	**Cast supplies, long leg cast, adult (11 years +), fiberglass**	A
B	**Q4031**	**Cast supplies, long leg cast, pediatric (0-10 years), plaster**	P
B	**Q4032**	**Cast supplies, long leg cast, pediatric (0-10 years), fiberglass**	P
B	**Q4033**	**Cast supplies, long leg cylinder cast, adult (11 years +), plaster**	A
B	**Q4034**	**Cast supplies, long leg cylinder cast, adult (11 years +), fiberglass**	A
B	**Q4035**	**Cast supplies, long leg cylinder cast, pediatric (0-10 years), plaster**	P
B	**Q4036**	**Cast supplies, long leg cylinder cast, pediatric (0-10 years), fiberglass**	P
B	**Q4037**	**Cast supplies, short leg cast, adult (11 years +), plaster**	A
B	**Q4038**	**Cast supplies, short leg cast, adult (11 years +), fiberglass**	A
B	**Q4039**	**Cast supplies, short leg cast, pediatric (0-10 years), plaster**	P
B	**Q4040**	**Cast supplies, short leg cast, pediatric (0-10 years), fiberglass**	P
B	**Q4041**	**Cast supplies, long leg splint, adult (11 years +), plaster**	A
B	**Q4042**	**Cast supplies, long leg splint, adult (11 years +), fiberglass**	A
B	**Q4043**	**Cast supplies, long leg splint, pediatric (0-10 years), plaster**	P
B	**Q4044**	**Cast supplies, long leg splint, pediatric (0-10 years), fiberglass**	P
B	**Q4045**	**Cast supplies, short leg splint, adult (11 years +), plaster**	A

Special Coverage Instructions	Noncovered by Medicare	Carrier Discretion	☑ Quantity Alert ● New Code ○ Reinstated Code ▲ Revised Code

B		Q4046	Cast supplies, short leg splint, adult (11 years +), fiberglass A
B		Q4047	Cast supplies, short leg splint, pediatric (0-10 years), plaster P
B		Q4048	Cast supplies, short leg splint, pediatric (0-10 years), fiberglass P
B		Q4049	Finger splint, static
B		Q4050	Cast supplies, for unlisted types and materials of casts
B		Q4051	Splint supplies, miscellaneous (includes thermoplastics, strapping, fasteners, padding and other supplies)

● A ☑ **Q4054** Injection, darbepoetin alfa, 1 mcg (for ESRD on dialysis) ⊘
Use this code for Aranesp.

MED: 100-4, 8, 60.4.2; 100-4, 8, 60.4.2.1

AHA: 1Q, '04, 12

● A ☑ **Q4055** Injection, epoetin alfa, 1000 units (for ESRD on dialysis) ⊘
MED: 100-4, 8, 60.4.2; 100-4, 8, 60.4.2.1

AHA: 1Q, '04, 12

N ☑ **Q4075** Injection, acyclovir, 5 mg ⊘
AHA: 4Q, '03, 5

N ☑ **Q4076** Injection, dopamine HCl, 40 mg ⊘
AHA: 4Q, '03, 5

N ☑ **Q4077** Injection, treprostinil, 1 mg ⊘
AHA: 4Q, '03, 5

DIAGNOSTIC RADIOLOGY SERVICES *R0000–R5999*

R codes are used for the transportation of portable x-ray and/or EKG equipment.

R codes fall under the jurisdiction of the local carrier.

Ⓝ ☑ **R0070** **Transportation of portable x-ray equipment and personnel to home or nursing home, per trip to facility or location, one patient seen**
Only a single, reasonable transportation charge is allowed for each trip the portable x-ray supplier makes to a location. When more than one patient is x-rayed at the same location, prorate the single allowable transport charge among all patients.

MED: 100-2, 15, 80.4; 100-4, 13, 90; 100-4, 13, 90

Ⓝ ☑ **R0075** **Transportation of portable x-ray equipment and personnel to home or nursing home, per trip to facility or location, more than one patient seen**
Only a single, reasonable transportation charge is allowed for each trip the portable x-ray supplier makes to a location. When more than one patient is x-rayed at the same location, prorate the single allowable transport charge among all patients.

MED: 100-2, 15, 80.4; 100-4, 13, 90; 100-4, 13, 90

Ⓝ ☑ **R0076** **Transportation of portable EKG to facility or location, per patient** ⊘
Only a single, reasonable transportation charge is allowed for each trip the portable EKG supplier makes to a location. When more than one patient is tested at the same location, prorate the single allowable transport charge among all patients.

MED: 100-1, 5, 90.2; 100-2, 15, 80.1; 100-2, 15, 80.4; 100-3, 20.15; 100-4, 13, 90; 100-4, 16, 10; 100-4, 16, 10.1; 100-4, 16, 110.4

Special Coverage Instructions	Noncovered by Medicare	Carrier Discretion	☑ Quantity Alert	● New Code	○ Reinstated Code	▲ Revised Code
2005 HCPCS	♀ Female Only	♂ Male Only ❶-❾ ASC Groups MED: Pub 100/NCD Reference	ᕀ DMEPOS Paid	⊘ SNF Excluded	**R Codes — 123**	

TEMPORARY NATIONAL CODES (NON–MEDICARE)
S0000–S9999

The S codes are used by the Blue Cross/Blue Shield Association (BCBSA) and the Health Insurance Association of America (HIAA) to report drugs, services, and supplies for which there are no national codes but for which codes are needed by the private sector to implement policies, programs, or claims processing. They are for the purpose of meeting the particular needs of the private sector. These codes are also used by the Medicaid program, but they are not payable by Medicare.

E ☑ **S0012** **Butorphanol tartrate, nasal spray, 25 mg**
Use this code for Stadol NS.

E ☑ **S0014** **Tacrine HCl, 10 mg**
Use this code for Cognex.

E ☑ **S0016** **Injection, amikacin sulfate, 500 mg**
Use this code for Amikin.

E ☑ **S0017** **Injection, aminocaproic acid, 5 grams**
Use this code for Amicar.

E ☑ **S0020** **Injection, bupivacaine HCl, 30 ml**
Use this code for Marcaine, Sensorcaine.

E ☑ **S0021** **Injection, cefoperazone sodium, 1 gram**
Use this code for Cefobid.

E ☑ **S0023** **Injection, cimetidine HCl, 300 mg**
Use this code for Tagament HCl.

E ☑ **S0028** **Injection, famotidine, 20 mg**
Use this code for Pepcid.

E ☑ **S0030** **Injection, metronidazole, 500 mg**
Use this code for Flagyl IV RTU.

E ☑ **S0032** **Injection, nafcillin sodium, 2 grams**
Use this code for Nallpen, Unipen.

E ☑ **S0034** **Injection, ofloxacin, 400 mg**
Use this code for Floxin IV.

E ☑ **S0039** **Injection, sulfamethoxazole and trimethoprim, 10 ml**
Use this code for Bactrim IV, Septra IV, SMZ-TMP, Sulfutrim.

E ☑ **S0040** **Injection, ticarcillin disodium and clavulanate potassium, 3.1 grams**
Use this code for Timentin.

E ☑ **S0071** **Injection, acyclovir sodium, 50 mg**
Use this code for Zovirax.

E ☑ **S0072** **Injection, amikacin sulfate, 100 mg**
Use this code for Amikin.

E ☑ **S0073** **Injection, aztreonam, 500 mg**
Use this code for Azactam.

E ☑ **S0074** **Injection, cefotetan disodium, 500 mg**
Use this code for Cefotan.

E ☑ **S0077** **Injection, clindamycin phosphate, 300 mg**
Use this code for Cleocin Phosphate.

E ☑ **S0078** **Injection, fosphenytoin sodium, 750 mg**
Use this code for Cerebryx.

E ☑ **S0080** **Injection, pentamidine isethionate, 300 mg**
Use this code for NebuPent, Pentam 300, Pentacarinat. See also code J2545.

E ☑ **S0081** **Injection, piperacillin sodium, 500 mg**
Use this code for Pipracil.

E ☑ **S0088** **Imatinib 100 mg**
Use this code for Gleevec.

E ☑ **S0090** **Sildenafil citrate, 25 mg**   ▲
Use this code for Viagra.

E ☑ **S0091** **Granisetron hydrochloride, 1 mg (for circumstances falling under the Medicare statute, use Q0166)**
Use this code for Kytril.

E ☑ **S0092** **Injection, hydromorphone hydrochloride, 250 mg (loading dose for infusion pump)**
Use this code for Dilaudid. Hydromophone. See also J1170.

E ☑ **S0093** **Injection, morphine sulfate, 500 mg (loading dose for infusion pump)**
Use this code for Duramorph, MS Contin, Morphine Sulfate. See also J2270, J2271, J2275.

E **S0104** **Zidovudine, oral 100 mg**
See also J3485 for Retrovir.

E ☑ **S0106** **Bupropion HCl sustained release tablet, 150 mg, per bottle of 60 tablets**
Use this code for Wellbutrin SR tablets.

E ☑ **S0107** **Injection, omalizumab, 25 mg**

E **S0108** **Mercaptopurine, oral, 50 mg**
Use this code for Purinethol oral.

● E ☑ **S0109** **Methadone, oral, 5mg**

E **S0114** **Injection, treprostinil sodium, 0.5 mg**
Use this code for Remodulin. See also K0455.

~~S0115~~   ~~Bortezomib, 3.5 mg~~

● E ☑ **S0116** **Bevacizumab, 100 mg**

● E ☑ **S0117** **Tretinoin, topical 5 grams**

E **S0122** **Injection, menotropins, 75 IU**
Use this code for Humegon, Pergonal.

E **S0126** **Injection, follitropin alfa, 75 IU**
Use this code for Gonal-F.

E **S0128** **Injection, follitropin beta, 75 IU**   ♀
Use this code for Follistim.

E **S0132** **Injection, ganirelix acetate, 250 mcg**   ♀

E ☑ **S0136** **Clozapine, 25 mg**

E ☑ **S0137** **Didanosine (ddi), 25 mg**

E ☑ **S0138** **Finasteride, 5 mg**   ♂
Use this code for Propecia (oral), Proscar (oral).

E ☑ **S0139** **Minoxidil, 10 mg**
Use this code for Loniten (oral).

E ☑ **S0140** **Saquinavir, 200 mg**
Use this code for Fortovase (oral).

E ☑ **S0141** **Zalcitabine (DDC), 0.375 mg**
Use this code for Hivid (oral).

E ☑ **S0155** **Sterile dilutant for epoprostenol, 50 ml**
Use this code for Flolan.

E ☑ **S0156** **Exemestane, 25 mg**
Use this code for Aromasin.

E ☑ **S0157** **Becaplermin gel 0.01%, 0.5 gm**
Use this code for Regraex Gel.

● E ☑ **S0158** **Injection, laronidase, 0.58 mg**
Use this code for Aldurazyme.

● E ☑ **S0159** **Injection, agalsidase beta, 35 mg**
Use this code for Fabrazyme.

● E ☑ **S0160** **Dextroamphetamine sulfate, 5 mg**

● E ☑ **S0161** **Calcitrol, 0.25 mcg**

| Special Coverage Instructions | Noncovered by Medicare | Carrier Discretion | ☑ Quantity Alert | ● New Code | ○ Reinstated Code | ▲ Revised Code |

2005 HCPCS   ♀ Female Only   ♂ Male Only   **1-9** ASC Groups   MED: Pub 100/NCD Reference   ᕃ DMEPOS Paid   Ⓢ SNF Excluded   **S Codes — 125**

● E ☑ **S0162** Injection, efalizumab, 125 mg
Use this code for Raptiva.

~~**S0163** Injection, risperidone, long acting, 12.5 mg~~

● E ☑ **S0164** Injection, pantoprazole sodium, 40 mg
Use this code for Protonix IV.

~~**S0165** Injection, abarelix, 100 mg~~

● E ☑ **S0166** Injection, olanzapine, 2.5 mg
Use this code for Zyprexa.

● E ☑ **S0167** Injection, apomorphine hydrochloride, 1 mg

● E ☑ **S0168** Injection, azacitidine, 100 mg
Use this code for Vidaza.

E ☑ **S0170** Anastrozole, oral, 1mg
Use this code for Arimidex.

E ☑ **S0171** Injection, bumetanide, 0.5 mg
Use this code for Bumex.

E ☑ **S0172** Chlorambucil, oral, 2 mg
Use this code for Leukeran.

E ☑ **S0173** Dexamethasone, oral, 4 mg
Use this code for Decadron, Dexone, Hexadrol.

E ☑ **S0174** Dolasetron mesylate, oral 50 mg (for circumstances falling under the Medicare statute, use Q0180)
Use this code for Anzemet.

E ☑ **S0175** Flutamide, oral, 125 mg
Use this code for Eulexin.

E ☑ **S0176** Hydroxyurea, oral, 500 mg
Use this code for Droxia.

E ☑ **S0177** Levamisole HCl, oral, 50 mg
Use this code for Ergamisol.

E ☑ **S0178** Lomustine, oral, 10 mg
Use this code for Ceenu.

E ☑ **S0179** Megestrol acetate, oral, 20 mg
Use this code for Megace.

E ☑ **S0181** Ondansetron HCl, oral, 4 mg (for circumstances falling under the Medicare statute, use Q0179)
Use this code for Zofran.

E ☑ **S0182** Procarbazine HCl, oral, 50 mg
Use this code for Matulane.

E ☑ **S0183** Prochlorperazine maleate, oral, 5 mg (for circumstances falling under the Medicare statute, use Q0164-Q0165)
Use this code for Compazine.

E ☑ **S0187** Tamoxifen citrate, oral, 10 mg
Use this code for Nolvadex.

E ☑ **S0189** Testosterone pellet, 75 mg

E ☑ **S0190** Mitepristone, oral, 200 mg   ♀
Use this code for Mifoprex 200 mg oral.

E ☑ **S0191** Misoprostol, oral, 200 mcg

● E ☑ **S0194** Dialysis/stress vitamin supplement, oral, 100 capsules

E **S0195** Pneumococcal conjugate vaccine, polyvalent, intramuscular, for children from five years to nine years of age who have not previously received the vaccine   P
Use this code for Pneumovax II.

● ☑ **S0196** Injectable poly-l-lactic acid, restorative implant, 1 ml, face (deep dermis, subcutaneous layers)

E **S0199** Medically induced abortion by oral ingestion of medication including all associated services and supplies (e.g., patient counseling, office visits, confirmation of pregnancy by HCG, ultrasound to confirm duration of pregnancy, ultrasound to confirm completion of abortion) except drugs   ♀

E **S0201** Partial hospitalization services, less than 24 hours, per diem

E **S0207** Paramedic intercept, non-hospital based ALS service (non-voluntary), non-transport

E **S0208** Paramedic intercept, hospital-based ALS service (non-voluntary), non-transport

E **S0209** Wheelchair van, mileage, per mile

E **S0215** Non-emergency transportation; mileage, per mile
See also codes A0021-A0999 for transportation.

E **S0220** Medical conference by a physician with interdisciplinary team of health professionals or representatives of community agencies to coordinate activities of patient care (patient is present); approximately 30 minutes

E **S0221** Medical conference by a physician with interdisciplinary team of health professionals or representatives of community agencies to coordinate activities of patient care (patient is present); approximately 60 minutes

E **S0250** Comprehensive geriatric assessment and treatment planning performed by assessment team   A

E **S0255** Hospice referral visit (advising patient and family of care options) performed by nurse, social worker, or other designated staff

● **S0257** Counseling and discussion regarding advance directives or end of life care planning and decisions, with patient and/or surrogate (list separately in addition to code for appropriate evaluation and management service)

E **S0260** History and physical (outpatient or office) related to surgical procedure (list separately in addition to code for appropriate evaluation and management service)

E **S0302** Completed early periodic screening diagnosis and treatment (EPSDT) service (list in addition to code for appropriate evaluation and management service)

E **S0310** Hospitalist services (list separately in addition to code for appropriate evaluation and management service)

E **S0315** Disease management program; initial assessment and initiation of the program

E **S0316** Follow-up/reassessment

E ☑ **S0317** Disease management program; per diem

E **S0320** Telephone calls by a registered nurse to a disease management program member for monitoring purposes; per month

E **S0340** Lifestyle modification program for management of coronary artery disease, including all supportive services; first quarter/stage

E **S0341** Lifestyle modification program for management of coronary artery disease, including all supportive services; second or third quarter/stage

E **S0342** Lifestyle modification program for management of coronary artery disease, including all supportive services; fourth quarter/stage

---

Special Coverage Instructions   Noncovered by Medicare   Carrier Discretion   ☑ Quantity Alert   ● New Code   ○ Reinstated Code   ▲ Revised Code

126 — S Codes   A Adult   M Maternity   P Pediatrics   I Infant   A-V APC Status Indicator   **2005 HCPCS**

E		S0390	Routine foot care; removal and/or trimming of corns, calluses and/or nails and preventive maintenance in specific medical conditions (e.g., diabetes), per visit See also CPT code 11719-11721.
E		S0395	Impression casting of a foot performed by a practitioner other than the manufacturer of the orthotic
E		S0400	Global fee for extracorporeal shock wave lithotripsy treatment of kidney stone(s) See CPT code 50590.
E	☑	S0500	Disposable contact lens, per lens
E	☑	S0504	Single vision prescription lens (safety, athletic, or sunglass), per lens
E	☑	S0506	Bifocal vision prescription lens (safety, athletic, or sunglass), per lens
E	☑	S0508	Trifocal vision prescription lens (safety, athletic, or sunglass), per lens
E	☑	S0510	Non-prescription lens (safety, athletic, or sunglass), per lens
E	☑	S0512	Daily wear specialty contact lens, per lens
E	☑	S0514	Color contact lens, per lens
● E		S0515	Scleral lens, liquid bandage device, per lens
E		S0516	Safety eyeglass frames
E		S0518	Sunglasses frames
E		S0580	Polycarbonate lens (list this code in addition to the basic code for the lens)
E		S0581	Nonstandard lens (list this code in addition to the basic code for the lens)
E		S0590	Integral lens service, miscellaneous services reported separately
E		S0592	Comprehensive contact lens evaluation
E		S0601	Screening proctoscopy ♂
E		S0605	Digital rectal examination, annual
E		S0610	Annual gynecological examination; new patient ♀
E		S0612	Annual gynecological examination; established patient ♀
● E		S0618	Audiometry for hearing aid evaluation to determine the level and degree of hearing loss
E		S0620	Routine ophthalmological examination including refraction; new patient
E		S0621	Routine ophthalmological examination including refraction; established patient
E		S0622	Physical exam for college, new or established patient (list separately in addition to appropriate evaluation and management code) ◮A
E		S0630	Removal of sutures by a physician other than the physician who originally closed the wound
E		S0800	Laser in situ keratomileusis (LASIK)
E		S0810	Photorefractive keratectomy (PRK)
E		S0812	Phototherapeutic keratectomy (PTK)
E		S0820	Computerized corneal topography, unilateral
E		S1001	Deluxe item, patient aware (list in addition to code for basic item)
E		S1002	Customized item (list in addition to code for basic item)
E		S1015	IV tubing extension set
E		S1016	Non-PVC (polyvinylchloride) intravenous administration set, for use with drugs that are not stable in PVC e.g., Paclitaxel
E		S1025	Inhaled nitric oxide for the treatment of hypoxic respiratory failure in the neonate; per diem
E		S1030	Continuous noninvasive glucose monitoring device, purchase (for physician interpretation of data, use CPT code)
E		S1031	Continuous noninvasive glucose monitoring device, rental, including sensor, sensor replacement, and download to monitor (for physician interpretation of data, use CPT code)
E		S1040	Cranial remolding orthosis, rigid, with soft interface material, custom fabricated, includes fitting and adjustment(s)
E		S2053	Transplantation of small intestine, and liver allografts
E		S2054	Transplantation of multivisceral organs
E		S2055	Harvesting of donor multivisceral organs, with preparation and maintenance of allografts; from cadaver donor
E		S2060	Lobar lung transplantation
E		S2061	Donor lobectomy (lung) for transplantation, living donor
E		S2065	Simultaneous pancreas kidney transplantation
E		S2070	Cystourethroscopy, with ureteroscopy and/or pyeloscopy; with endoscopic laser treatment of ureteral calculi (includes ureteral catheterization)
E		S2080	Laser-assisted uvulopalatoplasty (LAUP)
● E		S2082	Laparoscopy, surgical; gastric restrictive procedure, adjustable gastric band includes placement of subcutaneous port
● E		S2083	Adjustment of gastric band diameter via subcutanous port by injection or aspiration of saline
		S2085	~~Laparoscopy, gastric restrictive procedure, with gastric bypass for morbid obesity, with short limb (less than 100 cm) roux en y gastroenterostomy~~
E		S2090	Ablation, open, one or more renal tumor(s); cryosurgical
E		S2091	Ablation, percutaneous, one or more renal tumor(s); cryosurgical
E		S2095	Transcatheter occlusion or embolization for tumor destruction, percutaneous, any method, using yttrium 90 microspheres
E		S2102	Islet cell tissue transplant from pancreas; allogeneic
E		S2103	Adrenal tissue transplant to brain

Esophagus · Gastroesophageal sphincter · Diaphragm · Stomach · Duodenum

Esophagus · Diaphragm · Fundus · Adjustable gastric band

Special Coverage Instructions	Noncovered by Medicare	Carrier Discretion	☑ Quantity Alert	● New Code	○ Reinstated Code	▲ Revised Code

Temporary National Codes (Non–Medicare)

S2107 — S2370

E   **S2107**   Adoptive immunotherapy, i.e., development of specific anti-tumor reactivity (e.g., tumor-infiltrating lymphocyte therapy) per course of treatment

E   **S2112**   Arthroscopy, knee, surgical for harvesting of cartilage (chondrocyte cells)

~~S2113 Arthroscopy, knee, surgical for implantation of cultured analogous chondrocytes~~

E   **S2115**   Osteotomy, periacetabular, with internal fixation

E   **S2120**   Low density lipoprotein (LDL) apheresis using heparin-induced extracorporeal LDL precipitation

~~S2130 Endoluminal radiofrequency ablation of refluxing saphenous vein~~

~~S2131 Endovascular laser ablation of long or short saphenous vein, with or without proximal ligation or division~~

E   **S2135**   Neurolysis, by injection, of metatarsal neuroma/interdigital neuritis, any interspace of the foot

E   **S2140**   Cord blood harvesting for transplantation, allogeneic

E   **S2142**   Cord blood-derived stem-cell transplantation, allogeneic

▲ E   **S2150**   Bone marrow or blood-derived stem cells (peripheral or umbilical), allogeneic or autologous, harvesting, transplantation, and related complications; including: pheresis and cell preparation/storage; marrow ablative therapy; drugs, supplies, hospitalization with outpatient follow-up; medical/surgical, diagnostic, emergency, and rehabilitative services; and the number of days of pre-and post-transplant care in the global definition

● E   **S2152**   Solid organ(s), complete or segmental, single organ or combination of organs; deceased or living donor(s), procurement, transplantation, and related complications including: drugs; supplies; hospitalization with outpatient follow-up; medical/surgical, diagnostic, emergency, and rehabilitative services; and the number of days of pre- and post-transplant care in the global definition

E   **S2202**   Echosclerotherapy

E   **S2205**   Minimally invasive direct coronary artery bypass surgery involving mini-thoracotomy or mini-sternotomy surgery, performed under direct vision; using arterial graft(s), single coronary arterial graft

E   **S2206**   Minimally invasive direct coronary artery bypass surgery involving mini-thoracotomy or mini-sternotomy surgery, performed under direct vision; using arterial graft(s), two coronary arterial grafts

E   **S2207**   Minimally invasive direct coronary artery bypass surgery involving mini-thoracotomy or mini-sternotomy surgery, performed under direct vision; using venous graft only, single coronary venous graft

E   **S2208**   Minimally invasive direct coronary artery bypass surgery involving mini-thoracotomy or mini-sternotomy surgery, performed under direct vision; using single arterial and venous graft(s), single venous graft

E   **S2209**   Minimally invasive direct coronary artery bypass surgery involving mini-thoracotomy or mini-sternotomy surgery, performed under direct vision; using two arterial grafts and single venous graft

~~S2211 Transcatheter placement of intravascular stent(s), carotid artery, percutaneous, unilateral (if performed bilaterally, use 50 modifier)~~

E   **S2213**   Implantation of gastric electrical stimulation device

● E   **S2215**   Upper gastrointestinal endoscopy, including esophagus, stomach, and either the duodenum and/or jejunum as appropriate; with injection of implant material into and along the muscle of the lower esophageal sphincter for treatment of gastroesophageal reflux disease

E   **S2225**   Myringotomy, laser-assisted

E   **S2230**   Implantation of magnetic component of semi-implantable hearing device on ossicles in middle ear

E   **S2235**   Implantation of auditory brain stem implant

E   **S2250**   Uterine artery embolization for uterine fibroids   A ♀

~~S2255 Hysteroscopy, surgical; with occlusion of oviducts bilaterally by micro inserts for permanent sterilization~~

E   **S2260**   Induced abortion, 17 to 24 weeks, any surgical method   M ♀

E   **S2262**   Abortion for maternal indication, 25 weeks or greater   M ♀

E   **S2265**   Abortion for fetal indication, 25-28 weeks   M ♀

E   **S2266**   Abortion for fetal indication, 29-31 weeks   M ♀

E   **S2267**   Abortion for fetal indication, 32 weeks or greater   M ♀

E   **S2300**   Arthroscopy, shoulder, surgical; with thermally-induced capsulorrhaphy

E   **S2340**   Chemodenervation of abductor muscle(s) of vocal cord

E   **S2341**   Chemodenervation of adductor muscle(s) of vocal cord

E   **S2342**   Nasal endoscopy for post-operative debridement following functional endoscopic sinus surgery, nasal and/or sinus cavity(s), unilateral or bilateral

●   **S2348**   Decompression procedure, percutaneous, of nucleus pulposus of intervertebral disc, using radiofrequency energy, single or multiple levels, lumbar

E   **S2350**   Diskectomy, anterior, with decompression of spinal cord and/or nerve root(s), including osteophytectomy; lumbar, single interspace

E   **S2351**   Diskectomy, anterior, with decompression of spinal cord and/or nerve root(s), including osteophytectomy; lumbar, each additional interspace (list separately in addition to code for primary procedure)

E   **S2360**   Percutaneous vertebroplasty, one vertebral body, unilateral or bilateral injection; cervical

E   **S2361**   Each additional cervical vertebral body (list separately in addition to code for primary procedure)

E   **S2362**   Kyphoplasty, one vertebral body, unilateral or bilateral injection

E ☑   **S2363**   Kyphoplasty, one vertebral body, unilateral or bilateral injection; each additional vertebral body (list separately in addition to code for primary procedure)

E   **S2370**   Intradiscal electrothermal therapy, single interspace

Special Coverage Instructions   Noncovered by Medicare   Carrier Discretion   ☑ Quantity Alert   ● New Code   ○ Reinstated Code   ▲ Revised Code

128 — S Codes   A Adult   M Maternity   P Pediatrics   I Infant   A-Y APC Status Indicator   *2005 HCPCS*

E	☑	**S2371**	Each additional interspace (list separately in addition to code for primary procedure)
E		**S2400**	Repair, congenital diaphragmatic hernia in the fetus using temporary tracheal occlusion, procedure performed in utero ⓜ ♀ Repair, congenital diaphragmatic hernia in the fetus using temporary tracheal occlusion, procedure performed in utero.
E		**S2401**	Repair, urinary tract obstruction in the fetus, procedure performed in utero ⓜ ♀
E		**S2402**	Repair, congenital cystic adenomatoid malformation in the fetus, procedure performed in utero ⓜ ♀
E		**S2403**	Repair, extralobar pulmonary sequestration in the fetus, procedure performed in utero ⓜ ♀
E		**S2404**	Repair, myelomeningocele in the fetus, procedure performed in utero ⓜ ♀
E		**S2405**	Repair of sacrococcygeal teratoma in the fetus, procedure performed in utero ⓜ ♀
E		**S2409**	Repair, congenital malformation of fetus, procedure performed in utero, not otherwise classified ⓜ ♀
E		**S2411**	Fetoscopic laser therapy for treatment of twin-to-twin transfusion syndrome ⓜ ♀
E		**S3000**	Diabetic indicator; retinal eye exam, dilated, bilateral
E		**S3600**	STAT laboratory request (situations other than S3601)
E		**S3601**	Emergency STAT laboratory charge for patient who is homebound or residing in a nursing facility
E	☑	**S3620**	Newborn metabolic screening panel, includes test kit, postage and the laboratory tests specified by the state for inclusion in this panel (e.g., galactose; hemoglobin, electrophoresis; hydroxyprogesterone, 17-d; phenylanine (PKU); and thyroxine, total) Ⓟ
E		**S3625**	Maternal serum triple marker screen including alpha-fetoprotein (AFP), estriol, and human chorionic gonadotropin (hcG) ⓜ ♀
E		**S3630**	Eosinophil count, blood, direct
E		**S3645**	HIV-1 antibody testing of oral mucosal transudate
E		**S3650**	Saliva test, hormone level; during menopause Ⓐ ♀
E		**S3652**	Saliva test, hormone level; to assess preterm labor risk ⓜ ♀
E		**S3655**	Antisperm antibodies test (immunobead) Ⓐ ♀
E		**S3701**	Immunoassay for nuclear matrix protein 22 (NMP-22), quantitative
E		**S3708**	Gastrointestinal fat absorption study
E		**S3818**	Complete gene sequence analysis; BRCA 1 gene
E		**S3819**	Complete gene sequence analysis; BRCA 2 gene
E		**S3820**	Complete BRCA 1 and BRCA 2 gene sequence analysis for susceptibility to breast and ovarian cancer ♀
E		**S3822**	Single mutation analysis (in individual with a known BRCA 1 or BRCA 2 mutation in the family) for susceptibility to breast and ovarian cancer ♀
E		**S3823**	Three-mutation BRCA 1 and BRCA 2 analysis for susceptibility to breast and ovarian cancer in Ashkenazi individuals ♀
E		**S3828**	Complete gene sequence analysis; MLH 1 gene
E		**S3829**	Complete gene sequence analysis; MLH 2 gene
E		**S3830**	Complete MLH 1 and MLH 2 gene sequence analysis for hereditary nonpolyposis colorectal cancer (HNPCC) genetic testing
E		**S3831**	Single-mutation analysis (in individual with a known MLH 1 and MLH 2 mutation in the family) for hereditary nonpolyposis colorectal cancer (HNPCC) genetic testing
E		**S3833**	Complete APC gene sequence analysis for susceptibility to familial adenomatous polyposis (FAP) and attenuated FAP
E		**S3834**	Single-mutation analysis (in individual with a known APC mutation in the family) for susceptibility to familial adenomatous polyposis (FAP) and attenuated FAP
E		**S3835**	Complete gene sequence analysis for cystic fibrosis genetic testing
E		**S3837**	Complete gene sequence analysis for hemochromatosis genetic testing
E		**S3840**	DNA analysis for germline mutations of the RET proto-oncogene for susceptibility to multiple endocrine neoplasia type 2
E		**S3841**	Genetic testing for retinoblastoma
E		**S3842**	Genetic testing for Von Hippel-Lindau disease
E		**S3843**	DNA analysis of the F5 gene for susceptibility to factor V Leiden thrombophilia
E		**S3844**	DNA analysis of the connexin 26 gene (GJB2) for susceptibility to congenital, profound deafness
E		**S3845**	Genetic testing for alpha-thalassemia
E		**S3846**	Genetic testing for hemoglobin E beta-thalassemia
E		**S3847**	Genetic testing for Tay-Sachs disease
E		**S3848**	Genetic testing for Gaucher disease
E		**S3849**	Genetic testing for Niemann-Pick disease
E		**S3850**	Genetic testing for sickle cell anemia
E		**S3851**	Genetic testing for Canavan disease
E		**S3852**	DNA analysis for APOE epilson 4 allele for susceptibility to Alzheimer's disease
E		**S3853**	Genetic testing for myotonic muscular dystrophy
● E		**S3890**	DNA analysis, fecal, for colorectal cancer screening
E		**S3900**	Surface electromyography (EMG)
E		**S3902**	Ballistocardiogram
E		**S3904**	Masters two step
E		**S4005**	Interim labor facility global (labor occurring but not resulting in delivery) ⓜ ♀
E		**S4011**	In vitro fertilization; including but not limited to identification and incubation of mature oocytes, fertilization with sperm, incubation of embryo(s), and subsequent visualization for determination of development ⓜ ♀
E		**S4013**	Complete cycle, gamete intrafallopian transfer (GIFT), case rate ⓜ ♀
E		**S4014**	Complete cycle, zygote intrafallopian transfer (ZIFT), case rate ⓜ ♀
E		**S4015**	Complete in vitro fertilization cycle, not otherwise specified, case rate ⓜ ♀
E		**S4016**	Frozen in vitro fertilization cycle, case rate ♀
E		**S4017**	Incomplete cycle, treatment canceled prior to stimulation, case rate ♀
E		**S4018**	Frozen embryo transfer procedure canceled before transfer, case rate ♀
E		**S4020**	In vitro fertilization procedure canceled before aspiration, case rate ♀

Special Coverage Instructions � Noncovered by Medicare ▢ Carrier Discretion ☑ Quantity Alert ● New Code ○ Reinstated Code ▲ Revised Code

2005 HCPCS ♀ Female Only ♂ Male Only **1-9** ASC Groups **MED:** Pub 100/NCD Reference ⅋ DMEPOS Paid ⊘ SNF Excluded **S Codes — 129**

Ⓔ		S4021	In vitro fertilization procedure canceled after aspiration, case rate ♀
Ⓔ		S4022	Assisted oocyte fertilization, case rate ♀
Ⓔ		S4023	Donor egg cycle, incomplete, case rate ♀
Ⓔ		S4025	Donor services for in vitro fertilization (sperm or embryo), case rate Ⓐ
Ⓔ		S4026	Procurement of donor sperm from sperm bank Ⓐ
Ⓔ		S4027	Storage of previously frozen embryos
Ⓔ		S4028	Microsurgical epididymal sperm aspiration (MESA) Ⓐ♂
Ⓔ		S4030	Sperm procurement and cryopreservation services; initial visit Ⓐ♂
Ⓔ		S4031	Sperm procurement and cryopreservation services; subsequent visit Ⓐ♂
Ⓔ		S4035	Stimulated intrauterine insemination (IUI), case rate ♀
Ⓔ		S4036	Intravaginal culture (IVC), case rate ♀
Ⓔ		S4037	Cryopreserved embryo transfer, case rate ♀
Ⓔ		S4040	Monitoring and storage of cryopreserved embryos, per 30 days
●		S4042	Management of ovulation induction (interpretation of diagnostic tests and studies, non-face-to-face medical management of the patient), per cycle
Ⓔ		S4981	Insertion of levonorgestrel-releasing intrauterine system ♀
Ⓔ		S4989	Contraceptive intrauterine device (e.g., Progestacert IUD), including implants and supplies ♀
Ⓔ	☑	S4990	Nicotine patches, legend
Ⓔ	☑	S4991	Nicotine patches, non-legend
Ⓔ		S4993	Contraceptive pills for birth control ♀
Ⓔ		S4995	Smoking cessation gum
Ⓔ	☑	S5000	Prescription drug, generic
Ⓔ	☑	S5001	Prescription drug, brand name
Ⓔ	☑	S5010	5% dextrose and 45% normal saline, 1000 ml
Ⓔ	☑	S5011	5% dextrose in lactated ringer's, 1000 ml
Ⓔ	☑	S5012	5% dextrose with potassium chloride, 1000 ml
Ⓔ	☑	S5013	5% dextrose/45% normal saline with potassium chloride and magnesium sulfate, 1000 ml
Ⓔ	☑	S5014	5% dextrose/0.45% normal saline with potassium chloride and magnesium sulfate, 1500 ml
Ⓔ		S5035	Home infusion therapy, routine service of infusion device (e.g., pump maintenance)
Ⓔ		S5036	Home infusion therapy, repair of infusion device (e.g., pump repair)
Ⓔ		S5100	Day care services, adult; per 15 minutes Ⓐ
Ⓔ		S5101	Day care services, adult; per half day Ⓐ
Ⓔ		S5102	Day care services, adult; per diem Ⓐ
Ⓔ		S5105	Day care services, center-based; services not included in program fee, per diem
Ⓔ	☑	S5108	Home care training to home care client, per 15 minutes
Ⓔ	☑	S5109	Home care training to home care client, per session
Ⓔ		S5110	Home care training, family; per 15 minutes
Ⓔ		S5111	Home care training, family; per session
Ⓔ		S5115	Home care training, non-family; per 15 minutes
Ⓔ		S5116	Home care training, non-family; per session
Ⓔ		S5120	Chore services; per 15 minutes
Ⓔ		S5121	Chore services; per diem
Ⓔ		S5125	Attendant care services; per 15 minutes
Ⓔ		S5126	Attendant care services; per diem
Ⓔ		S5130	Homemaker service, NOS; per 15 minutes
Ⓔ		S5131	Homemaker service, NOS; per diem
Ⓔ		S5135	Companion care, adult (e.g., IADL/ADL); per 15 minutes Ⓐ
Ⓔ		S5136	Companion care, adult (e.g., IADL/ADL); per diem Ⓐ
Ⓔ		S5140	Foster care, adult; per diem Ⓐ
Ⓔ		S5141	Foster care, adult; per month Ⓐ
Ⓔ		S5145	Foster care, therapeutic, child; per diem Ⓟ
Ⓔ		S5146	Foster care, therapeutic, child; per month Ⓟ
Ⓔ		S5150	Unskilled respite care, not hospice; per 15 minutes
Ⓔ		S5151	Unskilled respite care, not hospice; per diem
Ⓔ		S5160	Emergency response system; installation and testing
Ⓔ		S5161	Emergency response system; service fee, per month (excludes installation and testing)
Ⓔ		S5162	Emergency response system; purchase only
Ⓔ		S5165	Home modifications; per service
Ⓔ		S5170	Home delivered meals, including preparation; per meal
Ⓔ		S5175	Laundry service, external, professional; per order
Ⓔ		S5180	Home health respiratory therapy, initial evaluation
Ⓔ		S5181	Home health respiratory therapy, NOS, per diem
Ⓔ		S5185	Medication reminder services, non-face-to-face; per month
Ⓔ		S5190	Wellness assessment, performed by nonphysician
Ⓔ		S5199	Personal care item, NOS, each
Ⓔ		S5497	Home infusion therapy, catheter care/maintenance, not otherwise classified; includes administrative services, professional pharmacy services, care coordination, and all necessary supplies and equipment (drugs and nursing visits coded separately), per diem
Ⓔ		S5498	Home infusion therapy, catheter care/maintenance, simple (single lumen), includes administrative services, professional pharmacy services, care coordination and all necessary supplies and equipment, (drugs and nursing visits coded separately), per diem
Ⓔ		S5501	Home infusion therapy, catheter care/maintenance, complex (more than one lumen), includes administrative services, professional pharmacy services, care coordination, and all necessary supplies and equipment (drugs and nursing visits coded separately), per diem
Ⓔ		S5502	Home infusion therapy, catheter care/maintenance, implanted access device, includes administrative services, professional pharmacy services, care coordination and all necessary supplies and equipment, (drugs and nursing visits coded separately), per diem (use this code for interim maintenance of vascular access not currently in use)
Ⓔ		S5517	Home infusion therapy, all supplies necessary for restoration of catheter patency or declotting

---

Special Coverage Instructions   Noncovered by Medicare   Carrier Discretion   ☑ Quantity Alert   ● New Code   ○ Reinstated Code   ▲ Revised Code

130 — S Codes   Ⓐ Adult   Ⓜ Maternity   Ⓟ Pediatrics   Ⓘ Infant   Ⓐ-Ⓨ APC Status Indicator   *2005 HCPCS*

E		**S5518**	Home infusion therapy, all supplies necessary for catheter repair
E		**S5520**	Home infusion therapy, all supplies (including catheter) necessary for a peripherally inserted central venous catheter (PICC) line insertion
E		**S5521**	Home infusion therapy, all supplies (including catheter) necessary for a midline catheter insertion
E		**S5522**	Home infusion therapy, insertion of peripherally inserted central venous catheter (PICC), nursing services only (no supplies or catheter included)
E		**S5523**	Home infusion therapy, insertion of midline central venous catheter, nursing services only (no supplies or catheter included)
E	☑	**S5550**	Insulin, rapid onset, 5 units
E	☑	**S5551**	Insulin, most rapid onset (Lispro or Aspart); 5 units
E	☑	**S5552**	Insulin, intermediate acting (NPH or LENTE); 5 units
E	☑	**S5553**	Insulin, long acting; 5 units
E	☑	**S5560**	Insulin delivery device, reusable pen; 1.5 ml size
E	☑	**S5561**	Insulin delivery device, reusable pen; 3 ml size
E	☑	**S5565**	Insulin cartridge for use in insulin delivery device other than pump; 150 units
E	☑	**S5566**	Insulin cartridge for use in insulin delivery device other than pump; 300 units
E	☑	**S5570**	Insulin delivery device, disposable pen (including insulin); 1.5 ml size
E	☑	**S5571**	Insulin delivery device, disposable pen (including insulin); 3 ml size
E		**S8004**	Radioimmunopharmaceutical localization of targeted cells; whole body
E		**S8030**	Scleral application of tantalum ring(s) for localization of lesions for proton beam therapy
E		**S8035**	Magnetic source imaging
E		**S8037**	Magnetic resonance cholangiopancreatography (MRCP)
E		**S8040**	Topographic brain mapping
E		**S8042**	Magnetic resonance imaging (MRI), low-field
E		**S8049**	Intraoperative radiation therapy (single administration)
E		**S8055**	Ultrasound guidance for multifetal pregnancy reduction(s), technical component (only to be used when the physician doing the reduction procedure does not perform the ultrasound. Guidance is included in the CPT code for multifetal pregnancy reduction - 59866) M ♀
E		**S8075**	Computer analysis of full-field digital mammogram and further physician review for interpretation, mammography (list separately in addition to code for primary procedure)
E		**S8080**	Scintimammography (radioimmunoscintigraphy of the breast), unilateral, including supply of radiopharmaceutical
E		**S8085**	Fluorine-18 fluorodeoxyglucose (F-18 FDG) imaging using dual-head coincidence detection system (non-dedicated PET scan)
E		**S8092**	Electron beam computed tomography (also known as Ultrafast CT, Cine CT)
● E		**S8093**	Computed tomographic angiography, coronary arteries, with contrast material(s)
E		**S8095**	Wig (for medically-induced or congenital hair loss)

E		**S8096**	Portable peak flow meter
E	☑	**S8097**	Asthma kit (including but not limited to portable peak expiratory flow meter, instructional video, brochure, and/or spacer)
E		**S8100**	Holding chamber or spacer for use with an inhaler or nebulizer; without mask
E		**S8101**	Holding chamber or spacer for use with an inhaler or nebulizer; with mask
E		**S8110**	Peak expiratory flow rate (physician services)
E	☑	**S8120**	Oxygen contents, gaseous, 1 unit equals 1 cubic foot
E	☑	**S8121**	Oxygen contents, liquid, 1 unit equals 1 pound
		~~S8182~~	~~Humidifier, heated, used with ventilator, non-servo controlled~~
		~~S8183~~	~~Humidifier, heated, used with ventilator, dual-servo controlled with temperature monitoring~~
E		**S8185**	Flutter device
E		**S8186**	Swivel adaptor
E	☑	**S8189**	Tracheostomy supply, not otherwise classified
E		**S8190**	Electronic spirometer (or microspirometer)
E		**S8210**	Mucus trap
E		**S8260**	Oral orthotic for treatment of sleep apnea, includes fitting, fabrication, and materials
E		**S8262**	Mandibular orthopedic repositioning device, each
E		**S8265**	Haberman Feeder for cleft lip/palate
● E		**S8301**	Infection control supplies, not otherwise specified
E	☑	**S8415**	Supplies for home delivery of infant M ♀
E		**S8420**	Gradient pressure aid (sleeve and glove combination), custom made
E	☑	**S8421**	Gradient pressure aid (sleeve and glove combination), ready made
E	☑	**S8422**	Gradient pressure aid (sleeve), custom made, medium weight
E	☑	**S8423**	Gradient pressure aid (sleeve), custom made, heavy weight
E	☑	**S8424**	Gradient pressure aid (sleeve), ready made
E	☑	**S8425**	Gradient pressure aid (glove), custom made, medium weight
E	☑	**S8426**	Gradient pressure aid (glove), custom made, heavy weight
E	☑	**S8427**	Gradient pressure aid (glove), ready made
E	☑	**S8428**	Gradient pressure aid (gauntlet), ready made
E	☑	**S8429**	Gradient pressure exterior wrap
E	☑	**S8430**	Padding for compression bandage, roll
E	☑	**S8431**	Compression bandage, roll
E	☑	**S8450**	Splint, prefabricated, digit (specify digit by use of modifier)
E	☑	**S8451**	Splint, prefabricated, wrist or ankle
E	☑	**S8452**	Splint, prefabricated, elbow
E		**S8460**	Camisole, postmastectomy
E	☑	**S8490**	Insulin syringes (100 syringes, any size)
E	☑	**S8948**	Application of a modality (requiring constant provider attendance) to one or more areas; low-level laser; each 15 minutes
E		**S8950**	Complex lymphedema therapy, each 15 minutes
E		**S8990**	Physical or manipulative therapy performed for maintenance rather than restoration

Special Coverage Instructions   Noncovered by Medicare   Carrier Discretion   ☑ Quantity Alert   ● New Code   ○ Reinstated Code   ▲ Revised Code

2005 HCPCS   ♀ Female Only   ♂ Male Only   **1**-**9** ASC Groups   **MED:** Pub 100/NCD Reference   ᕁ DMEPOS Paid   Ⓢ SNF Excluded   **S Codes — 131**

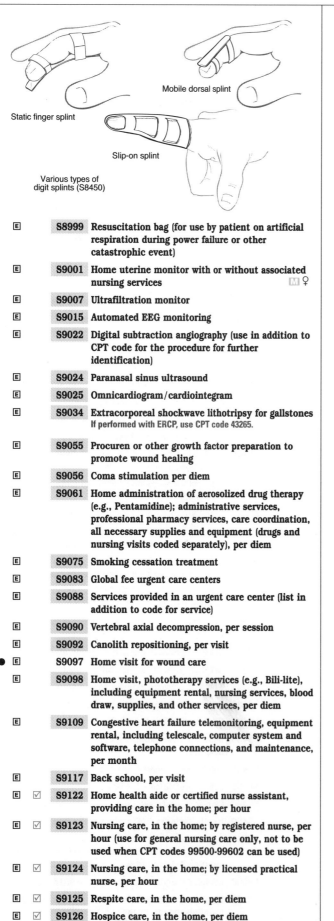

Static finger splint

Mobile dorsal splint

Slip-on splint

Various types of
digit splints (S8450)

E　**S8999**　Resuscitation bag (for use by patient on artificial respiration during power failure or other catastrophic event)

E　**S9001**　Home uterine monitor with or without associated nursing services　Ⓜ ♀

E　**S9007**　Ultrafiltration monitor

E　**S9015**　Automated EEG monitoring

E　**S9022**　Digital subtraction angiography (use in addition to CPT code for the procedure for further identification)

E　**S9024**　Paranasal sinus ultrasound

E　**S9025**　Omnicardiogram/cardiointegram

E　**S9034**　Extracorporeal shockwave lithotripsy for gallstones
If performed with ERCP, use CPT code 43265.

E　**S9055**　Procuren or other growth factor preparation to promote wound healing

E　**S9056**　Coma stimulation per diem

E　**S9061**　Home administration of aerosolized drug therapy (e.g., Pentamidine); administrative services, professional pharmacy services, care coordination, all necessary supplies and equipment (drugs and nursing visits coded separately), per diem

E　**S9075**　Smoking cessation treatment

E　**S9083**　Global fee urgent care centers

E　**S9088**　Services provided in an urgent care center (list in addition to code for service)

E　**S9090**　Vertebral axial decompression, per session

E　**S9092**　Canolith repositioning, per visit

● E　**S9097**　Home visit for wound care

E　**S9098**　Home visit, phototherapy services (e.g., Bili-lite), including equipment rental, nursing services, blood draw, supplies, and other services, per diem

E　**S9109**　Congestive heart failure telemonitoring, equipment rental, including telescale, computer system and software, telephone connections, and maintenance, per month

E　**S9117**　Back school, per visit

E ☑　**S9122**　Home health aide or certified nurse assistant, providing care in the home; per hour

E ☑　**S9123**　Nursing care, in the home; by registered nurse, per hour (use for general nursing care only, not to be used when CPT codes 99500-99602 can be used)

E ☑　**S9124**　Nursing care, in the home; by licensed practical nurse, per hour

E ☑　**S9125**　Respite care, in the home, per diem

E ☑　**S9126**　Hospice care, in the home, per diem

E ☑　**S9127**　Social work visit, in the home, per diem

E ☑　**S9128**　Speech therapy, in the home, per diem

E ☑　**S9129**　Occupational therapy, in the home, per diem

E　**S9131**　Physical therapy; in the home, per diem

E ☑　**S9140**　Diabetic management program, follow-up visit to non-MD provider

E ☑　**S9141**　Diabetic management program, follow-up visit to MD provider

E　**S9145**　Insulin pump initiation, instruction in initial use of pump (pump not included)

E　**S9150**　Evaluation by ocularist

E　**S9208**　Home management of preterm labor, including administrative services, professional pharmacy services, care coordination, and all necessary supplies or equipment (drugs and nursing visits coded separately), per diem (do not use this code with any home infusion per diem code)　Ⓜ ♀

E　**S9209**　Home management of preterm premature rupture of membranes (PPROM), including administrative services, professional pharmacy services, care coordination, and all necessary supplies or equipment (drugs and nursing visits coded separately), per diem (do not use this code with any home infusion per diem code)　Ⓜ ♀

E　**S9211**　Home management of gestational hypertension, includes administrative services, professional pharmacy services, care coordination and all necessary supplies and equipment (drugs and nursing visits coded separately); per diem (do not use this code with any home infusion per diem code)　Ⓜ ♀

E　**S9212**　Home management of postpartum hypertension, includes administrative services, professional pharmacy services, care coordination, and all necessary supplies and equipment (drugs and nursing visits coded separately), per diem (do not use this code with any home infusion per diem code)　♀

E　**S9213**　Home management of preeclampsia, includes administrative services, professional pharmacy services, care coordination, and all necessary supplies and equipment (drugs and nursing services coded separately); per diem (do not use this code with any home infusion per diem code)　Ⓜ ♀

E　**S9214**　Home management of gestational diabetes, includes administrative services, professional pharmacy services, care coordination, and all necessary supplies and equipment (drugs and nursing visits coded separately); per diem (do not use this code with any home infusion per diem code)　Ⓜ ♀

E　**S9325**　Home infusion therapy, pain management infusion; administrative services, professional pharmacy services, care coordination, and all necessary supplies and equipment, (drugs and nursing visits coded separately), per diem (do not use this code with S9326, S9327 or S9328)

E　**S9326**　Home infusion therapy, continuous (24 hours or more) pain management infusion; administrative services, professional pharmacy services, care coordination and all necessary supplies and equipment (drugs and nursing visits coded separately), per diem

Special Coverage Instructions　　Noncovered by Medicare　　Carrier Discretion　　☑ Quantity Alert　● New Code　○ Reinstated Code　▲ Revised Code

132 — S Codes　Ⓐ Adult　Ⓜ Maternity　Ⓟ Pediatrics　Ⓘ Infant　Ⓐ-Ⓨ APC Status Indicator　***2005 HCPCS***

E   **S9327** Home infusion therapy, intermittent (less than 24 hours) pain management infusion; administrative services, professional pharmacy services, care coordination, and all necessary supplies and equipment (drugs and nursing visits coded separately), per diem

E   **S9328** Home infusion therapy, implanted pump pain management infusion; administrative services, professional pharmacy services, care coordination, and all necessary supplies and equipment (drugs and nursing visits coded separately), per diem

E   **S9329** Home infusion therapy, chemotherapy infusion; administrative services, professional pharmacy services, care coordination, and all necessary supplies and equipment (drugs and nursing visits coded separately), per diem (do not use this code with S9330 or S9331)

E   **S9330** Home infusion therapy, continuous (24 hours or more) chemotherapy infusion; administrative services, professional pharmacy services, care coordination, and all necessary supplies and equipment (drugs and nursing visits coded separately), per diem

E   **S9331** Home infusion therapy, intermittent (less than 24 hours) chemotherapy infusion; administrative services, professional pharmacy services, care coordination, and all necessary supplies and equipment (drugs and nursing visits coded separately), per diem

E ☑   **S9335** Home therapy, hemodialysis; administrative services, professional pharmacy services, care coordination, and all necessary supplies and equipment (drugs and nursing services coded separately), per diem

E   **S9336** Home infusion therapy, continuous anticoagulant infusion therapy (e.g., heparin), administrative services, professional pharmacy services, care coordination and all necessary supplies and equipment (drugs and nursing visits coded separately), per diem

E   **S9338** Home infusion therapy, immunotherapy, administrative services, professional pharmacy services, care coordination, and all necessary supplies and equipment (drugs and nursing visits coded separately), per diem

E   **S9339** Home therapy; peritoneal dialysis, administrative services, professional pharmacy services, care coordination and all necessary supplies and equipment (drugs and nursing visits coded separately), per diem

E   **S9340** Home therapy; enteral nutrition; administrative services, professional pharmacy services, care coordination, and all necessary supplies and equipment (enteral formula and nursing visits coded separately), per diem

E   **S9341** Home therapy; enteral nutrition via gravity; administrative services, professional pharmacy services, care coordination, and all necessary supplies and equipment (enteral formula and nursing visits coded separately), per diem

E   **S9342** Home therapy; enteral nutrition via pump; administrative services, professional pharmacy services, care coordination, and all necessary supplies and equipment (enteral formula and nursing visits coded separately), per diem

E   **S9343** Home therapy; enteral nutrition via bolus; administrative services, professional pharmacy services, care coordination, and all necessary supplies and equipment (enteral formula and nursing visits coded separately), per diem

E   **S9345** Home infusion therapy, anti-hemophilic agent infusion therapy (e.g., factor VIII); administrative services, professional pharmacy services, care coordination, and all necessary supplies and equipment (drugs and nursing visits coded separately), per diem

E   **S9346** Home infusion therapy, alpha-1-proteinase inhibitor (e.g., Prolastin); administrative services, professional pharmacy services, care coordination, and all necessary supplies and equipment (drugs and nursing visits coded separately), per diem

E   **S9347** Home infusion therapy, uninterrupted, long-term, controlled rate intravenous or subcutaneous infusion therapy (e.g., Epoprostenol); administrative services, professional pharmacy services, care coordination, and all necessary supplies and equipment (drugs and nursing visits coded separately), per diem

E   **S9348** Home infusion therapy, sympathomimetic/inotropic agent infusion therapy (e.g., Dobutamine); administrative services, professional pharmacy services, care coordination, all necessary supplies and equipment (drugs and nursing visits coded separately), per diem

E   **S9349** Home infusion therapy, tocolytic infusion therapy; administrative services, professional pharmacy services, care coordination, and all necessary supplies and equipment (drugs and nursing visits coded separately), per diem   M ♀

E   **S9351** Home infusion therapy, continuous anti-emetic infusion therapy; administrative services, professional pharmacy services, care coordination, all necessary supplies and equipment (drugs and nursing visits coded separately), per diem

E   **S9353** Home infusion therapy, continuous insulin infusion therapy; administrative services, professional pharmacy services, care coordination, and all necessary supplies and equipment (drugs and nursing visits coded separately), per diem

E   **S9355** Home infusion therapy, chelation therapy; administrative services, professional pharmacy services, care coordination, and all necessary supplies and equipment (drugs and nursing visits coded separately), per diem

E   **S9357** Home infusion therapy, enzyme replacement intravenous therapy; (e.g., Imiglucerase); administrative services, professional pharmacy services, care coordination, and all necessary supplies and equipment (drugs and nursing visits coded separately), per diem

E   **S9359** Home infusion therapy, anti-tumor necrosis factor intravenous therapy; (e.g., Infliximab); administrative services, professional pharmacy services, care coordination, and all necessary supplies and equipment (drugs and nursing visits coded separately), per diem

E   **S9361** Home infusion therapy, diuretic intravenous therapy; administrative services, professional pharmacy services, care coordination, and all necessary supplies and equipment (drugs and nursing visits coded separately), per diem

Special Coverage Instructions   Noncovered by Medicare   Carrier Discretion   ☑ Quantity Alert   ● New Code   ○ Reinstated Code   ▲ Revised Code

2005 HCPCS   ♀ Female Only   ♂ Male Only   **1**-**9** ASC Groups   **MED:** Pub 100/NCD Reference   ⅃ DMEPOS Paid   ⊘ SNF Excluded   **S Codes — 133**

Temporary National Codes (Non–Medicare)

S9363 — S9452

▲ Ⓔ **S9363** Home infusion therapy, anti-spasmotic therapy; administrative services, professional pharmacy services, care coordination, and all necessary supplies and equipment (drugs and nursing visits coded separately), per diem

Ⓔ **S9364** Home infusion therapy, total parenteral nutrition (TPN); administrative services, professional pharmacy services, care coordination, and all necessary supplies and equipment including standard TPN formula (lipids, specialty amino acid formulas, drugs other than in standard formula and nursing visits coded separately), per diem (do not use with home infusion codes S9365-S9368 using daily volume scales)

Ⓔ **S9365** Home infusion therapy, total parenteral nutrition (TPN); 1 liter per day, administrative services, professional pharmacy services, care coordination, and all necessary supplies and equipment including standard TPN formula (lipids, specialty amino acid formulas, drugs other than in standard formula and nursing visits coded separately), per diem

Ⓔ **S9366** Home infusion therapy, total parenteral nutrition (TPN); more than 1 liter but no more than 2 liters per day, administrative services, professional pharmacy services, care coordination, and all necessary supplies and equipment including standard TPN formula (lipids, specialty amino acid formulas, drugs other than in standard formula and nursing visits coded separately), per diem

Ⓔ **S9367** Home infusion therapy, total parenteral nutrition (TPN); more than 2 liters but no more than 3 liters per day, administrative services, professional pharmacy services, care coordination, and all necessary supplies and equipment including standard TPN formula (lipids, specialty amino acid formulas, drugs other than in standard formula and nursing visits coded separately), per diem

Ⓔ **S9368** Home infusion therapy, total parenteral nutrition (TPN); more than 3 liters per day, administrative services, professional pharmacy services, care coordination, and all necessary supplies and equipment including standard TPN formula (lipids, specialty amino acid formulas, drugs other than in standard formula and nursing visits coded separately), per diem

Ⓔ **S9370** Home therapy, intermittent anti-emetic injection therapy; administrative services, professional pharmacy services, care coordination, and all necessary supplies and equipment (drugs and nursing visits coded separately), per diem

Ⓔ **S9372** Home therapy; intermittent anticoagulant injection therapy (e.g., heparin); administrative services, professional pharmacy services, care coordination, and all necessary supplies and equipment (drugs and nursing visits coded separately), per diem (do not use this code for flushing of infusion devices with heparin to maintain patency)

Ⓔ **S9373** Home infusion therapy, hydration therapy; administrative services, professional pharmacy services, care coordination, and all necessary supplies and equipment (drugs and nursing visits coded separately), per diem (do not use with hydration therapy codes S9374-S9377 using daily volume scales)

Ⓔ **S9374** Home infusion therapy, hydration therapy; 1 liter per day, administrative services, professional pharmacy services, care coordination, and all necessary supplies and equipment (drugs and nursing visits coded separately), per diem

Ⓔ **S9375** Home infusion therapy, hydration therapy; more than 1 liter but no more than 2 liters per day, administrative services, professional pharmacy services, care coordination, and all necessary supplies and equipment (drugs and nursing visits coded separately), per diem

Ⓔ **S9376** Home infusion therapy, hydration therapy; more than 2 liters but no more than 3 liters per day, administrative services, professional pharmacy services, care coordination, and all necessary supplies and equipment (drugs and nursing visits coded separately), per diem

Ⓔ **S9377** Home infusion therapy, hydration therapy; more than 3 liters per day, administrative services, professional pharmacy services, care coordination, and all necessary supplies (drugs and nursing visits coded separately), per diem

Ⓔ **S9379** Home infusion therapy, infusion therapy, not otherwise classified; administrative services, professional pharmacy services, care coordination, and all necessary supplies and equipment (drugs and nursing visits coded separately), per diem

Ⓔ **S9381** Delivery or service to high risk areas requiring escort or extra protection, per visit

Ⓔ **S9401** Anticoagulation clinic, inclusive of all services except laboratory tests, per session

Ⓔ **S9430** Pharmacy compounding and dispensing services

Ⓔ **S9434** Modified solid food supplements for inborn errors of metabolism

Ⓔ **S9435** Medical foods for inborn errors of metabolism

Ⓔ **S9436** Childbirth preparation/lamaze classes, nonphysician provider, per session   Ⓐ ♀

Ⓔ **S9437** Childbirth refresher classes, nonphysician provider, per session   Ⓐ ♀

Ⓔ **S9438** Cesarean birth classes, nonphysician provider, per session   Ⓐ ♀

Ⓔ **S9439** VBAC (vaginal birth after cesarean) classes, nonphysician provider, per session   Ⓐ ♀

Ⓔ **S9441** Asthma education, nonphysician provider, per session

Ⓔ **S9442** Birthing classes, nonphysician provider, per session   Ⓐ ♀

Ⓔ **S9443** Lactation classes, nonphysician provider, per session   Ⓐ ♀

Ⓔ **S9444** Parenting classes, nonphysician provider, per session   Ⓐ

Ⓔ **S9445** Patient education, not otherwise classified, nonphysician provider, individual, per session

Ⓔ **S9446** Patient education, not otherwise classified, nonphysician provider, group, per session

Ⓔ **S9447** Infant safety (including CPR) classes, nonphysician provider, per session

Ⓔ **S9449** Weight management classes, nonphysician provider, per session

Ⓔ **S9451** Exercise classes, nonphysician provider, per session

Ⓔ **S9452** Nutrition classes, nonphysician provider, per session

Special Coverage Instructions   Noncovered by Medicare   Carrier Discretion   ☑ Quantity Alert   ● New Code   ○ Reinstated Code   ▲ Revised Code

134 — S Codes   Ⓐ Adult   Ⓜ Maternity   Ⓟ Pediatrics   Ⓘ Infant   Ⓐ-Ⓨ APC Status Indicator   *2005 HCPCS*

| E | | S9453 | Smoking cessation classes, nonphysician provider, per session |

| E | | S9454 | Stress management classes, nonphysician provider, per session |

| E | | S9455 | Diabetic management program, group session |

| E | | S9460 | Diabetic management program, nurse visit |

| E | | S9465 | Diabetic management program, dietitian visit |

| E | | S9470 | Nutritional counseling, dietitian visit |

| E | | S9472 | Cardiac rehabilitation program, nonphysician provider, per diem |

| E | | S9473 | Pulmonary rehabilitation program, nonphysician provider, per diem |

| E | | S9474 | Enterostomal therapy by a registered nurse certified in enterostomal therapy, per diem |

| E | | S9475 | Ambulatory setting substance abuse treatment or detoxification services, per diem |

| E | ☑ | S9476 | Vestibular rehabilitation program, nonphysician provider, per diem |

| E | | S9480 | Intensive outpatient psychiatric services, per diem |

● | ☑ | S9482 | Family stabilization services, per 15 minutes

| E | | S9484 | Crisis intervention mental health services, per hour |

| E | | S9485 | Crisis intervention mental health services, per diem |

| E | | S9490 | Home infusion therapy, corticosteroid infusion; administrative services, professional pharmacy services, care coordination, and all necessary supplies and equipment (drugs and nursing visits coded separately), per diem |

| E | | S9494 | Home infusion therapy, antibiotic, antiviral, or antifungal therapy; administrative services, professional pharmacy services, care coordination, and all necessary supplies and equipment (drugs and nursing visits coded separately, per diem) (do not use this code with home infusion codes for hourly dosing schedules S9497-S9504) |

| E | | S9497 | Home infusion therapy, antibiotic, antiviral, or antifungal therapy; once every 3 hours; administrative services, professional pharmacy services, care coordination, and all necessary supplies and equipment (drugs and nursing visits coded separately), per diem |

| E | | S9500 | Home infusion therapy, antibiotic, antiviral, or antifungal therapy; once every 24 hours; administrative services, professional pharmacy services, care coordination, and all necessary supplies and equipment (drugs and nursing visits coded separately), per diem |

| E | | S9501 | Home infusion therapy, antibiotic, antiviral, or antifungal therapy; once every 12 hours; administrative services, professional pharmacy services, care coordination, and all necessary supplies and equipment (drugs and nursing visits coded separately), per diem |

| E | | S9502 | Home infusion therapy, antibiotic, antiviral, or antifungal therapy; once every 8 hours, administrative services, professional pharmacy services, care coordination, and all necessary supplies and equipment (drugs and nursing visits coded separately), per diem |

| E | | S9503 | Home infusion therapy, antibiotic, antiviral, or antifungal; once every 6 hours; administrative services, professional pharmacy services, care coordination, and all necessary supplies and equipment (drugs and nursing visits coded separately), per diem |

| E | | S9504 | Home infusion therapy, antibiotic, antiviral, or antifungal; once every 4 hours; administrative services, professional pharmacy services, care coordination, and all necessary supplies and equipment (drugs and nursing visits coded separately), per diem |

| E | | S9529 | Routine venipuncture for collection of specimen(s), single home bound, nursing home, or skilled nursing facility patient |

| E | | S9537 | Home therapy; hematopoietic hormone injection therapy (e.g., erythropoietin, G-CSF, GM-CSF); administrative services, professional pharmacy services, care coordination, and all necessary supplies and equipment (drugs and nursing visits coded separately), per diem |

| E | | S9538 | Home transfusion of blood product(s); administrative services, professional pharmacy services, care coordination and all necessary supplies and equipment (blood products, drugs, and nursing visits coded separately), per diem |

| E | | S9542 | Home injectable therapy, not otherwise classified, including administrative services, professional pharmacy services, care coordination, and all necessary supplies and equipment (drugs and nursing visits coded separately), per diem |

| E | | S9558 | Home injectable therapy; growth hormone, including administrative services, professional pharmacy services, care coordination, and all necessary supplies and equipment (drugs and nursing visits coded separately), per diem |

| E | | S9559 | Home injectable therapy, interferon, including administrative services, professional pharmacy services, care coordination, and all necessary supplies and equipment (drugs and nursing visits coded separately), per diem |

| E | | S9560 | Home injectable therapy; hormonal therapy (e.g., leuprolide, goserelin), including administrative services, professional pharmacy services, care coordination, and all necessary supplies and equipment (drugs and nursing visits coded separately), per diem |

| E | | S9562 | Home injectable therapy, palivizumab, including administrative services, professional pharmacy services, care coordination, and all necessary supplies and equipment (drugs and nursing visits coded separately), per diem |

| E | | S9590 | Home therapy, irrigation therapy (e.g., sterile irrigation of an organ or anatomical cavity); including administrative services, professional pharmacy services, care coordination, and all necessary supplies and equipment (drugs and nursing visits coded separately), per diem |

| E | | S9810 | Home therapy; professional pharmacy services for provision of infusion, specialty drug administration, and/or disease state management, not otherwise classified, per hour (do not use this code with any per diem code) |

| E | | S9900 | Services by authorized Christian Science practitioner for the process of healing, per diem; not to be used for rest or study; excludes inpatient services |

Special Coverage Instructions   Noncovered by Medicare   Carrier Discretion   ☑ Quantity Alert   ● New Code   ○ Reinstated Code   ▲ Revised Code

2005 HCPCS   ♀ Female Only   ♂ Male Only   **1-9** ASC Groups   **MED:** Pub 100/NCD Reference   ⅃. DMEPOS Paid   ⊘ SNF Excluded   **S Codes — 135**

Temporary National Codes (Non-Medicare)

S9970 — S9999

E	**S9970**	Health club membership, annual
E	**S9975**	Transplant related lodging, meals and transportation, per diem
● E	**S9976**	Lodging, per diem, not otherwise specified
● E	**S9977**	Meals, per diem not otherwise specified
E	**S9981**	Medical records copying fee, administrative
E	**S9982**	Medical records copying fee, per page
E	**S9986**	Not medically necessary service (patient is aware that service not medically necessary)
● E	**S9988**	Services provided as part of a Phase 1 clinical trial
E	**S9989**	Services provided outside of the United States of America (list in addition to code(s) for services(s))
E	**S9990**	Services provided as part of a Phase II clinical trial
E	**S9991**	Services provided as part of a Phase III clinical trial
E	**S9992**	Transportation costs to and from trial location and local transportation costs (e.g., fares for taxicab or bus) for clinical trial participant and one caregiver/companion
E	**S9994**	Lodging costs (e.g., hotel charges) for clinical trial participant and one caregiver/companion
E	**S9996**	Meals for clinical trial participant and one caregiver/companion
E	**S9999**	Sales tax

Special Coverage Instructions   Noncovered by Medicare   Carrier Discretion   ☑ Quantity Alert   ● New Code   ○ Reinstated Code   ▲ Revised Code

136 — S Codes   **A** Adult   **M** Maternity   **P** Pediatrics   **I** Infant   **A-Y** APC Status Indicator   *2005 HCPCS*

NATIONAL T CODES ESTABLISHED FOR STATE MEDICAID AGENCIES *T1000–T9999*

The T codes are designed for use by Medicaid state agencies to establish codes for items for which there are no permanent national codes but for which codes are necessary to administer the Medicaid program (T codes are not accepted by Medicare but can be used by private insurers). This range of codes describes nursing and home health-related services, substance abuse treatment, and certain training-related procedures.

These codes are not valid for Medicare.

E · **T1000** Private duty/independent nursing service(s) — licensed, up to 15 minutes

E · **T1001** Nursing assessment/evaluation

E · **T1002** RN services, up to 15 minutes

E · **T1003** LPN/LVN services, up to 15 minutes

E · **T1004** Services of a qualified nursing aide, up to 15 minutes

E · **T1005** Respite care services, up to 15 minutes

E · **T1006** Alcohol and/or substance abuse services, family/couple counseling

E · **T1007** Alcohol and/or substance abuse services, treatment plan development and/or modification

E · **T1009** Child sitting services for children of the individual receiving alcohol and/or substance abuse services

E · **T1010** Meals for individuals receiving alcohol and/or substance abuse services (when meals not included in the program)

E · **T1012** Alcohol and/or substance abuse services, skills development

E · **T1013** Sign language or oral interpretive services, per 15 minutes

E · **T1014** Telehealth transmission, per minute, professional services bill separately

E · **T1015** Clinic visit/encounter, all-inclusive

E · **T1016** Case management, each 15 minutes

E · **T1017** Targeted case management, each 15 minutes

E · **T1018** School-based individualized education program (IEP) services, bundled

E · **T1019** Personal care services, per 15 minutes, not for an inpatient or resident of a hospital, nursing facility, ICF/MR or IMD, part of the individualized plan of treatment (code may not be used to identify services provided by home health aide or certified nurse assistant)

E · **T1020** Personal care services, per diem, not for an inpatient or resident of a hospital, nursing facility, ICF/MR or IMD, part of the individualized plan of treatment (code may not be used to identify services provided by home health aide or certified nurse assistant)

E · **T1021** Home health aide or certified nurse assistant, per visit

E · **T1022** Contracted home health agency services, all services provided under contract, per day

E · **T1023** Screening to determine the appropriateness of consideration of an individual for participation in a specified program, project or treatment protocol, per encounter

E · **T1024** Evaluation and treatment by an integrated, specialty team contracted to provide coordinated care to multiple or severely handicapped children, per encounter P

E · **T1025** Intensive, extended multidisciplinary services provided in a clinic setting to children with complex medical, physical, mental and psychosocial impairments, per diem P

E · **T1026** Intensive, extended multidisciplinary services provided in a clinic setting to children with complex medical, physical, medical and psychosocial impairments, per hour P

E · **T1027** Family training and counseling for child development, per 15 minutes

E · **T1028** Assessment of home, physical and family environment, to determine suitability to meet patient's medical needs

E · **T1029** Comprehensive environmental lead investigation, not including laboratory analysis, per dwelling

E · **T1030** Nursing care, in the home, by registered nurse, per diem

E · **T1031** Nursing care, in the home, by licensed practical nurse, per diem

~~**T1500** Diaper/incontinent pant, reusable/washable, any size, each~~

E · **T1502** Administration of oral, intramuscular and/or subcutaneous medication by health care agency/professional, per visit

E · **T1999** Miscellaneous therapeutic items and supplies, retail purchases, not otherwise classified; identify product in remarks

E · **T2001** Non-emergency transportation; patient attendant/escort

E · **T2002** Non-emergency transportation; per diem

E · **T2003** Non-emergency transportation; encounter/trip

E · **T2004** Non-emergency transport; commercial carrier, multi-pass

▲ E · **T2005** Non-emergency transportation; stretcher van

E · **T2006** Ambulance response and treatment, no transport

E · **T2007** Transportation waiting time, air ambulance and non-emergency vehicle, one-half (1/2) hour increments

E ☑ **T2010** Preadmission screening and resident review (PASRR) level I identification screening, per screen

E · **T2011** Preadmission screening and resident review (PASRR) level II evaluation, per evaluation

E ☑ **T2012** Habilitation, educational; waiver, per diem

E ☑ **T2013** Habilitation, educational, waiver; per hour

E ☑ **T2014** Habilitation, prevocational, waiver; per diem

E ☑ **T2015** Habilitation, prevocational, waiver; per hour

E ☑ **T2016** Habilitation, residential, waiver; per diem

E ☑ **T2017** Habilitation, residential, waiver; 15 minutes

E ☑ **T2018** Habilitation, supported employment, waiver; per diem

E ☑ **T2019** Habilitation, supported employment, waiver; per 15 minutes

E ☑ **T2020** Day habilitation, waiver; per diem

E ☑ **T2021** Day habilitation, waiver; per 15 minutes

E ☑ **T2022** Case management, per month

E ☑ **T2023** Targeted case management; per month

E · **T2024** Service assessment/plan of care development, waiver

E · **T2025** Waiver services; not otherwise specified (NOS)

Special Coverage Instructions ▮   Noncovered by Medicare ▮   Carrier Discretion ▮   ☑ Quantity Alert   ● New Code   ○ Reinstated Code   ▲ Revised Code

2005 HCPCS   ♀ Female Only   ♂ Male Only   **1-9** ASC Groups   **MED:** Pub 100/NCD Reference   ⚕ DMEPOS Paid   ⊘ SNF Excluded   **T Codes — 137**

National T Codes

T2026 — T5999

E ☑ **T2026** Specialized childcare, waiver; per diem

E ☑ **T2027** Specialized childcare, waiver; per 15 minutes

E **T2028** Specialized supply, not otherwise specified, waiver

E **T2029** Specialized medical equipment, not otherwise specified, waiver

E ☑ **T2030** Assisted living, waiver; per month

E ☑ **T2031** Assisted living; waiver, per diem

E ☑ **T2032** Residential care, not otherwise specified (NOS), waiver; per month

E ☑ **T2033** Residential care, not otherwise specified (NOS), waiver; per diem

E ☑ **T2034** Crisis intervention, waiver; per diem

E **T2035** Utility services to support medical equipment and assistive technology/devices, waiver

E ☑ **T2036** Therapeutic camping, overnight, waiver; each session

E ☑ **T2037** Therapeutic camping, day, waiver; each session

E ☑ **T2038** Community transition, waiver; per service

E ☑ **T2039** Vehicle modifications, waiver; per service

E ☑ **T2040** Financial management, self-directed, waiver; per 15 minutes

E ☑ **T2041** Supports brokerage, self-directed, waiver; per 15 minutes

E ☑ **T2042** Hospice routine home care; per diem

E ☑ **T2043** Hospice continuous home care; per hour

E ☑ **T2044** Hospice inpatient respite care; per diem

E ☑ **T2045** Hospice general inpatient care; per diem

E ☑ **T2046** Hospice long term care, room and board only; per diem

E ☑ **T2048** Behavioral health; long-term care residential (non-acute care in a residential treatment program where stay is typically longer than 30 days), with room and board, per diem

● E ☑ **T2049** Non-emergency transportation; stretcher van, mileage; per mile

E **T2101** Human breast milk processing, storage and distribution only   ♀

● ☑ **T4521** Adult sized disposable incontinence product, brief/diaper, small, each
MED: 100-3, 230.10

● ☑ **T4522** Adult sized disposable incontinence product, brief/diaper, medium, each
MED: 100-3, 230.10

● ☑ **T4523** Adult sized disposable incontinence product, brief/diaper, large, each
MED: 100-3, 230.10

● ☑ **T4524** Adult sized disposable incontinence product, brief/diaper, extra large, each
MED: 100-3, 230.10

● ☑ **T4525** Adult sized disposable incontinence product, protective underwear/pull-on, small size, each
MED: 100-3, 230.10

● ☑ **T4526** Adult sized disposable incontinence product, protective underwear/pull-on, medium size, each
MED: 100-3, 230.10

● ☑ **T4527** Adult sized disposable incontinence product, protective underwear/pull-on, large size, each
MED: 100-3, 230.10

● ☑ **T4528** Adult sized disposable incontinence product, protective underwear/pull-on, extra large size, each
MED: 100-3, 230.10

● ☑ **T4529** Pediatric sized disposable incontinence product, brief/diaper, small/medium size, each
MED: 100-3, 230.10

● ☑ **T4530** Pediatric sized disposable incontinence product, brief/diaper, large size, each
MED: 100-3, 230.10

● ☑ **T4531** Pediatric sized disposable incontinence product, protective underwear/pull-on, small/medium size, each
MED: 100-3, 230.10

● ☑ **T4532** Pediatric sized disposable incontinence product, protective underwear/pull-on, large size, each
MED: 100-3, 230.10

● ☑ **T4533** Youth sized disposable incontinence product, brief/diaper, each
MED: 100-3, 230.10

● ☑ **T4534** Youth sized disposable incontinence product, protective underwear/pull-on, each
MED: 100-3, 230.10

● ☑ **T4535** Disposable liner/shield/guard/pad/undergarment, for incontinence, each
MED: 100-3, 230.10

● ☑ **T4536** Incontinence product, protective underwear/pull-on, reusable, any size, each
MED: 100-3, 230.10

● ☑ **T4537** Incontinence product, protective underpad, reusable, bed size, each
MED: 100-3, 230.10

● ☑ **T4538** Diaper service, reusable diaper, each diaper
MED: 100-3, 230.10

● ☑ **T4539** Incontinence product, diaper/brief, reusable, any size, each
MED: 100-3, 230.10

● ☑ **T4540** Incontinence product, protective underpad, reusable, chair size, each
MED: 100-3, 230.10

● ☑ **T4541** Incontinence product, disposable underpad, large, each

● ☑ **T4542** Incontinence product, disposable underpad, small size, each

E **T5001** Positioning seat for persons with special orthopedic needs, for use in vehicles

E **T5999** Supply, not otherwise specified

Special Coverage Instructions   Noncovered by Medicare   Carrier Discretion   ☑ Quantity Alert   ● New Code   ○ Reinstated Code   ▲ Revised Code

138 — T Codes   Ⓐ Adult   Ⓜ Maternity   Ⓟ Pediatrics   Ⓘ Infant   Ⓐ-Ⓨ APC Status Indicator   *2005 HCPCS*

VISION SERVICES *V0000–V2999*

These V codes include vision-related supplies, including spectacles, lenses, contact lenses, prostheses, intraocular lenses, and miscellaneous lenses.

FRAMES

V codes fall under the jurisdiction of the DME regional carrier, unless incident to other services or otherwise noted.

| Ⓐ | | **V2020** | Frames, purchases
MED: 100-2, 15, 120 | ♿ ⃠ |
| Ⓔ | | **V2025** | Deluxe frame
MED: 100-4, 1, 30.3.5 | ⃠ |

SPECTACLE LENSES

If procedure code 92390 or 92395 is reported, recode with the specific lens type listed below. For aphakic temporary spectacle correction, see 92358. See S0500–S0592 for temporary vision codes.

SINGLE VISION, GLASS, OR PLASTIC

Ⓐ	☑	**V2100**	Sphere, single vision, plano to plus or minus 4.00, per lens ♿
Ⓐ	☑	**V2101**	Sphere, single vision, plus or minus 4.12 to plus or minus 7.00d, per lens ♿
Ⓐ	☑	**V2102**	Sphere, single vision, plus or minus 7.12 to plus or minus 20.00d, per lens ♿
Ⓐ	☑	**V2103**	Spherocylinder, single vision, plano to plus or minus 4.00d sphere, 0.12 to 2.00d cylinder, per lens ♿
Ⓐ	☑	**V2104**	Spherocylinder, single vision, plano to plus or minus 4.00d sphere, 2.12 to 4.00d cylinder, per lens ♿
Ⓐ	☑	**V2105**	Spherocylinder, single vision, plano to plus or minus 4.00d sphere, 4.25 to 6.00d cylinder, per lens ♿
Ⓐ	☑	**V2106**	Spherocylinder, single vision, plano to plus or minus 4.00d sphere, over 6.00d cylinder, per lens ♿
Ⓐ	☑	**V2107**	Spherocylinder, single vision, plus or minus 4.25 to plus or minus 7.00 sphere, 0.12 to 2.00d cylinder, per lens ♿
Ⓐ	☑	**V2108**	Spherocylinder, single vision, plus or minus 4.25d to plus or minus 7.00d sphere, 2.12 to 4.00d cylinder, per lens ♿
Ⓐ	☑	**V2109**	Spherocylinder, single vision, plus or minus 4.25 to plus or minus 7.00d sphere, 4.25 to 6.00d cylinder, per lens ♿
Ⓐ	☑	**V2110**	Spherocylinder, single vision, plus or minus 4.25 to 7.00d sphere, over 6.00d cylinder, per lens ♿
Ⓐ	☑	**V2111**	Spherocylinder, single vision, plus or minus 7.25 to plus or minus 12.00d sphere, 0.25 to 2.25d cylinder, per lens ♿
Ⓐ	☑	**V2112**	Spherocylinder, single vision, plus or minus 7.25 to plus or minus 12.00d sphere, 2.25d to 4.00d cylinder, per lens ♿
Ⓐ	☑	**V2113**	Spherocylinder, single vision, plus or minus 7.25 to plus or minus 12.00d sphere, 4.25 to 6.00d cylinder, per lens ♿
Ⓐ	☑	**V2114**	Spherocylinder, single vision sphere over plus or minus 12.00d, per lens ♿
Ⓐ	☑	**V2115**	Lenticular (myodisc), per lens, single vision ♿
Ⓐ		**V2118**	Aniseikonic lens, single vision ♿

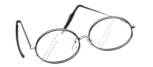

Monofocal spectacles (V2100-V2114)

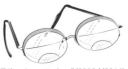

Trifocal spectacles (V2300-V2314)

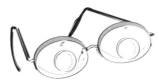

Low vision aids mounted to spectacles (V2610)

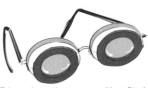

Telescopic or other compound lens fitted on spectacles as a low vision aid (V2615)

| Ⓐ | | **V2121** | Lenticular lens, per lens, single
MED: 100-2, 15, 120 ♿ |
| Ⓐ | | **V2199** | Not otherwise classified, single vision lens |

BIFOCAL, GLASS, OR PLASTIC

Ⓐ	☑	**V2200**	Sphere, bifocal, plano to plus or minus 4.00d, per lens ♿
Ⓐ	☑	**V2201**	Sphere, bifocal, plus or minus 4.12 to plus or minus 7.00d, per lens ♿
Ⓐ	☑	**V2202**	Sphere, bifocal, plus or minus 7.12 to plus or minus 20.00d, per lens ♿
Ⓐ	☑	**V2203**	Spherocylinder, bifocal, plano to plus or minus 4.00d sphere, 0.12 to 2.00d cylinder, per lens ♿
Ⓐ	☑	**V2204**	Spherocylinder, bifocal, plano to plus or minus 4.00d sphere, 2.12 to 4.00d cylinder, per lens ♿
Ⓐ	☑	**V2205**	Spherocylinder, bifocal, plano to plus or minus 4.00d sphere, 4.25 to 6.00d cylinder, per lens ♿
Ⓐ	☑	**V2206**	Spherocylinder, bifocal, plano to plus or minus 4.00d sphere, over 6.00d cylinder, per lens ♿
Ⓐ	☑	**V2207**	Spherocylinder, bifocal, plus or minus 4.25 to plus or minus 7.00 sphere, 0.12 to 2.00d cylinder, per lens ♿
Ⓐ	☑	**V2208**	Spherocylinder, bifocal, plus or minus 4.25 to plus or minus 7.00 sphere, 2.12 to 4.00d cylinder, per lens ♿
Ⓐ	☑	**V2209**	Spherocylinder, bifocal, plus or minus 4.25 to plus or minus 7.00 sphere, 4.25 to 6.00d cylinder, per lens ♿
Ⓐ	☑	**V2210**	Spherocylinder, bifocal, plus or minus 4.25 to plus or minus 7.00 sphere, over 6.00d cylinder, per lens ♿
Ⓐ	☑	**V2211**	Spherocylinder, bifocal, plus or minus 7.25 to plus or minus 12.00d sphere, 0.25 to 2.25d cylinder, per lens ♿
Ⓐ	☑	**V2212**	Spherocylinder, bifocal, plus or minus 7.25 to plus or minus 12.00d sphere, 2.25 to 4.00d cylinder, per lens ♿
Ⓐ	☑	**V2213**	Spherocylinder, bifocal, plus or minus 7.25 to plus or minus 12.00d sphere, 4.25 to 6.00d cylinder, per lens ♿
Ⓐ	☑	**V2214**	Spherocylinder, bifocal, sphere over plus or minus 12.00d, per lens ♿
Ⓐ	☑	**V2215**	Lenticular (myodisc), per lens, bifocal ♿
Ⓐ	☑	**V2218**	Aniseikonic, per lens, bifocal ♿
Ⓐ	☑	**V2219**	Bifocal seg width over 28mm ♿
Ⓐ	☑	**V2220**	Bifocal add over 3.25d ♿

| Special Coverage Instructions | | Noncovered by Medicare | | Carrier Discretion | | ☑ Quantity Alert | ● New Code | ○ Reinstated Code | ▲ Revised Code |

2005 HCPCS   ♀ Female Only   ♂ Male Only   **1**-**9** ASC Groups   MED: Pub 100/NCD Reference   ♿ DMEPOS Paid   ⃠ SNF Excluded   **V Codes — 139**

Vision Services

V2221 — V2625

[A]   **V2221**   Lenticular lens, per lens, bifocal   ♿
MED: 100-2, 15, 120

[A]   **V2299**   Specialty bifocal (by report)
Pertinent documentation to evaluate medical appropriateness should be included when this code is reported.

TRIFOCAL, GLASS, OR PLASTIC

[A] ☑ **V2300** Sphere, trifocal, plano to plus or minus 4.00d, per lens ♿

[A] ☑ **V2301** Sphere, trifocal, plus or minus 4.12 to plus or minus 7.00d per lens ♿

[A] ☑ **V2302** Sphere, trifocal, plus or minus 7.12 to plus or minus 20.00, per lens ♿

[A] ☑ **V2303** Spherocylinder, trifocal, plano to plus or minus 4.00d sphere, 0.12 to 2.00d cylinder, per lens ♿

[A] ☑ **V2304** Spherocylinder, trifocal, plano to plus or minus 4.00d sphere, 2.25 to 4.00d cylinder, per lens ♿

[A] ☑ **V2305** Spherocylinder, trifocal, plano to plus or minus 4.00d sphere, 4.25 to 6.00 cylinder, per lens ♿

[A] ☑ **V2306** Spherocylinder, trifocal, plano to plus or minus 4.00d sphere, over 6.00d cylinder, per lens ♿

[A] ☑ **V2307** Spherocylinder, trifocal, plus or minus 4.25 to plus or minus 7.00d sphere, 0.12 to 2.00d cylinder, per lens ♿

[A] ☑ **V2308** Spherocylinder, trifocal, plus or minus 4.25 to plus or minus 7.00d sphere, 2.12 to 4.00d cylinder, per lens ♿

[A] ☑ **V2309** Spherocylinder, trifocal, plus or minus 4.25 to plus or minus 7.00d sphere, 4.25 to 6.00d cylinder, per lens ♿

[A] ☑ **V2310** Spherocylinder, trifocal, plus or minus 4.25 to plus or minus 7.00d sphere, over 6.00d cylinder, per lens ♿

[A] ☑ **V2311** Spherocylinder, trifocal, plus or minus 7.25 to plus or minus 12.00d sphere, 0.25 to 2.25d cylinder, per lens ♿

[A] ☑ **V2312** Spherocylinder, trifocal, plus or minus 7.25 to plus or minus 12.00d sphere, 2.25 to 4.00d cylinder, per lens ♿

[A] ☑ **V2313** Spherocylinder, trifocal, plus or minus 7.25 to plus or minus 12.00d sphere, 4.25 to 6.00d cylinder, per lens ♿

[A] ☑ **V2314** Spherocylinder, trifocal, sphere over plus or minus 12.00d, per lens ♿

[A]   **V2315** Lenticular (myodisc), per lens, trifocal ♿

[A]   **V2318** Aniseikonic lens, trifocal ♿

[A] ☑ **V2319** Trifocal seg width over 28 mm ♿

[A] ☑ **V2320** Trifocal add over 3.25d ♿

[A]   **V2321** Lenticular lens, per lens, trifocal ♿
MED: 100-2, 15, 120

[A]   **V2399** Specialty trifocal (by report)
Pertinent documentation to evaluate medical appropriateness should be included when this code is reported.

VARIABLE ASPHERICITY LENS, GLASS, OR PLASTIC

[A] ☑ **V2410** Variable asphericity lens, single vision, full field, glass or plastic, per lens ♿

[A] ☑ **V2430** Variable asphericity lens, bifocal, full field, glass or plastic, per lens ♿

[A]   **V2499** Variable sphericity lens, other type

CONTACT LENS

If procedure code 92391 or 92396 is reported, recode with specific lens type listed below (per lens).

[A] ☑ **V2500** Contact lens, PMMA, spherical, per lens ♿

[A] ☑ **V2501** Contact lens, PMMA, toric or prism ballast, per lens ♿

[A] ☑ **V2502** Contact lens, PMMA, bifocal, per lens ♿

[A] ☑ **V2503** Contact lens, PMMA, color vision deficiency, per lens ♿

[A] ☑ **V2510** Contact lens, gas permeable, spherical, per lens ♿

[A] ☑ **V2511** Contact lens, gas permeable, toric, prism ballast, per lens ♿

[A] ☑ **V2512** Contact lens, gas permeable, bifocal, per lens ♿

[A] ☑ **V2513** Contact lens, gas permeable, extended wear, per lens ♿

[A] ☑ **V2520** Contact lens, hydrophilic, spherical, per lens ♿
Hydrophilic contact lenses are covered by Medicare only for aphakic patients. Local carrier if incident to physician services.
MED: 100-3, 80.1; 100-3, 80.4

[A] ☑ **V2521** Contact lens, hydrophilic, toric, or prism ballast, per lens ♿
Hydrophilic contact lenses are covered by Medicare only for aphakic patients. Local carrier if incident to physician services.
MED: 100-3, 80.1; 100-3, 80.4

[A] ☑ **V2522** Contact lens, hydrophilic, bifocal, per lens ♿
Hydrophilic contact lenses are covered by Medicare only for aphakic patients. Local carrier if incident to physician services.
MED: 100-3, 80.1; 100-3, 80.4

[A] ☑ **V2523** Contact lens, hydrophilic, extended wear, per lens ♿
Hydrophilic contact lenses are covered by Medicare only for aphakic patients.
MED: 100-3, 80.1; 100-3, 80.4

[A] ☑ **V2530** Contact lens, scleral, gas impermeable, per lens (for contact lens modification, see CPT Level I code 92325) ♿

[A] ☑ **V2531** Contact lens, scleral, gas permeable, per lens (for contact lens modification, see CPT Level I code 92325) ♿
MED: 100-3, 80.5

[A]   **V2599** Contact lens, other type ⊘
Local carrier if incident to physician services.

VISION AIDS

If procedure code 92392 is reported, recode with specific systems below.

[A]   **V2600** Hand held low vision aids and other nonspectacle mounted aids ⊘

[A]   **V2610** Single lens spectacle mounted low vision aids ⊘

[A]   **V2615** Telescopic and other compound lens system, including distance vision telescopic, near vision telescopes and compound microscopic lens system ⊘

PROSTHETIC EYE

[A]   **V2623** Prosthetic eye, plastic, custom ♿
MED: 100-2, 15, 120

[A]   **V2624** Polishing/resurfacing of ocular prosthesis ♿

[A]   **V2625** Enlargement of ocular prosthesis ♿

Special Coverage Instructions   Noncovered by Medicare   Carrier Discretion   ☑ Quantity Alert   ● New Code   ○ Reinstated Code   ▲ Revised Code

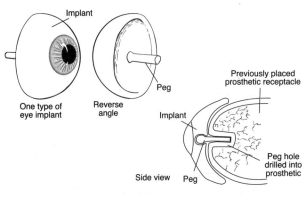

Implant

One type of eye implant

Reverse angle

Peg

Implant

Side view Peg

Previously placed prosthetic receptacle

Peg hole drilled into prosthetic

| A | | **V2626** | Reduction of ocular prosthesis | ᕦ |

| A | | **V2627** | Scleral cover shell | ᕦ |

A scleral shell covers the cornea and the anterior sclera. Medicare covers a scleral shell when it is prescribed as an artificial support to a shrunken and sightless eye or as a barrier in the treatment of severe dry eye.

MED: 100-3, 80.5

| A | | **V2628** | Fabrication and fitting of ocular conformer | ᕦ |

| A | | **V2629** | Prosthetic eye, other type | ⊘ |

INTRAOCULAR LENSES

| N | | **V2630** | Anterior chamber intraocular lens | ⊘ |

The IOL must be FDA-approved for reimbursement. Medicare payment for an IOL is included in the payment for ASC facility services. Medicare jurisdiction: local carrier.

MED: 100-2, 15, 120

| N | | **V2631** | Iris supported intraocular lens | ⊘ |

The IOL must be FDA-approved for reimbursement. Medicare payment for an IOL is included in the payment for ASC facility services. Medicare jurisdiction: local carrier.

MED: 100-2, 15, 120

| N | | **V2632** | Posterior chamber intraocular lens | ⊘ |

The IOL must be FDA-approved for reimbursement. Medicare payment for an IOL is included in the payment for ASC facility services. Medicare jurisdiction: local carrier.

MED: 100-2, 15, 120

MISCELLANEOUS

| A | ☑ | **V2700** | Balance lens, per lens | ᕦ |

| ● | | **V2702** | Deluxe lens feature | |
MED: 100-2, 15, 120

| A | ☑ | **V2710** | Slab off prism, glass or plastic, per lens | ᕦ |

| A | ☑ | **V2715** | Prism, per lens | ᕦ |

| A | ☑ | **V2718** | Press-on lens, Fresnel prism, per lens | ᕦ |

| A | ☑ | **V2730** | Special base curve, glass or plastic, per lens | ᕦ |

| A | ☑ | **V2744** | Tint, photochromatic, per lens | ᕦ |
MED: 100-2, 15, 120

| ▲ | A | ☑ | **V2745** | Addition to lens; tint, any color, solid, gradient or equal, excludes photochromatic, any lens material, per lens | ᕦ |
MED: 100-2, 15, 120

| A | ☑ | **V2750** | Antireflective coating, per lens | ᕦ |
MED: 100-2, 15, 120

| A | ☑ | **V2755** | U-V lens, per lens | ᕦ |
MED: 100-2, 15, 120

| E | | **V2756** | Eye glass case | ⊘ |

| A | ☑ | **V2760** | Scratch resistant coating, per lens | ᕦ |

| B | ☑ | **V2761** | Mirror coating, any type, solid, gradient or equal, any lens material, per lens | |
MED: 100-2, 15, 120

| A | ☑ | **V2762** | Polarization, any lens material, per lens | ᕦ |
MED: 100-2, 15, 120

| A | ☑ | **V2770** | Occluder lens, per lens | ᕦ |

| A | ☑ | **V2780** | Oversize lens, per lens | ᕦ |

| B | ☑ | **V2781** | Progressive lens, per lens | ⊘ |

| A | ☑ | **V2782** | Lens, index 1.54 to 1.65 plastic or 1.60 to 1.79 glass, excludes polycarbonate, per lens | ᕦ |
MED: 100-2, 15, 120

| A | ☑ | **V2783** | Lens, index greater than or equal to 1.66 plastic or greater than or equal to 1.80 glass, excludes polycarbonate, per lens | ᕦ |
MED: 100-2, 15, 120

| A | ☑ | **V2784** | Lens, polycarbonate or equal, any index, per lens | ᕦ |
MED: 100-2, 15, 120

| F | | **V2785** | Processing, preserving and transporting corneal tissue | ⊘ |
Medicare jurisdiction: local carrier.

| A | ☑ | **V2786** | Specialty occupational multifocal lens, per lens | ᕦ |
MED: 100-2, 15, 120

| N | | **V2790** | Amniotic membrane for surgical reconstruction, per procedure | ⊘ |
Medicare jurisdiction: local carrier.

| A | | **V2797** | Vision supply, accessory and/or service component of another HCPCS vision code | ⊘ |

| A | | **V2799** | Vision service, miscellaneous | ⊘ |
Determine if an alternative HCPCS Level II or a CPT code better describes the service being reported. This code should be used only if a more specific code is unavailable.

HEARING SERVICES *V5000–V5999*

This range of codes describes hearing tests and related supplies and equipment, speech-language pathology screenings, and repair of augmentative communicative system.

Hearing services fall under the jurisdiction of the local carrier unless incidental or otherwise noted.

| E | | **V5008** | Hearing screening | ⊘ |
MED: 100-2, 16, 90

| E | | **V5010** | Assessment for hearing aid | ⊘ |

| E | | **V5011** | Fitting/orientation/checking of hearing aid | ⊘ |

| E | | **V5014** | Repair/modification of a hearing aid | ⊘ |

| E | | **V5020** | Conformity evaluation | ⊘ |

| E | | **V5030** | Hearing aid, monaural, body worn, air conduction | ⊘ |

| E | | **V5040** | Hearing aid, monaural, body worn, bone conduction | ⊘ |

| E | | **V5050** | Hearing aid, monaural, in the ear | ⊘ |

| E | | **V5060** | Hearing aid, monaural, behind the ear | ⊘ |

| E | | **V5070** | Glasses, air conduction | ⊘ |

| E | | **V5080** | Glasses, bone conduction | ⊘ |

| E | | **V5090** | Dispensing fee, unspecified hearing aid | ⊘ |

| E | | **V5095** | Semi-implantable middle ear hearing prosthesis | |
Use this code for Vibrant Soundbridge Implantable Middle Ear Prosthesis.

| Special Coverage Instructions | Noncovered by Medicare | Carrier Discretion | ☑ Quantity Alert | ● New Code | ○ Reinstated Code | ▲ Revised Code |

2005 HCPCS ♀ Female Only ♂ Male Only **1-9** ASC Groups MED: Pub 100/NCD Reference ᕦ DMEPOS Paid ⊘ SNF Excluded **V Codes — 141**

Hearing Services

V5100 — V5364

E	V5100	Hearing aid, bilateral, body worn	⊘
E	V5110	Dispensing fee, bilateral	⊘
E	V5120	Binaural, body	⊘
E	V5130	Binaural, in the ear	⊘
E	V5140	Binaural, behind the ear	⊘
E	V5150	Binaural, glasses	⊘
E	V5160	Dispensing fee, binaural	⊘
E	V5170	Hearing aid, CROS, in the ear	⊘
E	V5180	Hearing aid, CROS, behind the ear	⊘
E	V5190	Hearing aid, CROS, glasses	⊘
E	V5200	Dispensing fee, CROS	⊘
E	V5210	Hearing aid, BICROS, in the ear	⊘
E	V5220	Hearing aid, BICROS, behind the ear	⊘
E	V5230	Hearing aid, BICROS, glasses	⊘
E	V5240	Dispensing fee, BICROS	⊘
E	V5241	Dispensing fee, monaural hearing aid, any type	
E	V5242	Hearing aid, analog, monaural, CIC (completely in the ear canal)	
E	V5243	Hearing aid, analog, monaural, ITC (in the canal)	
E	V5244	Hearing aid, digitally programmable analog, monaural, CIC	
E	V5245	Hearing aid, digitally programmable, analog, monaural, ITC	
E	V5246	Hearing aid, digitally programmable analog, monaural, ITE (in the ear)	
E	V5247	Hearing aid, digitally programmable analog, monaural, BTE (behind the ear)	
E	V5248	Hearing aid, analog, binaural, CIC	
E	V5249	Hearing aid, analog, binaural, ITC	
E	V5250	Hearing aid, digitally programmable analog, binaural, CIC	
E	V5251	Hearing aid, digitally programmable analog, binaural, ITC	
E	V5252	Hearing aid, digitally programmable, binaural, ITE	
E	V5253	Hearing aid, digitally programmable, binaural, BTE	
E	V5254	Hearing aid, digital, monaural, CIC	
E	V5255	Hearing aid, digital, monaural, ITC	

E	V5256	Hearing aid, digital, monaural, ITE	
E	V5257	Hearing aid, digital, monaural, BTE	
E	V5258	Hearing aid, digital, binaural, CIC	
	V5259	Hearing aid, digital, binaural, ITC	
	V5260	Hearing aid, digital, binaural, ITE	
	V5261	Hearing aid, digital, binaural, BTE	
	V5262	Hearing aid, disposable, any type, monaural	
☑	V5263	Hearing aid, disposable, any type, binaural	
☑	V5264	Ear mold/insert, not disposable, any type	
☑	V5265	Ear mold/insert, disposable, any type	
☑	V5266	Battery for use in hearing device	
☑	V5267	Hearing aid supplies/accessories	
☑	V5268	Assistive listening device, telephone amplifier, any type	
	V5269	Assistive listening device, alerting, any type	
	V5270	Assistive listening device, television amplifier, any type	
	V5271	Assistive listening device, television caption decoder	
	V5272	Assistive listening device, TDD	
	V5273	Assistive listening device, for use with cochlear implant	
	V5274	Assistive listening device, not otherwise specified	
	V5275	Ear impression, each	
	V5298	Hearing aid, not otherwise classified	
B	V5299	Hearing service, miscellaneous	

V5299 Determine if an alternative HCPCS Level II or a CPT code better describes the service being reported. This code should be used only if a more specific code is unavailable.

MED: 100-2, 16, 90

SPEECH-LANGUAGE PATHOLOGY SERVICES

E	V5336	Repair/modification of augmentative communicative system or device (excludes adaptive hearing aid)	⊘

V5336 Medicare jurisdiction: DME regional carrier.

E	V5362	Speech screening	
E	V5363	Language screening	
E	V5364	Dysphagia screening	

Special Coverage Instructions   Noncovered by Medicare   Carrier Discretion   ☑ Quantity Alert   ● New Code   ○ Reinstated Code   ▲ Revised Code

142 — V Codes   A Adult   M Maternity   P Pediatrics   I Infant   A-Y APC Status Indicator   *2005 HCPCS*

APPENDIX 1 — MODIFIERS

A1	Dressing for one wound
A2	Dressing for two wounds
A3	Dressing for three wounds
A4	Dressing for four wounds
A5	Dressing for five wounds
A6	Dressing for six wounds
A7	Dressing for seven wounds
A8	Dressing for eight wounds
A9	Dressing for nine or more wounds
AA	Anesthesia services performed personally by anesthesiologist
AD	Medical supervision by a physician: more than four concurrent anesthesia procedures
● AE	Registered dietician
● AF	Specialty physician
● AG	Primary physician
AH	Clinical psychologist
● AK	Non-participating physician
AM	Physician, team member service
AN	Determination of refractive state was not performed in the course of diagnostic
AP	Ophthalmological examination
● AR	Physician provider services in a physician scarcity area
AS	Physician assistant, nurse practitioner, or clinical nurse specialist services for assistant at surgery
AT	Acute treatment (this modifier should be used when reporting service 98940, at 98941, 98942)
AU	Item furnished in conjunction with a urological, ostomy, or tracheostomy supply
AV	Item furnished in conjunction with a prosthetic device, prosthetic or orthotic
AW	Item furnished in conjunction with a surgical dressing
AX	Item furnished in conjunction with dialysis services
BA	Item furnished in conjunction with parenteral enteral nutrition (pen) services
BO	Orally administered nutrition, not by feeding tube
BP	The beneficiary has been informed of the purchase and rental options and has elected to purchase the item
BR	The beneficiary has been informed of the purchase and rental options and has elected to rent the item
BU	The beneficiary has been informed of the purchase and rental options and after 30 days has not informed the supplier of his/her decision
CA	Procedure payable only in the inpatient setting when performed emergently on an outpatient who expires prior to admission
CB	Service ordered by a renal dialysis facility (RDF) physician as part of the ESRD beneficiary's dialysis

	benefit, is not part of the composite rate, and is separately reimbursable
CC	Procedure code change (use 'CC' when the procedure code submitted was changed either for administrative reasons or because an incorrect code was filed)
CD	AMCC test has been ordered by an ESRD facility or MCP physician that is part of the composite rate and is not separately billable
CE	AMCC test has been ordered by an ESRD facility or MCP physician that is a composite rate test but is beyond the normal frequency covered under the rate and is separately reimbursable based on medical necessity
CF	AMCC test has been ordered by an ESRD facility or MCP physician that is not part of the composite rate and is separately billable
CG	Innovator drug dispensed
E1	Upper left, eyelid
E2	Lower left, eyelid
E3	Upper right, eyelid
E4	Lower right, eyelid
EJ	Subsequent claims for a defined course of therapy, e.g., EPO, sodium hyaluronate, infliximab
EM	Emergency reserve supply (for ESRD benefit only)
EP	Service provided as part of Medicaid early periodic screening diagnosis and treatment (EPSDT) program
ET	Emergency services
EY	No physician or other licensed health care provider order for this item or service
F1	Left hand, second digit
F2	Left hand, third digit
F3	Left hand, fourth digit
F4	Left hand, fifth digit
F5	Right hand, thumb
F6	Right hand, second digit
F7	Right hand, third digit
F8	Right hand, fourth digit
F9	Right hand, fifth digit
FA	Left hand, thumb
▲ FP	Service provided as part of family planning program
G1	Most recent URR reading of less than 60
G2	Most recent URR reading of 60 to 64.9
G3	Most recent URR reading of 65 to 69.9
G4	Most recent URR reading of 70 to 74.9
G5	Most recent URR reading of 75 or greater
G6	ESRD patient for whom less than six dialysis sessions have been provided in a month
G7	Pregnancy resulted from rape or incest or pregnancy certified by physician as life threatening
G8	Monitored anesthesia care (MAC) for deep complex, complicated, or markedly invasive surgical procedure

G9	Monitored anesthesia care for patient who has history of severe cardio-pulmonary condition	HI	Integrated mental health and mental retardation/developmental disabilities program
GA	Waiver of liability statement on file	HJ	Employee assistance program
GB	Claim being re-submitted for payment because it is no longer covered under a global payment demonstration	HK	Specialized mental health programs for high-risk populations
GC	This service has been performed in part by a resident under the direction of a teaching physician	HL	Intern
		HM	Less than bachelor degree level
GE	This service has been performed by a resident without the presence of a teaching physician under the primary care exception	HN	Bachelors degree level
		HO	Masters degree level
		HP	Doctoral level
GF	Non-physician (e.g. nurse practitioner (NP), certified registered nurse anaesthetist (CRNA), certified registered nurse (CRN), clinical nurse specialist (CNS), physician assistant (PA) services in a critical access hospital	HQ	Group setting
		HR	Family/couple with client present
		HS	Family/couple without client present
		HT	Multi-disciplinary team
		HU	Funded by child welfare agency
GG	Performance and payment of a screening mammogram and diagnostic mammogram on the same patient, same day	HV	Funded state addictions agency
		HW	Funded by state mental health agency
		HX	Funded by county/local agency
GH	Diagnostic mammogram converted from screening mammogram on same day	HY	Funded by juvenile justice agency
		HZ	Funded by criminal justice agency
GJ	"Opt out" physician or practitioner emergency or urgent service	JW	Drug amount discarded/not administered to any patient
GK	Actual item/service ordered by physician, item associated with GA or GZ modifier	K0	Lower extremity prosthesis functional level 0 - does not have the ability or potential to ambulate or transfer safely with or without assistance and a prosthesis does not enhance their quality of life or mobility
GL	Medically unnecessary upgrade provided instead of standard item, no charge, no advance beneficiary notice (ABN)		
GM	Multiple patients on one ambulance trip	K1	Lower extremity prosthesis functional level 1 - has the ability or potential to use a prosthesis for transfers or ambulation on level surfaces at fixed cadence. Typical of the limited and unlimited household ambulatory
GN	Services delivered under an outpatient speech language pathology plan of care		
GO	Services delivered under an outpatient occupational therapy plan of care	K2	Lower extremity prosthesis functional level 2 - has the ability or potential for ambulation with the ability to traverse low level environmental barriers such as curbs, stairs or uneven surfaces. Typical of the limited community ambulator
GP	Services delivered under an outpatient physical therapy plan of care		
GQ	Via asynchronous telecommunications system		
GT	Via interactive audio and video telecommunication systems	K3	Lower extremity prosthesis functional level 3 - has the ability or potential for ambulation with variable cadence. Typical of the community ambulator who has the ability to transverse most environmental barriers and may have vocational, therapeutic, or exercise activity that demands prosthetic utilization beyond simple locomotion
GV	Attending physician not employed or paid under arrangement by the patient's hospice provider		
GW	Service not related to the hospice patient's terminal condition		
GY	Item or service statutorily excluded or does not meet the definition of any Medicare benefit	K4	Lower extremity prosthesis functional level 4 - has the ability or potential for prosthetic ambulation that exceeds the basic ambulation skills, exhibiting high impact, stress, or energy levels, typical of the prosthetic demands of the child, active adult, or athlete
GZ	Item or service expected to be denied as not reasonable and necessary		
H9	Court-ordered		
HA	Child/adolescent program		
HB	Adult program, non-geriatric	KA	Add on option/accessory for wheelchair
HC	Adult program, geriatric	KB	Beneficiary requested upgrade for ABN, more than 4 modifiers identified on claim
HD	Pregnant/parenting women's program		
HF	Substance abuse program		
HG	Opioid addiction treatment program	● KC	Replacement of special power wheelchair interface
HH	Integrated mental health/substance abuse program		

KD	Drug or biological infused through DME
● KF	Item designated by FDA as Class III device
KH	DMEPOS item, initial claim, purchase or first month rental
KI	DMEPOS item, second or third month rental
KJ	DMEPOS item, parenteral enteral nutrition (PEN) pump or capped rental, months four to fifteen
KM	Replacement of facial prosthesis including new impression/moulage
KN	Replacement of facial prosthesis using previous master model
KO	Single drug unit dose formulation
KP	First drug of a multiple drug unit dose formulation
KQ	Second or subsequent drug of a multiple drug unit dose formulation
KR	Rental item, billing for partial month
KS	Glucose monitor supply for diabetic beneficiary not treated with insulin
KX	Specific required documentation on file
KZ	New coverage not implemented by managed care
LC	Left circumflex coronary artery
LD	Left anterior descending coronary artery
LL	Lease/rental (use the 'LL' modifier when DME equipment rental is to be applied against the purchase price)
LR	Laboratory round trip
LS	FDA-monitored intraocular lens implant
LT	Left side (used to identify procedures performed on the left side of the body)
MS	Six month maintenance and servicing fee for reasonable and necessary parts and labor which are not covered under any manufacturer or supplier warranty
NR	New when rented (use the 'NR' modifier when DME which was new at the time of rental is subsequently purchased)
NU	New equipment
PL	Progressive addition lenses
Q2	HCFA/ORD demonstration project procedure/service
Q3	Live kidney donor surgery and related services
Q4	Service for ordering/referring physician qualifies as a service exemption
Q5	Service furnished by a substitute physician under a reciprocal billing arrangement
Q6	Service furnished by a locum tenens physician
Q7	One class A finding
Q8	Two class B findings
Q9	One class B and two class C findings
QA	FDA investigational device exemption
QB	Physician providing service in a rural HPSA
QC	Single channel monitoring

QD	Recording and storage in solid state memory by a digital recorder
QE	Prescribed amount of oxygen is less than 1 liter per minute (lpm)
QF	Prescribed amount of oxygen exceeds 4 liters per minute (lpm) and portable oxygen is prescribed
QG	Prescribed amount of oxygen is greater than 4 liters per minute(lpm)
QH	Oxygen conserving device is being used with an oxygen delivery system
QJ	Services/items provided to a prisoner or patient in state or local custody, however the state or local government, as applicable, meets the requirements in 42 cfr 411.4 (b)
QK	Medical direction of two, three, or four concurrent anesthesia procedures involving qualified individuals
QL	Patient pronounced dead after ambulance called
QM	Ambulance service provided under arrangement by a provider of services
QN	Ambulance service furnished directly by a provider of services
QP	Documentation is on file showing that the laboratory test(s) was ordered individually or ordered as a CPT-recognized panel other than automated profile codes 80002-80019, G0058, G0059, and G0060
QQ	Claim submitted with a written statement of intent
QS	Monitored anesthesia care service
QT	Recording and storage on tape by an analog tape recorder
QU	Physician providing service in an urban HPSA
QV	Item or service provided as routine care in a Medicare qualifying clinical trial
QW	CLIA waived test
QX	CRNA service: with medical direction by a physician
QY	Medical direction of one certified registered nurse anesthetist (CRNA) by an anesthesiologist
QZ	CRNA service: without medical direction by a physician
RC	Right coronary artery
RD	Drug provided to beneficiary, but not administered incident-to
RP	Replacement and repair RP may be used to indicate replacement of DME, orthotic and prosthetic devices which have been in use for sometime. The claim shows the code for the part, followed by the 'RP' modifier and the charge for the part
RR	Rental (use the 'RR' modifier when DME is to be rented)
RT	Right side (used to identify procedures performed on the right side of the body)
SA	Nurse practitioner rendering service in collaboration with a physician
SB	Nurse midwife
SC	Medically necessary service or supply

SD	Services provided by registered nurse with specialized, highly technical home infusion training
SE	State and/or federally-funded programs/services
SF	Second opinion ordered by a professional review organization (PRO) per section 9401, p.l. 99-272 (100% reimbursement - no Medicare deductible or coinsurance)
SG	Ambulatory surgical center (ASC) facility service
SH	Second concurrently administered infusion therapy
SJ	Third or more concurrently administered infusion therapy
SK	Member of high risk population (use only with codes for immunization)
SL	State supplied vaccine
SM	Second surgical opinion
SN	Third surgical opinion
SQ	Item ordered by home health
ST	Related to trauma or injury
SU	Procedure performed in physician's office (to denote use of facility and equipment)
SV	Pharmaceuticals delivered to patient's home but not utilized
● SW	Services provided by a certified diabetic educator
● SY	Persons who are in close contact with member of high-risk population (use only with codes for immunization)
T1	Left foot, second digit
T2	Left foot, third digit
T3	Left foot, fourth digit
T4	Left foot, fifth digit
T5	Right foot, great toe
T6	Right foot, second digit
T7	Right foot, third digit
T8	Right foot, fourth digit
T9	Right foot, fifth digit
TA	Left foot, great toe
TC	Technical component. Under certain circumstances, a charge may be made for the technical component alone. Under those circumstances the technical component charge is identified by adding modifier 'TC' to the usual procedure number. technical component charges are institutional charges and not billed separately by physicians. However, portable x-ray suppliers only bill for technical component and should utilize modifier TC. The charge data from portable x-ray suppliers will then be used to build customary and prevailing profiles
TD	RN
TE	LPN/LVN
TG	Complex/high tech level of care
TH	Obstetrical treatment/services, prenatal or postpartum
TJ	Program group, child and/or adolescent

TK	Extra patient or passenger, non-ambulance
TL	Early intervention/individualized family service plan (IFSP)
TM	Individualized education program (IEP)
TN	Rural/outside providers' customary service area
TP	Medical transport, unloaded vehicle
TQ	Basic life support transport by a volunteer ambulance provider
TR	School-based individualized education program (IEP) services provided outside the public school district responsible for the student
TS	Follow-up service
TT	Individualized service provided to more than one patient in same setting
TU	Special payment rate, overtime
TV	Special payment rates, holidays/weekends
TW	Back-up equipment
U1	Medicaid level of care 1, as defined by each state
U2	Medicaid level of care 2, as defined by each state
U3	Medicaid level of care 3, as defined by each state
U4	Medicaid level of care 4, as defined by each state
U5	Medicaid level of care 5, as defined by each state
U6	Medicaid level of care 6, as defined by each state
U7	Medicaid level of care 7, as defined by each state
U8	Medicaid level of care 8, as defined by each state
U9	Medicaid level of care 9, as defined by each state
UA	Medicaid level of care 10, as defined by each state
UB	Medicaid level of care 11, as defined by each state
UC	Medicaid level of care 12, as defined by each state
UD	Medicaid level of care 13, as defined by each state
UE	Used durable medical equipment
UF	Services provided in the morning
UG	Services provided in the afternoon
UH	Services provided in the evening
UJ	Services provided at night
UK	Services provided on behalf of the client to someone other than the client (collateral relationship)
UN	Two patients served
UP	Three patients served
UQ	Four patients served
UR	Five patients served
US	Six or more patients served
VP	Aphakic patient

CMS will no longer require the designation of the four PET Scan modifiers (N, E, P, S) and has made the determination that no paper documentation needs to be submitted up front with PET scan claims. Documentation requirements such as physician referral and medical necessity determination are to be maintained by the provider as part of the beneficiary's medical record. Review the expanded coverage of PET Scans and revised billing instructions. (PM AB-02-115 August 7, 2002)

APPENDIX 2 — ABBREVIATIONS AND ACRONYMS

HCPCS ABBREVIATIONS AND ACRONYMS

The following abbreviations and acronyms are used in the HCPCS descriptions:

/	or
<	less than
<=	less than equal to
>	greater than
>=	greater than equal to
AC	alternating current
AFO	ankle-foot orthosis
AICC	anti-inhibitor coagulant complex
AK	above the knee
AKA	above knee amputation
ALS	advanced life support
AMP	ampule
ART	artery
ART	Arterial
ASC	ambulatory surgery center
ATT	attached
A-V	Arteriovenous
AVF	arteriovenous fistula
BICROS	bilateral routing of signals
BK	below the knee
BLS	basic life support
BP	blood pressure
BTE	behind the ear (hearing aid)
CAPD	continuous ambulatory peritoneal dialysis
Carb	carbohydrate
CBC	complete blood count
cc	cubic centimeter
CCPD	continuous cycling peritoneal analysis
CHF	congestive heart failure
CIC	completely in the canal (hearing aid)
CIM	Coverage Issue Manual
Clsd	closed
cm	centimeter
CMN	certificate of medical necessity
CMS	Centers for Medicare and Medicaid Services
CMV	Cytomegalovirus
Conc	concentrate
Conc	concentrated
Cont	continuous
CP	clinical psychologist
CPAP	continuous positive airway pressure
CPT	Current Procedural Terminology
CRF	chronic renal failure

CRNA	certified registered nurse anesthetist
CROS	contralateral routing of signals
CSW	clinical social worker
CT	computed tomography
CTLSO	cervical-thoracic-lumbar-sacral orthosis
cu	cubic
DC	direct current
DI	diurnal rhythm
Dx	diagnosis
DLI	donor leukocyte infusion
DME	durable medical equipment
DMEPOS	Durable Medical Equipment, Prosthestics, Orthotics and Other Supplies
DMERC	durable medical equipment regional carrier
DR	diagnostic radiology
DX	diagnostic
e.g.	for example
Ea	each
ECF	extended care facility
EEG	electroencephalogram
EKG	electrocardiogram
EMG	electromyography
EO	elbow orthosis
EP	electrophysiologic
EPO	epoetin alfa
EPSDT	early periodic screening, diagnosis and treatment
ESRD	end-stage renal disease
Ex	extended
Exper	experimental
Ext	external
F	french
FDA	Food and Drug Administration
FDG-PET	Positron emission with tomography with 18 fluorodeoxyglucose
Fem	female
FO	finger orthosis
FPD	fixed partial denture
Fr	french
ft	foot
G-CSF	filgrastim (granulocyte colony-stimulating factor)
gm	gram (g)
H_2O	water
HCl	hydrochloric acid, hydrochloride
HCPCS	Healthcare Common Procedural Coding System
HCT	hematocrit
HFO	hand-finger orthosis
HHA	home health agency

HI	high	MESA	microsurgical epididymal sperm aspiration
HI-LO	high-low	mg	milligram
HIT	home infusion therapy	mgs	milligrams
HKAFO	hip-knee-ankle foot orthosis	MHT	megahertz
HLA	human leukocyte antigen	ml	milliliter
HMES	heat and moisture exchange system	mm	millimeter
HNPCC	hereditary non-polyposis colorectal cancer	mmHg	millimeters of Mercury
HO	hip orthosis	MRA	magnetic resonance angiography
HPSA	health professional shortage area	MRI	magnetic resonance imaging
ip	interphalangeal	NA	sodium
I-131	Iodine 131	NCI	National Cancer Institute
ICF	intermediate care facility	NEC	not elsewhere classified
ICU	intensive care facility	NG	nasogastric
IM	intramuscular	NH	nursing home
in	inch	NMES	neuromuscular electrical stimulation
INF	infusion	NOC	not otherwise classified
INH	inhalation solution	NOS	not otherwise specified
INJ	injection	O_2	oxygen
IOL	intraocular lens	OBRA	Omnibus Budget Reconciliation Act
IPD	intermittent peritoneal dialysis	OMT	osteopathic manipulation therapy
IPPB	intermittent positive pressure breathing	OPPS	outpatient prospective payment system
IT	intrathecal administration	OSA	obstructive sleep apnea
ITC	in the canal (hearing aid)	Ost	ostomy
ITE	in the ear (hearing aid)	OTH	other routes of administration
IU	international units	oz	ounce
IV	intravenous	PA	physician's assistant
IVF	in vitro fertilization	PAR	parenteral
KAFO	knee-ankle-foot orthosis	PCA	patient controlled analgesia
KO	knee orthosis	PCH	pouch
KOH	potassium hydroxide	PEN	parenteral and enteral nutrition
L	left	PENS	percutaneous electrical nerve stimulation
LASIK	laser in situ keratomileusis	PET	positron emission tomography
LAUP	laser assisted uvulopalatoplasty	PHP	pre-paid health plan
lbs	pounds	PHP	physician hospital plan
LDL	low density lipoprotein	PI	paramedic intercept
Lo	low	PICC	peripherally inserted central venous catheter
LPM	liters per minute	PKR	photorefractive keratotomy
LPN/LVN	Licensed Practical Nurse/Licensed Vocational Nurse	Pow	powder
LSO	lumbar-sacral orthosis	PRK	photoreactive keratectomy
mp	metacarpophalangeal	PRO	peer review organization
mcg	microgram	PSA	prostate specific antigen
mCi	millicurie	PTB	patellar tendon bearing
MCM	Medicare Carriers Manual	PTK	phototherapeutic keratectomy
MCP	metacarparpophalangeal joint	PVC	polyvinyl chloride
MCP	monthly capitation payment	R	right
mEq	milliequivalent	Repl	replace

RN	registered nurse
RP	retrograde pyelogram
Rx	prescription
SACH	solid ankle, cushion heel
SC	subcutaneous
SCT	specialty care transport
SEO	shoulder-elbow orthosis
SEWHO	shoulder-elbow-wrist-hand orthosis
SEXA	single energy x-ray absorptiometry
SGD	speech generating device
SGD	sinus rhythm
SM	samarium
SNCT	sensory nerve conduction test
SNF	skilled nursing facility
SO	sacroilliac othrosis
SO	shoulder orthosis
Sol	solution
SQ	square
SR	screen
ST	standard
ST	sustained release
Syr	syrup

TABS	tablets
Tc	Technetium
Tc 99m	technetium isotope
TENS	transcutaneous electrical nerve stimulator
THKAO	thoracic-hip-knee-ankle orthosis
TLSO	thoracic-lumbar-sacral-orthosis
TM	temporomandibular
TMJ	temporomandibular joint
TPN	total parenteral nutrition
U	unit
VAR	various routes of administration
w	with
w/	with
w/o	with or without
WAK	wearable artificial kidney
wc	wheelchair
WHFO	wrist-hand-finger orthotic
Wk	week
w/o	without
Xe	xenon (isotope mass of xenon 133)

APPENDIX 3 — TABLE OF DRUGS

INTRODUCTION AND DIRECTIONS

The *HCPCS 2005* Table of Drugs is designed to quickly and easily direct the user to drug names and their corresponding codes. Both generic and brand or trade names are alphabetically listed in the "Drug Name" column of the table. The associated A, C, J, K, Q, or S code is given only for the generic name of the drug. Brand or trade name drugs are cross-referenced to the appropriate generic drug name.

The "Amount" column lists the stated amount for the referenced generic drug as provided by CMS. "Up to" listings are inclusive of all quantities up to and including the listed amount. All other listings are for the amount of the drug as listed. The editors recognize that the availability of some drugs in the quantities listed is dependent on many variables beyond the control of the clinical ordering clerk. The availability in your area of regularly used drugs in the most cost-effective quantities should be relayed to your third-party payers.

The "Route of Administration" column addresses the most common methods of delivering the referenced generic drug as described in current pharmaceutical literature. The official definitions for Level II drug codes generally describe administration other than by oral method. Therefore, with a handful of exceptions, oral-delivered options for most drugs are omitted from the Route of Administration column. The following abbreviations and listings are used in the Route of Administration column:

IA — Intra-arterial administration

IV — Intravenous administration

IM — Intramuscular administration

IT — Intrathecal

SC — Subcutaneous administration

INH — Administration by inhaled solution

INJ — Injection not otherwise specified

VAR — Various routes of administration

OTH — Other routes of administration

ORAL — Administered orally

Intravenous administration includes all methods, such as gravity infusion, injections, and timed pushes. When several routes of administration are listed, the first listing is simply the first, or most common, method as described in current reference literature. The "VAR" posting denotes various routes of administration and is used for drugs that are commonly administered into joints, cavities, tissues, or topical applications, in addition to other parenteral administrations. Listings posted with "OTH" alert the user to other administration methods, such as suppositories or catheter injections.

Please be reminded that the Table of Drugs, as well as all HCPCS Level II national definitions and listings, constitutes a post-treatment medical reference for billing purposes only. Although the editors have exercised all normal precautions to ensure the accuracy of the table and related material, the use of any of this information to select medical treatment is entirely inappropriate.

Drug Name	Unit	Route	Code	Drug Name	Unit	Route	Code
5% DEXTROSE/NORMAL SALINE	5%	VAR	J7042	ALPHANATE	PER IU	IV	J7190
5% DEXTROSE/WATER	500 ML	IV	J7060	ALPHANINE SD	PER IU	IV	J7193
ABARELIX, 10 MG	10 MG	INJ	J0128	ALPROSTADIL	1.25 MCG	INJ	J0270
ABBOKINASE	250000 IU	IV	J3365	ALPROSTADIL	EA	OTH	J0275
ABBOKINASE	5000 IU	IV	J3364	ALTEPLASE RECOMBINANT	1 MG	IV	J2997
ABCIXIMAB	10 MG	IV	J0130	ALUPENT	10 MG	INH	J7668
ABELCET	10 MG	IV	J0287	AMANTADINE HYDROCHLORIDE	100 MG	ORAL	G9017
ACCUNEB	0.5 MG	INH	J7619	AMBISOME	10 MG	IV	J0289
ACETADOTE	1 G	INH	J7608	AMEVIVE	0.5 MG	INJ	J0215
ACETAZOLAMIDE SODIUM	500 MG	IM, IV	J1120	AMICAR	5 G	INJ	S0017
ACETYLCYSTEINE	0.5 MG	INH	J7610	AMIFOSTINE	500 MG	IV	J0207
ACETYLCYSTEINE	1 G	INH	J7608	AMIKACIN SULFATE	500 MG	INJ	S0016
ACTIMMUNE	0.25 MG	SC	J1830	AMIKIN	500 MG	INJ	S0016
ACTIMMUNE	3 MU	SC	J9216	AMINOCAPROIC ACID	5 G	INJ	S0017
ACTIVASE	1 MG	IV	J2997	AMINOPHYLLIN/AMINOPHYLLINE	250 MG	IV	J0280
ADALIMUMAB	20 MG	INJ	J0135	AMIODARONE HCL	30 MG	IV	J0282
ADBEON	4 MG	IM, IV	J0704	AMITRIPTYLINE HCL	20 MG	IM	J1320
ADENOCARD	6 MG	IV	J0150	AMOBARBITAL	125 MG	IM, IV	J0300
ADENOSCAN	30 MG	IV	J0152	AMPHOCIN	50 MG	IV	J0285
ADENOSINE	30 MG	IV	J0152	AMPHOTEC	10 MG	IV	J0288
ADENOSINE	6 MG	IV	J0150	AMPHOTERICIN B	50 MG	IV	J0285
ADRENALIN	1 MG	IM, IV, SC, VAR	J0170	AMPHOTERICIN B CHOLESTERYL SULFATE COMPLEX	10 MG	IV	J0288
ADRENALIN CHLORIDE	1 MG	IM, IV, SC, VAR	J0170	AMPHOTERICIN B LIPID COMPLEX	10 MG	IV	J0287
ADRIAMYCIN	10 MG	IV	J9000	AMPHOTERICIN B LIPOSOME	10 MG	IV	J0289
ADRUCIL	500 MG	IV	J9190	AMPICILLIN	500 MG	IM, IV	J0290
AEROBID	1 MG	INH	J7641	AMPICILLIN SODIUM	500 MG	IM, IV	J0290
AGALSIDASE BETA	1 MG	INJ	J0180	AMPICILLIN SODIUM/SULBACTAM SODIUM	1.5 G	IM, IV	J0295
AGGRASTAT	12.5 MG	IM, IV	J3246	AMYTAL SODIUM	125 MG	IM, IV	J0300
A-HYDROCORT	100 MG	IV, IM, SC	J1720	ANCEF	500 MG	IV, IM	J0690
ALATROFLOXACIN MESYLATE	100 MG	IV	J0200	ANDRO LA	200 MG	IM	J3130
ALBUTEROL	0.5 MG	INH	J7619	ANECTINE	20 MG	IM, IV	J0330
ALBUTEROL	5 MG	INH	J7621	ANGIOMAX	1 MG	INJ	J0583
ALBUTEROL CONCENETRATED FORM	1 MG	INH	J7611	ANISTREPLASE	30 UNITS	IV	J0350
ALBUTEROL SULFATE	0.5 MG	INH	J7619	ANTIFLEX	60 MG	IV, IM	J2360
ALBUTEROL UNIT DOSE FORM	1 MG	INH	J7613	ANTIHEMOPHILIC FACTOR HELIXATE	PER IU	IV	J7192
ALBUTEROL, UP TO 5 MG AND IPRATROPIUM BROMIDE, UP TO 1 MG, COMPOUNDED	5 MG	INH	J7616	ANTIHEMOPHILIC FACTOR HUMAN METHOD M MONOCLONAL PURIFIED	PER IU	IV	J7192
ALDESLEUKIN	1 VIAL	VAR	J9015	ANTIHEMOPHILIC FACTOR PORCINE	PER IU	IV	J7192
ALDOMET	250 MG	IV	J0210	ANTI-INHIBITOR	PER IU	IV	J7198
ALEFACEPT	7.5 MG	IM	C9212	ANTINAUS	50 MG	IM, IV	J2550
ALEFACEPT	0.5 MG	INJ	J0215	ANTITHROMBIN III THROMBATE III	PER IU	IV	J7197
ALEFACEPT	7.5 MG	IV	C9211	ANTI-THYMOCYTE GLOBULIN,EQUINE	250 MG	OTH	J7504
ALEMTUZUMAB	10 MG	INJ	J9010	ANZEMET	10 MG	IV	J1260
ALFERON N	250000 IU	IM	J9215	APREPITANT, ORAL, 5 MG	5 MG	ORAL	J8501
ALGLUCERASE	10 UNITS	IV	J0205	AQUAMEPHYTON	1 MG	IM, SC, IV	J3430
ALKERAN	50 MG	IV	J9245	ARALAST	10 MG	IV	J0256
ALKERAN	2 MG	ORAL	J8600	ARAMINE	10 MG	IV, IM, SC	J0380
ALPHA 1 - PROTEINASE INHIBITOR - HUMAN	10 MG	IV	J0256	ARANESP	5 MCG	IV	J0880

Drug Name	Unit	Route	Code
AREDIA	30 MG	IV	J2430
ARGATROBAN	30 MG	IV	J2430
ARISTOCORT	5 MG	IM	J3302
ARISTOSPAN	5 MG	VAR	J3303
ARIXTRA	0.5 MG	INJ	J1652
ARSENIC TRIOXIDE	1 MG	IV	J9017
ASPARAGINASE	10000 U	VAR	J9020
ASTRAMORPH PF	10 MG	IM, IV, SC	J2275
ATGAM	250 MG	OTH	J7504
ATIVAN	2 MG	IM, IV	J2060
ATROPEN	0.3 MG	IV, IM, SC	J0460
ATROPINE	PER MG	INH	J7636
ATROPINE SULFATE	0.3 MG	IV, IM, SC	J0460
AUROTHIOGLUCOSE	50 MG	IM	J2910
AUTOPLEX T	PER IU	IV	J7198
AVELOX	100 MG	INJ	J2280
AVONEX	33 MCG	IM	J1825
AZACITIDINE	1 MG	INJ	C9218
AZASAN	50 MG	ORAL	J7500
AZATHIOPRINE	50 MG	ORAL	J7500
AZATHIOPRINE	100 MG	OTH	J7501
AZATHIOPRINE SODIUM	100 MG	OTH	J7501
AZITHROMYCIN	500 MG	IV	J0456
AZTREONAM	500 MG	INJ	S0073
BACLOFEN	10 MG	IT	J0475
BACLOFEN	50 MCG	OTH	J0476
BACTERIOSTATIC WATER	5%	VAR	J7051
BACTOCILL	250 MG	IM, IV	J2700
BACTRAMYCIN	300 MG	IV	J2010
BAL	100 MG	IM	J0470
BANFLEX	60 MG	IV, IM	J2360
BARMINE	20 MG	IM	J0500
BAYGAM	1 CC	IM	J1460
BAYGAM	10 MG	IV	J1564
BAYRHO D	50 MCG	IM	J2788
BAYRHO-D	300 MCG	IM	J2790
BAYTET	250 U	IM	J1670
BCG VACCINE LIVE	PER VIAL	IV	J9031
BEBULIN VH	PER IU	IV	J7194
BECLOMETHASONE	1 MG	INH	J7622
BECLOVENT	1 MG	INH	J7622
BECONASE	1 MG	INH	J7622
BENADRYL	50 MG	IV, IM	J1200
BENEFIX	PER IU	IV	J7195
BENTYL	20 MG	IM	J0500
BENZTROPINE MESYLATE	1 MG	IM, IV	J0515
BETA-2	1 MG	INH	J7648
BETAMETHASONE ACETATE AND BETAMETHASONE SODIUM PHOSPHATE	3 MG, OF EACH	IM	J0702

Drug Name	Unit	Route	Code
BETAMETHASONE SODIUM PHOSPHATE	4 MG	IM, IV	J0704
BETAMETHASONE SODIUM PHOSPHATE	1 MG	INH	J7624
BETASERON	0.25 MG	SC	J1830
BETHANECHOL CHLORIDE, MYOTONACHOL OR URECHOLINE	5 MG	SC	J0520
BEVACIZUMAB	10 MG	INJ	J9035
BICILLIN CR	1200000 U	IM	J0540
BICILLIN CR	600000 U	IM	J0530
BICILLIN L A	1200000 U	IM	J0570
BICILLIN LA	600000 U	IM	J0560
BICNU	100 MG	IV	J9050
BITOLTEROL MESYLATE	PER MG	INH	J7628
BITOLTEROL MESYLATE	PER MG	INH	J7629
BIVALIRUDIN	1 MG	INJ	J0583
BLENOXANE	15 U	IM, IV, SC	J9040
BLEOMYCIN LYOPHILLIZED	15 U	IM, IV, SC	J9040
BLEOMYCIN SULFATE	15 U	IM, IV, SC	C9417
BLEOMYCIN SULFATE	15 U	IM, IV, SC	J9040
BORTEZOMIB	0.1 MG	INJ	J9041
BOTOX	1 U	IM	J0585
BOTOX BOTULINUM TOXIN TYPE A	1 U	IM	J0585
BOTULINUM TOXIN TYPE B	100 U	IM	J0587
BRETHINE	1 MG	SC, IV	J3105
BROM-A-COT	10 MG	IM, SC, IV	J0945
BROMPHENIRAMINE MALEATE	10 MG	IM, SC, IV	J0945
BRONCHO SALINE	5 CC	VAR	J7051
BUDESONIDE	0.25 MG	INH	J7633
BUDESONIDE	0.25-0.50 MG	INH	J7626
BUMETANIDE	0.5 MG	INJ	S0171
BUPRENEX	0.1 MG	INJ	J0592
BUPRENORPHINE HCL	0.1 MG	INJ	J0592
BUSULFAN	2 MG	ORAL	J8510
BUSULFEX	2 MG	ORAL	J8510
BUTORPHANOL TARTRATE	2 MG	IM, IV	J0595
CAFCIT	5 MG	IV	J0706
CAFFEINE CITRATE	5 MG	IV	J0706
CALCIJEX	0.1 MCG	IM	J0636
CALCITONIN SALMON	400 U	SC, IM	J0630
CALCITRIOL	0.1 MCG	IM	J0636
CALCIUM DISODIUM VERSENATE	1000 MG	IV, SC, IM	J0600
CALCIUM GLUCONATE	10 ML	IV	J0610
CALCIUM GLYCEROPHOSPHATE AND CALCIUM LACTATE	10 ML	IM, SC	J0620
CALPHOSAN	10 ML	IM, SC	J0620
CAMPATH	10 MG	INJ	J9010
CAMPTOSAR	20 MG	IV	J9206
CANCIDAS	5 MG	IV	J0637
CAPECITABINE	150 MG	ORAL	J8520
CARBACOT	10 ML	IV, IM	J2800
CARBOCAINE	10 ML	VAR	J0670

Drug Name	Unit	Route	Code
CARBOPLATIN	50 MG	IV	J9045
CARIMUNE	1 GM	IV	J1563
CARMUSTINE	100 MG	IV	J9050
CARNITOR	1 G	IV	J1955
CARTICEL		OTH	J7330
CASPOFUNGIN ACETATE	5 MG	IV	J0637
CATAPRES	1 MG	OTH	J0735
CAVERJECT	1.25 MCG	INJ	J0270
CEFAZOLIN	500 MG	IV, IM	J0690
CEFAZOLIN SODIUM	500 MG	IV, IM	J0690
CEFEPIME HCL	500 MG	IV	J0692
CEFIZOX	500 MG	IV, IM	J0715
CEFOTAN	500 MG	INJ	S0074
CEFOTAXIME	1 GM	IV, IM	J0698
CEFOTAXIME SODIUM	1 GM	IV, IM	J0698
CEFOTETAN DISODIUM	500 MG	INJ	S0074
CEFOXITIN	1 GM	IV, IM	J0694
CEFOXITIN SODIUM	1 GM	IV, IM	J0694
CEFTAZIDIME	500 MG	IM, IV	J0713
CEFTIZOXIME SODIUM	500 MG	IV, IM	J0715
CEFTRIAXONE	250 MG	IV, IM	J0696
CEFTRIAXONE SODIUM	250 MG	IV, IM	J0696
CEFUROXIME	750 MG	IM, IV	J0697
CEFUROXIME SODIUM STERILE	750 MG	IM, IV	J0697
CEFURXIME	750 MG	IM, IV	J0697
CELESTONE SOLUSPAN	3 MG, OF EACH	IM	J0702
CELLCEPT	250 MG	ORAL	J7517
CEPHALOTHIN SODIUM	1 G	IM, IV	J1890
CEPTAZ	500 MG	IM, IV	J0713
CEREDASE	10 UNITS	IV	J0205
CEREZYME	1 U	IV	J1785
CERUBIDINE	10 MG	IV	J9150
CETUXIMAB	10 MG	INJ	J9055
CHLORAMPHENICOL SODIUM SUCCINATE	1 G	IV	J0720
CHLORDIAZEPOXIDE HCL	100 MG	IM, IV	J1990
CHLOROPROCAINE HCL	30 ML	VAR	J2400
CHLOROTHIAZIDE SODIUM	500 MG	IV	J1205
CHLORPROMAZINE HCL	50 MG	IM, IV	J3230
CHOREX	1000 USP UNITS	IM	J0725
CHORIONIC GONADOTROPIN	1000 USP UNITS	IM	J0725
CIDOFOVIR	375 MG	IV	J0740
CILASTATIN SODIUM; IMIPENEM	250 MG	IV, IM	J0743
CIPRO	200 MG	IV	J0744
CIPROFLOXACIN FOR INTRAVENOUS INFUSION	200 MG	IV	J0744
CISPLATIN	10 MG	IV	C9418
CISPLATIN	10 MG	IV	J9060
CISPLATIN	10 MG	IV	J9060, C9418
CLADRIBINE	1 MG	IV	C9419

Drug Name	Unit	Route	Code
CLADRIBINE	1 MG	IV	J9065
CLAFORAN	1 GM	IV, IM	J0698
CLINAGEN LA	UP TO 40 MG	IM	J0970
CLINDAMYCIN PHOSPHATE	300 MG	INJ	S0077
CLONIDINE HCL	1 MG	OTH	J0735
COBAL	1000 MCG	IM, SC	J3420
CODEINE PHOSPHATE	30 MG	IM, IV, SC	J0745
COGENTIN	1 MG	IM, IV	J0515
COLCHICINE	1 MG	IV	J0760
COLHIST	10 MG	IM, SC, IV	J0945
COLISTIMETHATE SODIUM	150 MG	IM, IV	J0770
COLY-MYCIN M	150 MG	IM, IV	J0770
COMPAZINE	10 MG	IM, IV	J0780
CONTRACEPTIVE SUPPLY, HORMONE CONTAINING PATCH	EACH	OTH	J7304
COPAXONE	20 MG	INJ	J1595
COPPER T MODEL TCU380A IUD COPPER WIRE/COPPER COLLAR	EA	OTH	J7300
CORDARONE	30 MG	IV	J0282
CORTASTAT	1 MG	IM, IV, OTH	J1100
CORTASTAT LA	1 MG	IM	J1094
CORTICOTROPIN	40 U	IV, IM, SC	J0800
CORTIMED	80 MG	IM	J1040
CORTROSYN	0.25 MG	IM, IV	J0835
CORVERT	1 MG	IV	J1742
COSMEGEN	0.5 MG	IV	J9120
COSYNTROPIN	0.25 MG	IM, IV	J0835
COTOLONE	1 ML	IM	J2650
COTOLONE	5 MG	ORAL	J7510
CROMOLYN SODIUM	10 MG	INH	J7631
CRYSTAL B12	1000 MCG	IM, SC	J3420
CYANO	1000 MCG	IM, SC	J3420
CYANOCOBALAMIN	1000 MCG	IM, SC	J3420
CYCLOPHOSPHAMIDE	1 G	IV	J9096
CYCLOPHOSPHAMIDE	1 GM	IV	J9091
CYCLOPHOSPHAMIDE	100 MG	IV	C9420
CYCLOPHOSPHAMIDE	100 MG	IV	J9070
CYCLOPHOSPHAMIDE	100 MG	IV	J9093
CYCLOPHOSPHAMIDE	2 G	IV	J9097
CYCLOPHOSPHAMIDE	2 GM	IV	J9092
CYCLOPHOSPHAMIDE	200 MG	IV	J9080
CYCLOPHOSPHAMIDE	200 MG	IV	J9094
CYCLOPHOSPHAMIDE	500 MG	IV	J9090
CYCLOPHOSPHAMIDE	500 MG	IV	J9095
CYCLOPHOSPHAMIDE	25 MG	ORAL	J8530
CYCLOPHOSPHAMIDE LYOPHILIZED	100 MG	IV	C9421
CYCLOSPORINE	100 MG	ORAL	C9438
CYCLOSPORINE	100 MG	ORAL	J7502
CYCLOSPORINE	25 MG	ORAL	J7515
CYCLOSPORINE	250 MG	OTH	J7516

Drug Name	Unit	Route	Code
CYTARABINE	100 MG	SC, IV	C9422
CYTARABINE	100 MG	SC, IV	J9100
CYTARABINE	500 MG	SC, IV	J9110
CYTARABINE LIPOSOME	10 MG	IT	J9098
CYTOGAM	PER VIAL	IV	J0850
CYTOMEGALOVIRUS IMMUNE GLOB	PER VIAL	IV	J0850
CYTOVENE	500 MG	IV	J1570
CYTOXAN	25 MG	ORAL	J8530
CYTOXAN LYOPHILIZED	1 G	IV	J9096
CYTOXAN LYOPHILIZED	100 MG	IV	J9093
CYTOXAN LYOPHILIZED	2 G	IV	J9097
CYTOXAN LYOPHILIZED	200 MG	IV	J9094
CYTOXAN LYOPHILIZED	500 MG	IV	J9095
D.H.E.	1 MG	IM, IV	J1110
DACARBAZINE	100 MG	IV	C9423
DACARBAZINE	100 MG	IV	J9130
DACARBAZINE	200 MG	IV	J9140
DACLIZUMAB	25 MG	OTH	J7513
DACTINOMYCIN	0.5 MG	IV	J9120
DALALONE	1 MG	IM, IV, OTH	J1100
DALALONE LA	1 MG	IM	J1094
DALTEPARIN SODIUM	2500 IU	SC	J1645
DAPTOMYCIN	1 MG	INJ	J0878
DARBEPOETIN ALFA	1 MCG	IV	Q4054
DARBEPOETIN ALFA	1000 UNITS	IV	Q0137
DARBEPOETIN ALFA	5 MCG	IV	J0880
DAUNORUBICIN CITRATE	10 MG	IV	J9151
DAUNORUBICIN HCL	10 MG	IV	C9424
DAUNORUBICIN HCL	10 MG	IV	J9150
DAUNOXOME	10 MG	IV	J9151
DDAVP	1 MCG	IV, SC	J2597
DECADRON LA	1 MG	IM	J1094
DECADRON PHOSPHATE	1 MG	IM, IV, OTH	J1100
DECA-DURABOLIN	100 MG	IM	J2321
DECA-DURABOLIN	200 MG	IM	J2322
DEFEROXAMINE MESYLATE	500 MG	IM, SC, IV	J0895
DEFINITY	2 ML	INJ	C9112
DELATESTRYL	200 MG	IM	J3130
DELESTROGEN	10 MG	IM	J1380
DELESTROGEN	20 MG	IM	J1390
DELESTROGEN	UP TO 40 MG	IM	J0970
DELTASONE	5 MG	OTH	J7506
DEMADEX	10 MG	IV	J3265
DEMEROL	100 MG	IM, IV, SC	J2175
DEMEROL HCL	100 MG	IM, IV, SC	J2175
DENILEUKIN DIFTITOX	300 MCG	INJ	J9160
DEPANDRATE	1 CC, 200 MG	IM	J1080
DEPANDROGYN	1 ML	IM	J1060
DEPGYNOGEN	UP TO 5 MG	IM	J1000

Drug Name	Unit	Route	Code
DEPMEDALONE	40 MG	IM	J1030
DEPMEDALONE	80 MG	IM	J1040
DEPO ESTRADIOL CYPIONATE	UP TO 5 MG	IM	J1000
DEPO MEDROL	80 MG	IM	J1040
DEPO TESTADIOL	1 ML	IM	J1060
DEPO TESTOSTERONE CYPIONATE	UP TO 100 MG	IM	J1070
DEPOCYT	10 MG	IT	J9098
DEPO-ESTRADIOL	UP TO 5 MG	IM	J1000
DEPOGEN	UP TO 5 MG	IM	J1000
DEPO-MEDROL	40 MG	IM	J1030
DEPO-PROVERA	150 MG	IM	J1055
DEPO-PROVERA	50 MG	IM	J1051
DEPO-TESTOSTERONE	1 CC, 200 MG	IM	J1080
DEPO-TESTOSTERONE	UP TO 100 MG	IM	J1070
DEPTESTROGEN	UP TO 100 MG	IM	J1070
DERMAGRAFT	37.5 SQ CM	Oth	C9201
DERMAL AND EPIDERMAL, TISSUE OF NON-HUMAN ORIGIN, WITH OR WITHOUT OTHER BIOENGINEERED OR PROCESSED ELEMENTS, WITHOUT METABOLICALLY ACTIVE ELEMENTS	PER SQ CM	EA	J7343
DERMAL TISSUE, OF HUMAN ORIGIN, WITH OR WITHOUT OTHER BIOENGINEERED OR PROCESSED ELEMENTS, WITHOUT METABOLICALLY ACTIVE ELEMENTS	PER SQ CM	EA	J7344
DESFERAL	500 MG	IM, SC, IV	J0895
DESMOPRESSIN ACETATE	1 MCG	IV, SC	J2597
DEXAMETHASONE	PER MG	INH	J7637
DEXAMETHASONE	PER MG	INH	J7638
DEXAMETHASONE ACETATE	1 MG	IM	J1094
DEXAMETHASONE ACETATE ANHYDROUS	1 MG	IM	J1094
DEXAMETHASONE SODIUM PHOSPHATE	1 MG	IM, IV, OTH	J1100
DEXFERRUM	50 MG	VAR	J1750
DEXONE LA	1 MG	IM	J1094
DEXRAZOXANE	250 MG	IV	J1190
DEXRAZOXANE HYDROCHLORIDE	250 MG	IV	J1190
DEXRAZOXANE HYDROCHLORIDE	250 MG	IV	J1190, C9410
DEXTRAN 40	500 ML	IV	J7100
DEXTROSE	500 ML	IV	J7060
DEXTROSE	1000 CC	VAR	J7120
DEXTROSE/LACTATED RINGERS	1000 CC	VAR	J7120
DEXTROSE/SODIUM CHLORIDE	5%	VAR	J7042
DEXTROSE/THEOPHYLLINE	40 MG	IV	J2810
DIAMOX PARENTERAL	500 MG	IM, IV	J1120
DIASTAT	5 MG	IV, IM	J3360
DIAZEPAM	5 MG	IV, IM	J3360
DIAZOXIDE	300 MG	IV	J1730
DICYCLOMINE HCL	20 MG	IM	J0500
DIDRONEL	300 MG	IV	J1436
DIFLUCAN	200 MG	IV	J1450

Drug Name	Unit	Route	Code
DIGOXIN	0.5 MG	IM, IV	J1160
DIHYDROERGOTAMINE MESYLATE	1 MG	IM, IV	J1110
DILAUDID	4 MG	SC, IM, IV	J1170
DILAUDID-HP	4 MG	SC, IM, IV	J1170
DILOR	500 MG	IM	J1180
DIMENHYDRINATE	50 MG	IM, IV	J1240
DIMERCAPROL	100 MG	IM	J0470
DIMINE	50 MG	IV, IM	J1200
DIPHENHYDRAMINE HCL	50 MG	IV, IM	J1200
DIPYRIDAMOLE	10 MG	IV	J1245
DISOTATE	150 MG	IV	J3520
DIURIL	500 MG	IV	J1205
DIURIL SODIUM	500 MG	IV	J1205
DIZAC	5 MG	IV, IM	J3360
DMSO, DIMETHYL SULFOXIDE	50%, 50 ML	OTH	J1212
DOBUTAMINE	250 MG	IV	J1250
DOBUTAMINE HCL	250 MG	IV	J1250
DOCETAXEL	20 MG	IV	J9170
DOLASETRON MESYLATE	10 MG	IV	J1260
DOLOPHINE HCL	10 MG	IM, SC	J1230
DORNASE ALPHA	PER MG	INH	J7639
DOXERCALCIFEROL	1 MG	IV	J1270
DOXIL	10 MG	IV	J9001
DOXORUBICIN HCL	10 MG	IV	C9415
DOXORUBICIN HCL	10 MG	IV	J9000
DROPERIDOL	5 MG	IM, IV	J1790
DTIC-DOME	200 MG	IV	J9140
DUONEB	5 MG	INH	J7621
DUO-SPAN	1 ML	IM	J1060
DUO-SPAN II	1 ML	IM	J1060
DURACLON	1 MG	OTH	J0735
DURAMORPH	10 MG	IM, IV, SC	J2270
DURAMORPH	10 MG	IM, IV, SC	J2275
DURO CORT	80 MG	IM	J1040
DYPHYLLINE	500 MG	IM	J1180
EDETATE CALCIUM DISODIUM	1000 MG	IV, SC, IM	J0600
EDETATE DISODIUM	150 MG	IV	J3520
EDEX	1.25 MCG	INJ	J0270
ELAVIL	20 MG	IM	J1320
ELIGARD	1 MG	IM	J9218
ELITEK	50 MCG	IM	J2783
ELLENCE	2 MG	INJ	J9178
ELOXATIN	0.5 MG	INJ	J9263
ELSPAR	10000 U	VAR	J9020
EMINASE	30 UNITS	IV	J0350
ENBREL	25 MG	IM, IV	J1438
ENDOXAN-ASTA	1 GM	IV	J9091
ENDOXAN-ASTA	100 MG	IV	J9070
ENDOXAN-ASTA	200 MG	IV	J9080

Drug Name	Unit	Route	Code
ENDOXAN-ASTA	500 MG	IV	J9090
ENDRATE	150 MG	IV	J3520
ENOXAPARIN SODIUM	10 MG	SC	J1650
EPINEPHRINE HCL	1 MG	IM, IV, SC, VAR	J0170
EPINEPHRINE, ADRENALIN	1 MG	IM, IV, SC, VAR	J0170
EPIPEN	0.3 MG	IM	J0170
EPIRUBICIN HCL	2 MG	INJ	J9178
EPOPROSTENOL	0.5 MG	IV	J1325
EPSOM SALT	10 MG	IV	J3475
EPSO-PINE BATH	10 MG	IV	J3475
EPTIFIBATIDE	5 MG	IM, IV	J1327
ERGONOVINE MALEATE	0.2 MG	IM, IV	J1330
ERTAPENEM SODIUM	500 MG	IM, IV	J1335
ERYTHROCIN LACTOBIONATE	500 MG	IV	J1364
ESTRADIOL VALERATE	10 MG	IM	J1380
ESTRADIOL VALERATE	20 MG	IM	J1390
ESTRADIOL VALERATE	UP TO 40 MG	IM	J0970
ESTRAGYN	1 MG	IV, IM	J1435
ESTRO-A	1 MG	IV, IM	J1435
ESTROGEN CONJUGATED	25 MG	IV, IM	J1410
ESTRONE	1 MG	IV, IM	J1435
ETANERCEPT	25 MG	IM, IV	J1438
ETHYOL	500 MG	IV	J0207
ETIDRONATE DISODIUM	300 MG	IV	J1436
ETOPOSIDE	10 MG	IV	C9425
ETOPOSIDE	10 MG	IV	J9181
ETOPOSIDE	100 MG	IV	J9182
ETOPOSIDE	50 MG	ORAL	C9414
ETOPOSIDE	50 MG	ORAL	J8560
FACTOR IX NON-RECOMBINANT	PER IU	IV	J7193
FACTOR IX RECOMBINANT	PER IU	IV	J7195
FACTOR VIII PORCINE	PER IU	IV	J7191
FACTOR VIII RECOMBINANT	PER IU	IV	J7192
FACTOR VIII, HUMAN	PER IU	IV	J7190
FACTREL	100 MCG	SC, IV	J1620
FASLODEX	25 MG	INJ	J9395
FEIBA-VH IMMUNO	PER IU	IV	J7198
FENTANYL CITRATE	0.1 MG	IM, IV	J3010
FENTANYL CITRATE/SODIUM CHLORIDE	0.1 MG	IM, IV	J3010
FERRLECIT	12.5 MG	IV	J2916
FILGRASTIM	300 MCG	SC, IV	J1440
FILGRASTIM	480 MCG	SC, IV	J1441
FILGRASTIM (G-CSF)	300 MCG	SC, IV	J1440
FILGRASTIM (G-CSF)	480 MCG	SC, IV	J1441
FLAGYL	500 MG	INJ	S0030
FLEBOGAMMA	1 CC	IM	J1460
FLEBOGAMMA	1 G	IV	J1563
FLOLAN	0.5 MG	IV	J1325
FLOXURIDINE	500 MG	IV	C9426

Drug Name	Unit	Route	Code
FLOXURIDINE	500 MG	IV	J9200
FLUCONAZOLE	200 MG	IV	J1450
FLUDARA	50 MG	IV	J9185
FLUDARABINE PHOSPHATE	50 MG	IV	J9185
FLUNISOLIDE	1 MG	INH	J7641
FLUOROURACIL	500 MG	IV	J9190
FLUPHENAZINE DECANOATE	25 MG	INJ	J2680
FOMIVIRSEN SODIUM	1.65 MG	OTH	J1452
FONDAPARINUX SODIUM	0.5 MG	INJ	J1652
FORTAZ	500 MG	IM, IV	J0713
FOSCARNET SODIUM	1000 MG	IV	J1455
FOSCAVIR	1000 MG	IV	J1455
FRAGMIN	2500 IU	SC	J1645
FUDR	500 MG	IV	J9200
FULVESTRANT	25 MG	INJ	J9395
FUNGIZONE	50 MG	IV	J0285
FUROCOT	20 MG	IM, IV	J1940
FUROSEMIDE	20 MG	IM, IV	J1940
GALLIUM NITRATE	1 MG	INJ	J1457
GAMIMUNE N	1 G	IV	J1563
GAMMAGARD S/D	1 G	IV	J1563
GAMMAR P	1 G	IV	J1563
GAMUNEX	1 G	IV	J1563
GANCICLOVIR	4.5 MG	OTH	J7310
GANCICLOVIR SODIUM	500 MG	IV	J1570
GATIFLOXACIN	10 MG	IV	J1590
GEFITINIB	250 MG	ORAL	J8565
GEMCITABINE HCL	200 MG	IV	J9201
GEMTUZUMAB	5 MG	IV	J9300
GEMZAR	200 MG	IV	J9201
GENARC	PER IU	IV	J7192
GENGRAF	100 MG	ORAL	J7502
GENGRAF	25 MG	ORAL	J7515
GENOTROPIN	1 MG	SC	J2941
GENOTROPIN MINIQUICK	1 MG	SC	J2941
GENTAMICIN SULFATE/SODIUM CHLORIDE	80 MG	IM, IV	J1580
GENTAMICIN/GARAMYCIN	80 MG	IM, IV	J1580
GENTRAN	500 ML	IV	J7100
GEODON	10 MG	INJ	J3486
GESTERONE	50 MG	IM	J2675
GESTRIN	50 MG	IM	J2675
GLATIRAMER ACETATE	20 MG	INJ	J1595
GLUCAGON	1 MG	SC, IM, IV	J1610
GLYCOPYRROLATE	1 MG	INH	J7643
GOLD SODIUM THIOMALATE	50 MG	IM	J1600
GONADORELIN HCL	100 MCG	SC, IV	J1620
GOSERELIN ACETATE	3.6 MG	SC	J9202
GRANISETRON HCL	100 MCG	IV	J1626
GRANISETRON HYDROCHLORIDE	100 MCG	IM, IV	J1626

Drug Name	Unit	Route	Code
GYNOGEN LA	20 MG	IM	J1390
H.P. ACTHAR	40 U	VAR	J0800
HALDOL	5 MG	IM, IV	J1630
HALDOL DECANOATE	50 MG	IM	J1631
HALOPERIDOL	5 MG	IM, IV	J1630
HECTOROL	1 MG	IV	J1270
HELIXATE FS	PER IU	IV	J7192
HEMOFIL-M	PER IU	IV	J7190
HEP LOCK	10 UNITS	IV	J1642
HEPARIN	10 UNITS	IV	J1642
HEPARIN SODIUM	10 U	IV	J1642
HEPARIN SODIUM	1000 U	IV, SC	J1644
HERCEPTIN	10 MG	IV	J9355
HUMALOG	5 U	SC	S5551
HUMALOG	50 U	SC	J1817
HUMATROPE	1 MG	SC	J2941
HUMIRA	20 MG	INJ	J0135
HUMULIN	50 U	SC	J1817
HUMULIN R	5 U	SC	J1815
HUMULIN R U-500	5 U	SC	J1815
HYALGAN	20 MG	IA	J7317
HYALURONIC ACID	20 MG	IA	J7317
HYATE C	PER IU	IV	J7191
HYBOLIN DECANOATE	100 MG	IM	J2321
HYCAMTIN	4 MG	IV	J9350
HYDRALAZINE HCL	20 MG	IV, IM	J0360
HYDRATE	50 MG	IM, IV	J1240
HYDROCORTISONE ACETATE	25 MG	IV, IM, SC	J1700
HYDROCORTISONE SODIUM PHOSPHATE	50 MG	IV, IM, SC	J1710
HYDROCORTISONE SODIUM SUCCINATE	100 MG	IV, IM, SC	J1720
HYDROMORPHONE	4 MG	SC, IM, IV	J1170
HYDROMORPHONE HCL	4 MG	SC, IM, IV	J1170
HYDROXOCOBALAMIN	1000 MCG	IM, SC	J3420
HYDROXYCOBAL	1000 MCG	IM, SC	J3420
HYDROXYZINE HCL	25 MG	IM	J3410
HYLAN G-F 20	16 MG	IA	J7320
HYOSCYAMINE SULFATE	0.25 MG	SC, IM, IV	J1980
HYPERSTAT	300 MG	IV	J1730
HYREXIN	50 MG	IV, IM	J1200
HYZINE	25 MG	IM	J3410
IBUTILIDE FUMARATE	1 MG	IV	J1742
IDARUBICIN HCL	5 MG	IV	C9429
IDARUBICIN HCL	5 MG	IV	J9211
IFEX	1 G	IV	J9208
IFOSFAMIDE	1 G	IV	C9427
IFOSFAMIDE	1 G	IV	J9208
ILETIN II NPH PORK	50 U	SC	J1817
ILETIN II REGULAR PORK	5 U	SC	J1815
IMIGLUCERASE	1 U	IV	J1785

Drug Name	Unit	Route	Code
IMITREX	6 MG	SC	J3030
IMMUNE GLOBULIN	1 CC	IM	J1460
IMMUNE GLOBULIN	1 G	IV	J1563
IMMUNE GLOBULIN	10 MG	IV	J1564
IMURAN	50 MG	ORAL	J7500
IMURAN	100 MG	OTH	J7501
INAPSINE	5 MG	IM, IV	J1790
INDERAL	1 MG	IV	J1800
INFED	50 MG	IV, IM	J1750
INFERGEN	1 MCG	SC	J9212
INFLIXIMAB	100 MG	IV	J1745
INFUMORPH	10 MG	IM, IV, SC	J2270
INFUMORPH	10 MG	IM, IV, SC	J2275
INFUMORPH	100 MG	IM, IV, SC	J2271
INNOHEP	1000 IU	SC	J1655
INSULIN	5 U	SC	J1815
INSULIN	50 U	SC	J1817
INSULIN LISPRO	5 U	SC	S5551
INSULIN PURIFIED REGULAR PORK	5 U	SC	J1815
INTAL	10 MG	INH	J7631
INTEGRILIN	5 MG	IM, IV	J1327
INTERFERON ALFA-2A	3,000,000 UNITS	SC, IM	J9213
INTERFERON ALFA-2B	1,000,000 UNITS	SC, IM	J9214
INTERFERON ALFACON-1	1 MCG	SC	J9212
INTERFERON ALFA-N3	250000 IU	IM	J9215
INTERFERON BETA-1A	33 MCG	IM	J1825
INTERFERON BETA-1B	0.25 MG	SC	J1830
INTERFERON, ALFA-2A, RECOMBINANT	3,000,000 UNITS	SC, IM	J9213
INTERFERON, ALFA-2B, RECOMBINANT	1,000,000 UNITS	SC, IM	J9214
INTERFERON, ALFA-N3, (HUMAN LEUKOCYTE DERIVED)	250000 IU	IM	J9215
INTERFERON, GAMMA 1-B	3 MU	SC	J9216
INTRON A	1,000,000 UNITS	SC, IM	J9214
INVANZ	500 MG	IM, IV	J1335
IPRATROPIUM BROMIDE	1 MG	INH	J7644
IPRATROPIUN BROMIDE	1 MG	INH	J7645
IRINOTECAN	20 MG	IV	J9206
IRON DEXTRAN	50 MG	IV, IM	J1750
IRON SUCROSE	1 MG	IV	J1756
ISOCAINE	10 ML	VAR	J0670
ISOETHARINE HCL	1 MG	INH	J7649
ISOPROTERENOL HCL	1 MG	INH	J7659
ISOTONIC GENTAMICIN SULFATE	80 MG	IM, IV	J1580
ISUPREL	1 MG	INH	J7659
ITRACONAZOLE	50 MG	IV	J1835
IVEEGAM	1 G	IV	J1563
KABIKINASE	250000 IU	IV	J2995
KANAMYCIN	500 MG	IM, IV	J1840
KANTREX	500 MG	IM, IV	J1840

Drug Name	Unit	Route	Code
KEFUROX	750 MG	IM, IV	J0697
KEFZOL	500 MG	IV, IM	J0690
KENALOG-10	10 MG	IM	J3301
KESTRONE	1 MG	IV, IM	J1435
KETOROLAC	15 MG	IM, IV	J1885
KETOROLAC TROMETHAMINE	15 MG	IM, IV	J1885
KOATE-DVI	PER IU	IV	J7190
KOGENATE	PER IU	IV	J7190
KOGENATE FS	PER IU	IV	J7192
KONYNE	PER IU	IV	J7194
KUTAPRESSIN	20 MG	IM, IV	J1920
KYTRIL	100 MCG	IV	J1626
LANOXIN	0.5 MG	IM, IV	J1160
LANTUS	50 U	SC	J1817
LARONIDASE	0.1 MG	INJ	J1931
LASIX	20 MG	IM, IV	J1940
L-CARNITINE	1 G	IV	J1955
LENTE ILETIN I	5 U	SC	J1815
LEUCOVORIN CALCIUM	50 MG	IM, IV	J0640
LEUKINE	50 MCG	IV	J2820
LEUPROLIDE ACETATE	1 MG	IM	C9430
LEUPROLIDE ACETATE	1 MG	IM	J9218
LEUPROLIDE ACETATE	7.5 MG	IM	J9217
LEUPROLIDE ACETATE (FOR DEPOT SUSPENSION)	3.75 MG	IM	J1950
LEUPROLIDE ACETATE DEPOT	7.5 MG	IM	J9217
LEUSTATIN	1 MG	IV	J9065
LEVALBUTEROL CONCENTRATED FORM	0.5 MG	INH	J7612
LEVALBUTEROL UNIT FORM	0.5 MG	INH	J7614
LEVALBUTEROL, UP TO 2.5 MG AND IPRATROPIUM BROMIDE, UP TO 1 MG	2.5 MG	INH	J7617
LEVAQUIN	1 G	IV	J1956
LEVOCARNITINE	1 G	IV	J1955
LEVO-DROMORAN	2 MG	SC, IV	J1960
LEVOFLOXACIN	1 G	IV	J1956
LEVONORGESTREL	52 MG	OTH	J7302
LEVORPHANOL TARTRATE	2 MG	SC, IV	J1960
LEVSIN	0.25 MG	SC, IM, IV	J1980
LIBRIUM	100 MG	IM, IV	J1990
LIDOCAINE HCL	10 MG	IV	J2001
LINCOCIN HCL	300 MG	IV	J2010
LINEZOLID	200 MG	IV	J2020
LIORESAL INTRATHECAL REFILL	50 MCG	OTH	J0476
LIQUID PRED SYRUP	5 MG	OTH	J7506
LISPRO-PFC	50 U	SC	J1817
LORAZEPAM	2 MG	IM, IV	J2060
LOVENOX	10 MG	SC	J1650
LUMINAL SODIUM	120 MG	IM, IV	J2560
LUNELLE	5 MG/25 MG	IM	J1056
LUPRON	1 MG	IM	J9218

Drug Name	Unit	Route	Code
LUPRON DEPOT	7.5 MG	IM	J9217
LUPRON DEPOT	3.75 MG	INJ	J1950
LYMPHOCYTE IMMUNE GLOBULIN, ANTITHYMOCYTE GLOBULIN, EQUINE	250 MG	OTH	J7504
LYMPHOCYTE IMMUNE GLOBULIN, ANTITHYMOCYTE GLOBULIN, RABBIT	25 MG	OTH	J7511
MAGNESIUM SULFATE	10 MG	IV	J3475
MANNITOL	25% IN 50 ML	IV	J2150
MAXIPIME	500 MG	IV	J0692
MECHLORETHAMINE HYDROCHLORIDE	10 MG	IV	J9230
MEDROL	4 MG	ORAL	J7509
MEDROXYPROGESTERONE ACETATE	150 MG	IM	J1055
MEDROXYPROGESTERONE ACETATE	50 MG	IM	J1051
MEDROXYPROGESTERONE ACETATE/ ESTRADIOL CYPIONATE	5 MG/25 MG	IM	J1056
MEFOXIN	1 G	IV	J0694
MELPHALAN HCL	50 MG	IV	J9245
MELPHALAN HCL	2 MG	ORAL	J8600
MENADIONE	1 MG	IM, SC, IV	J3430
MEPERGAN	50 MG	IM, IV	J2180
MEPERIDINE AND PROMETHAZINE HCL	50 MG	IM, IV	J2180
MEPERIDINE HCL	100 MG	IM, IV, SC	J2175
MEPIVACAINE HCL	10 ML	VAR	J0670
MERITATE	150 MG	IV	J3520
MEROPENEM	100 MG	INJ	J2185
MERREM	100 MG	INJ	J2185
MESNA	200 MG	IV	C9428
MESNA	200 MG	IV	J9209
METAPREL	10 MG	INH	J7668
METARAMINOL BITARTRATE	10 MG	IV, IM, SC	J0380
METHACHOLINE CHLORIDE	1 MG	INH	J7674
METHADONE HCL	10 MG	IM, SC	J1230
METHERGINE	0.2 MG	IM, IV	J2210
METHOCARBAMOL	10 ML	IV, IM	J2800
METHOTREXATE	5 MG	IV, IM, IT, IA	J9250
METHOTREXATE	50 MG	IV, IM, IT, IA	J9260
METHOTREXATE SODIUM	5 MG	IV, IM, IT, IA	J9250
METHOTREXATE SODIUM	50 MG	IV, IM, IT, IA	J9260
METHOTREXATE SODIUM	2.5 MG	ORAL	J8610
METHYLCOTOLONE	80 MG	IM	J1040
METHYLDOPA HCL	250 MG	IV	J0210
METHYLDOPATE	5 MG	IV	J0210
METHYLDOPATE HCL	5 MG	IV	J0210
METHYLERGONOVINE MALEATE	0.2 MG	IM, IV	J2210
METHYLPRED	4 MG	ORAL	J7509
METHYLPREDNISOLONE	20 MG	IM	J1020
METHYLPREDNISOLONE	80 MG	IM	J1040
METHYLPREDNISOLONE	125 MG	IM, IV	J2930
METHYLPREDNISOLONE	40 MG	IM, IV	J2920
METHYLPREDNISOLONE	4 MG	ORAL	J7509

Drug Name	Unit	Route	Code
METHYLPREDNISOLONE ACETATE	20 MG	IM	J1020
METHYLPREDNISOLONE ACETATE	40 MG	IM	J1030
METHYLPREDNISOLONE ACETATE	80 MG	IM	J1040
METOCLOPRAMIDE	10 MG	IV	J2765
METRONIDAZOLE	500 MG	INJ	S0030
MIACALCIN	400 U	SC, IM	J0630
MICRHOGAM	50 MCG	IM	J2788
MICRHOGAM ULTRA-FILTERED	50 MCG	IM	J2788
MIDAZOLAM	1 MG	IM, IV	J2250
MIDAZOLAM HCI	1MG	IM, IV	J2250
MILRINONE LACTATE	5 MG	IV	J2260
MIO REL	60 MG	IV, IM	J2360
MIRENA	52 MG	OTH	J7302
MITHRACIN	2500 MCG	IV	J9270
MITOMYCIN	20 MG	IV	J9290
MITOMYCIN	40 MG	IV	J9291
MITOMYCIN	5 MG	IV	C9432
MITOMYCIN	5 MG	IV	J9280
MITOXANTRONE	5 MG	IV	J9293
MITOXANTRONE HYDROCHLORIDE	5 MG	IV	J9293
MONARC-M	PER IU	IV	J7190
MONOCLATE-P	PER IU	IV	J7190
MONONINE	PER IU	IV	J7193
MORPHINE SULFATE	10 MG	IM, IV, SC	J2270
MORPHINE SULFATE	100 MG	IM, IV, SC	J2271
MORPHINE SULFATE, PRESERVATIVE FREE, STERILE SOLUTION	10 MG	IM, IV, SC	J2275
MOXIFLOXACIN	100 MG	INJ	J2280
MUCOMYST	1 G	INH	J7608
MUROMONAB-CD3	5 MG	OTH	J7505
MUSE	EA	OTH	J0275
MUSTARGEN	10 MG	IV	J9230
MUTAMYCIN	20 MG	IV	J9290
MUTAMYCIN	40 MG	IV	J9291
MUTAMYCIN	5 MG	IV	J9280
MYCOPHENOLATE MOFETIL	250 MG	ORAL	J7517
MYCOPHENOLIC ACID	180 MG	ORAL	J7518
MYLERAN	2 MG	ORAL	J8510
MYLOTARG	5 MG	IV	J9300
MYOBLOC	100 U	IM	J0587
MYOCHRYSINE	50 MG	IM	J1600
MYOPHEN	60 MG	IV, IM	J2360
NALBUPHINE HCL	10 MG	IM, IV, SC	J2300
NALOXONE HCL	1 MG	IM, IV, SC	J2310
NANDROLONE DECANOATE	100 MG	IM	J2321
NANDROLONE DECANOATE	200 MG	IM	J2322
NANDROLONE DECANOATE	50 MG	IM	J2320
NARCAN	1 MG	IM, IV, SC	J2310
NAROPIN	1 MG	INJ	J2795

Drug Name	Unit	Route	Code
NATRECOR	0.5 MG	INJ	J2324
NAVELBINE	10 MG	IV	J9390
ND-STAT	10 MG	IM, SC, IV	J0945
NEBCIN	80 MG	IM, IV	J3260
NEBUPENT	300 MG	INH	J2545
NEMBUTAL SODIUM	120 MG	IM, IV	J2560
NEMBUTAL SODIUM	50 MG	IM, IV, OTH	J2515
NEO SYNEPHRINE HCL	1 ML	SC, IM, IV	J2370
NEORAL	100 MG	ORAL	J7502
NEORAL	25 MG	ORAL	J7515
NEOSAR	1 GM	IV	J9091
NEOSAR	2 GM	IV	J9092
NEOSAR	200 MG	IV	J9080
NEOSAR	500 MG	IV	J9090
NEOSTIGMINE METHYLSULFATE	250 MG	IM, IV	J2710
NESACAINE CHLOROPROCAINE HCL	30 ML	VAR	J2400
NESIRITIDE	0.5 MG	INJ	J2324
NEULASTA	6 MG	SC, SQ	J2505
NEUMEGA	5 MG	SC	J2355
NEUPOGEN	300 MCG	SC, IV	J1440
NEUPOGEN	480 MCG	SC, IV	J1441
NEUTREXIN	25 MG	IV	J3305
NIPENT	10 MG	IV	J9268
NOC DRUGS, INHALATION SOLUTION ADMINISTERED THROUGH DME	1 EA		J7699
NORDITROPIN	1 MG	SC	J2941
NORFLEX	60 MG	IV, IM	J2360
NORMAL SALINE	2 ML	IV	J2912
NOT OTHERWISE CLASSIFIED, ANTINEOPLASTIC DRUGS			J9999
NOVANTRONE	5 MG	IV	J9293
NOVAREL	1000 USP UNITS	IM	J0725
NOVOLIN	50 U	SC	J1817
NOVOLIN R	5 U	SC	J1815
NOVOLOG	50 U	SC	J1817
NOVOLOG FLEXPEN	50 U	SC	J1817
NOVOLOG MIX	50 U	SC	J1817
NOV-ONXOL	30 MG	IV	J9265
NUBAIN	10 MG	IM, IV, SC	J2300
NUMORPHAN	1 MG	IV, SC, IM	J2410
NUTRI-TWELVE	1000 MCG	IM, SC	J3420
NUTROPIN	1 MG	SC	J2941
NUVARING VAGINAL RING	EA	OTH	J7303
OCATMIDE PFS	10 MG	IV	J2765
OCTAGAM IMMUNE GLOBULIN	1 GM	IV	J1563
OCTREOTIDE ACETATE DEPOT	10 MG	IM	J2353
OCTREOTIDE, NON-DEPOT FORM	25 MCG	SC, IV	J2354
OMALIZUMAB	5 MG	INJ	J2357
ONCASPAR	PER VIAL	IM, IV	J9266
ONDANSETRON HYDROCHLORIDE	1 MG	IV	J2405

Drug Name	Unit	Route	Code
ONTAK	300 MCG	INJ	J9160
ONXOL	30 MG	IV	J9265
OPRELVEKIN	5 MG	SC	J2355
ORCEL	36 SQ CM	OTH	C9200
ORPHENADRINE CITRATE	60 MG	IV, IM	J2360
ORPHENATE	60 MG	IV, IM	J2360
ORTHOCLONE OKT3	5 MG	OTH	J7505
OSELTAMIVIR PHOSPHATE	75 MG	ORAL	G9019
OXACILLIN SODIUM	250 MG	IM, IV	J2700
OXALIPLATIN	0.5 MG	INJ	J9263
OXALIPLATIN	5 MG	INJ	C9205
OXYMORPHONE HCL	1 MG	IV, SC, IM	J2410
OXYTETRACYCLINE	50 MG	IM	J2460
OXYTETRACYCLINE HCL	50 MG	IM	J2460
OXYTOCIN	10 UNITS	IV, IM	J2590
PACLITAXEL	30 MG	IV	C9431
PACLITAXEL	30 MG	IV	J9265
PALIVIZUMAB	50 MG	IM	C9003
PALONOSETRON HCL	25 MCG	INJ	J2469
PAMIDRONATE DISODIUM	30 MG	IV	C9411
PAMIDRONATE DISODIUM	30 MG	IV	J2430
PANGLOBULIN	1 G	IV	J1563
PANTOPRAZOLE SODIUM	PER VIAL	INJ	C9113
PAPAVERINE HCL	60 MG	IV, IM	J2440
PARAPLANTIN	50 MG	IV	J9045
PARICALCITOL	1 MCG	IV, IM	J2501
PEDIAPRED	5 MG	ORAL	J7510
PEGASPARGASE	PER VIAL	IM, IV	J9266
PEMETREXED	10 MG	INJ	J9305
PEN G BENZ/PEN G PROCAINE	600000 U	IM	J0530
PENICILLIN G BENZATHINE	1200000 U	IM	J0570
PENICILLIN G BENZATHINE	600000 U	IM	J0560
PENICILLIN G BENZATHINE AND PENICILLIN G PROCAINE	1200000 U	IM	J0540
PENICILLIN G POTASSIUM	600000 U	IM, IV	J2540
PENICILLIN G PROCAINE	600,000 UNITS	IM, IV	J2510
PENTACARINAT	300 MG	INH	J2545
PENTAM	300 MG	INJ	J2545
PENTAMIDINE ISETHIONATE	300 MG	INH	J2545
PENTAZOCINE LACTATE	30 MG	IM, SC, IV	J3070
PENTOBARBITAL SODIUM	50 MG	IM, IV, OTH	J2515
PENTOSTATIN	10 MG	IV	J9268
PERFLEXANE LIPID MICROSPHERES	10 ML	INJ	C9203
PERFLUTREN LIPID MICROSPHERE	2 ML	INJ	C9112
PERPHENAZINE	5 MG	IM, IV	J3310
PHENERGAN	50 MG	IM, IV	J2550
PHENOBARBITAL SODIUM	120 MG	IM, IV	J2560
PHENTOLAMINE MESYLATE	5 MG	IM, IV	J2760
PHENYLEPHRINE HCL	1 ML	SC, IM, IV	J2370

Drug Name	Unit	Route	Code
PHENYTOIN SODIUM	50 MG	IM, IV	J1165
PHOTOFRIN	75 MG	IV	J9600
PHYTONADIONE	1 MG	IM, SC, IV	J3430
PIPERACILLIN SODIUM/TAZOBACTAM SODIUM	1 G/1.125 GM	IV	J2543
PITOCIN	10 UNITS	IV, IM	J2590
PLATINOL-AQ	10 MG	IV	J9060
PLICAMYCIN	2500 MCG	IV	J9270
POLOCAINE	10 ML	VAR	J0670
POLYGAM	10 MG	IV	J1564
POLYGAM S/D	1 G	IV	J1563
PORFIMER SODIUM	75 MG	IV	J9600
POTASSIUM CHLORIDE	2 MEQ	IV	J3480
PRALIDOXIME CHLORIDE	1 MG	IV, IM, SC	J2730
PREDACORT	1 ML	IM	J2650
PREDNISOLONE	5 MG	ORAL	J7510
PREDNISOLONE ACETATE	1 ML	IM	J2650
PREDNISONE	5 MG	ORAL	J7506
PREDNORAL	5 MG	ORAL	J7510
PREGNYL	1000 USP UNITS	IM	J0725
PRELONE	5 MG	ORAL	J7510
PREMARIN	25 MG	IV, IM	J1410
PRI-ANDRIOL LA	50 MG	IM	J2320
PRI-DEXTRA	50 MG	IV, IM	J1750
PRIMACOR	5 MG	IV	J2260
PRIMAXIN	250 MG	IV, IM	J0743
PRI-METHYLATE	80 MG	IM	J1040
PROCAINAMIDE HCL	1 G	IM, IV	J2690
PROCHLORPERAZINE	10 MG	IM, IV	J0780
PROCHLORPERAZINE MALEATE	10 MG	ORAL	Q0165
PROCHLORPERAZINE MALEATE	5 MG	ORAL	Q0164
PROFASI	1000 USP UNITS	IM	J0725
PROFILNINE SD	PER IU	IV	J7194
PROGESTERONE	50 MG	IM	J2675
PROGRAF	1 MG	ORAL	J7507
PROGRAF	5 MG	OTH	J7525
PROLASTIN	10 MG	IV	J0256
PROLEUKIN	1 VIAL	VAR	J9015
PROLIXIN DECANOATE	25 MG	INJ	J2680
PROMAZINE HCL	25 MG	IM	J2950
PROMETHAZINE HCL	50 MG	IM, IV	J2550
PROPLEX T	PER IU	IV	J7194
PROPRANOLOL HCL	1 MG	IV	J1800
PROREX	50 MG	IM, IV	J2550
PROSTAGLANDIN E1	1.25 MCG	INJ	J0270
PROSTIN VR	1.25 MCG	INJ	J0270
PROTAMINE SULFATE	10 MG	IV	J2720
PROTIRELIN	250 MCG	IV	J2725
PROTROPIN	1 MG	INJ	J2940

Drug Name	Unit	Route	Code
PROVENTIL	0.5 MG	INH	J7619
PULMICORT	0.25 MG	INH	J7633
PULMICORT RESPULES	0.25-0.50 MG	INH	J7626
PULMOZYME	1 MG	INH	J7639
PYRIDOXINE HCL	100 MG	INJ	J3415
QUELICIN	20 MG	IM, IV	J0330
QUINUPRISTIN/DALFOPRISTIN	500 MG	IV	J2770
RANITIDINE HCL	25 MG	INJ	J2780
RAPAMUNE	1 MG	ORAL	J7520
RASBURICASE	50 MCG	IM	J2783
REBIF	33 MCG	IM	J1825
RECOMBINATE	PER IU	IV	J7192
REFACTO	PER IU	IV	J7192
REGITINE	5 MG	IM, IV	J2760
REGLAN	10 MG	IV	J2765
RELAXIN	10 ML	IV, IM	J2800
RELION NOVOLIN	50 U	SC	J1817
RELION/NOVOLIN R	5 U	SC	J1815
REMICADE	10 MG	IV	J1745
REOPRO	10 MG	IV	J0130
RESP SYNCYTIAL VIR IMMUNE GLOB	50 MG	IV	J1565
RESPIGAM	50 MG	IV	J1565
RETAVASE	18.1 MG	IV	J2993
RETEPLASE	18.1 MG	IV	J2993
RETROVIR	10 MG	IV	J3485
RHO D IMMUNE GLOBULIN	50 MCG	IM	J2788
RHO D IMMUNE GLOBULIN	100 IU	IV	J2792
RHOGAM	300 MCG	IM	J2790
RHOPHYLAC	300 MCG	IM	J2790
RHOPHYLAC	100 IU	IV	J2792
RIMANTADINE HYDROCHLORIDE	100 MG	ORAL	G9020
RINGERS LACTATE INFUSION	1000 ML	VAR	J7120
RISPERIDONE, LONG ACTING	0.5 MG	INJ	J2794
RITUXAN	100 MG	IV	J9310
RITUXIMAB	100 MG	IV	J9310
ROBAXIN	10 ML	IV, IM	J2800
ROBINUL	1 MG	INH	J7643
ROCEPHIN	250 MG	IV, IM	J0696
ROFERON-A	3,000,000 UNITS	SC, IM	J9213
ROPIVACAINE HYDROCHLORIDE	1 MG	INJ	J2795
SAIZEN	1 MG	SC	J2941
SALINE	5 CC	VAR	J7051
SANDIMMUNE	100 MG	ORAL	J7502
SANDIMMUNE	25 MG	ORAL	J7515
SANDIMMUNE	250 MG	OTH	J7516
SANDOGLOBULIN	1 GM	IV	J1563
SANDOSTATIN	25 MCG	SC, IV	J2354
SANDOSTATIN LAR	10 MG	IM	J2353
SANGCYA	100 MG	ORAL	J7502

Drug Name	Unit	Route	Code
SANO DROL	80 MG	IM	J1040
SANO-DROL	40 MG	IM	J1030
SARGRAMOSTIM (GM-CSF)	50 MCG	IV	J2820
SEROSTIM	1 MG	INJ	J2941
SIROLIMUS	1 MG	ORAL	J7520
SODIUM CHLORIDE	2 ML	IV	J2912
SODIUM CHLORIDE	5 CC	VAR	J7051
SODIUM CHROMATE CR51	0.25 MCI	INJ	C9000
SODIUM FERRIC GLUCONATE COMPLEX IN SUCROSE	12.5 MG	IV	J2916
SODIUM HYALURONATE	20 MG	IA	C9413
SODIUM HYALURONATE	20 MG	IA	J7317
SOLGANAL	50 MG	IM	J2910
SOLU-CORTEF	100 MG	IV, IM, SC	J1720
SOLU-MEDROL	125 MG	IM, IV	J2930
SOLU-MEDROL	40 MG	IM, IV	J2920
SOLUREX	1 MG	IM, IV, OTH	J1100
SOMATREM	1 MG	INJ	J2940
SOMATROPIN	1 MG	SC	J2941
SONE	4 MG	IM, IV	J0704
SPECTINOMYCIN DIHYDROCHLORIDE	2 G	IM	J3320
SPORANOX	50 MG	IV	J1835
STADOL	1 MG	IM, IV	J0595
STERAPRED	5 MG	ORAL	J7506
STERILE SALINE OR WATER	5 CC	VAR	J7051
STREPTASE	250000 IU	IV	J2995
STREPTOKINASE	250000 IU	IV	J2995
STREPTOMYCIN	1 G	IM	J3000
STREPTOZOCIN	1 GM	IV	J9320
SUBLIMAZE	0.1 MG	IM, IV	J3010
SUCCINYLCHOLINE CHLORIDE	20 MG	IM, IV	J0330
SUMATRIPTAN SUCCINATE	6 MG	SC	J3030
SUPARTZ	20 MG	IA	J7317
SYNERCID	500 MG	IV	J2770
SYNVISC	16 MG	IA	J7320
SYREX	2 ML	IV	J2912
TACROLIMUS	1 MG	ORAL	J7507
TACROLIMUS	5 MG	OTH	J7525
TALWIN	30 MG	IM, SC, IV	J3070
TAXOL	30 MG	IV	J9265
TAXOTERE	20 MG	IV	J9170
TAZICEF	500 MG	IM, IV	J0713
TEMODAR	100 MG	ORAL	J8700
TEMOZOLOMIDE	100 MG	ORAL	J8700
TENECTEPLASE	50 MG	INJ	J3100
TEQUIN	10 MG	IV	J1590
TERBUTALINE SULFATE	1 MG	INH	J7681
TERBUTALINE SULFATE	1 MG	SC, IV	J3105
TERIPARATIDE	10 MCG	INJ	J3110

Drug Name	Unit	Route	Code
TESTERONE	50 MG	IM	J3140
TESTOSTERONE CYPIONATE	1 CC, 200 MG	IM	J1080
TESTOSTERONE CYPIONATE	UP TO 100 MG	IM	J1070
TESTOSTERONE CYPIONATE & ESTRADIOL CYPIONATE	1 ML	IM	J1060
TESTOSTERONE ENANTHATE	100 MG	IM	J3120
TESTOSTERONE ENANTHATE	200 MG	IM	J3130
TESTOSTERONE ENANTHATE AND ESTRADIOL VALERATE	UP TO 1 CC	IM	J0900
TESTOSTERONE PROPIONATE	100 MG	IM	J3150
TESTRO AQ	50 MG	IM	J3140
TETANUS IMMUNE GLOBULIN	250 U	IM	J1670
TETRACYCLINE HCL	250 MG	IV	J0120
THEOPHYLLINE	40 MG	IV	J2810
THERACYS	PER VIAL	IV	J9031
THIAMINE HCL	100 MG	INJ	J3411
THIETHYLPERAZINE MALEATE	10 MG	IM	J3280
THIETHYLPERAZINE MALEATE	10 MG	ORAL	Q0174
THIOTEPA	15 MG	IV	C9433
THIOTEPA	15 MG	IV	J9340
THORAZINE	50 MG	IM, IV	J3230
THROMBATE III	PER IU	IV	J7197
THYMOGLOBULIN	25 MG	OTH	J7511
THYROGEN	0.9 MG	IM, SC	J3240
THYROTROPIN ALPHA	0.9 MG	IM, SC	J3240
TIGAN	200 MG	IM	J3250
TINZAPARIN	1000 IU	SC	J1655
TIROFIBAN HCL	12.5 MG	IM, IV	J3246
TIROFIBAN HYDROCHLORIDE	12.5 MG	IM, IV	J3246
TNKASE	50 MG	INJ	J3100
TOBI	300 MG	INH	J7682
TOBRAMYCIN	300 MG	INH	J7682
TOBRAMYCIN SULFATE	80 MG	IM, IV	J3260
TOLAZOLINE HCL	25 MG	IV	J2670
TOPOSAR	100 MG	IV	J9182
TOPOTECAN	4 MG	IV	J9350
TORADOL IV/IM	15 MG	IM, IV	J1885
TORECAN	10 MG	IM	J3280
TORSEMIDE	10 MG	IV	J3265
TRASTUZUMAB	10 MG	IV	J9355
TRELSTAR DEPOT	3.75 MG	INJ	J3315
TRELSTAR LA	3.75 MG	INJ	J3315
TRIAMCINOLONE	1 MG	INH	J7684
TRIAMCINOLONE ACETONIDE	10 MG	IM	J3301
TRIAMCINOLONE DIACETATE	5 MG	IM	J3302
TRIAMCINOLONE HEXACETONIDE	5 MG	VAR	J3303
TRIMETHOBENZAMIDE HCL	200 MG	IM	J3250
TRIMETREXATE GLUCURONATE	25 MG	IV	J3305
TRIPTORELIN PAMOATE	3.75 MG	INJ	J3315
TRISENOX	1 MG	IV	J9017

Drug Name	Unit	Route	Code
TROBICIN	2 G	IM	J3320
TROVAN	100 MG	IV	J0200
TRUXADRYL	50 MG	IV, IM	J1200
TRYPTANOL	20 MG	IM	J1320
UNASYN	1.5 G	IM, IV	J0295
UNCLASSIFIED BIOLOGICS			J3590
UREA	40 G	IV	J3350
UROKINASE	250000 IU	IV	J3365
UROKINASE	5000 IU	IV	J3364
VALERGEN	20 MG	IM	J1390
VALERGEN	UP TO 40 MG	IM	J0970
VALIUM	5 MG	IV, IM	J3360
VALRUBICIN	200 MG	OTH	J9357
VALSTAR	200 MG	OTH	J9357
VANCOMYCIN HCL	500 MG	IV, IM	J3370
VELOSULIN BR	5 U	SC	J1815
VENOFER	1 MG	IV	J1756
VENOGLOBULIN-S	1 G	IV	J1563
VENTOLIN	0.5 MG	INH	J7619
VEPESID	10 MG	IV	J9181
VEPESID	100 MG	IV	J9182
VERTEPORFIN	0.1 MG	IV	J3396
VERTEPORFIN	15 MG	IV	J3395
VFEND	200 MG	INJ	J3465
VIADUR	1 MG	IM	J9219
VINBLASTINE SULFATE	1 MG	IV	J9360
VINCASAR PFS	1 MG	IV	J9370
VINCASAR PFS	2 MG	IV	J9375
VINCRISTINE SULFATE	1 MG	IV	J9370
VINCRISTINE SULFATE	2 MG	IV	J9375
VINORELBINE TARTRATE	10 MG	IV	J9390

Drug Name	Unit	Route	Code
VIRILON	1 CC, 200 MG	IM	J1080
VISTIDE	375 MG	IV	J0740
VISUDYNE	15 MG	IV	J3395
VITAMIN B-12 CYANOCOBALAMIN	1000 MCG	IM, SC	J3420
VITRASERT	4.5 MG	OTH	J7310
VITRAVENE	1.65 MG	OTH	J1452
VORICONAZOLE	200 MG	INJ	J3465
WATER	5 CC	VAR	J7051
WINRHO SDF	100 IU	IV	J2792
WYCILLIN	600,000 UNITS	IM, IV	J2510
XELODA	150 MG	ORAL	J8520
XOPENEX	0.5 MG	INH	J7619
XYLOCAINE	10 MG	IV	J2001
ZANAMIVIR	10 MG	INH	G9018
ZANOSAR	1 GM	IV	J9320
ZANTAC	25 MG	INJ	J2780
ZEMAIRA	10 MG	IV	J0256
ZEMPLAR	1 MCG	IV, IM	J2501
ZENAPAX	25 MG	OTH	J7513
ZIDOVUDINE	10 MG	IV	J3485
ZINACEF	750 MG	IM, IV	J0697
ZINECARD	250 MG	IV	J1190
ZIPRASIDONE MESYLATE	10 MG	INJ	J3486
ZITHROMAX	500 MG	IV	J0456
ZOFRAN	1 MG	IV	J2405
ZOLADEX	3.6 MG	SC	J9202
ZOLEDRONIC ACID	1 MG	INJ	J3487
ZOMETA	1 MG	INJ	J3487
ZORBTIVE	1 MG	SC	J2941
ZOSYN	1 G/1.125 GM	IV	J2543
ZYVOX	200 MG	IV	J2020

UNCLASSIFIED DRUGS

Drug Name	Unit	Route	Code
ACYCLOVIR	1 EA		J8499
ADRENALIN	1 EA		J7699
ALLOPURINOL SODIUM	300 MG	IV	J9999
ALOPRIM	300 MG	IV	J9999
ARIMIDEX	1 EA		J8999
AROMASIN	1 EA		J8999
BREVITAL SODIUM	1 EA		J3490
BUPIVACAINE HCL	1 EA		J3490
BUPIVACAINE SPINAL	1 EA		J3490
CEENU	1 EA		J8999
CIMETIDINE HCL	1 EA		J3490
DEXAMETHASONE	1 EA		J8499
DEXTROSE	1 EA		J7799
DEXTROSE HYPERTONIC	1 EA		J7799
DEXTROSE/SODIUM CHLORIDE	1 EA		J7799
DIPRIVAN	1 EA		J3490
DROXIA	1 EA		J8999
EPINEPHRINE HCL	1 EA		J7799
EULEXIN	1 EA		J8999
FAMOTIDINE	1 EA		J3490
FLUTAMIDE	1 EA		J8999
GLOFIL-125	1 EA		J3490
GONAL-F	1 EA		J3490
GONAL-F RFF	1 EA		J3490
HYDREA	1 EA		J8999
HYDROXYUREA	1 EA		J8999
INAMRINONE LACTATE	1 EA		J3490
KINERET	1 EA		J3490
LEUKERAN	1 EA		J8999
MANNITOL	1 EA		J7799
MARCAINE HCL	1 EA		J3490
MARCAINE SPINAL	1 EA		J3490
MATULANE	1 EA		J8999
MEGACE	1 EA		J8999

Drug Name	Unit	Route	Code
MEGESTROL ACETATE	1 EA		J8999
MERCAPTOPURINE	1 EA		J8999
METRONIDAZOLE	1 EA		J3490
MYLOCEL	1 EA		J8999
NABI-HB	1 EA		J3490
NAFCILLIN SODIUM	1 EA		J3490
NOLVADEX	1 EA		J8999
ORCEL	1 EA		J3490
OSMITROL	1 EA		J7799
PEGASYS	1 EA		J3490
PEG-INTRON	1 EA		J3490
PEPCID	1 EA		J3490
PHENYLEPHRINE HCL	1 EA		J7799
PIPERACILLIN	1 EA		J3490
PRESCRIPTION DRUG, ORAL, CHEMOTHERAPEUTIC, NOS	1 EA		J8999
PRESCRIPTION DRUG, ORAL, NON CHEMOTHERAPEUTIC, NOS	1 EA		J8499
PROPOFOL	1 EA		J3490
PROTONIX	1 EA		J3490
PURINETHOL	1 EA		J8999
PYRIDOXINE HCL	1 EA		J3490
REBETRON	1 EA		J3490
REGRANEX	1 EA		J3490
RESECTISOL	1 EA		J7799
SENSORCAINE	1 EA		J3490
SMZ-TMP	1 EA		J3490
SODIUM CHLORIDE	1 EA		J7699
SODIUM CHLORIDE	1 EA		J7799
STADOL	1 EA		J3490
SYNAGIS	1 EA		J3490
TAMOXIFEN	1 EA		J8999
TIMENTIN	1 EA		J3490
ZOVIRAX	1 EA		J8499

APPENDIX 4 — PUB 100/NCD REFERENCES

REVISIONS TO THE CMS MANUAL SYSTEM

The Centers for Medicare and Medicaid Services (CMS) initiated its long awaited transition from a paper-based manual system to a Web-based system on October 1, 2003, which updates and restructures all manual instructions. The new system, called the online CMS Manual system, combines all of the various program instructions into an electronic manual, which can be found at http://www.cms.hhs.gov/manuals.

Effective September 30, 2003, the former method of publishing program memoranda (PMs) to communicate program instructions was replaced by the following four templates:

One-time notification:

Manual revisions:

Business requirement:

Confidential requirements:

The Office of Strategic Operations and Regulatory Affairs (OSORA), Division of Issuances, will continue to communicate advanced program instructions to the regions and contractor community every Friday as it currently does. These instructions will also contain a transmittal sheet to identify changes pertaining to a specific manual, requirement, or notification.

The Web-based system has been organized by functional area (e.g., eligibility, entitlement, claims processing, benefit policy, program integrity) in an effort to eliminate redundancy within the manuals, simplify the updating process, and make CMS program instructions available in a more timely manner. The initial release will include Pub. 100, Pub. 100-02, Pub. 100-03, Pub. 100-04, Pub. 100-05, Pub. 100-09, Pub. 100-15, and Pub. 100-20.

The Web-based system contains the functional areas included in the table below:

Publication #	Title
Pub. 100	Introduction
Pub. 100-1	Medicare General Information, Eligibility, and Entitlement
Pub. 100-2	Medicare Benefit Policy (basic coverage rules)
Pub. 100-3	Medicare National Coverage Determinations (national coverage decisions)
Pub. 100-4	Medicare Claims Processing (includes appeals, contractor interface with CWF, and MSN)
Pub. 100-5	Medicare Secondary Payer
Pub. 100-6	Medicare Financial Management (includes Intermediary Desk Review and Audit)
Pub. 100-7	Medicare State Operations
Pub. 100-8	Medicare Program Integrity
Pub. 100-9	Medicare Contractor Beneficiary and Provider Communications
Pub. 100-10	Medicare Quality Improvement Organization
Pub. 100-11	Reserved
Pub. 100-12	State Medicaid
Pub. 100-13	Medicaid State Children's Health Insurance Program
Pub. 100-14	Medicare End Stage Renal Disease Network
Pub. 100-15	Medicare State Buy-In
Pub. 100-16	Medicare Managed Care
Pub. 100-17	Medicare Business Partners Systems Security
Pub. 100-18	Medicare Business Partners Security Oversight
Pub. 100-19	Demonstrations
Pub. 100-20	One-Time Notification

Table of Contents

The table below shows the paper-based manuals used to construct the Web-based system. Although this is just an overview, CMS is in the process of developing detailed crosswalks to guide you from a specific section of the old manuals to the appropriate area of the new manual, as well as to show how the information in each section was derived.

Paper-Based Manuals	Internet-Only Manuals
Pub. 06—Medicare Coverage Issues	Pub. 100-01—Medicare General Information, Eligibility, and Entitlement
Pub. 09—Medicare Outpatient Physical Therapy	Pub. 100-02—Medicare Benefit Policy
Pub. 10—Medicare Hospital	Pub. 100-03—Medicare National Coverage Determinations
Pub. 11—Medicare Home Health Agency	Pub. 100-04—Medicare Claims Processing
Pub. 12—Medicare Skilled Nursing Facility	Pub. 100-05—Medicare Secondary Payer
Pub. 13—Medicare Intermediary Manual, Parts 1, 2, 3, and 4	Pub. 100-06—Medicare Financial Management
Pub. 14—Medicare Carriers Manual, Parts 1, 2, 3, and 4	Pub. 100-08—Medicare Program Integrity
Pub. 21—Medicare Hospice	Pub. 100-09—Medicare Contractor Beneficiary and Provider Communications
Pub. 27—Medicare Rural Health Clinic and Federally Qualified Health Center	
Pub. 29—Medicare Renal Dialysis Facility	

Program Memoranda	
Pub. 60A—Intermediaries	
Pub. 60B—Carriers	
Pub. 60AB—Intermediaries/Carriers	
NOTE: Information derived from Pub. 06 to Pub. 60AB was used to develop Pub. 100-01 to Pub. 100-09 for the Internet-only manual.	
Pub. 19—Medicare Peer Review Organization	Pub. 100-10—Medicare Quality Improvement Organization
Pub. 07—Medicare State Operations	Pub. 100-07—Medicare State Operations
Pub. 45—State Medicaid	Pub. 100-12—State Medicaid
Pub. 81—Medicare End Stage Renal Disease Network Organizations	Pub. 100-13—Medicaid State Children's Health Insurance Program
Pub. 24—Medicare State Buy-In	Pub. 100-14—Medicare End Stage Renal Disease Network Organizations
Pub. 75—Health Maintenance Organization/Competitive Medical Plan	Pub. 100-15—Medicare State Buy-In
Pub. 76—Health Maintenance Organization/Competitive Medical Plan (PM)	Pub. 100-16—Medicare Managed Care
Pub. 77—Manual for Federally Qualified Health Maintenance Organizations	Pub. 100-17—Business Partners Systems Security
Pub. 13—Medicare Intermediaries Manual, Part 2	Pub. 100-18—Business Partners Security Oversight
Pub. 14—Medicare Carriers Manual, Part 2	Pub 100-19—Demonstrations
Pub. 13—Medicare Intermediaries Manual, Part 2	Pub 100-20—One-Time Notification
Pub. 14—Medicare Carriers Manual, Part 2	
Demonstrations (PMs)	
Program instructions that impact multiple manuals or have no manual impact.	

NATIONAL COVERAGE DETERMINATIONS MANUAL

The National Coverage Determinations Manual (NCD), which is the electronic replacement for the Coverage Issues Manual (CIM), is organized according to categories such as diagnostic services, supplies, and medical procedures. The table of contents lists each category and subject within that category. A revision transmittal sheet will identify any new material and recap the changes as well as provide an effective date for the change and any background information. At any time, one can refer to a transmittal indicated on the page of the manual to view this information.

By the time it is complete, the book will contain two chapters. Chapter 1 includes a description of national coverage determinations that have been made by CMS. When available, chapter 2 will contain a list of HCPCS codes related to each coverage determination. To make the manual easier to use, it is organized in accordance with CPT category sequences. Where there is no national coverage determination that affects a particular CPT category, the category is listed as reserved in the table of contents.

MEDICARE BENEFIT POLICY MANUAL

The Medicare Benefit Policy Manual replaces current Medicare general coverage instructions that are not national coverage determinations. As a general rule, in the past these instructions have been found in chapter II of the Medicare Carriers Manual, the Medicare Intermediary Manual, other provider manuals, and program memoranda. New instructions will be published in this manual. As new transmittals are included they will be identified.

On the CMS Web site, a crosswalk from the new manual to the source manual is provided with each chapter and may be accessed from the chapter table of contents. In addition, the crosswalk for each section is shown immediately under the section heading.

The list below is the table of contents for the Medicare Benefit Policy Manual:

Chapter	Title
One	Inpatient Hospital Services
Two	Inpatient Psychiatric Hospital Services
Three	Duration of Covered Inpatient Services
Four	Inpatient Psychiatric Benefit Days Reduction and Lifetime Limitation
Five	Lifetime Reserve Days
Six	Hospital Services Covered Under Part B
Seven	Home Health Services
Eight	Coverage of Extended Care (SNF) Services Under Hospital Insurance
Nine	Coverage of Hospice Services Under Hospital Insurance
Ten	Ambulance Services
Eleven	End Stage Renal Disease (ESRD)
Twelve	Comprehensive Outpatient Rehabilitation Facility (CORF) Coverage
Thirteen	Rural Health Clinic (RHC) and Federally Qualified Health Center (FQHC) Services
Fourteen	Medical Devices
Fifteen	Covered Medical and Other Health Services
Sixteen	General Exclusions from Coverage

MCM/CIM CROSSWALK TO PUB 100 REFERENCE

MCM	PUB 100
15016	100-4,12,100
15018	100-4,12,50
15020	100-4,12,60
15021.1	100-4,13,10
15022	100-4,12,70 ; 100-4,13,20 ; 100-4,13,90
15023	100-4,13,100
15026	100-4,12,80.3
15038	100-4,12,40.6
15050	100-4,12,200
15100	100-4,12,30.1
15200	100-4,12,30.2
15350	100-4,8,140 ; 100-4,8,170
15360	100-4,12,30.4
15400	100-4,12,30.5
15501	100-4,12,30.6
15504	100-4,12,30.6.8
15505	100-4,12,30.6.9
15505.1	100-4,12,30.6.9
15505.2	100-4,12,30.6.9
15514	100-4,12,30.6
2005.1	100-2,15,20.1
2005.2	100-2,15,20.2
2020	100-1,5,70 ; 100-2,15,30; 100-4,12,10
2020.26	100-1,5,70.6
2049	100-2,15,50
2050.3	100-2,15,60.3
2070	100-2,15,80
2070.1	100-1,5,90.2 ; 100-2,15,80.1; 100-4,16,10 ; 100-4,16,10.1 ; 100-4,16,110.4

2070.2	100-2,15,80.2; 100-4,12,160
2070.3	100-2,15,80.3
2070.4	100-2,15,80.4; 100-4,13,90
2079	100-2,15,100
2130	100-2,15,120
2136	100-2,15,150
2150	100-2,15,160; 100-4,12,160 ; 100-4,12,170 ; 100-4,12,170.1
2152	100-2,15,170; 100-4,12,150
2154	100-2,15,180
2210	100-2,15,230
2210.1	100-2,15,230.1
2210.2	100-2,15,230.2
2215	100-2,15,230.4; 100-4,5,10
2216	100-2,15,230.3
2265	100-2,15,260; 100-4,12,90.3 ; 100-4,14,10
2300	100-2,16,10
2300.1	100-2,16,180
2320	100-2,16,90
2329	100-2,16,120
2455	100-1,3,20.5 ; 100-1,3,20.5.2 ; 100-1,3,20.5.3
2470	100-1,3,30 ; 100-1,3,30.1 ; 100-1,3,30.2 ; 100-1,3,30.3 ; 100-4,12,210
2472.4	100-4,12,110.2
3045.4	100-4,1,30.3.5
3324	100-4,20,50.3
4137	100-4,12,50
4141	100-2,15,30
4146	100-1,3,30.2
4161	100-2,15,230.4
4172	100-4,12,140
4175	100-4,11,10 ; 100-4,11,40.1.3
4180	100-4,18,60
4182	100-4,18,50
4270	100-4,8,130 ; 100-4,8,70 ; 100-4,8,80 ; 100-4,8,90 ; 100-4,8,90.1 ; 100-4,8,90.3.2
4270.1	100-4,8,60.4.4 ; 100-4,8,90.1 ; 100-4,8,90.2 ; 100-4,8,90.2.2
4471.2	100-2,15,50.5
4601	100-4,18,20
4602	100-4,13,40 ; 100-4,13,40.1 ; 100-4,13,40.1.1 ; 100-4,18,20.7
4826	100-4,12,40.6
4827	100-4,12,40.7
4830	100-4,12,140.2
5112	100-4,12,160.1
5112.1	100-4,12,170
5249	100-4,8,120.1

The following table is the crosswalk of the NCD to the CIM. However, at this time, many of the NCD policies are not yet available. The CMS Web site also contains a crosswalk of the CIM to the NCD.

CIM	NCD
15049	100-3,80.2
35-10	100-3,20.29
35-100	100-3,80.2
35-101	100-3,250.4
35-11	100-3,230.3
35-12	100-3,140.4
35-13	100-3,150.7
35-14	100-3,70.1; 100-3,70.2
35-15	100-3,240.7
35-16	100-3,40.50; 100-3,80.11
35-17	100-3,160.1
35-19	100-3,30.6; 100-3,110.10
35-2	100-3,150.1
35-20	100-3,160.2; 100-3,130.6; 100-3,130.5; 100-3,40.50; 100-3,230.1
35-21	100-3,10.3
35-21.1	100-3,10.4; 100-3,130.2
35-22	100-3,10.3; 100-3,130.1; 100-3,130.2
35-22.1	100-3,10.4; 100-3,130.2
35-22.2	100-3,160.2; 100-3,130.6
35-22.3	100-3,160.2; 100-3,130.6; 100-3,130.5
35-23	100-3,130.3
35-23.1	100-3,130.4
35-24	100-3,230.4
35-25	100-3,20.10
35-26	100-3,40.50
35-26.1	100-3,40.50
35-27	100-3,30.1; 100-3,30.1.1

35-3	100-3,240.3
35-30	100-3,110.8
35-30.1	100-3,110.8.1
35-31	100-3,250.4; 100-3,160.2; 100-3,270.4; 100-3,250.1
35-32	100-3,20.1
35-33	100-3,100.8; 100-3,10.4
35-34	100-3,20.23
35-35	100-3,20.28
35-38	100-3,110.15; 100-3,230.14
35-39	100-3,80.6
35-40	100-3,100.1
35-41	100-3,150.5
35-42	100-3,130.7
35-44	100-3,10.1
35-45	100-3,20.25
35-46	100-3,160.7.1
35-47	100-3,140.2
35-48	100-3,150.2
35-49	100-3,110.1
35-5	100-3,30.8
35-51	100-3,130.8
35-52	100-3,140.5
35-53	100-3,260.1
35-53.1	100-3,260.2
35-54	100-3,80.7
35-55	100-3,240.6
35-57	100-3,160.8
35-57.1	100-3,160.9
35-58	100-3,20.3
35-59	100-3,100.2
35-60	100-3,110.14
35-61	100-3,140.3
35-64	100-3,20.21
35-66	100-3,250.4; 100-3,40.50; 100-3,250.1
35-7	100-3,20.18
35-71	100-3,110.16
35-72	100-3,160.15
35-73	100-3,100.10
35-75	100-3,20.11
35-77	100-3,160.12
35-78	100-3,20.12
35-79	100-3,20.8.3
35-8	100-3,30.3
35-81	100-3,230.1
35-82	100-3,260.3
35-83	100-3,100.3
35-84	100-3,160.4
35-85	100-3,20.4
35-87	100-3,260.9
35-88	100-3,110.4
35-89	100-3,170.3
35-9	100-3,80.10
35-90	100-3,20.5
35-91	100-3,100.13
35-92	100-3,30.5
35-94	100-3,20.6
35-96	100-3,230.9
35-98	100-3,35-102
35-99	100-3,140.1
40-1	100-3,190.12
40-10	100-3,190.21
40-11	100-3,190.22
40-12	100-3,190.23
40-13	100-3,190.24
40-14	100-3,190.25
40-15	100-3,190.26
40-16	100-3,190.27
40-17	100-3,190.28
40-18	100-3,190.29
40-19	100-3,190.30
40-2	100-3,190.13
40-20	100-3,190.31
40-21	100-3,190.32
40-22	100-3,190.33
40-23	100-3,190.34
40-3	100-3,190.14
40-4	100-3,190.15
40-5	100-3,190.16
40-6	100-3,190.17
40-7	100-3,190.18
40-8	100-3,190.19
40-9	100-3,190.20
4281	100-3,70.2.1
45-1	100-3,160.17
45-10	100-3,30.7
45-11	100-3,10.5
45-12	100-3,270.5
45-16	100-3,110.2
45-17	100-3,160.20
45-18	100-3,110.5
45-19	100-3,10.2; 100-3,280.13
45-20	100-3,20.22
45-21	100-3,110.6
45-22	100-3,260.7
45-23	100-3,230.12
45-24	100-3,110.3; 100-3,110.3
45-25	100-3,160.13
45-27	100-3,110.7
45-28	100-3,110.9
45-30	100-3,80.3; 100-3,80.3
45-4	100-3,150.6
45-7	100-3,80.1; 100-3,80.4
50-1	100-3,20.8.1; 100-3,20.8
50-10	100-3,230.6
50-12	100-3,220.1
50-13	100-3,220.2; 100-3,220.3
50-14	100-3,220.3
50-15	100-3,20.15
50-17	100-3,190.10
50-18	100-3,190.4
50-20	100-3,190.2
50-20.1	100-3,210.2
50-21	100-3,220.4
50-22	100-3,50-22
50-23	100-3,190.1
50-24	100-3,190.6
50-25	100-3,100.4
50-27	100-3,220.7
50-29	100-3,190.3
50-3	100-3,20.13
50-30	100-3,220.8
50-31	100-3,160.10
50-32	100-3,20.7
50-33	100-3,230.2
50-34	100-3,300.1
50-35	100-3,190.5
50-36	100-3,220.6
50-37	100-3,20.17
50-38	100-3,80.8
50-39	100-3,160.21
50-39.1	100-3,160.22
50-40	100-3,160.5
50-42	100-3,20.19
50-44	100-3,150.3
50-45	100-3,190.8
50-49	100-3,80.9
50-5	100-3,220.11
50-51	100-3,100.5
50-52	100-3,190.9
50-53	100-3,110.11
50-54	100-3,20.16
50-55	100-3,210.1
50-58	100-3,220.12
50-59	100-3,20.7; 100-3,220.13
50-6	100-3,20.14
50-7	100-3,220.5
50-8	100-3,70.2
50-9	100-3,100.12
55-3	100-3,110.15; 100-3,230.14
60-14	100-3,280.14
60-20	100-3,280.13
60-22	100-3,160.18

60-23	100-3,50.1
60-25	100-3,270.2
60-7	100-3,20.8.2
65-14	100-3,50.3
65-5	100-3,100-3
65-6	100-3,20.8.1; 100-3,20.8
65-8	100-3,160.7
65-9	100-3,230.10
80-2	100-3,40.1
80-3	100-3,180.1

PUB 100 REFERENCES

Pub. 100-1, Chapter 3, Section 20.5

Blood Deductibles (Part A and Part B)

Program payment may not be made for the first 3 pints of whole blood or equivalent units of packed red cells received under Part A and Part B combined in a calendar year. However, blood processing (e.g., administration, storage) is not subject to the deductible.

The blood deductibles are in addition to any other applicable deductible and coinsurance amounts for which the patient is responsible.

The deductible applies only to the first 3 pints of blood furnished in a calendar year, even if more than one provider furnished blood.

Pub. 100-1, Chapter 3, Section 20.5.2

Part B Blood Deductible

Blood is furnished on an outpatient basis or is subject to the Part B blood deductible and is counted toward the combined limit. It should be noted that payment for blood may be made to the hospital under Part B only for blood furnished in an outpatient setting. Blood is not covered for inpatient Part B services.

Pub. 100-1, Chapter 3, Section 20.5.3

Items Subject to Blood Deductibles

The blood deductibles apply only to whole blood and packed red cells. The term whole blood means human blood from which none of the liquid or cellular components have been removed. Where packed red cells are furnished, a unit of packed red cells is considered equivalent to a pint of whole blood. Other components of blood such as platelets, fibrinogen, plasma, gamma globulin, and serum albumin are not subject to the blood deductible. However, these components of blood are covered as biologicals.

Pub. 100-1, Chapter 5, Section 90.2

Laboratory Defined

Laboratory means a facility for the biological, microbiological, serological, chemical, immuno-hematological, hematological, biophysical, cytological, pathological, or other examination of materials derived from the human body for the purpose of providing information for the diagnosis, prevention, or treatment of any disease or impairment of, or the assessment of the health of, human beings. These examinations also include procedures to determine, measure, or otherwise describe the presence or absence of various substances or organisms in the body. Facilities only collecting or preparing specimens (or both) or only serving as a mailing service and not performing testing are not considered laboratories.

Pub. 100-2, Chapter 10, Section 10.1

Vehicle and Crew Requirement

(Rev. 1, 10-01-03)

B3-2120.1, A3-3114, HO-236.1

Pub. 100-2, Chapter 10, Section 20

Coverage Guidelines for Ambulance Service Claims

(Rev. 1, 10-01-03)

B3-2125

Payment may be made for expenses incurred by a patient for ambulance service provided conditions l, 2, and 3 in the left-hand column have been met. The right-hand column indicates the documentation needed to establish that the condition has been met.

Conditions	Review Action
1. Patient was transported by an approved supplier of ambulance services.	1. Ambulance supplier is listed in the table of approved ambulance companies (§10.1.3)
2. The patient was suffering from an illness or injury, which contraindicated transportation by other means. (§10.2)	2. (a) The contractor presumes the requirement was met if the submitted documentation indicates that the patient: • Was transported in an emergency situation, e.g., as a result of an accident, injury or acute illness, or • Needed to be restrained to prevent injury to the beneficiary or others; or • Was unconscious or in shock; or • Required oxygen or other emergency treatment during transport to the nearest appropriate facility; or • Exhibits signs and symptoms of acute respiratory distress or cardiac distress such as shortness of breath or chest pain; or • Exhibits signs and symptoms that indicate the possibility of acute stroke; or • Had to remain immobile because of a fracture that had not been set or the possibility of a fracture; or • Was experiencing severe hemorrhage; or • Could be moved only by stretcher; or • Was bed-confined before and after the ambulance trip.
	(b) In the absence of any of the conditions listed in (a)above additional documentation should be obtained to establish medical need where the evidence indicates the existence of the circumstances listed below: (i) Patient's condition would not ordinarily require movement by stretcher, or (ii) The individual was not admitted as a hospital inpatient (except in accident cases), or (iii) The ambulance was used solely because other means of transportation were unavailable, or (iv) The individual merely needed assistance in getting from his room or home to a vehicle. (c) Where the information indicates a situation not listed in 2(a) or 2(b) above, refer the case to your supervisor.
3. The patient was transported from and to points listed below. (a) From patient's residence (or other place where need arose) to hospital or skilled nursing facility.	3. Claims should show the ZIP code of the point of pickup. (a) i. Condition met if trip began within the institution's service area as shown in the carrier's locality guide ii. Condition met where the trip began outside the institution's service area if the institution was the nearest one with appropriate facilities.
NOTE: A patient's residence is the place where he or she makes his/her home and dwells permanently, or for an extended period of time. A skilled nursing facility is one, which is listed in the Directory of Medical Facilities as a participating SNF or as an institution which meets §1861(j)(1) of the Act. NOTE: A claim for ambulance service to a participating hospital or skilled nursing facility should not be denied on the grounds that there is a nearer nonparticipating institution having appropriate facilities.	
(b) Skilled nursing facility to a hospital or hospital to a skilled nursing facility.	(b) (i) Condition met if the ZIP code of the pickup point is within the service area of the destination as shown in the carrier's locality guide. (ii) Condition met where the ZIP code of the pickup point is outside the service area of the destination if the destination institution was the nearest appropriate facility.
(c) Hospital to hospital or skilled nursing facility to skilled nursing facility.	(c) Condition met if the discharging institution was not an appropriate facility and the admitting institution was the nearest appropriate facility.
(d) From a hospital or skilled nursing facility to patient's residence.	(d) (i) Condition met if patient's residence is within the institution's service area as shown in the carrier's locality guide. (ii) Condition met where the patient's residence is outside the institution's service area if the institution was the nearest appropriate facility.
(e) Round trip for hospital or participating skilled nursing facility inpatients to the nearest hospital or nonhospital treatment facility	(e) Condition met if the reasonable and necessary diagnostic or therapeutic service required by patient's condition is not available at the institution where the beneficiary is an inpatient.

Conditions, cont.	Review Action, cont.
NOTE: Ambulance service to a physician's office or a physician-directed clinic is not covered. See §10.3.7 above, where a stop is made at a physician's office en route to a hospital and §10.3.3 for additional exceptions.)	
4. Ambulance services involving hospital admissions in Canada or Mexico are covered (Medicare Claims Processing Manual, Chapter 1, "General Billing Requirements," §§10.1.3.) if the following conditions are met:	(a) The foreign hospitalization has been determined to be covered; and (b) The ambulance service meets the coverage requirements set forth in §§10-10.3. If the foreign hospitalization has been determined to be covered on the basis of emergency services (See the Medicare Claims Processing Manual, Chapter 1, "General Billing Requirements," §10.1.3), the necessity requirement (§10.2) and the destination requirement (§10.3) are considered met
5. The carrier will make partial payment for otherwise covered ambulance service, which exceeded limits defined in item 6. The carrier will base the payment on the amount payable had the patient been transported:	(a) From the pickup point to the nearest appropriate facility, or (b) From the nearest appropriate facility to the beneficiary's residence where he or she is being returned home from a distant institution.

Pub. 100-2, Chapter 11, Section 130.1

Inpatient Dialysis in Nonparticipating Hospitals
(Rev. 1, 10-01-03)

A3-3173.3

Emergency inpatient dialysis services provided by a nonparticipating U.S. hospital are covered if the requirements in §130 above are met.

Pub. 100-2, Chapter 15, Section 50

Drugs and Biologicals
B3-2049, A3-3112.4.B, HO-230.4.B

The Medicare program provides limited benefits for outpatient drugs. The program covers drugs that are furnished "incident to" a physician's service provided that the drugs are not usually self-administered by the patients who take them.

Generally, drugs and biologicals are covered only if all of the following requirements are met:

They meet the definition of drugs or biologicals (see §50.1);

They are of the type that are not usually self-administered. (see §50.2);

They meet all the general requirements for coverage of items as incident to a physician's services (see §§50.1 and 50.3);

They are reasonable and necessary for the diagnosis or treatment of the illness or injury for which they are administered according to accepted standards of medical practice (see §50.4);

They are not excluded as noncovered immunizations (see §50.4.4.2); and

They have not been determined by the FDA to be less than effective. (See §§50.4.4).

Medicare Part B does generally not cover drugs that can be self-administered, such as those in pill form, or are used for self-injection. However, the statute provides for the coverage of some self-administered drugs. Examples of self-administered drugs that are covered include blood-clotting factors, drugs used in immunosuppressive therapy, erythropoietin for dialysis patients, osteoporosis drugs for certain homebound patients, and certain oral cancer drugs. (See §110.3 for coverage of drugs, which are necessary to the effective use of Durable Medical Equipment (DME) or prosthetic devices.)

Pub. 100-2, Chapter 15, Section 50.2

Determining Self-Administration of Drug or Biological
(Rev. 1, 10-01-03)

AB-02-072, AB-02-139, B3-2049.2

The Medicare program provides limited benefits for outpatient prescription drugs. The program covers drugs that are furnished "incident to" a physician's service provided that the drugs are not usually self-administered by the patients who take them. Section 112 of the Benefits, Improvements & Protection Act of 2000 (BIPA) amended sections 1861(s)(2)(A) and 1861(s)(2)(B) of the Act to redefine this exclusion. The prior statutory language referred to those drugs "which cannot be self-administered." Implementation of the BIPA provision requires interpretation of the phrase "not usually self-administered by the patient".

A - Policy

Fiscal intermediaries and carriers are instructed to follow the instructions below when applying the exclusion for drugs that are usually self-administered by the patient. Each individual contractor must make its own individual determination on each drug. Contractors must continue to apply the policy that not only the drug is medically reasonable and necessary for any individual claim, but also that the route of administration is medically reasonable and necessary. That is, if a drug is available in both oral and injectable forms, the injectable form of the drug must be medically reasonable and necessary as compared to using the oral form.

For certain injectable drugs, it will be apparent due to the nature of the condition(s) for which they are administered or the usual course of treatment for those conditions, they are, or are not, usually self-administered. For example, an injectable drug used to treat migraine headaches is usually self-administered. On the other hand, an injectable drug, administered at the same time as chemotherapy, used to treat anemia secondary to chemotherapy is not usually self-administered.

B - Administered

The term "administered" refers only to the physical process by which the drug enters the patient's body. It does not refer to whether the process is supervised by a medical professional (for example, to observe proper technique or side-effects of the drug). Only injectable (including intravenous) drugs are eligible for inclusion under the "incident to" benefit. Other routes of administration including, but not limited to, oral drugs, suppositories, topical medications are all considered to be usually self-administered by the patient.

C - Usually

For the purposes of applying this exclusion, the term "usually" means more than 50 percent of the time for all Medicare beneficiaries who use the drug. Therefore, if a drug is self-administered by more than 50 percent of Medicare beneficiaries, the drug is excluded from coverage and the contractor may not make any Medicare payment for it. In arriving at a single determination as to whether a drug is usually self-administered, contractors should make a separate determination for each indication for a drug as to whether that drug is usually self-administered.

After determining whether a drug is usually self-administered for each indication, contractors should determine the relative contribution of each indication to total use of the drug (i.e., weighted average) in order to make an overall determination as to whether the drug is usually self-administered. For example, if a drug has three indications, is not self-administered for the first indication, but is self administered for the second and third indications, and the first indication makes up 40 percent of total usage, the second indication makes up 30 percent of total usage, and the third indication makes up 30 percent of total usage, then the drug would be considered usually self-administered.

Reliable statistical information on the extent of self-administration by the patient may not always be available. Consequently, CMS offers the following guidance for each contractor's consideration in making this determination in the absence of such data:

1. Absent evidence to the contrary, presume that drugs delivered intravenously are not usually self-administered by the patient.

2. Absent evidence to the contrary, presume that drugs delivered by intramuscular injection are not usually self-administered by the patient. (Avonex, for example, is delivered by intramuscular injection, not usually self-administered by the patient.) The contractor may consider the depth and nature of the particular intramuscular injection in applying this presumption. In applying this presumption, contractors should examine the use of the particular drug and consider the following factors:

3. Absent evidence to the contrary, presume that drugs delivered by subcutaneous injection are self-administered by the patient. However, contractors should examine the use of the particular drug and consider the following factors:

A. Acute Condition - Is the condition for which the drug is used an acute condition? If so, it is less likely that a patient would self-administer the drug. If the condition were longer term, it would be more likely that the patient would self-administer the drug.

B. Frequency of Administration - How often is the injection given? For example, if the drug is administered once per month, it is less likely to be self-administered by the patient. However, if it is administered once or more per week, it is likely that the drug is self-administered by the patient.

In some instances, carriers may have provided payment for one or perhaps several doses of a drug that would otherwise not be paid for because the drug is usually self-administered. Carriers may have exercised this discretion for limited coverage, for example, during a brief time when the patient is being trained under the supervision of a physician in the proper technique for self-administration. Medicare will no longer pay for such doses. In addition, contractors may no longer pay for any drug when it is administered on an outpatient emergency basis, if the drug is excluded because it is usually self-administered by the patient.

D – Definition of Acute Condition

For the purposes of determining whether a drug is usually self-administered, an acute condition means a condition that begins over a short time period, is likely to be of short duration and/or the expected course of treatment is for a short, finite interval. A course of treatment consisting of scheduled injections lasting less than two weeks, regardless of frequency or route of administration, is considered acute. Evidence to support this may include Food and Drug administration (FDA) approval language, package inserts, drug compendia, and other information.

E - By the Patient

The term "by the patient" means Medicare beneficiaries as a collective whole. The carrier includes only the patients themselves and not other individuals (that is, spouses, friends, or other care-givers are not considered the patient). The determination is based on whether the drug is self-administered by the patient a majority of the time that the drug is used on an outpatient basis by Medicare beneficiaries for medically necessary indications. The carrier ignores all instances when the drug is administered on an inpatient basis.

The carrier makes this determination on a drug-by-drug basis, not on a beneficiary-by-beneficiary basis. In evaluating whether beneficiaries as a collective whole self-administer, individual beneficiaries who do not have the capacity to self-administer any drug due to a condition other than the condition for which they are taking the drug in question are not considered. For example, an individual afflicted with paraplegia or advanced dementia would not have the capacity to self-administer any injectable drug, so such individuals would not be included in the population upon which the determination for self-administration by the patient was based. Note that some individuals afflicted with a less severe stage of an otherwise debilitating condition would be included in the population upon which the determination for "self-administered by the patient" was based; for example, an early onset of dementia.

F - Evidentiary Criteria

Contractors are only required to consider the following types of evidence: peer reviewed medical literature, standards of medical practice, evidence-based practice guidelines, FDA approved label, and package inserts. Contractors may also consider other evidence submitted by interested individuals or groups subject to their judgment.

Contractors should also use these evidentiary criteria when reviewing requests for making a determination as to whether a drug is usually self-administered, and requests for reconsideration of a pending or published determination.

Please note that prior to the August 1, 2002, one of the principal factors used to determine whether a drug was subject to the self-administered exclusion was whether the FDA label contained instructions for self-administration. However, CMS notes that under the new standard, the fact that the FDA label includes instructions for self-administration is not, by itself, a determining factor that a drug is subject to this exclusion.

G - Provider Notice of Noncovered Drugs

Contractors must describe on their Web site the process they will use to determine whether a drug is usually self-administered and thus does not meet the "incident to" benefit category. Contractors must publish a list of the injectable drugs that are subject to the self-administered exclusion on their Web site, including the data and rationale that led to the determination. Contractors will report the workload associated with developing new coverage statements in CAFM 21208.

Contractors must provide notice 45 days prior to the date that these drugs will not be covered. During the 45-day time period, contractors will maintain existing medical review and payment procedures. After the 45-day notice, contractors may deny payment for the drugs subject to the notice.

Contractors must not develop local medical review policies (LMRPs) for this purpose because further elaboration to describe drugs that do not meet the 'incident to' and the 'not usually self-administered' provisions of the statute are unnecessary. Current LMRPs based solely on these provisions must be withdrawn. LMRPs that address the self-administered exclusion and other information may be reissued absent the self-administered drug exclusion material. Contractors will report this workload in CAFM 21206. However, contractors may continue to use and write LMRPs to describe reasonable and necessary uses of drugs that are not usually self-administered.

H - Conferences Between Contractors

Contractors' Medical Directors may meet and discuss whether a drug is usually self-administered without reaching a formal consensus. Each contractor uses its discretion as to whether or not it will participate in such discussions. Each contractor must make its own individual determinations, except that fiscal intermediaries may, at their discretion, follow the determinations of the local carrier with respect to the self-administered exclusion.

I - Beneficiary Appeals

If a beneficiary's claim for a particular drug is denied because the drug is subject to the "self-administered drug" exclusion, the beneficiary may appeal the denial. Because it is a "benefit category" denial and not a denial based on medical necessity, an Advance Beneficiary Notice (ABN) is not required. A "benefit category" denial (i.e., a denial based on the fact that there is no benefit category under which the drug may be covered) does not trigger the financial liability protection provisions of Limitation On Liability (under §1879 of the Act). Therefore, physicians or providers may charge the beneficiary for an excluded drug.

J - Provider and Physician Appeals

A physician accepting assignment may appeal a denial under the provisions found in Chapter 29 of the Medicare Claims Processing Manual.

K - Reasonable and Necessary

Carriers and fiscal intermediaries will make the determination of reasonable and necessary with respect to the medical appropriateness of a drug to treat the patient's condition. Contractors will continue to make the determination of whether the intravenous or injection form of a drug is appropriate as opposed to the oral form. Contractors will also continue to make the determination as to whether a physician's office visit was reasonable and necessary. However, contractors should not make a determination of whether it was reasonable and necessary for the patient to choose to have his or her drug administered in the physician's office or outpatient hospital setting. That is, while a physician's office visit may not be reasonable and necessary in a specific situation, in such a case an injection service would be payable.

L - Reporting Requirements

Each carrier and intermediary must report to CMS, every September 1 and March 1, its complete list of injectable drugs that the contractor has determined are excluded when furnished incident to a physician's service on the basis that the drug is usually self-administered. The CMS anticipates that contractors will review injectable drugs on a rolling basis and publish their list of excluded drugs as it is developed. For example, contractors should not wait to publish this list until every drug has been reviewed. Contractors must send their exclusion list to the following e-mail address: drugdata@cms.hhs.gov a template that CMS will provide separately, consisting of the following data elements in order:

1. Carrier Name
2. State
3. Carrier ID#
4. HCPCS
5. Descriptor
6. Effective Date of Exclusion
7. End Date of Exclusion
8. Comments

Any exclusion list not provided in the CMS mandated format will be returned for correction.

To view the presently mandated CMS format for this report, open the file located at: http://cms.hhs.gov/manuals/pm_trans/AB02_139a.zip

Pub. 100-2, Chapter 15, Section 50.4

Reasonableness and Necessity
(Rev. 1, 10-01-03)

B3-2049.4

100-2,15, Chapter 15, Section 50.4.2

Unlabeled Use of Drug
(Rev. 1, 10-01-03)

B3-2049.3

An unlabeled use of a drug is a use that is not included as an indication on the drug's label as approved by the FDA. FDA approved drugs used for indications other than what is indicated on the official label may be covered under Medicare if the carrier determines the use to be medically accepted, taking into consideration the major drug compendia, authoritative medical literature and/or accepted standards of medical practice. In the case of drugs used in an anti-cancer chemotherapeutic regimen, unlabeled uses are covered for a medically accepted indication as defined in §50.5.

These decisions are made by the contractor on a case-by-case basis.

Pub. 100-2, Chapter 15, Section 50.5

Self-Administered Drugs and Biologicals
B3-2049.5

Medicare Part B does not cover drugs that are usually self-administered by the patient unless the statute provides for such coverage. The statute explicitly provides coverage, for blood clotting factors, drugs used in immunosuppressive therapy, erythropoietin for dialysis patients, certain oral anti-cancer drugs and anti-emetics used in certain situations.

Pub. 100-2, Chapter 15, Section 80.1

Clinical Laboratory Services

B3-2070.1

Section 1833 and 1861 of the Act provides for payment of clinical laboratory services under Medicare Part B. Clinical laboratory services involve the biological, microbiological, serological, chemical, immunohematological, hematological, biophysical, cytological, pathological, or other examination of materials derived from the human body for the diagnosis, prevention, or treatment of a disease or assessment of a medical condition. Laboratory services must meet all applicable requirements of the Clinical Laboratory Improvement Amendments of 1988 (CLIA), as set forth in 42 CFR part 493. Section 1862(a)(1)(A) of the Act provides that Medicare payment may not be made for services that are not reasonable and necessary. Clinical laboratory services must be ordered and used promptly by the physician who is treating the beneficiary as described in 42 CFR 410.32(a), or by a qualified nonphysician practitioner, as described in 42 CFR 410.32(a)(3).

See the Medicare Claims Processing Manual Chapter 16 for related claims processing instructions.

Pub. 100-2, Chapter 15, Section 80.4

Coverage of Portable X-Ray Services Not Under the Direct Supervision of a Physician

B3-2070.4

Pub. 100-2, Chapter 15, Section 100

Surgical Dressings, Splints, Casts, and Other Devices Used for Reductions of Fractures and Dis

B3-2079, A3-3110.3, HO-228.3,

Surgical dressings are limited to primary and secondary dressings required for the treatment of a wound caused by, or treated by, a surgical procedure that has been performed by a physician or other health care professional to the extent permissible under State law. In addition, surgical dressings required after debridement of a wound are also covered, irrespective of the type of debridement, as long as the debridement was reasonable and necessary and was performed by a health care professional acting within the scope of his/her legal authority when performing this function. Surgical dressings are covered for as long as they are medically necessary.

Primary dressings are therapeutic or protective coverings applied directly to wounds or lesions either on the skin or caused by an opening to the skin. Secondary dressing materials that serve a therapeutic or protective function and that are needed to secure a primary dressing are also covered. Items such as adhesive tape, roll gauze, bandages, and disposable compression material are examples of secondary dressings. Elastic stockings, support hose, foot coverings, leotards, knee supports, surgical leggings, gauntlets, and pressure garments for the arms and hands are examples of items that are not ordinarily covered as surgical dressings. Some items, such as transparent film, may be used as a primary or secondary dressing.

If a physician, certified nurse midwife, physician assistant, nurse practitioner, or clinical nurse specialist applies surgical dressings as part of a professional service that is billed to Medicare, the surgical dressings are considered incident to the professional services of the health care practitioner. (See §§60.1, 180, 190, 200, and 210.) When surgical dressings are not covered incident to the services of a health care practitioner and are obtained by the patient from a supplier (e.g., a drugstore, physician, or other health care practitioner that qualifies as a supplier) on an order from a physician or other health care professional authorized under State law or regulation to make such an order, the surgical dressings are covered separately under Part B.

Splints and casts, and other devices used for reductions of fractures and dislocations are covered under Part B of Medicare. This includes dental splints.

Pub. 100-2, Chapter 15, Section 110

Durable Medical Equipment - General

(Rev. 1, 10-01-03)

B3-2100, A3-3113, HO-235, HHA-220

Expenses incurred by a beneficiary for the rental or purchases of durable medical equipment (DME) are reimbursable if the following three requirements are met:

- The equipment meets the definition of DME (§110.1);

- The equipment is necessary and reasonable for the treatment of the patient's illness or injury or to improve the functioning of his or her malformed body member (§110.1); and

- The equipment is used in the patient's home.

The decision whether to rent or purchase an item of equipment generally resides with the beneficiary, but the decision on how to pay rests with CMS. For some DME, program payment policy calls for lump sum payments and in others for periodic payment. Where covered DME is furnished to a beneficiary by a supplier of services other than a provider of services, the DMERC makes the reimbursement. If a provider of services furnishes the equipment, the intermediary makes the reimbursement. The payment method is identified in the annual fee schedule update furnished by CMS.

The CMS issues quarterly updates to a fee schedule file that contains rates by HCPCS code and also identifies the classification of the HCPCS code within the following categories.

Category Code	Definition
IN	Inexpensive and Other Routinely Purchased Items
FS	Frequently Serviced Items
CR	Capped Rental Items
OX	Oxygen and Oxygen Equipment
OS	Ostomy, Tracheostomy & Urological Items
SD	Surgical Dressings
PO	Prosthetics & Orthotics
SU	Supplies
TE	Transcutaneous Electrical Nerve Stimulators

The DMERCs, carriers, and intermediaries, where appropriate, use the CMS files to determine payment rules. See the Medicare Claims Processing Manual, Chapter 20, "Durable Medical Equipment, Surgical Dressings and Casts, Orthotics and Artificial Limbs, and Prosthetic Devices," for a detailed description of payment rules for each classification.

Payment may also be made for repairs, maintenance, and delivery of equipment and for expendable and nonreusable items essential to the effective use of the equipment subject to the conditions in §110.2.

See the Medicare Benefit Policy Manual, Chapter 11, "End Stage Renal Disease," for hemodialysis equipment and supplies.

Pub. 100-2, Chapter 15, Section 110.1

Definition of Durable Medical Equipment

(Rev. 1, 10-01-03)

B3-2100.1, A3-3113.1, HO-235.1, HHA-220.1, B3-2100.2, A3-3113.2, HO-235.2, HHA-220.2

Durable medical equipment is equipment which:

- Can withstand repeated use;

- Is primarily and customarily used to serve a medical purpose;

- Generally is not useful to a person in the absence of an illness or injury; and

- Is appropriate for use in the home.

All requirements of the definition must be met before an item can be considered to be durable medical equipment.

The following describes the underlying policies for determining whether an item meets the definition of DME and may be covered.

A - Durability

An item is considered durable if it can withstand repeated use, i.e., the type of item that could normally be rented. Medical supplies of an expendable nature, such as incontinent pads, lambs wool pads, catheters, ace bandages, elastic stockings, surgical facemasks, irrigating kits, sheets, and bags are not considered "durable" within the meaning of the definition. There are other items that, although durable in nature, may fall into other coverage categories such as supplies, braces, prosthetic devices, artificial arms, legs, and eyes.

B - Medical Equipment

Medical equipment is equipment primarily and customarily used for medical purposes and is not generally useful in the absence of illness or injury. In most instances, no development will be needed to determine whether a specific item of equipment is medical in nature. However, some cases will require development to determine whether the item constitutes medical equipment. This development would include the advice of local medical organizations (hospitals, medical schools, medical societies) and specialists in the field of physical medicine and rehabilitation. If the equipment is new on the market, it may be necessary, prior to seeking professional advice, to obtain information from the supplier or manufacturer explaining the design, purpose, effectiveness and method of using the equipment in the home as well as the results of any tests or clinical studies that have been conducted.

1. Equipment Presumptively Medical - Items such as hospital beds, wheelchairs, hemodialysis equipment, iron lungs, respirators, intermittent positive pressure breathing machines, medical regulators, oxygen tents, crutches, canes, trapeze bars, walkers, inhalators, nebulizers, commodes, suction machines, and traction equipment presumptively constitute medical equipment. (Although hemodialysis equipment is covered as a prosthetic device (§120), it also meets the definition of DME, and reimbursement for the rental or purchase of such equipment for use in the beneficiary's home will be made only under the provisions for payment applicable to DME. See the Medicare Benefit Policy Manual, Chapter 11, "End Stage Renal Disease," §30.1, for coverage of home use of hemodialysis.) NOTE: There is a wide variety in types of respirators and suction machines. The DMERC's medical staff should determine whether the apparatus specified in the claim is appropriate for home use.

2. Equipment Presumptively Nonmedical - Equipment which is primarily and customarily used for a nonmedical purpose may not be considered "medical" equipment for which payment can be made under the medical insurance program. This is true even though the item has some remote medically related use. For example, in the case of a cardiac patient, an air conditioner might possibly be used to lower room temperature to reduce fluid loss in the patient and to restore an environment conducive to maintenance of the proper fluid balance. Nevertheless, because the primary and customary use of an air conditioner is a nonmedical one, the air conditioner cannot be deemed to be medical equipment for which payment can be made.

Other devices and equipment used for environmental control or to enhance the environmental setting in which the beneficiary is placed are not considered covered DME. These include, for example, room heaters, humidifiers, dehumidifiers, and electric air cleaners. Equipment which basically serves comfort or convenience functions or is primarily for the convenience of a person caring for the patient, such as elevators, stairway elevators, and posture chairs, do not constitute medical equipment. Similarly, physical fitness equipment (such as an exercycle), first-aid or precautionary-type equipment (such as preset portable oxygen units), self-help devices (such as safety grab bars), and training equipment (such as Braille training texts) are considered nonmedical in nature.

3. Special Exception Items - Specified items of equipment may be covered under certain conditions even though they do not meet the definition of DME because they are not primarily and customarily used to serve a medical purpose and/or are generally useful in the absence of illness or injury. These items would be covered when it is clearly established that they serve a therapeutic purpose in an individual case and would include:

a. Gel pads and pressure and water mattresses (which generally serve a preventive purpose) when prescribed for a patient who had bed sores or there is medical evidence indicating that they are highly susceptible to such ulceration; and

b. Heat lamps for a medical rather than a soothing or cosmetic purpose, e.g., where the need for heat therapy has been established.

In establishing medical necessity for the above items, the evidence must show that the item is included in the physician's course of treatment and a physician is supervising its use.

NOTE: The above items represent special exceptions and no extension of coverage to other items should be inferred

C - Necessary and Reasonable

Although an item may be classified as DME, it may not be covered in every instance. Coverage in a particular case is subject to the requirement that the equipment be necessary and reasonable for treatment of an illness or injury, or to improve the functioning of a malformed body member. These considerations will bar payment for equipment which cannot reasonably be expected to perform a therapeutic function in an individual case or will permit only partial therapeutic function in an individual case or will permit only partial payment when the type of equipment furnished substantially exceeds that required for the treatment of the illness or injury involved.

See the Medicare Claims Processing Manual, Chapter 1, "General Billing Requirements;" §60, regarding the rules for providing advance beneficiary notices (ABNs) that advise beneficiaries, before items or services actually are furnished, when Medicare is likely to deny payment for them. ABNs allow beneficiaries to make an informed consumer decision about receiving items or services for which they may have to pay out-of-pocket and to be more active participants in their own health care treatment decisions.

1 - Necessity for the Equipment

Equipment is necessary when it can be expected to make a meaningful contribution to the treatment of the patient's illness or injury or to the improvement of his or her malformed body member. In most cases the physician's prescription for the equipment and other medical information available to the DMERC will be sufficient to establish that the equipment serves this purpose.

2 - Reasonableness of the Equipment

Even though an item of DME may serve a useful medical purpose, the DMERC or intermediary must also consider to what extent, if any, it would be reasonable for the

Medicare program to pay for the item prescribed. The following considerations should enter into the determination of reasonableness:

1. Would the expense of the item to the program be clearly disproportionate to the therapeutic benefits which could ordinarily be derived from use of the equipment?

2. Is the item substantially more costly than a medically appropriate and realistically feasible alternative pattern of care?

3. Does the item serve essentially the same purpose as equipment already available to the beneficiary?

3 - Payment Consistent With What is Necessary and Reasonable

Where a claim is filed for equipment containing features of an aesthetic nature or features of a medical nature which are not required by the patient's condition or where there exists a reasonably feasible and medically appropriate alternative pattern of care which is less costly than the equipment furnished, the amount payable is based on the rate for the equipment or alternative treatment which meets the patient's medical needs.

The acceptance of an assignment binds the supplier-assignee to accept the payment for the medically required equipment or service as the full charge and the supplier-assignee cannot charge the beneficiary the differential attributable to the equipment actually furnished.

4 - Establishing the Period of Medical Necessity

Generally, the period of time an item of durable medical equipment will be considered to be medically necessary is based on the physician's estimate of the time that his or her patient will need the equipment. See the Medicare Program Integrity Manual, Chapters 5 and 6, for medical review guidelines.

D - Definition of a Beneficiary's Home

B3-2100.3, A3-3113.6, HO-235.6, HHA-220.3

For purposes of rental and purchase of DME a beneficiary's home may be his/her own dwelling, an apartment, a relative's home, a home for the aged, or some other type of institution. However, an institution may not be considered a beneficiary's home if it:

• Meets at least the basic requirement in the definition of a hospital, i.e., it is primarily engaged in providing by or under the supervision of physicians, to inpatients, diagnostic and therapeutic services for medical diagnosis, treatment, and care of injured, disabled, and sick persons, or rehabilitation services for the rehabilitation of injured, disabled, or sick persons; or

• Meets at least the basic requirement in the definition of a skilled nursing facility, i.e., it is primarily engaged in providing to inpatients skilled nursing care and related services for patients who require medical or nursing care, or rehabilitation services for the rehabilitation of injured, disabled, or sick persons.

Thus, if an individual is a patient in an institution or distinct part of an institution which provides the services described in the bullets above, the individual is not entitled to have separate Part B payment made for rental or purchase of DME. This is because such an institution may not be considered the individual's home. The same concept applies even if the patient resides in a bed or portion of the institution not certified for Medicare.

If the patient is at home for part of a month and, for part of the same month is in an institution that cannot qualify as his or her home, or is outside the U.S., monthly payments may be made for the entire month. Similarly, if DME is returned to the provider before the end of a payment month because the beneficiary died in that month or because the equipment became unnecessary in that month, payment may be made for the entire month.

Pub. 100-2, Chapter 15, Section 110.2

Repairs, Maintenance, Replacement, and Delivery
(Rev. 1, 10-01-03)

B3-2100.4, A3-3113.3, HO-235.3, HHA-220.4

Under the circumstances specified below, payment may be made for repair, maintenance, and replacement of medically required DME which the beneficiary owns or is purchasing, including equipment which had been in use before the user enrolled in Part B of the program.

A - Repairs

B3-2100.4, A3-3113.3A, HO-235.3A

Repairs to equipment, which a beneficiary is purchasing or already owns are covered when necessary to make the equipment serviceable. A service charge may include the use of "loaner" equipment where this is required. If the expense for repairs exceeds the estimated expense of purchasing or renting another item of equipment for the remaining period of medical need, no payment can be made for the amount of the excess. (See subsection C where claims for repairs suggest malicious damage or culpable neglect.)

B - Maintenance

B3-2100.4, A3-3113.3.B, HO-235.3.B

Routine periodic servicing, such as testing, cleaning, regulating, and checking of the beneficiary's equipment, is not covered. The owner is expected to perform such routine maintenance rather than a retailer or some other person who charges the beneficiary. Normally, purchasers of DME are given operating manuals which describe the type of servicing an owner may perform to properly maintain the equipment. Thus, hiring a third party to do such work is for the convenience of the beneficiary and is not covered.

However, more extensive maintenance which, based on the manufacturers' recommendations, is to be performed by authorized technicians, is covered as repairs. This might include, for example, breaking down sealed components and performing tests which require specialized testing equipment not available to the beneficiary.

For capped rental items which have reached the 15-month rental cap, contractors pay claims for maintenance and servicing fees after 6 months have passed from the end of the final paid rental month or from the end of the period the item is no longer covered under the supplier's or manufacturer's warranty, whichever is later. See the Medicare Claims Processing Manual, Chapter 20, "Durable Medical Equipment, Prosthetics and Orthotics, and Supplies (DMEPOS)," for additional instruction and an example.

C - Replacement

B3-2100.4, A3-3113.3.C, HO-235.3.C

Replacement of equipment is covered in cases which the beneficiary owns or is purchasing is covered in cases of loss or irreparable damage or wear and when required because of a change in the patient's condition. Expenses for replacement required because of loss or irreparable damage may be reimbursed without a physician's order when in the judgment of the DMERC the equipment as originally ordered, considering the age of the order, still fills the patient's medical needs. However, claims involving replacement equipment necessitated because of wear or a change in the patient's condition must be supported by a current physician's order.

If a capped rental item of equipment has been in continuous use by the patient, on either a rental or purchase basis, for the equipment's useful lifetime or if the item is lost or irreparably damaged, the patient may elect to obtain a new piece of equipment. The contractor determines the reasonable useful lifetime for capped rental equipment but in no case can it be less than five years. Computation of the useful lifetime is based on when the equipment is delivered to the beneficiary, not the age of the equipment.

Payment may not be made for items covered under a manufacturer's or supplier's warranty. (See the Medicare Claims Processing Manual, Chapter 20, "Durable Medical Equipment, Prosthetics and Orthotics, and Supplies (DMEPOS)," and the Medicare Benefit Policy Manual, Chapter 16, "General Exclusions from Coverage," in regard to payment for equipment replaced under a warranty.) Cases suggesting malicious damage, culpable neglect, or wrongful disposition of equipment should be investigated and denied where the DMERC determines that it is unreasonable to make program payment under the circumstances. DMERCs refer such cases to the program integrity specialist in the RO.

D - Delivery

B3-2100.4, A3-3113.3.D, HO-235.3.D

Delivery and service charges are covered, but the related payment is included in the fee schedule for the related item. Separate payment is not made.

However, where special circumstances apply, e.g., beneficiary lives in remote area, or equipment could not be obtained from a local dealer special consideration can be applied at the discretion of the DMERC/intermediary.

Pub. 100-2, Chapter 15, Section 110.3

Coverage of Supplies and Accessories
(Rev. 1, 10-01-03)

B3-2100.5, A3-3113.4, HO-235.4, HHA-220.5

Payment may be made for supplies, e.g., oxygen, that are necessary for the effective use of durable medical equipment. Such supplies include those drugs and biologicals which must be put directly into the equipment in order to achieve the therapeutic benefit of the durable medical equipment or to assure the proper functioning of the equipment, e.g., tumor chemotherapy agents used with an infusion pump or heparin used with a home dialysis system. However, the coverage of such drugs or biologicals does not preclude the need for a determination that the drug or biological itself is reasonable and necessary for treatment of the illness or injury or to improve the functioning of a malformed body member.

In the case of prescription drugs, other than oxygen, used in conjunction with durable medical equipment, prosthetic, orthotics, and supplies (DMEPOS) or prosthetic devices, the entity that dispenses the drug must furnish it directly to the patient for whom a prescription is written. The entity that dispenses the drugs must have a Medicare supplier number, must possess a current license to dispense prescription drugs in the State in which the drug is dispensed, and must bill and receive payment in its own

name. A supplier that is not the entity that dispenses the drugs cannot purchase the drugs used in conjunction with DME for resale to the beneficiary. Reimbursement may be made for replacement of essential accessories such as hoses, tubes, mouthpieces, etc., for necessary DME, only if the beneficiary owns or is purchasing the equipment.

Pub. 100-2, Chapter 15, Section 120

Prosthetic Devices

B3-2130, A3-3110.4, HO-228.4, A3-3111, HO-229

A - General

Prosthetic devices (other than dental) which replace all or part of an internal body organ (including contiguous tissue), or replace all or part of the function of a permanently inoperative or malfunctioning internal body organ are covered when furnished on a physician's order. This does not require a determination that there is no possibility that the patient's condition may improve sometime in the future. If the medical record, including the judgment of the attending physician, indicates the condition is of long and indefinite duration, the test of permanence is considered met. (Such a device may also be covered under §60.l as a supply when furnished incident to a physician's service.)

Examples of prosthetic devices include artificial limbs, parenteral and enteral (PEN) nutrition, cardiac pacemakers, prosthetic lenses (see subsection B), breast prostheses (including a surgical brassiere) for postmastectomy patients, maxillofacial devices, and devices which replace all or part of the ear or nose. A urinary collection and retention system with or without a tube is a prosthetic device replacing bladder function in case of permanent urinary incontinence. The foley catheter is also considered a prosthetic device when ordered for a patient with permanent urinary incontinence. However, chucks, diapers, rubber sheets, etc., are supplies that are not covered under this provision. Although hemodialysis equipment is a prosthetic device, payment for the rental or purchase of such equipment in the home is made only for use under the provisions for payment applicable to durable medical equipment.

An exception is that if payment cannot be made on an inpatient's behalf under Part A, hemodialysis equipment, supplies, and services required by such patient could be covered under Part B as a prosthetic device, which replaces the function of a kidney. See the Medicare Benefit Policy Manual, Chapter 11, "End Stage Renal Disease," for payment for hemodialysis equipment used in the home. See the Medicare Benefit Policy Manual, Chapter 1, "Inpatient Hospital Services," §10, for additional instructions on hospitalization for renal dialysis.

NOTE: Medicare does not cover a prosthetic device dispensed to a patient prior to the time at which the patient undergoes the procedure that makes necessary the use of the device. For example, the carrier does not make a separate Part B payment for an intraocular lens (IOL) or pacemaker that a physician, during an office visit prior to the actual surgery, dispenses to the patient for his or her use. Dispensing a prosthetic device in this manner raises health and safety issues. Moreover, the need for the device cannot be clearly established until the procedure that makes its use possible is successfully performed. Therefore, dispensing a prosthetic device in this manner is not considered reasonable and necessary for the treatment of the patient's condition.

Colostomy (and other ostomy) bags and necessary accouterments required for attachment are covered as prosthetic devices. This coverage also includes irrigation and flushing equipment and other items and supplies directly related to ostomy care, whether the attachment of a bag is required.

Accessories and/or supplies which are used directly with an enteral or parenteral device to achieve the therapeutic benefit of the prosthesis or to assure the proper functioning of the device may also be covered under the prosthetic device benefit subject to the additional guidelines in the Medicare National Coverage Determinations Manual.

Covered items include catheters, filters, extension tubing, infusion bottles, pumps (either food or infusion), intravenous (I.V.) pole, needles, syringes, dressings, tape, Heparin Sodium (parenteral only), volumetric monitors (parenteral only), and parenteral and enteral nutrient solutions. Baby food and other regular grocery products that can be blenderized and used with the enteral system are not covered. Note that some of these items, e.g., a food pump and an I.V. pole, qualify as DME. Although coverage of the enteral and parenteral nutritional therapy systems is provided on the basis of the prosthetic device benefit, the payment rules relating to lump sum or monthly payment for DME apply to such items.

The coverage of prosthetic devices includes replacement of and repairs to such devices as explained in subsection D.

Finally, the Benefits Improvement and Protection Act of 2000 amended §1834(h)(1) of the Act by adding a provision (1834 (h)(1)(G)(i)) that requires Medicare payment to be made for the replacement of prosthetic devices which are artificial limbs, or for the replacement of any part of such devices, without regard to continuous use or useful lifetime restrictions if an ordering physician determines that the replacement device, or replacement part of such a device, is necessary.

PUB 100 REFERENCES

Payment may be made for the replacement of a prosthetic device that is an artificial limb, or replacement part of a device if the ordering physician determines that the replacement device or part is necessary because of any of the following:

1. A change in the physiological condition of the patient;

2. An irreparable change in the condition of the device, or in a part of the device; or

3. The condition of the device, or the part of the device, requires repairs and the cost of such repairs would be more than 60 percent of the cost of a replacement device, or, as the case may be, of the part being replaced.

This provision is effective for items replaced on or after April 1, 2001. It supersedes any rule that that provided a 5-year or other replacement rule with regard to prosthetic devices.

B - Prosthetic Lenses

The term "internal body organ" includes the lens of an eye. Prostheses replacing the lens of an eye include post-surgical lenses customarily used during convalescence from eye surgery in which the lens of the eye was removed. In addition, permanent lenses are also covered when required by an individual lacking the organic lens of the eye because of surgical removal or congenital absence. Prosthetic lenses obtained on or after the beneficiary's date of entitlement to supplementary medical insurance benefits may be covered even though the surgical removal of the crystalline lens occurred before entitlement.

1 - Prosthetic Cataract Lenses

One of the following prosthetic lenses or combinations of prosthetic lenses furnished by a physician (see §30.4 for coverage of prosthetic lenses prescribed by a doctor of optometry) may be covered when determined to be reasonable and necessary to restore essentially the vision provided by the crystalline lens of the eye:

Prosthetic bifocal lenses in frames;

Prosthetic lenses in frames for far vision, and prosthetic lenses in frames for near vision; or

When a prosthetic contact lens(es) for far vision is prescribed (including cases of binocular and monocular aphakia), make payment for the contact lens(es) and prosthetic lenses in frames for near vision to be worn at the same time as the contact lens(es), and prosthetic lenses in frames to be worn when the contacts have been removed.

Lenses which have ultraviolet absorbing or reflecting properties may be covered, in lieu of payment for regular (untinted) lenses, if it has been determined that such lenses are medically reasonable and necessary for the individual patient.

Medicare does not cover cataract sunglasses obtained in addition to the regular (untinted) prosthetic lenses since the sunglasses duplicate the restoration of vision function performed by the regular prosthetic lenses.

2 - Payment for Intraocular Lenses (IOLs) Furnished in Ambulatory Surgical Centers (ASCs)

Effective for services furnished on or after March 12, 1990, payment for intraocular lenses (IOLs) inserted during or subsequent to cataract surgery in a Medicare certified ASC is included with the payment for facility services that are furnished in connection with the covered surgery.

Refer to the Medicare Claims Processing Manual, Chapter 14, "Ambulatory Surgical Centers," for more information.

3 - Limitation on Coverage of Conventional Lenses

One pair of conventional eyeglasses or conventional contact lenses furnished after each cataract surgery with insertion of an IOL is covered.

C - Dentures

Dentures are excluded from coverage. However, when a denture or a portion of the denture is an integral part (built-in) of a covered prosthesis (e.g., an obturator to fill an opening in the palate), it is covered as part of that prosthesis.

D - Supplies, Repairs, Adjustments, and Replacement

Supplies are covered that are necessary for the effective use of a prosthetic device (e.g., the batteries needed to operate an artificial larynx). Adjustment of prosthetic devices required by wear or by a change in the patient's condition is covered when ordered by a physician. General provisions relating to the repair and replacement of durable medical equipment in §110.2 for the repair and replacement of prosthetic devices are applicable. (See the Medicare Benefit Policy Manual, Chapter 16, "General Exclusions from Coverage," §40.4, for payment for devices replaced under a warranty.) Replacement of conventional eyeglasses or contact lenses furnished in accordance with §120.B.3 is not covered.

Necessary supplies, adjustments, repairs, and replacements are covered even when the device had been in use before the user enrolled in Part B of the program, so long as the device continues to be medically required.

Pub. 100-2, Chapter 15, Section 140

Therapeutic Shoes for Individuals with Diabetes
(Rev. 1, 10-01-03)

B3-2134

Coverage of therapeutic shoes (depth or custom-molded) along with inserts for individuals with diabetes is available as of May 1, 1993. These diabetic shoes are covered if the requirements as specified in this section concerning certification and prescription are fulfilled. In addition, this benefit provides for a pair of diabetic shoes even if only one foot suffers from diabetic foot disease. Each shoe is equally equipped so that the affected limb, as well as the remaining limb, is protected. Claims for therapeutic shoes for diabetics are processed by the Durable Medical Equipment Regional Carriers (DMERCs).

Therapeutic shoes for diabetics are not DME and are not considered DME nor orthotics, but a separate category of coverage under Medicare Part B. (See §1861(s)(12) and §1833(o) of the Act.)

A - Definitions

The following items may be covered under the diabetic shoe benefit:

1 - Custom-Molded Shoes

Custom-molded shoes are shoes that:

- Are constructed over a positive model of the patient's foot;

- Are made from leather or other suitable material of equal quality;

- Have removable inserts that can be altered or replaced as the patient's condition warrants; and

- Have some form of shoe closure.

2 - Depth Shoes

Depth shoes are shoes that:

- Have a full length, heel-to-toe filler that, when removed, provides a minimum of 3/16 inch of additional depth used to accommodate custom-molded or customized inserts;

- Are made from leather or other suitable material of equal quality;

- Have some form of shoe closure; and

- Are available in full and half sizes with a minimum of three widths so that the sole is graded to the size and width of the upper portions of the shoes according to the American standard last sizing schedule or its equivalent. (The American standard last sizing schedule is the numerical shoe sizing system used for shoes sold in the United States.)

3 - Inserts

Inserts are total contact, multiple density, removable inlays that are directly molded to the patient's foot or a model of the patient's foot and that are made of a suitable material with regard to the patient's condition.

B - Coverage

1 - Limitations

For each individual, coverage of the footwear and inserts is limited to one of the following within one calendar year:

- No more than one pair of custom-molded shoes (including inserts provided with such shoes) and two additional pairs of inserts; or

- No more than one pair of depth shoes and three pairs of inserts (not including the noncustomized removable inserts provided with such shoes).

2 - Coverage of Diabetic Shoes and Brace

Orthopedic shoes, as stated in the Medicare Claims Processing Manual, Chapter 20, "Durable Medical Equipment, Surgical Dressings and Casts, Orthotics and Artificial Limbs, and Prosthetic Devices," generally are not covered. This exclusion does not apply to orthopedic shoes that are an integral part of a leg brace. In situations in which an individual qualifies for both diabetic shoes and a leg brace, these items are covered separately. Thus, the diabetic shoes may be covered if the requirements for this section are met, while the brace may be covered if the requirements of §130 are met.

3 - Substitution of Modifications for Inserts

An individual may substitute modification(s) of custom-molded or depth shoes instead of obtaining a pair(s) of inserts in any combination. Payment for the modification(s) may not exceed the limit set for the inserts for which the individual is entitled. The following is a list of the most common shoe modifications available, but it is not meant as an exhaustive list of the modifications available for diabetic shoes:

- Rigid Rocker Bottoms - These are exterior elevations with apex positions for 51 percent to 75 percent distance measured from the back end of the heel. The apex is a narrowed or pointed end of an anatomical structure. The apex must be

National Coverage Determinations Manual

positioned behind the metatarsal heads and tapered off sharply to the front tip of the sole. Apex height helps to eliminate pressure at the metatarsal heads. Rigidity is ensured by the steel in the shoe. The heel of the shoe tapers off in the back in order to cause the heel to strike in the middle of the heel;

• Roller Bottoms (Sole or Bar) - These are the same as rocker bottoms, but the heel is tapered from the apex to the front tip of the sole;

• Metatarsal Bars - An exterior bar is placed behind the metatarsal heads in order to remove pressure from the metatarsal heads. The bars are of various shapes, heights, and construction depending on the exact purpose;

• Wedges (Posting) - Wedges are either of hind foot, fore foot, or both and may be in the middle or to the side. The function is to shift or transfer weight bearing upon standing or during ambulation to the opposite side for added support, stabilization, equalized weight distribution, or balance; and

• Offset Heels - This is a heel flanged at its base either in the middle, to the side, or a combination, that is then extended upward to the shoe in order to stabilize extreme positions of the hind foot.

Other modifications to diabetic shoes include, but are not limited to flared heels, Velcro closures, and inserts for missing toes.

4 - Separate Inserts

Inserts may be covered and dispensed independently of diabetic shoes if the supplier of the shoes verifies in writing that the patient has appropriate footwear into which the insert can be placed. This footwear must meet the definitions found above for depth shoes and custom-molded shoes.

C - Certification

The need for diabetic shoes must be certified by a physician who is a doctor of medicine or a doctor of osteopathy and who is responsible for diagnosing and treating the patient's diabetic systemic condition through a comprehensive plan of care. This managing physician must:

• Document in the patient's medical record that the patient has diabetes;

• Certify that the patient is being treated under a comprehensive plan of care for diabetes, and that the patient needs diabetic shoes; and

• Document in the patient's record that the patient has one or more of the following conditions:

—Peripheral neuropathy with evidence of callus formation;

—History of pre-ulcerative calluses;

—History of previous ulceration;

—Foot deformity;

—Previous amputation of the foot or part of the foot; or

—Poor circulation.

D - Prescription

Following certification by the physician managing the patient's systemic diabetic condition, a podiatrist or other qualified physician who is knowledgeable in the fitting of diabetic shoes and inserts may prescribe the particular type of footwear necessary.

E - Furnishing Footwear

The footwear must be fitted and furnished by a podiatrist or other qualified individual such as a pedorthist, an orthotist, or a prosthetist. The certifying physician may not furnish the diabetic shoes unless the certifying physician is the only qualified individual in the area. It is left to the discretion of each carrier to determine the meaning of "in the area."

Pub. 100-2, Chapter 15, Section 150

Dental Services

B3-2136

As indicated under the general exclusions from coverage, items and services in connection with the care, treatment, filling, removal, or replacement of teeth or structures directly supporting the teeth are not covered. "Structures directly supporting the teeth" means the periodontium, which includes the gingivae, dentogingival junction, periodontal membrane, cementum of the teeth, and alveolar process.

In addition to the following, see Pub 100-1, the Medicare General Information, Eligibility, and Entitlement Manual, Chapter 5, Definitions and Pub 3, the Medicare National Coverage Determinations Manual for specific services which may be covered when furnished by a dentist. If an otherwise noncovered procedure or service is performed by a dentist as incident to and as an integral part of a covered procedure or service performed by the dentist, the total service performed by the dentist on such an occasion is covered.

EXAMPLE 1

The reconstruction of a ridge performed primarily to prepare the mouth for dentures is a noncovered procedure. However, when the reconstruction of a ridge is performed as a result of and at the same time as the surgical removal of a tumor (for other than dental purposes), the totality of surgical procedures is a covered service.

EXAMPLE 2

Medicare makes payment for the wiring of teeth when this is done in connection with the reduction of a jaw fracture.

The extraction of teeth to prepare the jaw for radiation treatment of neoplastic disease is also covered. This is an exception to the requirement that to be covered, a noncovered procedure or service performed by a dentist must be an incident to and an integral part of a covered procedure or service performed by the dentist. Ordinarily, the dentist extracts the patient's teeth, but another physician, e.g., a radiologist, administers the radiation treatments.

When an excluded service is the primary procedure involved, it is not covered, regardless of its complexity or difficulty. For example, the extraction of an impacted tooth is not covered. Similarly, an alveoplasty (the surgical improvement of the shape and condition of the alveolar process) and a frenectomy are excluded from coverage when either of these procedures is performed in connection with an excluded service, e.g., the preparation of the mouth for dentures. In a like manner, the removal of a torus palatinus (a bony protuberance of the hard palate) may be a covered service. However, with rare exception, this surgery is performed in connection with an excluded service, i.e., the preparation of the mouth for dentures. Under such circumstances, Medicare does not pay for this procedure.

Dental splints used to treat a dental condition are excluded from coverage under 1862(a)(12) of the Act. On the other hand, if the treatment is determined to be a covered medical condition (i.e., dislocated upper/lower jaw joints), then the splint can be covered.

Whether such services as the administration of anesthesia, diagnostic x-rays, and other related procedures are covered depends upon whether the primary procedure being performed by the dentist is itself covered. Thus, an x-ray taken in connection with the reduction of a fracture of the jaw or facial bone is covered. However, a single x-ray or x-ray survey taken in connection with the care or treatment of teeth or the periodontium is not covered.

Medicare makes payment for a covered dental procedure no matter where the service is performed. The hospitalization or nonhospitalization of a patient has no direct bearing on the coverage or exclusion of a given dental procedure.

Payment may also be made for services and supplies furnished incident to covered dental services. For example, the services of a dental technician or nurse who is under the direct supervision of the dentist or physician are covered if the services are included in the dentist's or physician's bill.

Pub. 100-2, Chapter 15, Section 230

Payable Rehabilitation Services

B3-2210

A - General

To be covered PT, OT or speech-language pathology services, the services must relate directly and specifically to an active written treatment regimen established by the physician or non-physician practitioner after any needed consultation with the qualified PT, OT, or speech-language pathologist and must be reasonable and necessary to the treatment of the individual's illness or injury. The physician, non-physician practitioner or the qualified therapist providing such services may establish a plan of treatment for outpatient PT, OT, or speech-language pathology services.

There is a limit for the amount of therapy expenses that is recognized as payable for some years. See the Medicare Claims Processing Manual, Chapter 5, §10.2, for a complete description of this financial limitation.

B - Reasonable and Necessary

To be considered reasonable and necessary the following conditions must be met:

The services must be considered under accepted standards of medical practice to be a specific and effective treatment for the patient's condition;

The services must be of such a level of complexity and sophistication or the condition of the patient must be such that the services required can be safely and effectively performed only by a qualified PT, OT, or speech language pathologist or under the therapist's supervision. Services which do not require the performance or supervision of a therapist are not considered reasonable or necessary PT, OT or speech-language pathology services, even if they are performed or supervised by a therapist. (When the carrier determines the services furnished were of a type that could have been safely and related to the maintenance of function (see subsection D) do not require the skills of a qualified physical therapist.

PUB 100 REFERENCES

Pub. 100-2, Chapter 15, Section 290

Foot Care

A3-3158, B3-2323, HO-260.9, B3-4120.1

A - Treatment of Subluxation of Foot

Subluxations of the foot are defined as partial dislocations or displacements of joint surfaces, tendons ligaments, or muscles of the foot. Surgical or nonsurgical treatments undertaken for the sole purpose of correcting a subluxated structure in the foot as an isolated entity are not covered.

However, medical or surgical treatment of subluxation of the ankle joint (talo-crural joint) is covered. In addition, reasonable and necessary medical or surgical services, diagnosis, or treatment for medical conditions that have resulted from or are associated with partial displacement of structures is covered. For example, if a patient has osteoarthritis that has resulted in a partial displacement of joints in the foot, and the primary treatment is for the osteoarthritis, coverage is provided

B - Exclusions from Coverage

The following foot care services are generally excluded from coverage under both Part A and Part B. (See §290.F and §290.G for instructions on applying foot care exclusions.)

1 - Treatment of Flat Foot

The term "flat foot" is defined as a condition in which one or more arches of the foot have flattened out. Services or devices directed toward the care or correction of such conditions, including the prescription of supportive devices, are not covered.

2 - Routine Foot Care

Except as provided above, routine foot care is excluded from coverage. Services that normally are considered routine and not covered by Medicare include the following:

The cutting or removal of corns and calluses;

The trimming, cutting, clipping, or debriding of nails; and

Other hygienic and preventive maintenance care, such as cleaning and soaking the feet, the use of skin creams to maintain skin tone of either ambulatory or bedfast patients, and any other service performed in the absence of localized illness, injury, or symptoms involving the foot.

3 - Supportive Devices for Feet

Orthopedic shoes and other supportive devices for the feet generally are not covered. However, this exclusion does not apply to such a shoe if it is an integral part of a leg brace, and its expense is included as part of the cost of the brace. Also, this exclusion does not apply to therapeutic shoes furnished to diabetics.

C - Exceptions to Routine Foot Care Exclusion

1 - Necessary and Integral Part of Otherwise Covered Services

In certain circumstances, services ordinarily considered to be routine may be covered if they are performed as a necessary and integral part of otherwise covered services, such as diagnosis and treatment of ulcers, wounds, or infections.

2 - Treatment of Warts on Foot

The treatment of warts (including plantar warts) on the foot is covered to the same extent as services provided for the treatment of warts located elsewhere on the body.

3 - Presence of Systemic Condition

The presence of a systemic condition such as metabolic, neurologic, or peripheral vascular disease may require scrupulous foot care by a professional that in the absence of such condition(s) would be considered routine (and, therefore, excluded from coverage). Accordingly, foot care that would otherwise be considered routine may be covered when systemic condition(s) result in severe circulatory embarrassment or areas of diminished sensation in the individual's legs or feet. (See subsection A.

In these instances, certain foot care procedures that otherwise are considered routine (e.g., cutting or removing corns and calluses, or trimming, cutting, clipping, or debriding nails) may pose a hazard when performed by a nonprofessional person on patients with such systemic conditions. (See §290.G for procedural instructions.)

4 - Mycotic Nails

In the absence of a systemic condition, treatment of mycotic nails may be covered.

The treatment of mycotic nails for an ambulatory patient is covered only when the physician attending the patient's mycotic condition documents that (1) there is clinical evidence of mycosis of the toenail, and (2) the patient has marked limitation of ambulation, pain, or secondary infection resulting from the thickening and dystrophy of the infected toenail plate.

The treatment of mycotic nails for a nonambulatory patient is covered only when the physician attending the patient's mycotic condition documents that (1) there is clinical evidence of mycosis of the toenail, and (2) the patient suffers from pain or secondary infection resulting from the thickening and dystrophy of the infected toenail plate.

For the purpose of these requirements, documentation means any written information that is required by the carrier in order for services to be covered. Thus, the information submitted with claims must be substantiated by information found in the patient's medical record. Any information, including that contained in a form letter, used for documentation purposes is subject to carrier verification in order to ensure that the information adequately justifies coverage of the treatment of mycotic nails.

D - Systemic Conditions That Might Justify Coverage

Although not intended as a comprehensive list, the following metabolic, neurologic, and peripheral vascular diseases (with synonyms in parentheses) most commonly represent the underlying conditions that might justify coverage for routine foot care.

Diabetes mellitus*

Arteriosclerosis obliterans (A.S.O., arteriosclerosis of the extremities, occlusive peripheral arteriosclerosis)

Buerger's disease (thromboangiitis obliterans)

Chronic thrombophlebitis *

Peripheral neuropathies involving the feet -

Associated with malnutrition and vitamin deficiency *

Malnutrition (general, pellagra)

Alcoholism

Malabsorption (celiac disease, tropical sprue)

Pernicious anemia

Associated with carcinoma *

Associated with diabetes mellitus *

Associated with drugs and toxins *

Associated with multiple sclerosis *

Associated with uremia (chronic renal disease) *

Associated with traumatic injury

Associated with leprosy or neurosyphilis

Associated with hereditary disorders

Hereditary sensory radicular neuropathy

Angiokeratoma corporis diffusum (Fabry's)

Amyloid neuropathy

When the patient's condition is one of those designated by an asterisk (*), routine procedures are covered only if the patient is under the active care of a doctor of medicine or osteopathy who documents the condition.

E - Supportive Devices for Feet

Orthopedic shoes and other supportive devices for the feet generally are not covered. However, this exclusion does not apply to such a shoe if it is an integral part of a leg brace, and its expense is included as part of the cost of the brace. Also, this exclusion does not apply to therapeutic shoes furnished to diabetics.

F - Presumption of Coverage

In evaluating whether the routine services can be reimbursed, a presumption of coverage may be made where the evidence available discloses certain physical and/or clinical findings consistent with the diagnosis and indicative of severe peripheral involvement. For purposes of applying this presumption the following findings are pertinent:

Class A Findings

Nontraumatic amputation of foot or integral skeletal portion thereof.

Class B Findings

Absent posterior tibial pulse;

Advanced trophic changes as: hair growth (decrease or absence) nail changes (thickening) pigmentary changes (discoloration) skin texture (thin, shiny) skin color (rubor or redness) (Three required); and

Absent dorsalis pedis pulse.

Class C Findings

Claudication;

Temperature changes (e.g., cold feet);

Edema;

Paresthesias (abnormal spontaneous sensations in the feet); and

Burning.

The presumption of coverage may be applied when the physician rendering the routine foot care has identified:

1. A Class A finding;

2. Two of the Class B findings; or

3. One Class B and two Class C findings.

Cases evidencing findings falling short of these alternatives may involve podiatric treatment that may constitute covered care and should be reviewed by the intermediary's medical staff and developed as necessary.

For purposes of applying the coverage presumption where the routine services have been rendered by a podiatrist, the contractor may deem the active care requirement met if the claim or other evidence available discloses that the patient has seen an M.D. or D.O. for treatment and/or evaluation of the complicating disease process during the 6-month period prior to the rendition of the routine-type services. The intermediary may also accept the podiatrist's statement that the diagnosing and treating M.D. or D.O. also concurs with the podiatrist's findings as to the severity of the peripheral involvement indicated.

Services ordinarily considered routine might also be covered if they are performed as a necessary and integral part of otherwise covered services, such as diagnosis and treatment of diabetic ulcers, wounds, and infections.

G - Application of Foot Care Exclusions to Physician's Services

The exclusion of foot care is determined by the nature of the service. Thus, payment for an excluded service should be denied whether performed by a podiatrist, osteopath, or a doctor of medicine, and without regard to the difficulty or complexity of the procedure.

When an itemized bill shows both covered services and noncovered services not integrally related to the covered service, the portion of charges attributable to the noncovered services should be denied. (For example, if an itemized bill shows surgery for an ingrown toenail and also removal of calluses not necessary for the performance of toe surgery, any additional charge attributable to removal of the calluses should be denied.)

In reviewing claims involving foot care, the carrier should be alert to the following exceptional situations:

1. Payment may be made for incidental noncovered services performed as a necessary and integral part of, and secondary to, a covered procedure. For example, if trimming of toenails is required for application of a cast to a fractured foot, the carrier need not allocate and deny a portion of the charge for the trimming of the nails. However, a separately itemized charge for such excluded service should be disallowed. When the primary procedure is covered the administration of anesthesia necessary for the performance of such procedure is also covered.

2. Payment may be made for initial diagnostic services performed in connection with a specific symptom or complaint if it seems likely that its treatment would be covered even though the resulting diagnosis may be one requiring only noncovered care.

The name of the M.D. or D.O. who diagnosed the complicating condition must be submitted with the claim. In those cases, where active care is required, the approximate date the beneficiary was last seen by such physician must also be indicated.

NOTE: Section 939 of P.L. 96-499 removed "warts" from the routine foot care exclusion effective July 1, 1981.

Relatively few claims for routine-type care are anticipated considering the severity of conditions contemplated as the basis for this exception. Claims for this type of foot care should not be paid in the absence of convincing evidence that nonprofessional performance of the service would have been hazardous for the beneficiary because of an underlying systemic disease. The mere statement of a diagnosis such as those mentioned in §D above does not of itself indicate the severity of the condition. Where development is indicated to verify diagnosis and/or severity the carrier should follow existing claims processing practices which may include review of carrier's history and medical consultation as well as physician contacts.

The rules in §290.F concerning presumption of coverage also apply.

Codes and policies for routine foot care and supportive devices for the feet are not exclusively for the use of podiatrists. These codes must be used to report foot care services regardless of the specialty of the physician who furnishes the services. Carriers must instruct physicians to use the most appropriate code available when billing for routine foot care.

Pub. 100-2, Chapter 16, Section 10

General Exclusions From Coverage
A3-3150, HO-260, HHA-232, B3-2300

No payment can be made under either the hospital insurance or supplementary medical insurance program for certain items and services, when the following conditions exist:

Not reasonable and necessary (§20);

No legal obligation to pay for or provide (§40);

Paid for by a governmental entity (§50);

Not provided within United States (§60);

Resulting from war (§70);

Personal comfort (§80);

Routine services and appliances (§90);

Custodial care (§110);

Cosmetic surgery (§120);

Charges by immediate relatives or members of household (§130);

Dental services (§140);

Paid or expected to be paid under workers' compensation (§150);

Nonphysician services provided to a hospital inpatient that were not provided directly or arranged for by the hospital (§170);

Services Related to and Required as a Result of Services Which are not Covered Under Medicare (§180);

Excluded foot care services and supportive devices for feet (§30); or

Excluded investigational devices (See Chapter 14, §30).

Pub. 100-2, Chapter 16, Section 20

Services Not Reasonable and Necessary
(Rev. 1, 10-01-03)

A3-3151, HO-260.1, B3-2303, AB-00-52 - 6/00

Items and services which are not reasonable and necessary for the diagnosis or treatment of illness or injury or to improve the functioning of a malformed body member are not covered, e.g., payment cannot be made for the rental of a special hospital bed to be used by the patient in their home unless it was a reasonable and necessary part of the patient's treatment. See also §80.

A health care item or service for the purpose of causing, or assisting to cause, the death of any individual (assisted suicide) is not covered. This prohibition does not apply to the provision of an item or service for the purpose of alleviating pain or discomfort, even if such use may increase the risk of death, so long as the item or service is not furnished for the specific purpose of causing death.

Pub. 100-2, Chapter 16, Section 90

Routine Services and Appliances
A3-3157, HO-260.7, B3-2320, R-1797A3 - 5/00

Routine physical checkups; eyeglasses, contact lenses, and eye examinations for the purpose of prescribing, fitting, or changing eyeglasses; eye refractions by whatever practitioner and for whatever purpose performed; hearing aids and examinations for hearing aids; and immunizations are not covered.

The routine physical checkup exclusion applies to (a) examinations performed without relationship to treatment or diagnosis for a specific illness, symptom, complaint, or injury; and (b) examinations required by third parties such as insurance companies, business establishments, or Government agencies.

If the claim is for a diagnostic test or examination performed solely for the purpose of establishing a claim under title IV of Public Law 91-173, "Black Lung Benefits," the service is not covered under Medicare and the claimant should be advised to contact their Social Security office regarding the filing of a claim for reimbursement under the "Black Lung" program.

The exclusions apply to eyeglasses or contact lenses, and eye examinations for the purpose of prescribing, fitting, or changing eyeglasses or contact lenses for refractive errors. The exclusions do not apply to physicians' services (and services incident to a physicians' service) performed in conjunction with an eye disease, as for example, glaucoma or cataracts, or to post-surgical prosthetic lenses which are customarily used during convalescence from eye surgery in which the lens of the eye was removed, or to permanent prosthetic lenses required by an individual lacking the organic lens of the eye, whether by surgical removal or congenital disease. Such prosthetic lens is a replacement for an internal body organ - the lens of the eye. (See the Medicare Benefit Policy Manual, Chapter 15, "Covered Medical and Other Health Services," §120).

Expenses for all refractive procedures, whether performed by an ophthalmologist (or any other physician) or an optometrist and without regard to the reason for performance of the refraction, are excluded from coverage.

A - Immunizations

Vaccinations or inoculations are excluded as immunizations unless they are either

Directly related to the treatment of an injury or direct exposure to a disease or condition, such as antirabies treatment, tetanus antitoxin or booster vaccine, botulin antitoxin, antivenin sera, or immune globulin.(In the absence of injury or direct exposure, preventive immunization (vaccination or inoculation) against such diseases as smallpox, polio, diphtheria, etc., is not covered.); or

National Coverage Determinations Manual

Specifically covered by statute, as described in the Medicare Benefit Policy Manual, Chapter 15, "Covered Medical and Other Health Services," §50.

B - Antigens

Prior to the Omnibus Reconciliation Act of 1980, a physician who prepared an antigen for a patient could not be reimbursed for that service unless the physician also administered the antigen to the patient. Effective January 1, 1981, payment may be made for a reasonable supply of antigens that have been prepared for a particular patient even though they have not been administered to the patient by the same physician who prepared them if:

The antigens are prepared by a physician who is a doctor of medicine or osteopathy, and

The physician who prepared the antigens has examined the patient and has determined a plan of treatment and a dosage regimen.

A reasonable supply of antigens is considered to be not more than a 12-week supply of antigens that has been prepared for a particular patient at any one time. The purpose of the reasonable supply limitation is to assure that the antigens retain their potency and effectiveness over the period in which they are to be administered to the patient. (See the Medicare Benefit Policy Manual, Chapter 15, "Covered Medical and Other Health Services," §50.4.4.2)

Pub. 100-2, Chapter 16, Section 140

Dental Services Exclusion

(Rev. 1, 10-01-03)

A3-3162, HO-260.13, B3-2336

Items and services in connection with the care, treatment, filling, removal, or replacement of teeth, or structures directly supporting the teeth are not covered. Structures directly supporting the teeth mean the periodontium, which includes the gingivae, dentogingival junction, periodontal membrane, cementum, and alveolar process. However, payment may be made for certain other services of a dentist. (See the Medicare Benefit Policy Manual, Chapter 15, "Covered Medical and Other Health Services," §150.)

The hospitalization or nonhospitalization of a patient has no direct bearing on the coverage or exclusion of a given dental procedure.

When an excluded service is the primary procedure involved, it is not covered regardless of its complexity or difficulty. For example, the extraction of an impacted tooth is not covered. Similarly, an alveoplasty (the surgical improvement of the shape and condition of the alveolar process) and a frenectomy are excluded from coverage when either of these procedures is performed in connection with an excluded service, e.g., the preparation of the mouth for dentures. In like manner, the removal of the torus palatinus (a bony protuberance of the hard palate) could be a covered service. However, with rare exception, this surgery is performed in connection with an excluded service, i.e., the preparation of the mouth for dentures. Under such circumstances, reimbursement is not made for this purpose.

The extraction of teeth to prepare the jaw for radiation treatments of neoplastic disease is also covered. This is an exception to the requirement that to be covered, a noncovered procedure or service performed by a dentist must be an incident to and an integral part of a covered procedure or service performed by the dentist. Ordinarily, the dentist extracts the patient's teeth, but another physician, e.g., a radiologist, administers the radiation treatments.

Whether such services as the administration of anesthesia, diagnostic x-rays, and other related procedures are covered depends upon whether the primary procedure being performed by the dentist is covered. Thus, an x-ray taken in connection with the reduction of a fracture of the jaw or facial bone is covered. However, a single x-ray or x-ray survey taken in connection with the care or treatment of teeth or the periodontium is not covered.

See also the Medicare Benefit Policy Manual, Chapter 1, "Inpatient Hospital Services," §70, and Chapter 15, "Covered Medical and Other Health Services," §150 for additional information on dental services.

Pub. 100-3, Section 20.9

Artificial Hearts And Related Devices

(Rev. 2, 10-17-03)

A ventricular assist device (VAD) or left ventricular assist device (LVAD) is used to assist a damaged or weakened heart in pumping blood. These devices are used for support of blood circulation post-cardiotomy, as a bridge to a heart transplant, or as destination therapy.

A - Covered Indications

1. Postcardiotomy (effective for services performed on or after October 18, 1993)

   Post-cardiotomy is the period following open-heart surgery. VADs used for support of blood circulation post-cardiotomy are covered only if they have received

approval from the Food and Drug Administration (FDA) for that purpose, and the VADs are used according to the FDA- approved labeling instructions.

2. Bridge-to-Transplant (effective for services performed on or after January 22, 1996)

   The VADs used for bridge-to-transplant are covered only if they have received approval from the FDA for that purpose, and the VADs are used according to the FDA-approved labeling instructions. All of the following criteria must be fulfilled in order for Medicare coverage to be provided for a VAD used as a bridge-to-transplant:

   a. The patient is approved and listed as a candidate for heart transplantation by a Medicare-approved heart transplant center; and

   b. The implanting site, if different than the Medicare-approved transplant center, must receive written permission from the Medicare-approved heart transplant center under which the patient is listed prior to implantation of the VAD.

   The Medicare-approved heart transplant center should make every reasonable effort to transplant patients on such devices as soon as medically reasonable. Ideally, the Medicare-approved heart transplant centers should determine patient-specific timetables for transplantation, and should not maintain such patients on VADs if suitable hearts become available.

3. Destination Therapy (effective for services performed on or after October 1, 2003)

   Destination therapy is for patients that require permanent mechanical cardiac support. The VADs used for destination therapy are covered only if they have received approval from the FDA for that purpose, and the device is used according to the FDA-approved labeling instructions. VADs are covered for patients who have chronic end-stage heart failure (New York Heart Association Class IV end-stage left ventricular failure for at least 90 days with a life expectancy of less than 2 years), are not candidates for heart transplantation, and meet all of the following conditions:

   a. The patient's Class IV heart failure symptoms have failed to respond to optimal medical management, including dietary salt restriction, diuretics, digitalis, beta-blockers, and ACE inhibitors (if tolerated) for at least 60 of the last 90 days;

   b. The patient has a left ventricular ejection fraction (LVEF) < 25%;

   c. The patient has demonstrated functional limitation with a peak oxygen consumption of < 12 ml/kg/min; or the patient has a continued need for intravenous inotropic therapy owing to symptomatic hypotension, decreasing renal function, or worsening pulmonary congestion; and,

   d. The patient has the appropriate body size ($\geq$ 1.5 m_) to support the VAD implantation.

In addition, the Centers for Medicare & Medicaid Services (CMS) has determined that VAD implantation as destination therapy is reasonable and necessary only when the procedure is performed in a Medicare-approved heart transplant facility that, between January 1, 2001, and September 30, 2003, implanted at least 15 VADs as a bridge-to-transplant or as destination therapy. These devices must have been approved by the FDA for destination therapy or as a bridge-to-transplant, or have been implanted as part of an FDA investigational device exemption (IDE) trial for one of these two indications.

The VADs implanted for other investigational indications or for support of blood circulation post-cardiotomy do not satisfy the volume requirement for this purpose. Since the relationship between volume and outcomes has not been well-established for VAD use, facilities that have minimal deficiencies in meeting this standard may apply and include a request for an exception based upon additional factors. Some of the factors CMS will consider are geographic location of the center, number of destination procedures performed, and patient outcomes from VAD procedures completed.

Also, this facility must be an active, continuous member of a national, audited registry that requires submission of health data on all VAD destination therapy patients from the date of implantation throughout the remainder of their lives. This registry must have the ability to accommodate data related to any device approved by the FDA for destination therapy regardless of manufacturer. The registry must also provide such routine reports as may be specified by CMS, and must have standards for data quality and timeliness of data submissions such that hospitals failing to meet them will be removed from membership. The CMS believes that the registry sponsored by the International Society for Heart and Lung Transplantation is an example of a registry that meets these characteristics.

Hospitals also must have in place staff and procedures that ensure that prospective VAD recipients receive all information necessary to assist them in giving appropriate informed consent for the procedure so that they and their families are fully aware of the aftercare requirements and potential limitations, as well as benefits, following VAD implantation.

The CMS plans to develop accreditation standards for facilities that implant VADs and, when implemented, VAD implantation will be considered reasonable and necessary only at accredited facilities.

A list of facilities eligible for Medicare reimbursement for VADs as destination therapy will be maintained on our Web site and available at www.cms.hhs.gov/coverage/lvadfacility.asp. In order to be placed on this list, facilities must submit a letter to the Director, Coverage and Analysis Group, 7500 Security Blvd, Mailstop C1-09-06, Baltimore, MD 21244. This letter must be received by CMS within 90 days of the issue date on this transmittal. The letter must include the following information: Facility's name and complete address;

- Facility's Medicare provider number;

- List of all implantations between Jan. 1, 2001, and Sept. 30, 2003, with the following information:

  —Date of implantation,

  —Indication for implantation (only destination and bridge-to-transplant can be reported; post-cardiotomy VAD implants are not to be included),

  —Device name and manufacturer, and,

  —Date of device removal and reason (e.g., transplantation, recovery, device malfunction), or date and cause of patient's death;

    • Point-of-contact for questions with telephone number;

    • Registry to which patient information will be submitted; and,

    • Signature of a senior facility administrative official.

Facilities not meeting the minimal standards and requesting exception should, in addition to supplying the information above, include the factors that they deem critical in requesting the exception to the standards.

The CMS will review the information contained in the above letters. When the review is complete, all necessary information is received, and criteria are met, CMS will include the name of the newly Medicare-approved facility on the CMS web site. No reimbursement for destination therapy will be made for implantations performed before the date the facility is added to the CMS web site. Each newly approved facility will also receive a formal letter from CMS stating the official approval date it was added to the list.

  B. Noncovered Indications (effective for services performed on or after May 19, 1986)

    1. Artificial Heart

    Since there is no authoritative evidence substantiating the safety and effectiveness of a VAD used as a replacement for the human heart, Medicare does not cover this device when used as an artificial heart.

    2. All other indications for the use of VADs not otherwise listed remain noncovered, except in the context of Category B IDE clinical trials (42 CFR 405) or as a routine cost in clinical trials defined under section 310.1 of the NCD manual (old CIM 30-1).

Pub 100-3, Section 20.15

Electrocardiographic Services

Reimbursement may be made under Part B for electrocardiographic (EKG) services rendered by a physician or incident to his/her services or by an approved laboratory or an approved supplier of portable X-ray services. Since there is no coverage for EKG services of any type rendered on a screening basis or as part of a routine examination, the claim must indicate the signs and symptoms or other clinical reason necessitating the services.

A separate charge by an attending or consulting physician for EKG interpretation is allowed only when it is the normal practice to make such charge in addition to the regular office visit charge. No payment is made for EKG interpretations by individuals other than physicians.

On a claim involving EKG services furnished by a laboratory or portable x-ray supplier, identify the physician ordering the service and, when the charge includes both the taking of the tracing and its interpretation, include the identity of the physician making the interpretation. No separate bill for the services of a physician is paid unless it is clear that he/she was the patient's attending physician or was acting as a consulting physician. The taking of an EKG in an emergency, i.e., when the patient is or may be experiencing what is commonly referred to as a heart attack, is covered as a laboratory service or a diagnostic service by a portable X-ray supplier only when the evidence shows that a physician was in attendance at the time the service was performed or immediately thereafter.

The documentation required in the various situations mentioned above must be furnished not only when the laboratory or portable X-ray supplier bills the patient or carrier for its service, but also when such a facility bills the attending physician who, in turn, bills the patient or carrier for the EKG services.(In addition to the evidence required to document the claim, the laboratory or portable x-ray supplier must maintain in its records the referring physician 's written order and the identity of the employee taking the tracing.)

Long Term EKG Monitoring, also referred to as long-term EKG recording, Holter recording, or dynamic electrocardiography, is a diagnostic procedure which provides a continuous record of the electrocardiographic activity of a patient's heart while he is engaged in his daily activities.

The basic components of the long-term EKG monitoring systems are a sensing element, the design of which may provide either for the recording of electrocardiographic information on magnetic tape or for detecting significant variations in rate or rhythm as they occur, and a component for either graphically recording the electrocardiographic data or for visual or computer assisted analysis of the information recorded on magnetic tape. The long-term EKG permits the examination in the ambulant or potentially ambulant patient of as many as 70,000 heartbeats in a 12-hour recording while the standard EKG which is obtained in the recumbent position, yields information on only 50 to 60 cardiac cycles and provides only a limited data base on which diagnostic judgments may be made.

Many patients with cardiac arrhythmias are unaware of the presence of an irregularity in heart rhythm. Due to the transient nature of many arrhythmias and the short intervals in which the rhythm of the heart is observed by conventional standard EKG techniques, the offending arrhythmias can go undetected. With the extended examination provided by the long-term EKG, the physician is able not only to detect but also to classify various types of rhythm disturbances and waveform abnormalities and note the frequency of their occurrence. The knowledge of the reaction of the heart to daily activities with respect to rhythm, rate, conduction disturbances, and changes are of great assistance in directing proper therapy and

This modality is valuable in both inpatient and outpatient diagnosis and therapy. Long-term monitoring of ambulant or potentially ambulant inpatients provides significant potential for reducing the length of stay for post-coronary infarct patients in the intensive care setting and may result in earlier discharge from the hospital with greater assurance of safety to the patients. The indications for the use of this technique, noted below, are similar for both inpatients and outpatients.

The long-term EKG has proven effective in detecting transient episodes of cardiac dysrhythmia and in permitting the correlation of these episodes with cardiovascular symptomatology.It is also useful for patients who have symptoms of obscure etiology suggestive of cardiac arrhythmia.Examples of such symptoms include palpitations, chest pain, dizziness, light-headedness, near syncope, syncope, transient ischemic episodes, dyspnea, and shortness of breath.

This technique would also be appropriate at the time of institution of any arrhythmic drug therapy and may be performed during the course of therapy to evaluate response.It is also appropriate for evaluating a change of dosage and may be indicated shortly before and after the discontinuation of anti-arrhythemic medication.The therapeutic response to a drug whose duration of action and peak of effectiveness is defined in hours cannot be properly assessed by examining 30-40 cycles on a standard EKG rhythm strip.The knowledge that all patients placed on anti-arrhythmic medication do not respond to therapy and the known toxicity of anti-arrhythmic agents clearly indicate that proper assessment should be made on an individual basis to determine whether medication should be continued and at what dosage level.

The long-term EKG is also valuable in the assessment of patients with coronary artery disease. It enables the documentation of etiology of such symptoms as chest pain and shortness of breath.Since the standard EKG is often normal during the intervals between the episodes of precordial pain, it is essential to obtain EKG information while the symptoms are occurring. The long-term EKG has enabled the correlation of chest symptoms with the objective evidence of ST-segment abnormalities.It is appropriate for patients who are recovering from an acute mycardial infarction or coronary insufficiency before and after discharge from the hospital, since it is impossible to predict which of these patients is subject to ventricular arrhythmias on the basis of the presence or absence of rhythm disturbances during the period of initial coronary care. The long-term EKG enables the physician to identify patients who are at a higher risk of dying suddenly in the period following an acute myocardial infarction.It may also be reasonable and necessary where the high-risk patient with known cardiovascular disease advances to a substantially higher level of activity which might trigger increased or new types of arrhythmias necessitating treatment. Such a high-risk case would be one in which there is documentation that acute phase arrhythmias have not totally disappeared during the period of convalescence.

The use of the long-term EKG for routine assessment of pacemaker function can no longer be justified (see §20.8.1). Its use for the patient with an internal pacemaker would be covered only when he has symptoms suggestive of arrhythmia not revealed by the standard EKG or rhythm strip.

These guidelines are intended as a general outline of the circumstances under which the use of this diagnostic procedure would be warranted. Each patient receiving a long-term EKG should be evaluated completely, prior to performance of this diagnostic study. A complete history and physical examination should be obtained and the referring physician should review the indications for use of the long-term EKG.

The performance of a long-term EKG does not necessarily require the prior performance of a standard EKG. Nor does the demonstration of a normal standard EKG preclude the need for a long- term EKG. Finally, the demonstration of an abnormal standard EKG does not obviate the need for a long-term EKG if there is suspicion that the dysrhythmia is transient in nature.

PUB 100 REFERENCES

A period of recording of up to 24 hours would normally be adequate to detect most transient arrhythmias and provide essential diagnostic information. The medical necessity for longer periods of monitoring must be documented.

Medical documentation for adjudicating claims for the use of the long-term EKG should be similar to other EKG services, X-ray services, and laboratory procedures. Generally, a statement of the diagnostic impression of the referring physician with an indication of the patient's relevant signs and symptoms should be sufficient for purposes of making a determination regarding the reasonableness and medical necessity for the use of this procedure. However, the intermediaries or carriers should require whatever additional documentation their medical consultants deem necessary to properly adjudicate the individual claim where the information submitted is not adequate.

It should be noted that the recording device furnished to the patient is simply one component of the diagnostic system and a separate charge for it will not be recognized under the durable medical equipment benefit.

Patient-Activated EKG Recorders, distributed under a variety of brand names, permit the patient to record an EKG upon manifestation of symptoms, or in response to a physician's order (e.g., immediately following strong exertion).Most such devices also permit the patient to simultaneously voice-record in order to describe symptoms and/or activity. In addition, some of these devices permit transtelephonic transmission of the recording to a physician's office, clinic, hospital, etc., having a decoder/recorder for review and analysis, thus eliminating the need to physically transport the tape. Some of these devices also permit a "time sampling" mode of operation. However, the "time sampling" mode is not covered—only the patient-activated mode of operation, when used for the indications described below, is covered at this time.

Services in connection with patient-activated EKG recorders are covered when used as an alternative to the long-term EKG monitoring (described above) for similar indications—detecting and characterizing symptomatic arrhythmias, regulation of anti-arrhythmic drug therapy, etc. Like long- term EKG monitoring, use of these devices is covered for evaluating patients with symptoms of obscure etiology suggestive of cardiac arrhythmia such as palpitations, chest pain, dizziness, lightheadedness, near syncope, syncope, transient ischemic episodes, dyspnea and shortness of breath.

As with long-term EKG monitors, patient-activated EKG recorders may be useful for both inpatient and outpatient diagnosis and therapy.While useful for assessing some post-coronary infarct patients in the hospital setting, these devices should not, however, be covered for outpatient monitoring of recently discharged post-infarct patients.

Computer Analyzed Electrocardiograms-Computer interpretation of EKG's is recognized as a valid and effective technique which will improve the quality and availability of cardiology services. Reimbursement may be made for such computer service when furnished in the setting and under the circumstances required for coverage of other electrocardiographic services. Where either a laboratory's or a portable x-ray supplier's charge for EKG services includes the physician review and certification of the printout as well as the computer interpretation, the certifying physician must be identified on the HCFA-1490 before the entire charge can be considered a reimbursable charge. Where the laboratory's (or portable x-ray supplier's) reviewing physician is not identified, the carrier should conclude that no professional component is involved and make its charge determination accordingly. If the supplying laboratory (or portable x-ray supplier when supplied by such a facility) does not include professional review and certification of the hard copy, a charge by the patient's physician may be recognized for the service. In any case the charge for the physician component should be substantially less than that for physician interpretation of the conventional EKG tracing in view of markedly reduced demand on the physician's time where computer interpretation is involved. Considering the unit cost reduction expected of this innovation, the total charge for the complete EKG service (taking of tracing and interpretation) when computer interpretation is employed should never exceed that considered reasonable for the service when physician interpretation is involved.

Transtelephonic Electrocardiographic Transmissions (Formerly Referred to as EKG Telephone Reporter Systems) is extended to include the use of transtelephonic electrocardiographic (EKG) transmissions as a diagnostic service for the indications described below, when performed with equipment meeting the standards described below, subject to the limitations and conditions specified below. Coverage is further limited to the amounts payable with respect to the physician's service in interpreting the results of such transmissions, including charges for rental of the equipment. The device used by the beneficiary is part of a total diagnostic system and is not considered durable medical equipment.

1. Covered Uses

The use of transtelephonic EKGs is covered for the following uses:

To detect, characterize, and document symptomatic transient arrhythmias;

To overcome problems in regulating antiarrhythmic drug dosage;

To carry out early posthospital monitoring of patients discharged after myocardial infarction; (only if 24-hour coverage is provided, see 4. below).

Since cardiology is a rapidly changing field, some uses other than those specified above may be covered if, in the judgment of the contractor's medical consultants, such a use was justifiable in the particular case.The enumerated uses above represent uses for which a firm coverage determination has been made, and for which contractors may make payment without extensive claims development or review.

2. Specifications for Devices

The devices used by the patient are highly portable (usually pocket-sized) and detect and convert the normal EKG signal so that it can be transmitted via ordinary telephone apparatus to a receiving station. At the receiving end, the signal is decoded and transcribed into a conventional EKG. There are numerous devices available which transmit EKG readings in this fashion. For purposes of Medicare coverage, however, the transmitting devices must meet at least the following criteria:

They must be capable of transmitting EKG Leads, I, II, or III;

These lead transmissions must be sufficiently comparable to readings obtained by a conventional EKG to permit proper interpretation of abnormal cardiac rhythms.

3. Potential for Abuse - Need for Screening Guidelines

While the use of these devices may often compare favorably with more costly alternatives, this is the case only where the information they contribute is actively utilized by a knowledgeable practitioner as part of overall medical management of the patient. Consequently, it is vital that contractors be aware of the potential for abuse of these devices, and adopt necessary screening and physician education policies to detect and halt potentially abusive situations. For example, use of these devices to diagnose and treat suspected arrhythmias as a routine substitute for more conventional methods of diagnosis, such as a careful history, physical examination, and standard EKG and rhythm strip would not be appropriate. Moreover, contractors should require written justification for use of such devices in excess of 30 consecutive days in cases involving detection of transient arrhythmias.

Contractors may find it useful to review claims for these devices with a view toward detecting patterns of practice which may be useful in developing schedules which may be adopted for screening such claims in the future.

4. Twenty-four Hour Coverage

No payment may be made for the use of these devices to carry out early posthospital monitoring of patients discharged after myocardial infarction unless provision is made for 24 hour coverage in the manner described below.

Twenty-four hour coverage means that there must be, at the monitoring site (or sites) an experienced EKG technician receiving calls; tape recording devices do not meet this requirement. Further, such technicians should have immediate access to a physician, and have been instructed in when and how to contact available facilities to assist the patient in case of emergencies.

Pub 100-3, Section 20.16

Cardiac Output Monitoring by Thoracic Electrical Bioimpedance (TEB)

A. Covered Indications

1. TEB is covered for the following uses:

a. Differentiation of cardiogenic from pulmonary causes of acute dyspnea when medical history, physical examination, and standard assessment tools provide insufficient information, and the treating physician has determined that TEB hemodynamic data are necessary for appropriate management of the patient.

b. Optimization of atrioventricular (A/V) interval for patients with A/V sequential cardiac pacemakers when medicalhistory, physical examination, and standard assessment tools provide insufficient information, and the treating physician has determined that TEB hemodynamic data are necessary for appropriate management of the patient.

c. Monitoring of continuous inotropic therapy for patients with terminal congestive heart failure, when those patients have chosen to die with comfort at home, or for patients waiting at home for a heart transplantd.

d. Evaluation for rejection in patients with a heart transplant as a predetermined alternative to a myocardial biopsy. Medical necessity must be documented should a biopsy be performed after TEB.

e. Optimization of fluid management in patients with congestive heart failure when medical history, physical examination, and standard assessment tools provide insufficient information, and the treating physician has determined that TEB hemodynamic data are necessary for appropriate management of the patient.

2. Contractors have discretion to determine whether the use of TEB for the management of drug-resistant hypertension is reasonable and necessary. Drug resistant hypertension is defined as failure to achieve goal BP in patients who are adhering to full doses of an appropriate three-drug regimen that includes a diuretic.

B. Noncovered Indications

1. TEB is noncovered when used for patients:

a. With proven or suspected disease involving severe regurgitation of the aorta;

b. With minute ventilation (MV) sensor function pacemakers, since the device may adversely affect the functioning of that type of pacemaker;

c. During cardiac bypass surgery; or

d. In the management of all forms of hypertension (with the exception of drug-resistant hypertension as outlined above).

2. All other uses of TEB not otherwise specified remain non-covered. (This NCD last reviewed January 2004.)

Pub 100-3, Section 20.19

Ambulatory Blood Pressure Monitoring

ABPM must be performed for at least 24 hours to meet coverage criteria.

ABPM is only covered for those patients with suspected white coat hypertension. Suspected white coat hypertension is defined as

1) office blood pressure >140/90 mm Hg on at least three separate clinic/office visits with two separate measurements made at each visit;

2) at least two documented blood pressure measurements taken outside the office which are less than 140/90 mm Hg; and

3) no evidence of end-organ damage.

The information obtained by ABPM is necessary in order to determine the appropriate management of the patient. ABPM is not covered for any other uses. In the rare circumstance that ABPM needs to be performed more than once in a patient, the qualifying criteria described above must be met for each subsequent ABPM test.

For those patients that undergo ABPM and have an ambulatory blood pressure of less than 135/85 with no evidence of end-organ damage, it is likely that their cardiovascular risk is similar to that of normotensives. They should be followed over time. Patients for which ABPM demonstrates a blood pressure of >135/85 may be at increased cardiovascular risk, and a physician may wish to consider antihypertensive therapy.

Pub. 100-3, Section 20.20

External Counterpulsation (ECP) for Severe Angina
(Rev. 1, 10-03-03)

CIM 35-74

Covered

External counterpulsation (ECP), commonly referred to as enhanced external counterpulsation, is a noninvasive outpatient treatment for coronary artery disease refractory to medical and/or surgical therapy. Although ECP devices are cleared by the Food and Drug Administration (FDA) for use in treating a variety of cardiac conditions, including stable or unstable angina pectoris, acute myocardial infarction and cardiogenic shock, the use of this device to treat cardiac conditions other than stable angina pectoris is not covered, since only that use has developed sufficient evidence to demonstrate its medical effectiveness. Noncoverage of hydraulic versions of these types of devices remains in force.

Coverage is provided for the use of ECP for patients who have been diagnosed with disabling angina (Class III or Class IV, Canadian Cardiovascular Society Classification or equivalent classification) who, in the opinion of a cardiologist or cardiothoracic surgeon, are not readily amenable to surgical intervention, such as PTCA or cardiac bypass because:

1. Their condition is inoperable, or at high risk of operative complications or post-operative failure;

2. Their coronary anatomy is not readily amenable to such procedures; or

3. They have co-morbid states that create excessive risk.

A full course of therapy usually consists of 35 one-hour treatments which may be offered once or twice daily, usually five days per week. The patient is placed on a treatment table where their lower trunk and lower extremities are wrapped in a series of three compressive air cuffs which inflate and deflate in synchronization with the patient's cardiac cycle.

During diastole, the three sets of air cuffs are inflated sequentially (distal to proximal) compressing the vascular beds within the muscles of the calves, lower thighs and upper thighs. This action results in an increase in diastolic pressure, generation of retrograde arterial blood flow and an increase in venous return. The cuffs are deflated simultaneously just prior to systole which produces a rapid drop in vascular impedance, a decrease in ventricular workload and an increase in cardiac output.

The augmented diastolic pressure and retrograde aortic flow appear to improve myocardial perfusion, while systolic unloading appears to reduce cardiac workload and oxygen requirements. The increased venous return coupled with enhanced systolic flow appears to increase cardiac output. As a result of this treatment, most patients experience increased time until onset of ischemia, increased exercise tolerance, and a reduction in the number and severity of anginal episodes. Evidence was presented that

this effect lasted well beyond the immediate post-treatment phase, with patients symptom-free for several months to two years.

This procedure must be done under direct supervision of a physician.

Pub. 100-3, Section 20.24

Displacement Cardiography
(Rev. 1, 10-03-03)

CIM 50-50

Displacement cardiography, including cardiokymography and photokymography, is a noninvasive diagnostic test used in evaluating coronary artery disease.

A - Cardiokymography

Cardiokymography is covered for services rendered on or after October 12, 1988.

Cardiokymography is a covered service only when it is used as an adjunct to electrocardiographic stress testing in evaluating coronary artery disease and only when the following clinical indications are present:

• For male patients, atypical angina pectoris or nonischemic chest pain; or

• For female patients, angina, either typical or atypical.

B - Photokymography - Not Covered

Photokymography remains excluded from coverage.

Pub 100-3, Section 20.21

Chelation Therapy for Treatment of Atherosclerosis
The application of chelation therapy using ethylenediamine-tetra-acetic acid (EDTA) for the treatment and prevention of atherosclerosis is controversial. There is no widely accepted rationale to explain the beneficial effects attributed to this therapy. Its safety is questioned and its clinical effectiveness has never been established by well designed, controlled clinical trials. It is not widely accepted and practiced by American physicians. EDTA chelation therapy for atherosclerosis is considered experimental. For these reasons, EDTA chelation therapy for the treatment or prevention of atherosclerosis is not covered.

Some practitioners refer to this therapy as chemoendarterectomy and may also show a diagnosis other than atherosclerosis, such as arteriosclerosis or calcinosis. Claims employing such variant terms should also be denied under this section.

Pub 100-3, Section 20.22

Ethylenediamine-Tetra-Acetic (EDTA) Chelation Therapy for Treatment of Atherosclerosis
The use of EDTA as a chelating agent to treat atherosclerosis, arteriosclerosis, calcinosis, or similar generalized condition not listed by the FDA as an approved use is not covered. Any such use of EDTA is considered experimental.

Pub 100-3, Section 20.23

Fabric Wrapping of Abdominal Aneurysms
Fabric wrapping of abdominal aneurysms is not a covered Medicare procedure. This is a treatment for abdominal aneurysms which involves wrapping aneurysms with cellophane or fascia lata. This procedure has not been shown to prevent eventual rupture. In extremely rare instances, external wall reinforcement may be indicated when the current accepted treatment (excision of the aneurysm and reconstruction with synthetic materials) is not a viable alternative, but external wall reinforcement is not fabric wrapping. Accordingly, fabric wrapping of abdominal aneurysms is not considered reasonable and necessary within the meaning of §1862(a)(1) of the Act.

Pub 100-3, Section 20.29

Hyperbaric Oxygen Therapy
A. Covered Conditions.—Program reimbursement for HBO therapy will be limited to that which is administered in a chamber (including the one man unit) and is limited to the following conditions:

1. Acute carbon monoxide intoxication, (ICD-9-CM diagnosis 986).

2. Decompression illness, (ICD-9-CM diagnosis 993.2, 993.3).

3. Gas embolism, (ICD-9-CM diagnosis 958.0, 999.1).

4. Gas gangrene, (ICD-9-CM diagnosis 0400).

5. Acute traumatic peripheral ischemia. HBO therapy is a valuable adjunctive treatment to be used in combination with accepted standard therapeutic measures when loss of function, limb, or life is threatened. (ICD-9-CM diagnosis 902.53, 903.01, 903.1, 904.0, 904.41.)

6. Crush injuries and suturing of severed limbs. As in the previous conditions, HBO therapy would be an adjunctive treatment when loss of function, limb, or life is threatened. (ICD-9-CM diagnosis 927.00-927.03, 927.09-927.11, 927.20-927.21, 927.8-927.9, 928.00-928.01, 928.10-928.11, 928.20-928.21, 928.3, 928.8-928.9, 929.0, 929.9, 996.90- 996.99.)

7. Progressive necrotizing infections (necrotizing fasciitis), (ICD-9-CM diagnosis 728.86).

8. Acute peripheral arterial insufficiency, (ICD-9-CM diagnosis 444.21, 444.22, 81).

9. Preparation and preservation of compromised skin grafts (not for primary management of wounds), (ICD-9CM diagnosis 996.52; excludes artificial skin graft).

10. Chronic refractory osteomyelitis, unresponsive to conventional medical and surgical management, (ICD-9-CM diagnosis 730.10-730.19).

11. Osteoradionecrosis as an adjunct to conventional treatment, (ICD-9-CM diagnosis 526.89).

12. Soft tissue radionecrosis as an adjunct to conventional treatment, (ICD-9-CM diagnosis 990).

13. Cyanide poisoning, (ICD-9-CM diagnosis 987.7, 989.0).

14. Actinomycosis, only as an adjunct to conventional therapy when the disease process is refractory to antibiotics and surgical treatment, (ICD-9-CM diagnosis 039.0-039.4, 039.8, 039.9).

15. Diabetic wounds of the lower extremities in patients who meet the following three criteria:

    a. Patient has type I or type II diabetes and has a lower extremity wound that is due to diabetes;

    b. Patient has a wound classified as Wagner grade III or higher; and

    c. Patient has failed an adequate course of standard wound therapy.

The use of HBO therapy is covered as adjunctive therapy only after there are no measurable signs of healing for at least 30 - days of treatment with standard wound therapy and must be used in addition to standard wound care. Standard wound care in patients with diabetic wounds includes: assessment of a patient's vascular status and correction of any vascular problems in the affected limb if possible, optimization of nutritional status, optimization of glucose control, debridement by any means to remove devitalized tissue, maintenance of a clean, moist bed of granulation tissue with appropriate moist dressings, appropriate off-loading, and necessary treatment to resolve any infection that might be present. Failure to respond to standard wound care occurs when there are no measurable signs of healing for at least 30 consecutive days. Wounds must be evaluated at least every 30 days during administration of HBO therapy. Continued treatment with HBO therapy is not covered if measurable signs of healing have not been demonstrated within any 30-day period of treatment.

B. Noncovered Conditions.—All other indications not specified under §35-10(A) are not covered under the Medicare program. No program payment may be made for any conditions other than those listed in §35-10 (A).

No program payment may be made for HBO in the treatment of the following conditions:

    1. Cutaneous, decubitus, and stasis ulcers.

    2. Chronic peripheral vascular insufficiency.

    3. Anaerobic septicemia and infection other than clostridial.

    4. Skin burns (thermal).

    5. Senility.

    6. Myocardial infarction.

    7. Cardiogenic shock.

    8. Sickle cell anemia.

    9. Acute thermal and chemical pulmonary damage, i.e., smoke inhalation with pulmonary insufficiency.

    10. Acute or chronic cerebral vascular insufficiency.

    11. Hepatic necrosis.

    12. Aerobic septicemia.

    13. Nonvascular causes of chronic brain syndrome (Pick's disease, Alzheimer's disease, Korsakoff's disease).

    14. Tetanus.

    15. Systemic aerobic infection.

    16. Organ transplantation.

    17. Organ storage.

    18. Pulmonary emphysema.

    19. Exceptional blood loss anemia.

    20. Multiple Sclerosis.

    21. Arthritic Diseases.

    22. Acute cerebral edema.

C. Topical Application of Oxygen.

This method of administering oxygen does not meet the definition of HBO therapy as stated above. Also, its clinical efficacy has not been established. Therefore, no Medicare reimbursement may be made for the topical application of oxygen.

Pub 100-3, Section 20.8

Cardiac Pacemakers

Cardiac pacemakers are covered as prosthetic devices under the Medicare program, subject to the following conditions and limitations. While cardiac pacemakers have been covered under Medicare for many years, there were no specific guidelines for their use other than the general Medicare requirement that covered services be reasonable and necessary for the treatment of the condition. Services rendered for cardiac pacing on or after the effective dates of this instruction are subject to these guidelines, which are based on certain assumptions regarding the clinical goals of cardiac pacing. While some uses of pacemakers are relatively certain or unambiguous, many other uses require considerable expertise and judgment.

Consequently, the medical necessity for permanent cardiac pacing must be viewed in the context of overall patient management. The appropriateness of such pacing may be conditional on other diagnostic or therapeutic modalities having been undertaken. Although significant complications and adverse side effects of pacemaker use are relatively rare, they cannot be ignored when considering the use of pacemakers for dubious medical conditions, or marginal clinical benefit.

These guidelines represent current concepts regarding medical circumstances in which permanent cardiac pacing may be appropriate or necessary. As with other areas of medicine, advances in knowledge and techniques in cardiology are expected. Consequently, judgments about the medical necessity and acceptability of new uses for cardiac pacing in new classes of patients may change as more more conclusive evidence becomes available. This instruction applies only to permanent cardiac pacemakers, and does not address the use of temporary, non-implanted pacemakers.

The two groups of conditions outlined below deal with the necessity for cardiac pacing for patients in general. These are intended as guidelines in assessing the medical necessity for pacing therapies, taking into account the particular circumstances in each case. However, as a general rule, the two groups of current medical concepts may be viewed as representing:

Group I: Single-Chamber Cardiac Pacemakers - a) conditions under which single chamber pacemaker claims may be considered covered without further claims development; and b) conditions under which single-chamber pacemaker claims would be denied unless further claims development shows that they fall into the covered category, or special medical circumstances exist of the sufficiency to convince the contractor that the claim should be paid.

Group II: Dual-Chamber Cardiac Pacemakers - a) conditions under which dual-chamber pacemaker claims may be considered covered without further claims development, and b) conditions under which dual-chamber pacemaker claims would be denied unless further claims development shows that they fall into the covered categories for single- and dual-chamber pacemakers, or special medical circumstances exist sufficient to convince the contractor that the claim should be paid.

CMS opened the NCD on Cardiac Pacemakers to afford the public an opportunity to comment on the proposal to revise the language contained in the instruction. The revisions transfer the focus of the NCD from the actual pacemaker implantation procedure itself to the reasonable and necessary medical indications that justify cardiac pacing. This is consistent with our findings that pacemaker implantation is no longer considered routinely harmful or an experimental procedure.

Group I: Single-Chamber Cardiac Pacemakers (Effective March 16, 1983)

A. Nationally Covered Indications

Conditions under which cardiac pacing is generally considered acceptable or necessary, provided that the conditions are chronic or recurrent and not due to transient causes such as acute myocardial infarction, drug toxicity, or electrolyte imbalance. (In cases where there is a rhythm disturbance, if the rhythm disturbance is chronic or recurrent, a single episode of a symptom such as syncope or seizure is adequate to establish medical necessity.)

    1. Acquired complete (also referred to as third-degree) AV heart block.

    2. Congenital complete heart block with severe bradycardia (in relation to age), or significant physiological deficits or significant symptoms due to the bradycardia.

    3. Second-degree AV heart block of Type II (i.e., no progressive prolongation of P-R interval prior to each blocked beat. P-R interval indicates the time taken for an impulse to travel from the atria to the ventricles on an electrocardiogram).

    4. Second-degree AV heart block of Type I (i.e., progressive prolongation of P-R interval prior to each blocked beat) with significant symptoms due to hemodynamic instability associated with the heart block.

    5. Sinus bradycardia associated with major symptoms (e.g., syncope, seizures, congestive heart failure); or substantial sinus bradycardia (heart rate less than 50)

associated with dizziness or confusion. The correlation between symptoms and bradycardia must be documented, or the symptoms must be clearly attributable to the bradycardia rather than to some other cause.

6. In selected and few patients, sinus bradycardia of lesser severity (heart rate 50-59) with dizziness or confusion. The correlation between symptoms and bradycardia must be documented, or the symptoms must be clearly attributable to the bradycardia rather than to some other cause.

7. Sinus bradycardia is the consequence of long-term necessary drug treatment for which there is no acceptable alternative when accompanied by significant symptoms (e.g., syncope, seizures, congestive heart failure, dizziness or confusion). The correlation between symptoms and bradycardia must be documented, or the symptoms must be clearly attributable to the bradycardia rather than to some other cause.

8. Sinus node dysfunction with or without tachyarrhythmias or AV conduction block (i.e., the bradycardia-tachycardia syndrome, sino-atrial block, sinus arrest) when accompanied by significant symptoms (e.g., syncope, seizures, congestive heart failure, dizziness or confusion).

9. Sinus node dysfunction with or without symptoms when there are potentially life-threatening ventricular arrhythmias or tachycardia secondary to the bradycardia (e.g., numerous premature ventricular contractions, couplets, runs of premature ventricular contractions, or ventricular tachycardia).

10. Bradycardia associated with supraventricular tachycardia (e.g., atrial fibrillation, atrial flutter, or paroxysmal atrial tachycardia) with high-degree AV block which is unresponsive to appropriate pharmacological management and when the bradycardia is associated with significant symptoms (e.g., syncope, seizures, congestive heart failure, dizziness or confusion).

11. The occasional patient with hypersensitive carotid sinus syndrome with syncope due to bradycardia and unresponsive to prophylactic medical measures.

12. Bifascicular or trifascicular block accompanied by syncope which is attributed to transient complete heart block after other plausible causes of syncope have been reasonably excluded.

13. Prophylactic pacemaker use following recovery from acute myocardial infarction during which there was temporary complete (third-degree) and/or Mobitz Type II second-degree AV block in association with bundle branch block.

14. In patients with recurrent and refractory ventricular tachycardia, "overdrive pacing" (pacing above the basal rate) to prevent ventricular tachycardia.

(Effective May 9, 1985)

15. Second-degree AV heart block of Type I with the QRS complexes prolonged.

B. Nationally Noncovered Indications

Conditions which, although used by some physicians as a basis for permanent cardiac pacing, are considered unsupported by adequate evidence of benefit and therefore should not generally be considered appropriate uses for single-chamber pacemakers in the absence of the above indications. Contractors should review claims for pacemakers with these indications to determine the need for further claims development prior to denying the claim, since additional claims development may be required. The object of such further development is to establish whether the particular claim actually meets the conditions in a) above. In claims where this is not the case or where such an event appears unlikely, the contractor may deny the claim

1. Syncope of undetermined cause.

2. Sinus bradycardia without significant symptoms.

3. Sino-atrial block or sinus arrest without significant symptoms.

4. Prolonged P-R intervals with atrial fibrillation (without third-degree AV block) or with other causes of transient ventricular pause.

5. Bradycardia during sleep.

6. Right bundle branch block with left axis deviation (and other forms of fascicular or bundle branch block) without syncope or other symptoms of intermittent AV block).

7. Asymptomatic second-degree AV block of Type I unless the QRS complexes are prolonged or electrophysiological studies have demonstrated that the block is at or beyond the level of the His bundle (a component of the electrical conduction system of the heart).

Effective October 1, 2001

8. Asymptomatic bradycardia in post-myocardial infarction patients about to initiate long-term beta-blocker drug therapy.

Group II: Dual-Chamber Cardiac Pacemakers - (Effective May 9, 1985)

A. Nationally Covered Indications

Conditions under dual-chamber cardiac pacing are considered acceptable or necessary in the general medical community unless conditions 1 and 2 under Group II. B., are present:

1. Patients in who single-chamber (ventricular pacing) at the time of pacemaker insertion elicits a definite drop in blood pressure, retrograde conduction, or discomfort.

2. Patients in whom the pacemaker syndrome (atrial ventricular asynchrony), with significant symptoms, has already been experienced with a pacemaker that is being replaced.

3. Patients in whom even a relatively small increase in cardiac efficiency will importantly improve the quality of life, e.g., patients with congestive heart failure despite adequate other medical measures.

4. Patients in whom the pacemaker syndrome can be anticipated, e.g., in young and active people, etc.

Dual-chamber pacemakers may also be covered for the conditions, as listed in Group I. A., if the medical necessity is sufficiently justified through adequate claims development. Expert physicians differ in their judgments about what constitutes appropriate criteria for dual-chamber pacemaker use. The judgment that such a pacemaker is warranted in the patient meeting accepted criteria must be based upon the individual needs and characteristics of that patient, weighing the magnitude and likelihood of anticipated benefits against the magnitude and likelihood of disadvantages to the patient.

B. Nationally Noncovered Indications

Whenever the following conditions (which represent overriding contraindications) are present, dual-chamber pacemakers are not covered:

1. Ineffective atrial contractions (e.g., chronic atrial fibrillation or flutter, or giant left atrium.

2. Frequent or persistent supraventricular tachycardias, except where the pacemaker is specifically for the control of the tachycardia.

3. A clinical condition in which pacing takes place only intermittently and briefly, and which is not associated with a reasonable likelihood that pacing needs will become prolonged, e.g., the occasional patient with hypersensitive carotid sinus syndrome with syncope due to bradycardia and unresponsive to prophylactic medical measures.

4. Prophylactic pacemaker use following recovery from acute myocardial infarction during which there was temporary complete (third-degree) and/or Type II second-degree AV block in association with bundle branch block.

C. Other

All other indications for dual-chamber cardiac pacing for which CMS has not specifically indicated coverage remain nationally noncovered, ecept for Category B IDE clinical trails, or as routine costs of dual-chamber cardiac pacing associated with clinical trials, in accordance with section 310.1 of the NCD Manual..

(This NCD last reviewed June 2004.)

Pub 100-3, Section 20.8.1

Cardiac Pacemaker Evaluation Services

Medicare covers a variety of services for the post-implant follow-up and evaluation of implanted cardiac pacemakers. The following guidelines are designed to assist contractors in identifying and processing claims for such services.

NOTE: These new guidelines are limited to lithium battery-powered pacemakers, because mercury-zinc battery-powered pacemakers are no longer being manufactured and virtually all have been replaced by lithium units. Contractors still receiving claims for monitoring such units should continue to apply the guidelines published in 1980 to those units until they are replaced.

One fact of which contractors should be aware is that many dual-chamber units may be programmed to pace only the ventricles; this may be done either at the time the pacemaker is implanted or at some time afterward. In such cases, a dual-chamber unit, when programmed or reprogrammed for ventricular pacing, should be treated as a single-chamber pacemaker in applying screening guidelines.

The decision as to how often any patient's pacemaker should be monitored is the responsibility of the patient's physician who is best able to take into account the condition and circumstances of the individual patient. These may vary over time, requiring modifications of the frequency with which the patient should be monitored. In cases where monitoring is done by some entity other than the patient's physician, such as a commercial monitoring service or hospital outpatient department, the physician's prescription for monitoring is required and should be periodically renewed (at least annually) to assure that the frequency of monitoring is proper for the patient. When a patient is monitered both during clinica visits and transtelephonically, the contractor should be sure to include frequency data on both ypes of monitoring in evaluating the reasonableness of the frequency of monitoring services received by the patient.

Since there are over 200 pacemaker models in service at any given point, and a variety of patient conditions that give rise to the need for pacemakers, the question of the appropriate frequency of monitorings is a complex one. Nevertheless, it is possible to develop guidelines within which the vast majority of pacemaker monitorings will fall and contractors should do this, using their own data and experience, as well as the frequency guidelines which follow, in order to limit extensive claims development to those cases requiring special attention.

Pub 100-3, Section 20.8.2

Self-Contained Pacemaker Monitors

Self-contained pacemaker monitors are accepted devices for monitoring cardiac pacemakers. Accordingly, program payment may be made for the rental or purchase of either of the following pacemaker monitors when it is prescribed by a physician for a patient with a cardiac pacemaker:

A. Digital Electronic Pacemaker Monitor.—This device provides the patient with an instantaneous digital readout of his pacemaker pulse rate. Use of this device does not involve professional services until there has been a change of five pulses (or more) per minute above or below the initial rate of the pacemaker; when such change occurs, the patient contacts his physician.

B. Audible/Visible Signal Pacemaker Monitor.—This device produces an audible and visible signal which indicates the pacemaker rate. Use of this device does not involve professional services until a change occurs in these signals; at such time, the patient contacts his physician.

NOTE: The design of the self-contained pacemaker monitor makes it possible for the patient to monitor his pacemaker periodically and minimizes the need for regular visits to the outpatient department of the provider. Therefore, documentation of the medical necessity for pacemaker evaluation in the outpatient department of the provider should be obtained where such evaluation is employed in addition to the self-contained pacemaker monitor used by the patient in his home.

Pub 100-3, Section 30.1

Biofeedback Therapy

Biofeedback therapy is covered under Medicare only when it is reasonable and necessary for the individual patient for muscle re-education of specific muscle groups or for treating pathological muscle abnormalities of spasticity, incapacitating muscle spasm, or weakness, and more conventional treatments (heat, cold, massage, exercise, support) have not been successful. This therapy is not covered for treatment of ordinary muscle tension states or for psychosomatic conditions. (See the Medicare Benefit Policy Manual, Chapter 15, for general coverage requirements about physical therapy requirements.)

Pub 100-3, Section 30.1.1

Biofeedback Therapy for the Treatment of Urinary Incontinence

This policy applies to biofeedback therapy rendered by a practitioner in an office or other facility setting.

Biofeedback is covered for the treatment of stress and/or urge incontinence in cognitively intact patients who have failed a documented trial of pelvic muscle exercise (PME) training. Biofeedback is not a treatment, per se, but a tool to help patients learn how to perform PME. Biofeedback-assisted PME incorporates the use of an electronic or mechanical device to relay visual and/or auditory evidence of pelvic floor muscle tone, in order to improve awareness of pelvic floor musculature and to assist patients in the performance of PME.

A failed trial of PME training is defined as no clinically significant improvement in urinary incontinence after completing 4 weeks of an ordered plan of pelvic muscle exercises to increase periurethral muscle strength.

Contractors may decide whether or not to cover biofeedback as an initial treatment modality.

Home use of biofeedback therapy is not covered.

Pub 100-3, Section 30.7

Laetrile and Related Substances

The FDA has determined that neither Laetrile nor any other drug called by the various terms mentioned above, nor any other product which might be characterized as a "nitriloside" is generally recognized (by experts qualified by scientific training and experience to evaluate the safety and effectiveness of drugs) to be safe and effective for any therapeutic use. Therefore, use of this drug cannot be considered to be reasonable and necessary within the meaning of §1862(a)(1) of the Act and program payment may not be made for its use or any services furnished in connection with its administration.

A hospital stay only for the purpose of having laetrile (or any other drug called by the terms mentioned above) administered is not covered. Also, program payment may not be made for laetrile (or other drug noted above) when it is used during the course of an otherwise covered hospital stay, since the FDA has found such drugs to not be safe and effective for any therapeutic purpose.

Pub 100-3, Section 30.8

Cellular Therapy

Accordingly, cellular therapy is not considered reasonable and necessary within the meaning of section 1862(a)(1) of the law.

Pub. 100-3, Section 40.2

Home Blood Glucose Monitors

(Rev. 1, 10-03-03)

CIM 60-11

There are several different types of blood glucose monitors that us e reflectance meters to determine blood glucose levels. Medicare coverage of these devices varies, with respect to both the type of device and the medical condition of the patient for whom the device is prescribed.

Reflectance colorimeter devices used for measuring blood glucose levels in clinical settings are not covered as durable medical equipment for use in the home because their need for frequent professional re-calibration makes them unsuitable for home use. However, some types of blood glucose monitors which use a reflectance meter specifically designed for home use by diabetic patients may be covered as durable medical equipment, subject to the conditions and limitations described below.

Blood glucose monitors are meter devices that read color changes produced on specially treated reagent strips by glucose concentrations in the patient's blood. The patient, using a disposable sterile lancet, draws a drop of blood, places it on a reagent strip and, following instructions which may vary with the device used, inserts it into the device to obtain a reading. Lancets, reagent strips, and other supplies necessary for the proper functioning of the device are also covered for patients for whom the device is indicated. Home blood glucose monitors enable certain patients to better control their blood glucose levels by frequently checking and appropriately contacting their attending physician for advice and treatment. Studies indicate that the patient's ability to carefully follow proper procedures is critical to obtaining satisfactory results with these devices. In addition, the cost of the devices, with their supplies, limits economical use to patients who must make frequent checks of their blood glucose levels. Accordingly, coverage of home blood glucose monitors is limited to patients meeting the following conditions:

1. The patient has been diagnosed as having diabetes;

2. The patient's physician states that the patient is capable of being trained to use the particular device prescribed in an appropriate manner. In some cases, the patient may not be able to perform this function, but a responsible individual can be trained to use the equipment and monitor the patient to assure that the intended effect is achieved. This is permissible if the record is properly documented by the patient's physician; and

3. The device is designed for home rather than clinical use.

There is also a blood glucose monitoring system designed especially for use by those with visual impairments. The monitors used in such systems are identical in terms of reliability and sensitivity to the standard blood glucose monitors described above. They differ by having such features as voice synthesizers, automatic timers, and specially designed arrangements of supplies and materials to enable the visually impaired to use the equipment without assistance.

These special blood glucose monitoring systems are covered under Medicare if the following conditions are met:

- The patient and device meet the three conditions listed above for coverage of standard home blood glucose monitors; and

- The patient's physician certifies that he or she has a visual impairment severe enough to require use of this special monitoring system.

The additional features and equipment of these special systems justify a higher reimbursement amount than allowed for standard blood glucose monitors. Separately identify claims for such devices and establish a separate reimbursement amount for them. For those carriers using HCPCS, the procedure code and definitions are E2100 (Blood glucose monitor with integrated voice synthesizer) and E2101 (Blood glucose monitor with integrated lancing/blood sample).

Pub 100-3, Section 50.1

Speech Generating Devices

Effective January 1, 2001, augmentative and alternative communication devices or communicators, which are hereafter referred to as "speech generating devices" are now considered to fall within the DME benefit category established by §1861(n) of the Social Security Act. They may be covered if the contractor's medical staff determines that the patient suffers from a severe speech impairment and that the medical condition warrants the use of a device based on the following definitions.

Pub 100-3, Section 50.2

Electronic Speech Aids

Electronic speech aids are covered under Part B as prosthetic devices when the patient has had a laryngectomy or his larynx is permanently inoperative. There are two types of speech aids. One operates by placing a vibrating head against the throat; the other amplifies sound waves through a tube which is inserted into the user's mouth. A patient who has had radical neck surgery and/or extensive radiation to the anterior part of the neck would generally be able to use only the "oral tube" model or one of the more sensitive and more expensive "throat contact" devices.

Cross-reference: The Medicare Benefit Policy Manual, Chapter 15, "Covered Medical and Other Health Services," §120.

Pub 100-3, Section 50.3

Cochlear Implantation

Medicare coverage is provided only for those patients who meet all of the following selection guidelines.

A. General

Diagnosis of bilateral severe-to-profound sensorineural hearing impairment with limited benefit from appropriate hearing (or vibrotactile) aids;

Cognitive ability to use auditory clues and a willingness to undergo an extended program of rehabilitation;

Freedom from middle ear infection, an accessible cochlear lumen that is structurally suited to implantation, and freedom from lesions in the auditory nerve and acoustic areas of the central nervous system;

No contraindications to surgery; and

The device must be used in accordance withe the FDA-approved labeling.

B-Adults

Cochlear implants may be covered for adults (over age 18) for prelinguistically, perilinguistically, and postlinguistically deafened adults. Postlinguistically deafened adults must demonstrate test scores of 30 percent or less on sentence recognition scores from tape recorded tests in the patient's best listening condition.

C-Children

Cochlear implants may be covered for prelinguistically and postlinguistically deafened children aged 2 through 17. Bilateral profound sensorineural deafness must be demonstrated by the inability to improve on age appropriate closed-set word identification tasks with amplification.

Pub. 100-3, Section 50.4

Tracheostomy Speaking Valve

(Rev. 1, 10-03-03)

CIM 65-16

A trachea tube has been determined to satisfy the definition of a prosthetic device, and the tracheostomy speaking valve is an add on to the trachea tube which may be considered a medically necessary accessory that enhances the function of the tube. In other words, it makes the system a better prosthesis. As such, a tracheostomy speaking valve is covered as an element of the trachea tube which makes the tube more effective.

Pub 100-3, Section 70.2.1

Services Provided for the Diagnosis and Treatment of Diabetic Sensory Neuropathy with Loss of Protective Sensation (AKA Diabetic Peripheral Neuropathy

Diabetic sensory neuropathy with LOPS is a localized illness of the feet and falls within the regulation's exception to the general exclusionary rule [see 42 CFR §411.15(l)(1)(i)]. Foot exams for people with diabetic sensory neuropathy with LOPS are reasonable and necessary to allow for early intervention in serious complications that typically afflict diabetics with the disease.

Effective for services furnished on or after July 1, 2002, Medicare covers, as a physician service, an evaluation (examination and treatment) of the feet no more often than every six months for individuals with a documented diagnosis of diabetic sensory neuropathy and LOPS, as long as the beneficiary has not seen a foot care specialist for some other reason in the interim. LOPS shall be diagnosed through sensory testing with the 5.07 monofilament using established guidelines, such as those developed by the National Institute of Diabetes and Digestive and Kidney Diseases guidelines. Five sites should be tested on the plantar surface of each foot, according to the National Institute of Diabetes and Digestive and Kidney Diseases guidelines. The areas must be tested randomly since the loss of protective sensation may be patchy in distribution, and the patient may get clues if the test is done rhythmically. Heavily callused areas should be avoided. As suggested by the American Podiatric Medicine Association, an absence of sensation at two or more sites out of 5 tested on either foot when tested with the 5.07

Semmes-Weinstein monofilament must be present and documented to diagnose peripheral neuropathy with loss of protective sensation.

A The examination includes:
1) a patient history, and

2) a physical examination that must consist of at least the following elements:

a. visual inspection of forefoot and hindfoot (including toe web spaces);

b. evaluation of protective sensation;

c. evaluation of foot structure and biomechanics;

d. evaluation of vascular status and skin integrity;

e. evaluation of the need for special footwear; and

3) patient education.

B. Treatment includes, but is not limited to:

1) local care of superficial wounds;

2) debridement of corns and calluses; and

3) trimming and debridement of nails.

The diagnosis of diabetic sensory neuropathy with LOPS should be established and documented prior to coverage of foot care. Other causes of peripheral neuropathy should be considered and investigated by the primary care physician prior to initiating or referring for foot care for persons with LOPS.

Pub 100-3, Section 80.1

Hydrophilic Contact Lens For Corneal Bandage

Payment may be made under §1861(s)(2) of the Act for a hydrophilic contact les approved by the Food and Drug Administration (FDA) and used as a supply incident to a pphysician's service. Payment for the lens is included in the payment for the physician's service to which the lens is incident. Contractors are authorized to accept an FDA letter of approval or other FDA published material as evidence of FDA approval. (See §80.4 of the NCD Manual for coverage of a hydrophilic contact lens as prosthetic device.)

Pub 100-3, Section 80.2

Ocular Photodynamic Therapy

OPT is only covered when used in conjunction with verteporfin.

Effective July 1, 2001, OPT with verteporfin was approved for a diagnosis of neovascular AMD with predominantly classic subfoveal choroidal neovascularization (CNV) lesions (where the area of classic CNV occupies ,â• 50% of the area of the entire lesion) at the initial visit as determined by a fluorescein angiogram.

On October 17, 2001, CMS announced its "intent to cover" OPT with verteporfin for AMD patients with occult and no classic subfoveal CNV as determined by a fluorescein angiogram. The October 17, 2001, decision was never implemented.

On March 28, 2002, after thorough review and reconsideration of the October 17, 2001, intent to cover policy, CMS determined that the current noncoverage policy for OPT for verteporfin for AMD patients with occult and no classic subfoveal CNV as determined by a fluorescein angiogram should remain in effect.

Effective August 20, 2002, CMS issued a noncovered instruction for OPT with verteporfin for AMD patients with occult and no classic subfoveal CNV as determined by a fluorescein angiogram.

Covered Indications

Effective April 1, 2004, OPT with verteporfin continues to be approved for a diagnosis of neovascular AMD with predominantly classic subfoveal CNV lesions (where the area of classic CNV occupies ,â• 50% of the area of the entire lesion) at the initial visit as determined by a fluorescein angiogram. (CNV lesions are comprised of classic and/or occult components.) Subsequent follow-up visits require a fluorescein angiogram prior to treatment. There are no requirements regarding visual acuity, lesion size, and number of re-treatments when treating predominantly classic lesions.

In addition, after thorough review and reconsideration of the August 20, 2002, noncoverage policy, CMS determines that the evidence is adequate to conclude that OPT with verteporfin is reasonable and necessary for treating:

1. Subfoveal occult with no classic CNV associated with AMD; and,

2. Subfoveal minimally classic CNV (where the area of classic CNV occupies less than 50% of the area of the entire lesion) associated with AMD.

The above 2 indications are considered reasonable and necessary only when:

1. The lesions are small (4 disk areas or less in size) at the time of initial treatment or within the 3 months prior to initial treatment; and,

2. The lesions have shown evidence of progression within the 3 months prior to initial treatment. Evidence of progression must be documented by deterioration of visual acuity (at least 5 letters on a standard eye examination chart), lesion growth (an

increase in at least 1 disk area), or the appearance of blood associated with the lesion.

Noncovered Indications

Other uses of OPT with verteporfin to treat AMD not already addressed by CMS will continue to be noncovered. These include, but are not limited to, the following AMD indications:

Juxtafoveal or extrafoveal CNV lesions (lesions outside the fovea),:

Inability to obtain a fluorescein angiogram,:

Atrophic or "dry" AMD.

Other

OPT with verteporfin for other ocular indications, such as pathologic myopia or presumed ocular histoplasmosis syndrome, continue to be eligible for local coverage determinations through individual contractor discretion.

(This NCD last reviewed March 2004.)

Pub 100-3, Section 80.3

Photosensitive Drugs
Verteporfin

Verteporfin, a benzoporphyrin derivative, is an intravenous lipophilic photosensitive drug with an absorption peak of 690 nm. This drug was first approved by the Food and Drug Administration (FDA) on April 12, 2000, and subsequently, approved for inclusion in the United States Pharmacopoeia on July 18, 2000, meeting Medicare's definition of a drug as defined under §1861(t)(1) of the Social Security Act. Effective July 1, 2001, Verteporfin is only covered when used in conjunction with ocular photodynamic therapy (see §35-100 PHOTODYNAMIC THERAPY) when furnished intravenously incident to a physician's service. For patients with age-related macular degeneration, Verteporfin is only covered with a diagnosis of neovascular age-related macular degeneration (ICD-9-CM 362.52) with predominately classic subfoveal choroidal neovascular (CNV) lesions (where the area of classic CNV occupies = 50% of the area of the entire lesion) at the initial visit as determined by a fluorescein angiogram (CPT code 92235). Subsequent follow-up visits will require a fluorescein angiogram prior to treatment. OPT with verteporfin is covered for the above indication and will remain noncovered for all other indications related to AMD (see CIM § CIM § 35-100). OPT with Verteporfin for use in non-AMD conditions is eligible for coverage through individual contractor discretion.

Pub 100-3, Section 80.3

Verteporfin
Covered Indications

Effective April 1, 2004, OPT with verteporfin is covered for patients with a diagnosis of neovascular age-related macular degeneration (AMD) with:

Predominately classic subfoveal choroidal neovascularization (CNV) lesions (where the area of classic CNV occupies ,â• 50% of the area of the entire lesion) at the initial visit as determined by a fluorescein angiogram. (CNV lesions are comprised of classic and/or occult components.) Subsequent follow-up visits require a fluorescein angiogram prior to treatment. There are no requirements regarding visual acuity, lesion size, and number of retreatments when treating predominantly classic lesions.

Subfoveal occult with no classic associated with AMD.

Subfoveal minimally classic CNV CNV (where the area of classic CNV occupies less than 50% of the area of the entire lesion) associated with AMD.

The above 2 indications are considered reasonable and necessary only when:

1. The lesions are small (4 disk areas or less in size) at the time of initial treatment or within the 3 months prior to initial treatment; and,

2. The lesions have shown evidence of progression within the 3 months prior to initial treatment. Evidence of progression must be documented by deterioration of visual acuity (at least 5 letters on a standard eye examination chart), lesion growth (an increase in at least 1 disk area), or the appearance of blood associated with the lesion.

Noncovered Indications

Other uses of OPT with verteporfin to treat AMD not already addressed by CMS will continue to be noncovered. These include, but are not limited to, the following AMD indications: juxtafoveal or extrafoveal CNV lesions (lesions outside the fovea), inability to obtain a fluorescein angiogram, or atrophic or "dry" AMD.

Other

OPT with verteporfin for other ocular indications, such as pathologic myopia or presumed ocular histoplasmosis syndrome, continue to be eligible for local coverage determinations through individual contractor discretion.

(This NCD last reviewed March 2004.)

Pub 100-3, Section 80.4

Hydrophilic Contact Lenses

Hydrophilic contact lenses are eyeglasses within the meaning of the exclusion in §1862(a)(7) of the Act and are not covered when used in the treatment of nondiseased eyes with spherical ametrophia, refractive astigmatism, and/or corneal astigmatism. Payment may be made under the prosthetic device benefit, however, for hydrophilic contact lenses when prescribed for an aphakic patient.

Contractors are authorized to accept an FDA letter of approval or other FDA published material as evidence of FDA approval. (See §80.1 of the NCD Manual for coverage of a hydrophilic lens as a corneal bandage.)

Pub 100-3, Section 80.5

Scleral Shell

A scleral shell fits over the entire exposed surface of the eye as opposed to a corneal contact lens which covers only the central non-white area encompassing the pupil and iris. Where an eye has been rendered sightless and shrunken by inflammatory disease, a scleral shell may, among other things, obviate the need for surgical enucleation and prosthetic implant and act to support the surrounding orbital tissue.

In such a case, the device serves essentially as an artificial eye. In this situation, payment may be made for a scleral shell under §1861(s)(8) of the law.

Scleral shells are occasionally used in combination with artificial tears in the treatment of "dry eye" of diverse etiology. Tears ordinarily dry at a rapid rate, and are continually replaced by the lacrimal gland. When the lacrimal gland fails, the half-life of artificial tears may be greatly prolonged by the use of the scleral contact lens as a protective barrier against the drying action of the atmosphere. Thus, the difficult and sometimes hazardous process of frequent installation of artificial tears may be avoided. The lens acts in this instance to substitute, in part, for the functioning of the diseased lacrimal gland and would be covered as a prosthetic device in the rare case when it is used in the treatment of "dry eye."

Pub. 100-3, Section 100.6

Gastric Freezing
(Rev. 1, 10-03-03)

CIM 35-65

Gastric freezing for chronic peptic ulcer disease is a non-surgical treatment which was popular about 20 years ago but now is seldom done. It has been abandoned due to a high complication rate, only temporary improvement experienced by patients, and lack of effectiveness when tested by double-blind, controlled clinical trials. Since the procedure is now considered obsolete, it is not covered.

Pub 100-3, Section 110.2

Certain Drugs Distributed by the National Cancer Institute

A physician is eligible to receive Group C drugs from the Divison of Cancer Treatment only if the following requirements are met:

A physician must be registered with the NCI as an investigator by having completed an FD-Form 1573;

A written request for the drug, indicating the disease to be treated, must be submitted to the NCI;

The use of the drug must be limited to indications outlined in the NCI's guidelines; and

All adverse reactions must be reported to the Investigational Drug Branch of the Division of Cancer Treatment.

In view of these NCI controls on distribution and use of Group C drugs, intermediaries may assume, in the absence of evidence to the contrary, that a Group C drug and the related hospital stay are covered if all other applicable coverage requirements are satisfied.

If there is reason to question coverage in a particular case, the matter should be resolved with the assistance of the Quality improvemetn organization (QIO), or if there is none, the assistance of your medical consultants.

Information regarding those drugs which are classified as Group C drugs may be obtained from:

Office of the Chief, Investigational Drug BranchDivision of Cancer Treatment, CTEP, Landow BuildingRoom 4C09, National Cancer InstituteBethesda, Maryland 20205

Pub 100-3, Section 110.3

Anti-Inhibitor Coagulant Complex (AICC)

Anti-inhibitor coagulant complex, AICC, is a drug used to treat hemophilia in patients with factor VIII inhibitor antibodies. AICC has been shown to be safe and effective and has Medicare coverage when furnished to patients with hemophilia A and inhibitor antibodies to factor VIII who have major bleeding episodes and who fail to respond to other, less expensive therapies.

Pub 100-3, Section 110.8

Blood Platelet Transfusions

Blood platelet transplants are safe and effective for the correction of thrombocytopenia and other blood defects. It is covered under Medicare when treatment is reasonable and necessary for the individual patient.

Pub 100-3, Section 130.5

Treatment of Alcoholism and Drug Abuse in a Freestanding Clinic

Coverage is available for alcoholism or drug abuse treatment services (such as drug therapy, psychotherapy, and patient education) that are provided incident to a physician's professional service in a freestanding clinic to patients who, for example, have been discharged from an inpatient hospital stay for the treatment of alcoholism or drug abuse or to individuals who are not in the acute stages of alcoholism or drug abuse but require treatment. The coverage available for these services is subject to the same rules generally applicable to the coverage of clinic services. (See HCFA-Pub. 14-3, §§2020ff., and §§2050 ff.) Of course, the services also must be reasonable and necessary for the diagnosis or treatment of the individual's alcoholism or drug abuse. The Part B psychiatric limitation (see HCFA-Pub. 14-3, §2470) would apply to alcoholism or drug abuse treatment services furnished by physicians to individuals who are not hospital inpatients.

Pub 100-3, Section 130.6

Treatment of Drug Abuse (Chemical Dependency)

Accordingly, when it is medically necessary for a patient to receive detoxification and/or rehabilitation for drug substance abuse as a hospital inpatient, coverage for care in that setting is available. Coverage is also available for treatment services that are provided in the outpatient department of a hospital to patients who, for example, have been discharged from an inpatient stay for the treatment of drug substance abuse or who require treatment but do not require the availability and intensity of services found only in the inpatient hospital setting. The coverage available for these services is subject to the same rules generally applicable to the coverage of outpatient hospital services. The services must also be reasonable and necessary for treatment of the individual's condition. Decisions regarding reasonableness and necessity of treatment, the need for an inpatient hospital level of care, and length of treatment should be made by intermediaries based on accepted medical practice with the advice of their medical consultant. (In hospitals under PSRO review, PSRO determinations of medical necessity of services and appropriateness of the level of care at which services are provided are binding on the title XVIII fiscal intermediaries for purposes of adjudicating claims for payment.)

Pub 100-3, Section 140.2

Breast Reconstruction Following Mastectomy

Reconstruction of the affected and the contralateral unaffected breast following a medically necessary mastectomy is considered a relatively safe and effective noncosmetic procedure. Accordingly, program payment may be made for breast reconstruction surgery following removal of a breast for any medical reason.

Program payment may not be made for breast reconstruction for cosmetic reasons. (Cosmetic surgery is excluded from coverage under §I862(a)(I0) of the Social Security Act.)

Pub 100-3, Section 150.2

Osteogenic Stimulation

1. Noninvasive Stimulator.—The noninvasive stimulator device is covered only for the following indications:

   Nonunion of long bone fractures;

   Failed fusion, where a minimum of nine months has elapsed since the last surgery;

   Congenital pseudarthroses; and:

   As an adjunct to spinal fusion surgery for patients at high risk of pseudarthrosis due to previously failed spinal fusion at the same site or for those undergoing multiple level fusion. A multiple level fusion involves 3 or more vertebrae (e.g., L3-L5, L4-S1, etc).

2. Invasive (Implantable) Stimulator.—The invasive stimulator device is covered only for the following indications:

   Nonunion of long bone fractures; and:

   As an adjunct to spinal fusion surgery for patients at high risk of pseudarthrosis due to previously failed spinal fusion at the same site or for those undergoing multiple level fusion.

A multiple level fusion involves 3 or more vertebrae (e.g., L3-L5, L4-S1, etc.).

Effective for services performed on or after September 15, 1980, nonunion of long bone fractures, for both noninvasive and invasive devices, is considered to exist only after 6 or more months have elapsed without healing of the fracture.

Effective for services performed on or after April 1, 2000, nonunion of long bone fractures, for both noninvasive and invasive devices, is considered to exist only when serial radiographs have confirmed that fracture healing has ceased for three or more months prior to starting treatment with the electrical osteogenic stimulator. Serial radiographs must include a minimum of two sets of radiographs, each including multiple views of the fracture site, separated by a minimum of 90 days.

B. Ultrasonic Osteogenic Stimulators.—An ultrasonic osteogenic stimulator is a non-invasive device that emits low intensity, pulsed ultrasound. The ultrasound signal is applied to the skin surface at the fracture location via ultrasound, conductive gel in order to stimulate fracture healing.

Effective for services performed on or after January 1, 2001, ultrasonic osteogenic stimulators are covered as medically reasonable and necessary for the treatment of non-union fractures. In demonstrating nonunion of fractures, we would expect:

1. A minimum of two sets of radiographs obtained prior to starting treatment with the osteogenic stimulator, separated by a minimum of 90 days. Each radiograph must include multiple views of the fracture site accompanied with a written interpretation by a physician stating that there has been no clinically significant evidence of fracture healing between the two sets of radiographs.

2. Indications that the patient failed at least one surgical intervention for the treatment of the fracture.

Non-unions of the skull, vertebrae, and those that are tumor-related are excluded from coverage. The ultrasonic osteogenic stimulator may not be used concurrently with other non-invasive osteogenic devices. The national non-coverage policy related to ultrasonic osteogenic stimulators for fresh fractures and delayed unions remains in place. This policy relates only to non-union as defined above.

Pub 100-3, Section 150.3

Bone (Mineral) Density Studies

The Following Bone (Mineral) Density Studies Are Covered Under Medicare:

A. Single Photon Absorptiometry

A non-invasive radiological technique that measures absorption of a monochromatic photon beam by bone material. The device is placed directly on the patient, uses a low dose of radionuclide, and measures the mass absorption efficiency of the energy used. It provides a quantitative measurement of the bone mineral of cortical and trabecular bone, and is used in assessing an individual's treatment response at appropriate intervals.

Single photon absorptiometry is covered under Medicare when used in assessing changes in bone density of patients with osteodystrophy or osteoporosis when performed on the same individual at intervals of 6 to 12 months.

B. Bone Biopsy

A physiologic test which is a surgical, invasive procedure. A small sample of bone (usually from the ilium) is removed, generally by a biopsy needle. The biopsy sample is then examined histologically, and provides a qualitative measurement of the bone mineral of trabecular bone. This procedure is used in ascertaining a differential diagnosis of bone disorders and is used primarily to differentiate osteomalacia from osteoporosis.

Bone biopsy is covered under Medicare when used for the qualitative evaluation of bone no more than four times per patient, unless there is special justification given. When used more than four times on a patient, bone biopsy leaves a defect in the pelvis and may produce some patient discomfort.

C. Photodensitometry(radiographic absorptiometry)

A noninvasive radiological procedure that attempts to assess bone mass by measuring the optical density of extremity radiographs with a photodensitometer, usually with a reference to a standard density wedge placed on the film at the time of exposure. This procedure provides a quantitative measurement of the bone mineral of bone, and is used for monitoring gross bone change.

The Following Bone (Mineral) Density Study Is Not Covered Under Medicare:

D. Dual Photon Absorptiometry

A noninvasive radiological technique that measures absorption of a dichromatic beam by bone material. This procedure is not covered under Medicare because it is still considered to be in the investigational stage.

Pub 100-3, Section 150.6

Vitamin B12 Injections to Strengthen Tendons, Ligaments, etc., of the Foot

Vitamin B12 injections to strengthen tendons, ligaments, etc., of the foot are not covered under Medicare because (1) there is no evidence that vitamin B12 injections are effective for the purpose of strengthening weakened tendons and ligaments, and (2) this is nonsurgical treatment under the subluxation exclusion. Accordingly, vitamin B12 injections are not considered reasonable and necessary within the meaning of §1862(a)(1) of the Act.

Pub 100-3, Section 150.7

Prolotherapy, Joint Sclerotherapy, and Ligamentous Injections with Sclerosing Agents

The medical effectiveness of the above therapies has not been verified by scientifically controlled studies. Accordingly, reimbursement for these modalities should be denied on the ground that they are not reasonable and necessary as required by §1862(a)(1) of the Act.

Pub 100-3, Section 160.12

Neuromuscular Electrical Stimulaton (NMES)

Treatment of Muscle Atrophy

Coverage of NMES to treat muscle atrophy is limited to the treatment of patients with disuse atrophy where the nerve supply to the muscle is intact, including brain, spinal cord and peripheral nerves and other non-neurological reasons for disuse atrophy. Examples include casting or splinting of a limb, contracture due to scarring of soft tissue as in burn lesions, and hip replacement surgery (until orthotic training begins). (See CIM 45-25 for an explanation of coverage of medically necessary supplies for the effective use of NMES).

Use for Walking in Patients with Spinal Cord Injury (SCI)

The type of NMES that is used to enhance the ability to walk of SCI patients is commonly referred to as functional electrical stimulation (FES). These devices are surface units that use electrical impulses to activate paralyzed or weak muscles in precise sequence. Coverage for the use of NMES/FES is limited to SCI patients, for walking, who have completed a training program, which consists of at least 32 physical therapy sessions with the device over a period of 3 months. The trial period of physical therapy will enable the physician treating the patient for his or her spinal cord injury to properly evaluate the person's ability to use these devices frequently and for the long term. Physical therapy sessions are only covered in the inpatient hospital, outpatient hospital, comprehensive outpatient rehabilitation facilities, and outpatient rehabilitation facilities. The physical therapy necessary to perform this training must be directly performed by the physical therapist as part of a one-on-one training program; this service cannot be done unattended.

The goal of physical therapy must be to train SCI patients on the use of NMES/FES devices to achieve walking, not to reverse or retard muscle atrophy.

Coverage for NMES/FES for walking will be limited to SCI patients with all of the following characteristics:

1) persons with intact lower motor units (L1 and below) (both muscle and peripheral nerve);

2) persons with muscle and joint stability for weight bearing at upper and lower extremities that can demonstrate balance and control to maintain an upright support posture independently;

3) persons that demonstrate brisk muscle contraction to NMES and have sensory perception of electrical stimulation sufficient for muscle contraction;

4) persons that possess high motivation, commitment and cognitive ability to use such devices for walking;

5) persons that can transfer independently and can demonstrate independent standing tolerance for at least 3 minutes;

6) persons that can demonstrate hand and finger function to manipulate controls;

7) persons with at least 6-month post recovery spinal cord injury and restorative surgery;

8) persons without hip and knee degenerative disease and no history of long bone fracture secondary to osteoporosis; and

9) persons who have demonstrated a willingness to use the device long-term.

NMES/FES for walking will not be covered in SCI patients with any of the following:

1) persons with cardiac pacemakers;

2) severe scoliosis or severe osteoporosis;

3) skin disease or cancer at area of stimulation;

4) irreversible contracture; or

5) autonomic dysreflexia.

The only settings where therapists with the sufficient skills to provide these services are employed, are inpatient hospitals, outpatient hospitals, comprehensive outpatient rehabilitation facilities and outpatient rehabilitation facilities. The physical therapy necessary to perform this training must be part of a one-on-one training program.

Additional therapy after the purchase of the DME would be limited by our general policies on coverage of skilled physical therapy.

All other uses of NMES remain non-covered.

Pub 100-3, Section 160.13

Supplies Used in the Delivery of Transcutaneous Electrical Nerve Stimulation (TENS) and Neuromuscular Electrical Stimulation (NMES)

A form-fitting conductive garment (and medically necessary related supplies) may be covered under the program only when:

1. It has received permission or approval for marketing by the Food and Drug Administration;

2. It has been prescribed by a physician for use in delivering covered TENS or NMES treatment; and

3. One of the medical indications outlined below is met:

    The patient cannot manage without the conductive garment because there is such a large area or so many sites to be stimulated and the stimulation would have to be delivered so frequently that it is not feasible to use conventional electrodes, adhesive tapes and lead wires;

    The patient cannot manage without the conductive garment for the treatment of chronic intractable pain because the areas or sites to be stimulated are inaccessible with the use of conventional electrodes, adhesive tapes and lead wires;

    The patient has a documented medical condition such as skin problems that preclude the application of conventional electrodes, adhesive tapes and lead wires;

    The patient requires electrical stimulation beneath a cast either to treat disuse atrophy, where the nerve supply to the muscle is intact, or to treat chronic intractable pain; or

    The patient has a medical need for rehabilitation strengthening (pursuant to a written plan of rehabilitation) following an injury where the nerve supply to the muscle is intact.

A conductive garment is not covered for use with a TENS device during the trial period specified in §35-46 unless:

4. The patient has a documented skin problem prior to the start of the trial period; and

5. The carrier's medical consultants are satisfied that use of such an item is medically necessary for the patient.

Pub 100-3, Section 160.2

Treatment of Motor Function Disorders with Electric Nerve Stimulation

Where electric nerve stimulation is employed to treat motor function disorders, no reimbursement may be made for the stimulator or for the services related to its implantation since this treatment cannot be considered reasonable and necessary.

NOTE: For Medicare coverage of deep brain stimulation for essential tremor and Parkinson's disease, see §65-19.

Pub. 100-3, Section 160.23

Sensory Nerve Conduction Threshold Tests (sNCTs) (Effective April 1, 2004)
(Rev.15, 06-18-04)

A. General

The sNCT is a psychophysical assessment of both central and peripheral nerve functions. It measures the detection threshold of accurately calibrated sensory stimuli. This procedure is intended to evaluate and quantify function in both large and small caliber fibers for the purpose of detecting neurologic disease. Sensory perception and threshold detection are dependent on the integrity of both the peripheral sensory apparatus and peripheral-central sensory pathways. In theory, an abnormality detected by this procedure may signal dysfunction anywhere in the sensory pathway from the receptors, the sensory tracts, the primary sensory cortex, to the association cortex.

This procedure is different and distinct from assessment of nerve conduction velocity, amplitude and latency. It is also different from short-latency somatosensory evoked potentials.

Effective October 1, 2002, CMS initially concluded that there was insufficient scientific or clinical evidence to consider the sNCT test and the device used in performing this test reasonable and necessary within the meaning of section 1862(a)(1)(A) of the law. \

Therefore, sNCT was noncovered.

Effective April 1, 2004, based on a reconsideration of current Medicare policy for sNCT, CMS concludes that the use of any type of sNCT device (e.g., "current output" type device used to perform current perception threshold (CPT), pain perception threshold (PPT), or pain tolerance threshold (PTT) testing or "voltage input" type device used for voltage-nerve conduction threshold (v-NCT) testing to diagnose sensory neuropathies or radiculopathies in Medicare beneficiaries is not reasonable and necessary.

B. Nationally Covered Indications

Not applicable.

C. Nationally Noncovered Indications

All uses of sNCT to diagnose sensory neuropathies or radiculopathies are noncovered.

(This NCD last reviewed June 2004.)

Pub. 100-3, Section 160.6

Carotid Sinus Nerve Stimulator

(Rev. 1, 10-03-03)

CIM 65-4

Implantation of the carotid sinus nerve stimulator is indicated for relief of angina pectoris in carefully selected patients who are refractory to medical therapy and who after undergoing coronary angiography study either are poor candidates for or refuse to have coronary bypass surgery. In such cases, Medicare reimbursement may be made for this device and for the related services required for its implantation.

However, the use of the carotid sinus nerve stimulator in the treatment of paroxysmal supraventricular tachycardia is considered investigational and is not in common use by the medical community. The device and related services in such cases cannot be considered as reasonable and necessary for the treatment of an illness or injury or to improve the functioning of a malformed body member as required by §1862(a)(1) of the Act.

Cross-reference:

The Medicare Benefit Policy Manual, Chapter 15, "Covered Medical and Other Services," §120

The Medicare Benefit Policy Manual, Chapter 1, "Inpatient Hospital Services," §40 and §120.

Pub 100-3, Section 160.7

Electrical Nerve Stimulators

Two general classifications of electrical nerve stimulators are employed to treat chronic intractable pain: peripheral nerve stimulators and central nervous system stimulators.

A-Implanted Peripheral Nerve Stimulators

Payment may be made under the prosthetic device benefit for implanted peripheral nerve stimulators. Use of this stimulator involves implantation of electrodes around a selected peripheral nerve. The stimulating electrode is connected by an insulated lead to a receiver unit which is implanted under the skin at a depth not greater than 1/2 inch. Stimulation is induced by a generator connected to an antenna unit which is attached to the skin surface over the receiver unit. Implantation of electrodes requires surgery and usually necessitates an operating room.

NOTE: Peripheral nerve stimulators may also be employed to assess a patient's suitability for continued treatment with an electric nerve stimulator. As explained in §160.7.1, such use of the stimulator is covered as part of the total diagnostic service furnished to the beneficiary rather than as a prosthesis.

B-Central Nervous System Stimulators (Dorsal Column and Depth Brain Stimulators). The implantation of central nervous system stimulators may be covered as therapies for the relief of chronic intractable pain, subject to the following conditions:

1- Types of Implantations

There are two types of implantations covered by this instruction:

Dorsal Column (Spinal Cord) Neurostimulation.—The surgical implantation of neurostimulator electrodes within the dura mater (endodural) or the percutaneous insertion of electrodes in the epidural space is covered.

Depth Brain Neurostimulation.—The stereotactic implantation of electrodes in the deep brain (e.g., thalamus and periaqueductal gray matter) is covered.

2- Conditions for Coverage

No payment may be made for the implantation of dorsal column or depth brain stimulators or services and supplies related to such implantation, unless all of the conditions listed below have been met:

The implantation of the stimulator is used only as a late resort (if not a last resort) for patients with chronic intractable pain;

With respect to item a, other treatment modalities (pharmacological, surgical, physical, or psychological therapies) have been tried and did not prove satisfactory, or are judged to be unsuitable or contraindicated for the given patient;

Patients have undergone careful screening, evaluation and diagnosis by a multidisciplinary team prior to implantation. (Such screening must include psychological, as well as physical evaluation);

All the facilities, equipment, and professional and support personnel required for the proper diagnosis, treatment training, and followup of the patient (including that required to satisfy item c) must be available; and

Demonstration of pain relief with a temporarily implanted electrode precedes permanent implantation. Contractors may find it helpful to work with QIOs to obtain the information needed to apply these conditions to claims.

Pub 100-3, Section 160.7.1

Assessing Patient's Suitability for Electrical Nerve Stimulation Therapy

Electrical nerve stimulation is an accepted modality for assessing a patient's suitability for ongoing treatment with a transcutaneous or an implanted nerve stimulator. Accordingly, program payment may be made for the following techniques when used to determine the potential therapeutic usefulness of an electrical nerve stimulator:

A. Transcutaneous Electrical Nerve Stimulation (TENS).

This technique involves attachment of a transcutaneous nerve stimulator to the surface of the skin over the peripheral nerve to be stimulated. It is used by the patient on a trial basis and its effectiveness in modulating pain is monitored by the physician, or physical therapist. Generally, the physician or physical therapist is able to determine whether the patient is likely to derive a significant therapeutic benefit from continuous use of a transcutaneous stimulator within a trial period of 1 month; in a few cases this determination may take longer to make. Document the medical necessity for such services which are furnished beyond the first month. (See §45-25 for an explanation of coverage of medically necessary supplies for the effective use of TENS.)

If TENS significantly alleviates pain, it may be considered as primary treatment; if it produces no relief or greater discomfort than the original pain electrical nerve stimulation therapy is ruled out. However, where TENS produces incomplete relief, further evaluation with percutaneous electrical nerve stimulation may be considered to determine whether an implanted peripheral nerve stimulator would provide significant relief from pain. (See §35-46B.)

Usually, the physician or physical therapist providing the services will furnish the equipment necessary for assessment. Where the physician or physical therapist advises the patient to rent the TENS from a supplier during the trial period rather than supplying it himself/herself, program payment may be made for rental of the TENS as well as for the services of the physician or physical therapist who is evaluating its use. However, the combined program payment which is made for the physician's or physical therapist's services and the rental of the stimulator from a supplier should not exceed the amount which would be payable for the total service, including the stimulator, furnished by the physician or physical therapist alone.

B. Percutaneous Electrical Nerve Stimulation (PEN)

This diagnostic procedure which involves stimulation of peripheral nerves by a needle electrode inserted through the skin is performed only in a physician's office, clinic, or hospital outpatient department. Therefore, it is covered only when performed by a physician or incident to physician's service. If pain is effectively controlled by percutaneous stimulation, implantation of electrodes is warranted.

As in the case of TENS (described in subsection A), generally the physician should be able to determine whether the patient is likely to derive a significant therapeutic benefit from continuing use of an implanted nerve stimulator within a trial period of 1 month. In a few cases, this determination may take longer to make. The medical necessity for such diagnostic services which are furnished beyond the first month must be documented.

NOTE: Electrical nerve stimulators do not prevent pain but only alleviate pain as it occurs. A patient can be taught how to employ the stimulator, and once this is done, can use it safely and effectively without direct physician supervision. Consequently, it is inappropriate for a patient to visit his/her physician, physical therapist, or an outpatient clinic on a continuing basis for treatment of pain with electrical nerve stimulation. Once it is determined that electrical nerve stimulation should be continued as therapy and the patient has been trained to use the stimulator, it is expected that a stimulator will be implanted or the patient will employ the TENS on a continual basis in his/her home. Electrical nerve stimulation treatments furnished by a physician in his/her office, by a physical therapist or outpatient clinic are excluded from coverage by §1862(a)(1) of the Act. (See §65-8 for an explanation of coverage of the therapeutic use of implanted peripheral nerve stimulators under the prosthetic devices benefit. See §60-20 for an explanation of coverage of the therapeutic use of TENS under the durable medical equipment benefit.)

PUB 100 REFERENCES

Pub. 100-3, Section 180.2

Enteral and Parenteral Nutritional Therapy

(Rev. 1, 10-03-03)

CIM 65-10

Covered As Prosthetic Device

There are patients who, because of chronic illness or trauma, cannot be sustained through oral feeding. These people must rely on either enteral or parenteral nutritional therapy, depending upon the particular nature of their medical condition.

Coverage of nutritional therapy as a Part B benefit is provided under the prosthetic device benefit provision which requires that the patient must have a permanently inoperative internal body organ or function thereof. Therefore, enteral and parenteral nutritional therapy are not covered under Part B in situations involving temporary impairments.

Coverage of such therapy, however, does not require a medical judgment that the impairment giving rise to the therapy will persist throughout the patient's remaining years. If the medical record, including the judgment of the attending physician, indicates that the impairment will be of long and indefinite duration, the test of permanence is considered met.

If the coverage requirements for enteral or parenteral nutritional therapy are met under the prosthetic device benefit provision, related supplies, equipment and nutrients are also covered under the conditions in the following paragraphs and the Medicare Benefit Policy Manual, Chapter 15, "Covered Medical and Other Health Services," §120.

Parenteral Nutrition Therapy Daily parenteral nutrition is considered reasonable and necessary for a patient with severe pathology of the alimentary tract which does not allow absorption of sufficient nutrients to maintain weight and strength commensurate with the patient's general condition.

Since the alimentary tract of such a patient does not function adequately, an indwelling catheter is placed percutaneously in the subclavian vein and then advanced into the superior vena cava where intravenous infusion of nutrients is given for part of the day. The catheter is then plugged by the patient until the next infusion. Following a period of hospitalization which is required to initiate parenteral nutrition and to train the patient in catheter care, solution preparation, and infusion technique, the parenteral nutrition can be provided safely and effectively in the patient's home by nonprofessional persons who have undergone special training. However, such persons cannot be paid for their services, nor is payment available for any services furnished by nonphysician professionals except as services furnished incident to a physician's service.

For parenteral nutrition therapy to be covered under Part B, the claim must contain a physician's written order or prescription and sufficient medical documentation to permit an independent conclusion that the requirements of the prosthetic device benefit are met and that parenteral nutrition therapy is medically necessary. An example of a condition that typically qualifies for coverage is a massive small bowel resection resulting in severe nutritional deficiency in spite of adequate oral intake. However, coverage of parenteral nutrition therapy for this and any other condition must be approved on an individual, case-by-case basis initially and at periodic intervals of no more than three months by the carrier's medical consultant or specially trained staff, relying on such medical and other documentation as the carrier may require. If the claim involves an infusion pump, sufficient evidence must be provided to support a determination of medical necessity for the pump. Program payment for the pump is based on the reasonable charge for the simplest model that meets the medical needs of the patient as established by medical documentation.

Nutrient solutions for parenteral therapy are routinely covered. However, Medicare pays for no more than one month's supply of nutrients at any one time. Payment for the nutrients is based on the reasonable charge for the solution components unless the medical record, including a signed statement from the attending physician, establishes that the beneficiary, due to his/her physical or mental state, is unable to safely or effectively mix the solution and there is no family member or other person who can do so. Payment will be on the basis of the reasonable charge for more expensive premixed solutions only under the latter circumstances.

Enteral Nutrition Therapy

Enteral nutrition is considered reasonable and necessary for a patient with a functioning gastrointestinal tract who, due to pathology to, or nonfunction of, the structures that normally permit food to reach the digestive tract, cannot maintain weight and strength commensurate with his or her general condition. Enteral therapy may be given by nasogastric, jejunostomy, or gastrostomy tubes and can be provided safely and effectively in the home by nonprofessional persons who have undergone special training. However, such persons cannot be paid for their services, nor is payment available for any services furnished by nonphysician professionals except as services furnished incident to a physician's service.

Typical examples of conditions that qualify for coverage are head and neck cancer with reconstructive surgery and central nervous system disease leading to interference with the neuromuscular mechanisms of ingestion of such severity that the beneficiary cannot be maintained with oral feeding. However, claims for Part B coverage of enteral nutrition therapy for these and any other conditions must be approved on an individual, case-by-case basis. Each claim must contain a physician's written order or prescription and sufficient medical documentation (e.g., hospital records, clinical findings from the attending physician) to permit an independent conclusion that the patient's condition meets the requirements of the prosthetic device benefit and that enteral nutrition therapy is medically necessary. Allowed claims are to be reviewed at periodic intervals of no more than 3 months by the contractor's medical consultant or specially trained staff, and additional medical documentation considered necessary is to be obtained as part of this review.

Medicare pays for no more than one month's supply of enteral nutrients at any one time.

If the claim involves a pump, it must be supported by sufficient medical documentation to establish that the pump is medically necessary, i.e., gravity feeding is not satisfactory due to aspiration, diarrhea, dumping syndrome. Program payment for the pump is based on the reasonable charge for the simplest model that meets the medical needs of the patient as established by medical documentation.

Nutritional Supplementation

Some patients require supplementation of their daily protein and caloric intake. Nutritional supplements are often given as a medicine between meals to boost protein-caloric intake or the mainstay of a daily nutritional plan. Nutritional supplementation is not covered under Medicare Part B.

Pub 100-3, Section 190.2

Diagnostic Pap Smears

A diagnostic pap smear and related medically necessary services are covered under Medicare Part B when ordered by a physician under one of the following conditions:

Previous cancer of the cervix, uterus, or vagina that has been or is presently being treated;

Previous abnormal pap smear;

Any abnormal findings of the vagina, cervix, uterus, ovaries, or adnexa;

Any significant complaint by the patient referable to the female reproductive system; or

Any signs or symptoms that might in the physician's judgment reasonably be related to a gynecologic disorder.

Pub 100-3, Section 190.6

Hair Analysis

Hair analysis to detect mineral traces as an aid in diagnosing human disease is not a covered service under Medicare.

The correlation of hair analysis to the chemical state of the whole body is not possible at this time, and therefore this diagnostic procedure cannot be considered to be reasonable and necessary under §1862(a)(1) of the Act.

Pub 100-3, Section 210.1

Prostate Cancer Screening Tests

A. General.—Section 4103 of the Balanced Budget Act of 1997 provides for coverage of certain prostate cancer screening tests subject to certain coverage, frequency, and payment limitations. Effective for services furnished on or after January 1, 2000. Medicare will cover prostate cancer screening tests/procedures for the early detection of prostate cancer. Coverage of prostate cancer screening tests includes the following procedures furnished to an individual for the early detection of prostate cancer:

Screening digital rectal examination; and:

Screening prostate specific antigen blood test:

B. Screening Digital Rectal Examinations.—Screening digital rectal examinations (HCPCS code G0102) are covered at a frequency of once every 12 months for men who have attained age 50 (at least 11 months have passed following the month in which the last Medicare-covered screening digital rectal examination was performed). Screening digital rectal examination means a clinical examination of an individual's prostate for nodules or other abnormalities of the prostate. This screening must be performed by a doctor of medicine or osteopathy (as defined in §1861(r)(1) of the Act), or by a physician assistant, nurse practitioner, clinical nurse specialist, or certified nurse midwife (as defined in §1861(aa) and §1861(gg) of the Act) who is authorized under State law to perform the examination, fully knowledgeable about the beneficiary's medical condition, and would be responsible for using the results of any examination performed in the overall management of the beneficiary's specific medical problem.

C. Screening Prostate Specific Antigen Tests.—Screening prostate specific antigen tests (code G0103) are covered at a frequency of once every 12 months for men who have attained age 50 (at least 11 months have passed following the month in which the last Medicare-covered screening prostate specific antigen test was performed). Screening prostate specific antigen tests (PSA) means a test to detect the marker for adenocarcinoma of prostate. PSA is a reliable immunocytochemical marker for primary and metastatic adenocarcinoma of prostate. This screening must be ordered by the beneficiary's physician or by the beneficiary's physician assistant, nurse practitioner, clinical nurse specialist, or certified nurse midwife (the term "attending physician" is defined in §1861(r)(1) of the Act to mean a doctor of medicine or osteopathy and the terms "physician assistant, nurse practitioner, clinical nurse specialist, or certified nurse midwife" are defined in §1861(aa) and §1861(gg) of the Act) who is fully knowledgeable about the beneficiary's medical condition, and who would be responsible for using the results of any examination (test) performed in the overall management of the beneficiary's specific medical problem.

Pub 100-3, Section 220.6

Dementia and Neurodegenerative Diseases
(Effective September 15, 2004)

(Rev. 24, Issued: 10-01-04, Effective: 09-15-04, Implementation: 10-04-2004)

A. General

Medicare covers FDG-PET scans for either the differential diagnosis of fronto-temporal dementia (FTD) and Alzheimer's disease (AD) under specific requirements; OR, its use in a Centers for Medicare & Medicaid Services (CMS)-approved practical clinical trial focused on the utility of FDG-PET in the diagnosis or treatment of dementing neurodegenerative diseases. Specific requirements for each indication are clarified below:

B. Nationally Covered Indications

1. FDG-PET Requirements for Coverage in the Differential Diagnosis of AD and FTD:

An FDG-PET scan is considered reasonable and necessary in patients with a recent diagnosis of dementia and documented cognitive decline of at least 6 months, who meet diagnostic criteria for both AD and FTD. These patients have been evaluated for specific alternate neurodegenerative diseases or other causative factors, but the cause of the clinical symptoms remains uncertain.

The following additional conditions must be met before an FDG-PET scan will be covered:

a. The patient's onset, clinical presentation, or course of cognitive impairment is such that FTD is suspected as an alternative neurodegenerative cause of the cognitive decline. Specifically, symptoms such as social disinhibition, awkwardness, difficulties with language, or loss of executive function are more prominent early in the course of FTD than the memory loss typical of AD;

b. The patient has had a comprehensive clinical evaluation (as defined by the American Academy of Neurology (AAN)) encompassing a medical history from the patient and a well-acquainted informant (including assessment of activities of daily living), physical and mental status examination (including formal documentation of cognitive decline occurring over at least 6 months) aided by cognitive scales or neuropsychological testing, laboratory tests, and structural imaging such as magnetic resonance imaging (MRI) or computed tomography (CT);

c. The evaluation of the patient has been conducted by a physician experienced in the diagnosis and assessment of dementia;

d. The evaluation of the patient did not clearly determine a specific neurodegenerative disease or other cause for the clinical symptoms, and information available through FDG-PET is reasonably expected to help clarify the diagnosis between FTD and AD and help guide future treatment;

e. The FDG-PET scan is performed in a facility that has all the accreditation necessary to operate nuclear medicine equipment. The reading of the scan should be done by an expert in nuclear medicine, radiology, neurology, or psychiatry, with experience interpreting such scans in the presence of dementia;

f. A brain single photon emission computed tomography (SPECT) or FDG-PET scan has not been obtained for the same indication.

(The indication can be considered to be different in patients who exhibit important changes in scope or severity of cognitive decline, and meet all other qualifying criteria listed above and below (including the judgment that the likely diagnosis remains uncertain). The results of a prior SPECT or FDG-PET scan must have been inconclusive or, in the case of SPECT, difficult to interpret due to immature or inadequate technology. In these instances, an FDG-PET scan may be covered after one year has passed from the time the first SPECT or FDG-PET scan was performed.)

g. The referring and billing provider(s) have documented the appropriate evaluation of the Medicare beneficiary. Providers should establish the medical necessity of an FDG-PET scan by ensuring that the following information has been collected and is maintained in the beneficiary medical record:

Date of onset of symptoms;

Diagnosis of clinical syndrome (normal aging; mild cognitive impairment or MCI; mild, moderate or severe dementia);

Mini mental status exam (MMSE) or similar test score;

Presumptive cause (possible, probable, uncertain AD);

Any neuropsychological testing performed;

Results of any structural imaging (MRI or CT) performed;

Relevant laboratory tests (B12, thyroid hormone); and,

Number and name of prescribed medications.

The billing provider must furnish a copy of the FDG-PET scan result for use by CMS and its contractors upon request. These verification requirements are consistent with federal requirements set forth in 42 Code of Federal Regulations section 410.32 generally for diagnostic x-ray tests, diagnostic laboratory tests, and other tests. In summary, section 410.32 requires the billing physician and the referring physician to maintain information in the medical record of each patient to demonstrate medical necessity [410.32(d) (2)] and submit the information demonstrating medical necessity to CMS and/or its agents upon request [410.32(d)(3)(I)] (OMB number 0938-0685).

2. FDG-PET Requirements for Coverage in the Context of a CMS-approved Practical Clinical Trial Utilizing a Specific Protocol to Demonstrate the Utility of FDG-PET in the Diagnosis, and Treatment of Neurodegenerative Dementing Diseases

An FDG-PET scan is considered reasonable and necessary in patients with mild cognitive impairment or early dementia (in clinical circumstances other than those specified in subparagraph 1) only in the context of an approved clinical trial that contains patient safeguards and protections to ensure proper administration, use and evaluation of the FDG-PET scan.

The clinical trial must compare patients who do and do not receive an FDG-PET scan and have as its goal to monitor, evaluate, and improve clinical outcomes. In addition, it must meet the following basic criteria:

a. Written protocol on file;

b. Institutional Review Board review and approval;

c. Scientific review and approval by two or more qualified individuals who are not part of the research team; and,

d. Certification that investigators have not been disqualified.

C. Nationally Noncovered Indications

All other uses of FDG-PET for patients with a presumptive diagnosis of dementia-causing neurodegenerative disease (e.g., possible or probable AD, clinically typical FTD, dementia of Lewy bodies, or Creutzfeld-Jacob disease) for which CMS has not specifically indicated coverage continue to be noncovered.

D. Other

Not applicable.

(This NCD last reviewed September 2004.)

Pub 100-3, Section 230.1

Treatment of Kidney Stones

In addition to the traditional surgical/endoscopic techniques for the treatment of kidney stones, the following lithotripsy techniques are also covered for services rendered on or after March 15, 1985.

A. Extracorporeal Shock Wave Lithotripsy.—Extracorporeal Shock Wave Lithotripsy (ESWL) is a non-invasive method of treating kidney stones using a device called a lithotriptor. The lithotriptor uses shock waves generated outside of the body to break up upper urinary tract stones. It focuses the shock waves specifically on stones under X-ray visualization, pulverizing them by repeated shocks. ESWL is covered under Medicare for use in the treatment of upper urinary tract kidney stones.

B. Percutaneous Lithotripsy.—Percutaneous lithotripsy (or nephrolithotomy) is an invasive method of treating kidney stones by using ultrasound, electrohydraulic or mechanical lithotripsy. A probe is inserted through an incision in the skin directly over the kidney and applied to the stone. A form of lithotripsy is then used to fragment the stone. Mechanical or electrohydraulic lithotripsy may be used as an alternative or adjunct to ultrasonic lithotripsy. Percutaneous lithotripsy of kidney stones by ultrasound or by the related techniques of electrohydraulic or mechanical lithotripsy is covered under Medicare.

The following is covered for services rendered on or after January 16, 1988.

C. Transurethral Ureteroscopic Lithotripsy.—Transurethral ureteroscopic lithotripsy is a method of fragmenting and removing ureteral and renal stones through a cystoscope. The cystoscope is inserted through the urethra into the bladder. Catheters are passed through the scope into the opening where the ureters enter the bladder. Instruments passed through this opening into the ureters are used to manipulate and ultimately disintegrate stones, using either mechanical crushing, transcystoscopic electrohydraulic shock waves, ultrasound or laser. Transurethral ureteroscopic lithotripsy for the treatment of urinary tract stones of the kidney or ureter is covered under Medicare.

PUB 100 REFERENCES

Pub. 100-3, Section 230.5

Gravlee Jet Washer

(Rev. 1, 10-03-03)

CIM 50-4

The Gravlee Jet Washer is a sterile, disposable, diagnostic device for detecting endometrial cancer. The use of this device is indicated where the patient exhibits clinical symptoms or signs suggestive of endometrial disease, such as irregular or heavy vaginal bleeding.

Program payment cannot be made for the washer or the related diagnostic services when furnished in connection with the examination of an asymptomatic patient. Payment for routine physical checkups is precluded under the statute. (See §1862(a)(7) of the Act.)

(See the Medicare Benefit Policy Manual, Chapter 16, "General Exclusions From Coverage," §90).

Pub. 100-3, Section 230.7

Water Purification and Softening Systems Used in Conjunction with Home Dialysis

(Rev. 1, 10-03-03)

CIM 55-1

A - Water Purification Systems

Water used for home dialysis should be chemically free of heavy trace metals and/or organic contaminants that could be hazardous to the patient. It should also be as free of bacteria as possible but need not be biologically sterile. Since the characteristics of natural water supplies in most areas of the country are such that some type of water purification system is needed, such a system used in conjunction with a home dialysis (either peritoneal or hemodialysis) unit is covered under Medicare.

There are two types of water purification systems that will satisfy these requirements:

- Deionization - The removal of organic substances, mineral salts of magnesium and calcium (causing hardness), compounds of fluoride and chloride from tap water using the process of filtration and ion exchange; or

- Reverse Osmosis - The process used to remove impurities from tap water utilizing pressure to force water through a porous membrane.

Use of both a deionization unit and reverse osmosis unit in series, theoretically to provide the advantages of both systems, has been determined medically unnecessary since either system can provide water which is both chemically and bacteriologically pure enough for acceptable use in home dialysis. In addition, spare deionization tanks are not covered since they are essentially a precautionary supply rather than a current requirement for treatment of the patient.

Activated carbon filters used as a component of water purification systems to remove unsafe concentrations of chlorine and chloramines are covered when prescribed by a physician.

B - Water Softening System

Except as indicated below, a water softening system used in conjunction with home dialysis is excluded from coverage under Medicare as not being reasonable and necessary within the meaning of §1862(a)(1) of the Act. Such a system, in conjunction with a home dialysis unit, does not adequately remove the hazardous heavy metal contaminants (such as arsenic) which may be present in trace amounts.

A water softening system may be covered when used to pretreat water to be purified by a reverse osmosis (RO) unit for home dialysis where:

The manufacturer of the RO unit has set standards for the quality of water entering the RO (e.g., the water to be purified by the RO must be of a certain quality if the unit is to perform as intended);

The patients water is demonstrated to be of a lesser quality than required; and

The softener is used only to soften water entering the RO unit, and thus, used only for dialysis. (The softener need not actually be built into the RO unit, but must be an integral part of the dialysis system.)

C - Developing Need When a Water Softening System is Replaced with a Water

Purification Unit in an Existing Home Dialysis System

The medical necessity of water purification units must be care fully developed when they replace water softening systems in existing home dialysis systems. A purification system may be ordered under these circumstances for a number of reasons. For example, changes in the medical community's opinions regarding the quality of water necessary for safe dialysis may lead the physician to decide the quality of water previously used should be improved, or the water quality itself may have deteriorated. Patients may have dialyzed using only an existing water softener previous to Medicare ESRD coverage because of inability to pay for a purification system. On the other hand, in some cases, the installation of a purification system is not medically necessary. Thus,

when such a case comes to the contractor's attention, the contractor asks the physician to furnish the reason for the changes. Supporting documentation, such as the suppliers recommendations or water analysis, may be required. All such cases should be reviewed by the contractor's medical consultants.

Cross reference:

The Medicare Benefit Policy Manual, Chapter 15, "Covered Medical and Other Health Services," §110.

Pub. 100-3, Section 230.8

Non-Implantable Pelvic Flood Electrical Stimulator

(Rev. 1, 10-03-03)

CIM 60-24

Non-implantable pelvic floor electrical stimulators provide neuromuscular electrical stimulation through the pelvic floor with the intent of strengthening and exercising pelvic floor musculature. Stimulation is generally delivered by vaginal or anal probes connected to an external pulse generator.

The methods of pelvic floor electrical stimulation vary in location, stimulus frequency (Hz), stimulus intensity or amplitude (mA), pulse duration (duty cycle), treatments per day, number of treatment days per week, length of time for each treatment session, overall time period for device use and between clinic and home settings. In general, the stimulus frequency and other parameters are chosen based on the patient's clinical diagnosis.

Pelvic floor electrical stimulation with a non-implantable stimulator is covered for the treatment of stress and/or urge urinary incontinence in cognitively intact patients who have failed a documented trial of pelvic muscle exercise (PME) training.

A failed trial of PME training is defined as no clinically significant improvement in urinary continence after completing 4 weeks of an ordered plan of pelvic muscle exercises designed to increase periurethral muscle strength.

Pub 100-3, Section 230.10

Incontinence Control Devices

A. Mechanical/Hydraulic Incontinence Control Devices.—Mechanical/hydraulic incontinence control devices are accepted as safe and effective in the management of urinary incontinence in patients with permanent anatomic and neurologic dysfunctions of the bladder. This class of devices achieves control of urination by compression of the urethra. The materials used and the success rate may vary somewhat from device to device. Such a device is covered when its use is reasonable and necessary for the individual patient.

B. Collagen Implant.—A collagen implant, which is injected into the submucosal tissues of the urethra and/or the bladder neck and into tissues adjacent to the urethra, is a prosthetic device used in the treatment of stress urinary incontinence resulting from intrinsic sphincter deficiency (ISD). ISD is a cause of stress urinary incontinence in which the urethral sphincter is unable to contract and generate sufficient resistance in the bladder, especially during stress maneuvers.

Prior to collagen implant therapy, a skin test for collagen sensitivity must be administered and evaluated over a 4 week period.

In male patients, the evaluation must include a complete history and physical examination and a simple cystometrogram to determine that the bladder fills and stores properly. The patient then is asked to stand upright with a full bladder and to cough or otherwise exert abdominal pressure on his bladder. If the patient leaks, the diagnosis of ISD is established.

In female patients, the evaluation must include a complete history and physical examination (including a pelvic exam) and a simple cystometrogram to rule out abnormalities of bladder compliance and abnormalities of urethral support. Following that determination, an abdominal leak point pressure (ALLP) test is performed. Leak point pressure, stated in cm H2O, is defined as the intra-abdominal pressure at which leakage occurs from the bladder (around a catheter) when the bladder has been filled with a minimum of 150 cc fluid. If the patient has an ALLP of less than 100 cm H2O, the diagnosis of ISD is established.

To use a collagen implant, physicians must have urology training in the use of a cystoscope and must complete a collagen implant training program.

Coverage of a collagen implant, and the procedure to inject it, is limited to the following types of patients with stress urinary incontinence due to ISD:

Male or female patients with congenital sphincter weakness secondary to conditions such as myelomeningocele or epispadias;

Male or female patients with acquired sphincter weakness secondary to spinal cord lesions;

Male patients following trauma, including prostatectomy and/or radiation; and

Female patients without urethral hypermobility and with abdominal leak point pressures of 100 cm H2O or less.

Patients whose incontinence does not improve with 5 injection procedures (5 separate treatment sessions) are considered treatment failures, and no further treatment of urinary incontinence by collagen implant is covered. Patients who have a reoccurrence of incontinence following successful treatment with collagen implants in the past (e.g., 6-12 months previously) may benefit from additional treatment sessions. Coverage of additional sessions may be allowed but must be supported by medical justification.

C. Non-Implantable Pelvic Floor Electrical Stimulator.—(See §60-24.)

Pub 100-3, Section 230.12

Dimethyl Sulfoxide (DMSO)

The Food and Drug Administration has determined that the only purpose for which DMSO is safe and effective for humans is in the treatment of the bladder condition, interstitial cystitis. Therefore, the use of DMSO for all other indications is not considered to be reasonable and necessary. Payment may be made for its use only when reasonable and necessary for a patient in the treatment of interstitial cystitis.

Pub. 100-3, Section 230.16

Bladder Stimulators (Pacemakers)

(Rev. 1, 10-03-03)

CIM 65-11

Not Covered

There are a number of devices available to induce emptying of the urinary bladder by using electrical current which forces the muscles of the bladder to contract. These devices (commonly known as bladder stimulators or pacemakers) are characterized by the implantation of electrodes in the wall of the bladder, the rectal cones, or the spinal cord. While these treatments may effectively empty the bladder, the issue of safety involving the initiation of infection, erosion, placement, and material selection has not been resolved. Further, some facilities previously using electronic emptying have stopped using this method due to the pain experienced by the patient.

The use of spinal cord electrical stimulators, rectal electrical stimulators, and bladder wall stimulators is not considered reasonable and necessary. Therefore, no program payment may be made for these devices or for their implant.

Pub. 100-3, Section 230.17

Urinary Drainage Bags

(Rev. 1, 10-03-03)

CIM 65-17

Urinary collection and retention system are covered as prosthetic devices that replace bladder function in the case of permanent urinary incontinence. Urinary drainage bags that can be used either as bedside or leg drainage bags may be either multi-use or single use systems. Both the multi-use and the single use bags have a system that prevents urine backflow. However, the single use system is non-drainable. There is insufficient evidence to support the medical necessity of a single use system bag rather than the multi-use bag. Therefore, a single use drainage system is subject to the same coverage parameters as the multi-use drainage bags.

Pub 100-3, Section 230.6

Vabra Aspirator

Program payment cannot be made for the aspirator or the related diagnostic services when furnished in connection with the examination of an asymptomatic patient. Payment for routine physical checkups is precluded under the statute (§1862(a)(7) of the Act).

Pub. 100-3, Section 240.1

Lung Volume Reduction Surgery (Reduction Pneumoplasty)

(Rev. 3, 11-04-03)

Lung volume reduction surgery (LVRS) or reduction pneumoplasty, also referred to as lung shaving or lung contouring, is performed on patients with severe emphysema in order to allow the remaining compressed lung to expand, and thus, improve respiratory function.

Covered Indications

Medicare-covered LVRS approaches are limited to bilateral excision of a damaged lung with stapling performed via median sternotomy or video-assisted thoracoscopic surgery.

1. National Emphysema Treatment Trial (NETT) participants (effective for services performed on or after August 11, 1997):

Medicare provides coverage to those beneficiaries who are participating in the NETT trial for all services integral to the study and for which the Medicare statute does not prohibit coverage.

2. Medicare will only consider LVRS reasonable and necessary when all of the following requirements are met (effective for services performed on or after January 1, 2004):

a. The patient satisfies all the criteria outlined below:

Assessment	Criteria
History and physical examination	Consistent with emphysema BMI, $\leq$ 31.1 kg/m2 (men) or $\leq$ 32.3 kg/m2 (women) Stable with $\leq$20 mg prednisone (or equivalent) qd
Radiographic	High Resolution Computer Tomography (HRCT) scan evidence of bilateral emphysema
Pulmonary function (pre-rehabilitation)	Forced expiratory volume in one second (FEV1) $\leq$ 45% predicted ($\geq$ 15% predicted if age $\geq$ 70 years) Total lung capacity (TLC) $\geq$ 100% predicted post-bronchodilator Residual volume (RV) $\geq$ 150% predicted post-bronchodilator
Arterial blood gas level (pre-rehabilitation)	PCO2, $\leq$ 60 mm Hg (PCO2, $\leq$ 55 mm Hg if 1-mile above sea level) PO2, $\geq$ 45 mm Hg on room air (PO2, $\geq$ 30 mm Hg if 1-mile above sea level)
Cardiac assessment	Approval for surgery by cardiologist if any of the following are present: Unstable angina; left-ventricular ejection fraction (LVEF) cannot be estimated from the echocardiogram; LVEF < 45%; dobutamine-radionuclide cardiac scan indicates coronary artery disease or ventricular dysfunction; arrhythmia (> 5 premature ventricular contractions per minute; cardiac rhythm other than sinus; premature ventricular contractions on EKG at rest)
Surgical assessment	Approval for surgery by pulmonary physician, thoracic surgeon, and anesthesiologist post-rehabilitation
Exercise	Post-rehabilitation 6-min walk of $\geq$140 m; able to complete 3 min unloaded pedaling in exercise tolerance test (pre- and post-rehabilitation)
Consent	Signed consents for screening and rehabilitation
Smoking	Plasma cotinine level $\leq$ 13.7 ng/mL (or arterial carboxyhemoglobin $\leq$ 2.5% if using nicotine products) Nonsmoking for 4 months prior to initial interview and throughout evaluation for surgery
Preoperative diagnostic and therapeutic program adherence	Must complete assessment for and program of preoperative services in preparation for surgery

In addition, the patient must have:

• Severe upper lobe predominant emphysema (as defined by radiologist assessment of upper lobe predominance on CT scan), or

• Severe non-upper lobe emphysema with low exercise capacity.

Patients with low exercise capacity are those whose maximal exercise capacity is at or below 25 watts for women and 40 watts (w) for men after completion of the preoperative therapeutic program in preparation for LVRS. Exercise capacity is measured by incremental, maximal, symptom-limited exercise with a cycle ergometer utilizing 5 or 10 watt/minute ramp on 30% oxygen after 3 minutes of unloaded pedaling.

c. The surgery must be performed at facilities that were identified by the National Heart, Lung, and Blood Institute to meet the thresholds for participation in the NETT, and at sites that have been approved by Medicare as lung transplant facilities. These facilities are listed on our Web site at www.cms.hhs.gov/coverage/lvrsfacility.pdf. The CMS is currently working to develop accreditation standards for facilities to perform LVRS and when implemented, will consider LVRS to be reasonable and necessary only at accredited facilities.

d. The surgery must be preceded and followed by a program of diagnostic and therapeutic services consistent with those provided in the NETT and designed to maximize the patient's potential to successfully undergo and recover from surgery. The program must include a 6- to 10-week series of at least 16, and no more than 20, preoperative sessions, each lasting a minimum of 2 hours. It must also include at least 6, and no more than 10, postoperative sessions, each lasting a minimum of 2 hours, within 8 to 9 weeks of the LVRS. This program must be consistent with the care plan developed by the treating physician following performance of a comprehensive evaluation of the patient's medical, psychosocial and nutritional needs, be consistent with the preoperative and postoperative services provided in the NETT, and arranged, monitored, and performed under the coordination of the facility where the surgery takes place.

Noncovered Indications

1. LVRS is not covered in any of the following clinical circumstances:

a. Patient characteristics carry a high risk for perioperative morbidity and/or mortality;

b. The disease is unsuitable for LVRS;

c. Medical conditions or other circumstances make it likely that the patient will be unable to complete the preoperative and postoperative pulmonary diagnostic and therapeutic program required for surgery;

d. The patient presents with FEV₁ £ 20% of predicted value, and either homogeneous distribution of emphysema on CT scan, or carbon monoxide diffusing capacity of £ 20% of predicted value (high-risk group identified October 2001 by the NETT); or

e. The patient satisfies the criteria outlined above in section 2(a), and has severe, non-upper lobe emphysema with high exercise capacity. High exercise capacity is defined as a maximal workload at the completion of the preoperative diagnostic and therapeutic program that is above 25 w for women and 40 w for men (under the measurement conditions for cycle ergometry specified above).

2. All other indications for LVRS not otherwise specified remain noncovered.

Pub. 100-3, Section 240.2

Home Use of Oxygen

(Rev. 1, 10-03-03)

CIM 60-4

A - General

Medicare coverage of home oxygen and oxygen equipment under the durable medical equipment (DME) benefit (see §1861(s)(6)of the Act) is considered reasonable and necessary only for patients with significant hypoxemia who meet the medical documentation, laboratory evidence, and health conditions specified in subsections B, C, and D. This section also includes special coverage criteria for portable oxygen systems. Finally, a statement on the absence of coverage of the professional services of a respiratory therapist under the DME benefit is included in subsection F.

B - Medical Documentation

Initial claims for oxygen services must include a completed Form CMS-484 (Certificate of Medical Necessity: Oxygen) to establish whether coverage criteria are met and to ensure that the oxygen services provided are consistent with the physician's prescription or other medical documentation. The treating physician's prescription or other medical documentation must indicate that other forms of treatment (e.g., medical and physical therapy directed at secretions, bronchospasm and infection) have been tried, have not been sufficiently successful, and oxygen therapy is still required. While there is no substitute for oxygen therapy, each patient must receive optimum therapy before long-term home oxygen therapy is ordered. Use Form CMS-484 for recertifications. (See the Medicare Program Integrity Manual, Chapter 5, for completion of Form CMS-484.)

The medical and prescription information in section B of Form CMS-484 can be completed only by the treating physician, the physician's employee, or another clinician (e.g., nurse, respiratory therapist, etc.) as long as that person is not the DME supplier. Although hospital discharge coordinators and medical social workers may assist in arranging for physician-prescribed home oxygen, they do not have the authority to prescribe the services. Suppliers may not enter this information. While this section may be completed by non-physician clinician or a physician employee, it must be reviewed and the Form CMS-484 signed by the attending physician.

A physician's certification of medical necessity for oxygen equipment must include the results of specific testing before coverage can be determined.

Claims for oxygen must also be supported by medical documentation in the patient's record. Separate documentation is used with electronic billing. This documentation may be in the form of a prescription written by the patient's attending physician who has recently examined the patient (normally within a month of the start of therapy) and must specify:

- A diagnosis of the disease requiring home use of oxygen;

- The oxygen flow rate; and

- An estimate of the frequency, duration of use (e.g., 2 liters per minute, 10 minutes per hour, 12 hours per day), and duration of need (e.g., 6 months or lifetime).

NOTE: A prescription for "Oxygen PRN" or "Oxygen as needed" does not meet this last requirement. Neither provides any basis for determining if the amount of oxygen is reasonable and necessary for the patient.

A member of the carrier's medical staff should review all claims with oxygen flow rates of more than four liters per minute before payment can be made.

The attending physician specifies the type of oxygen delivery system to be used (i.e., gas, liquid, or concentrator) by signing the completed Form CMS-484. In addition, the supplier or physician may use the space in section C for written confirmation of additional details of the physician's order. The additional order information contained in section C may include the means of oxygen delivery (mask, nasal, cannula, etc.), the specifics of varying flow rates, and/or the noncontinuous use of oxygen as appropriate. The physician confirms this order information with their signature in section D.

New medical documentation written by the patient's attending physician must be submitted to the carrier in support of revised oxygen requirements when there has been a change in the patient's condition and need for oxygen therapy.

Carriers are required to conduct periodic, continuing medical necessity reviews on patients whose conditions warrant these reviews and on patients with indefinite or extended periods of necessity as described in the Medicare Program Integrity Manual, Chapter 5, "Items and Services Having Special DMERC Review Considerations." When indicated, carriers may also request documentation of the results of a repeat arterial blood gas or oximetry study.

NOTE: Section 4152 of OBRA 1990 requires earlier recertification and retesting of oxygen patients who begin coverage with an arterial blood gas result at or above a partial pressure of 55 or an arterial oxygen saturation percentage at or above 89. (See the Medicare Claims Processing Manual, Chapter 20, "Durable Medical Equipment, Prosthetics and Orthotics, and Supplies (DMEPOS)," §100.2.3, for certification and retesting schedules.)

C - Laboratory Evidence

Initial claims for oxygen therapy must also include the results of a blood gas study that has been ordered and evaluated by the attending physician. This is usually in the form of a measurement of the partial pressure of oxygen (PO2) in arterial blood. A measurement of arterial oxygen saturation obtained by ear or pulse oximetry, however, is also acceptable when ordered and evaluated by the attending and performed under his or her supervision or when performed by a qualified provider or supplier of laboratory services.

When the arterial blood gas and the oximetry studies are both used to document the need for home oxygen therapy and the results are conflicting, the arterial blood gas study is the preferred source of documenting medical need. A DME supplier is not considered a qualified provider or supplier of laboratory services for purposes of these guidelines.

This prohibition does not extend to the results of blood gas test conducted by a hospital certified to do such tests. The conditions under which the laboratory tests are performed must be specified in writing and submitted with the initial claim, i.e., at rest, during exercise, or during sleep.

The preferred sources of laboratory evidence are, existing physician and/or hospital records that reflect the patient's medical condition. Since it is expected that virtually all patients who qualify for home oxygen coverage for the first time under these guidelines have recently been discharged from a hospital where they submitted to arterial blood gas tests, the carrier needs to request that such test results be submitted in support of their initial claims for home oxygen. If more than one arterial blood gas test is performed during the patient's hospital stay, the test result obtained closest to, but no earlier than two days prior to the hospital discharge date is required as evidence of the need for home oxygen therapy.

For those patients whose initial oxygen prescription did not originate during a hospital stay, blood gas studies should be done while the patient is in the chronic stable state, i.e., not during a period of an acute illness or an exacerbation of their underlying disease.

Carriers may accept an attending physician's statement of recent hospital test results for a particular patient, when appropriate, in lieu of copies of actual hospital records.

A repeat arterial blood gas study is appropriate when evidence indicates that an oxygen recipient has undergone a major change in their condition relevant to home use of oxygen. If the carrier has reason to believe that there has been a major change in the patient's physical condition, it may ask for documentation of the results of another blood gas or oximetry study.

D - Health Conditions

Coverage is available for patients with significant hypoxemia in the chronic stable state, i.e, not during a period of acute illness or an exacerbation of their underlying disease, if:

1. The attending physician has determined that the patient has a health condition outlined in subsection D.1,

2. The patient meets the blood gas evidence requirements specified in subsection D.3, and

3. The patient has appropriately tried other treatment without complete success. (See subsection B.)

1 - Conditions for Which Oxygen Therapy May Be Covered

- A severe lung disease, such as chronic obstructive pulmonary disease, diffuse interstitial lung disease, cystic fibrosis, bronchiectasis, widespread pulmonary neoplasm, or

- Hypoxia-related symptoms or findings that might be expected to improve with oxygen therapy. Examples of these symptoms and findings are pulmonary hypertension, recurring congestive heart failure due to chronic cor pulmonale, erythrocytosis, impairment of the cognitive process, nocturnal restlessness, and morning headache.

2 - Conditions for Which Oxygen Therapy Is Not Covered

- Angina pectoris in the absence of hypoxemia. This condition is generally not the result of a low oxygen level in the blood, and there are other preferred treatments;

- Breathlessness without cor pulmonale or evidence of hypoxemia. Although intermittent oxygen use is sometimes prescribed to relieve this condition, it is potentially harmful and psychologically addicting;

- Severe peripheral vascular disease resulting in clinically evident desaturation in one or more extremities. There is no evidence that increased PO2 improves the oxygenation of tissues with impaired circulation; or

- Terminal illnesses that do not affect the lungs.

3 - Covered Blood Gas Values

If the patient has a condition specified in subsection D.1, the carrier must review the medical documentation and laboratory evidence that has been submitted for a particular patient (see subsections B and C) and determine if coverage is available under one of the three group categories outlined below.

(a) - Group I - Except as modified in subsection d, coverage is provided for patients with significant hypoxemia evidenced by any of the following:

- An arterial PO2 at or below 55 mm Hg, or an arterial oxygen saturation at or below 88 percent, taken at rest, breathing room air.

- An arterial PO2 at or below 55 mm Hg, or an arterial oxygen saturation at or below 88 percent, taken during sleep for a patient who demonstrates an arterial PO2 at or above 56 mm Hg, or an arterial oxygen saturation at or above 89 percent, while awake; or a greater than normal fall in oxygen level during sleep (a decrease in arterial PO2 more than 10 mm Hg, or decrease in arterial oxygen saturation more than 5 percent) associated with symptoms or signs reasonably attributable to hypoxemia (e.g., impairment of cognitive processes and nocturnal restlessness or insomnia). In either of these cases, coverage is provided only for use of oxygen during sleep, and then only one type of unit will be covered. Portable oxygen ,therefore, would not be covered in this situation.

- An arterial PO2 at or below 55 mm Hg or an arterial oxygen saturation at or below 88 percent, taken during exercise for a patient who demonstrates an arterial PO2 at or above 56 mm Hg, or an arterial oxygen saturation at or above 89 percent, during the day while at rest. In this case, supplemental oxygen is provided for during exercise if there is evidence the use of oxygen improves the hypoxemia that was demonstrated during exercise when the patient was breathing room air.

(b) - Group II - Except as modified in subsection d, coverage is available for patients whose arterial PO2 is 56-59 mm Hg or whose arterial blood oxygen saturation is 89 percent, if there is evidence of:

- Dependent edema suggesting congestive heart failure;

- Pulmonary hypertension or cor pulmonale, determined by measurement of pulmonary artery pressure, gated blood pool scan, echocardiogram, or "P" pulmonale on EKG (P wave greater than 3 mm in standard leads II, III, or AVF); or

- Erythrocythemia with a hematocrit greater than 56 percent.

(c) - Group III - Except as modified in subsection d, carriers must apply a rebuttable presumption that a home program of oxygen use is not medically necessary for patients with arterial PO2 levels at or above 60 mm Hg, or arterial blood oxygen saturation at or above 90 percent. In order for claims in this category to be reimbursed, the carrier's reviewing physician needs to review any documentation submitted in rebuttal of this presumption and grant specific approval of the claims.

The CMS expects few claims to be approved for coverage in this category.

(d) - Variable Factors That May Affect Blood Gas Values - In reviewing the arterial PO2 levels and the arterial oxygen saturation percentages specified in subsections D. 3.a, b and c, the carrier's medical staff must take into account variations in oxygen measurements that may result from such factors as the patient's age, the altitude level, or the patient's decreased oxygen carrying capacity.

E - Portable Oxygen Systems

A patient meeting the requirements specified below may qualify for coverage of a portable oxygen system either (1) by itself or (2) to use in addition to a stationary oxygen system. Portable oxygen is not covered when it is provided only as a backup to a stationary oxygen system. A portable oxygen system is covered for a particular patient if:

- The claim meets the requirements specified in subsections A-D, as appropriate; and

- The medical documentation indicates that the patient is mobile in the home and would benefit from the use of a portable oxygen system in the home. Portable oxygen systems are not covered for patients who qualify for oxygen solely based on blood gas studies obtained during sleep

F - Respiratory Therapists

Respiratory therapists' services are not covered under the provisions for coverage of oxygen services under the Part B durable medical equipment benefit as outlined above.

This benefit provides for coverage of home use of oxygen and oxygen equipment, but does not include a professional component in the delivery of such services.

(See §280.1, and the Medicare Benefit Policy Manual, Chapter 15, "Covered Medical and Other Health Services," §110)

Pub. 100-3, Section 240.4

Continuous Positive Airway Pressure (CPAP)
(Rev. 1, 10-03-03)

CIM 60-17

The CPAP is a noninvasive technique for providing single levels of air pressure from a flow generator, via a nose mask, through the nares. The purpose is to prevent the collapse of the oropharyngeal walls and the obstruction of airflow during sleep which occurs in obstructive sleep apnea (OSA).

The diagnosis of OSA requires documentation of at least 30 episodes of apnea, each lasting a minimum of 10 seconds, during 6-7 hours of recorded sleep. The use of CPAP is covered under Medicare when used in adult patients with moderate or severe OSA for whom surgery is a likely alternative to CPAP.

Initial claims must be supported by medical documentation (separate documentation where electronic billing is used), such as a prescription written by the patient's attending physician, that specifies:

- A diagnosis of moderate or severe obstructive sleep apnea, and

- Surgery is a likely alternative.

- The claim must also certify that the documentation supporting a diagnosis of OSA (described above) is available.

The use of CPAP devices are covered under Medicare when ordered and prescribed by the licensed treating physician to be used in adult patients with OSA if either of the following criteria using the Apnea-Hyopopnea Index (AHI) are met:

- AHI ≥ 15 events per hour, or

- AHI ≥ 5 and ≤ 14 events per hour with documented symptoms of excessive daytime sleepiness, impaired cognition, mood disorders or insomnia, or documented hypertension, ischemic heart disease or history of stroke.

The AHI is equal to the average number of episodes of apnea and hyponea per hour and must be based on a minimum of two hours of sleep recorded by polysomnography using actual recorded hours of sleep (i.e., the AHI may not be extrapolated or projected).

Apnea is defined as a cessation of airflow for at least 10 seconds. Hypopnea is defined as an abnormal respiratory event lasting at least 10 seconds with at least a 30 percent reduction in thoracoabdominal movement or airflow as compared to baseline, and with at least a 4 percent oxygen desaturation.

The polysomnography must be performed in a facility - based sleep study laboratory, and not in the home or in a mobile facility.

Initial claims for CPAP devices must be supported by information contained in the medical record indicating that the patient meets Medicare's stated coverage criteria.

Cross References: §280.1.

Pub. 100-3, Section 240.5

Intrapulmonary Percussive Ventilator (IPV)
(Rev. 1, 10-03-03)

CIM 60-21

Not Covered

IPV is a mechanized form of chest physical therapy. Instead of a therapist clapping or slapping the patient's chest wall, the IPV delivers mini-bursts (more than 200 per minute) of respiratory gasses to the lungs via a mouthpiece. Its intended purpose is to mobilize endobronchial secretions and diffuse patchy atelectasis. The patient controls variables such as inspiratory time, peak pressure and delivery rates.

Studies do not demonstrate any advantage of IPV over that achieved with good pulmonary care in the hospital environment and there are no studies in the home setting. There are no data to support the effectiveness of the device. Therefore, IPV in the home setting is not covered.

Pub 100-3, Section 260.3

Pancreas Transplants
Medicare has had a policy of not covering pancreas transplantation for many years as the safety and effectiveness of the procedure had not been demonstrated. The Office of Health Technology Assessment performed an assessment on pancreas-kidney transplantation in 1994. They found reasonable graft survival outcomes for patients receiving either simultaneous pancreas-kidney transplantation and pancreas after kidney transplantation.

Effective July 1, 1999, Medicare will cover whole organ pancreas transplantation (ICD-9-CM code 52.80, or 52.82, CPT code 48554) only when it is performed simultaneous with or after a kidney transplant (ICD-9-CM code 55.69, CPT code 50360, or 50365). If the pancreas transplant occurs after the kidney transplant, immunosuppressive therapy will begin with the date of discharge from the inpatient stay for the pancreas transplant.

Pancreas transplantation for diabetic patients who have not experienced end stage renal failure secondary to diabetes continues to be excluded from Medicare coverage. Medicare also excludes coverage of transplantation of partial pancreatic tissue or islet cells. There is not sufficient evidence at this time to support a determination that these procedures are reasonable and necessary.

Pub 100-3, Section 260.7

Lymphocyte Immune Globulin, Anti-Thymocyte Globulin (Equine)

The FDA has approved one lymphocyte immune globulin preparation for marketing, lymphocyte immune globulin, anti-thymocyte globulin (equine). This drug is indicated for the management of allograft rejection episodes in renal transplantation. It is covered under Medicare when used for this purpose. Other forms of lymphocyte globulin preparation which the FDA approves for this indication in the future may be covered under Medicare.

Pub 100-3, Section 270.2

Noncontact Normothermic Wound Therapy (NNWT)

There is insufficient scientific or clinical evidence to consider this device as reasonable and necessary for the treatment of wounds within the meaning of §1862(a)(1)(A) of the Social Security Act and will not be covered by Medicare.

Pub. 100-3, Section 280.1

Durable Medical Equipment Reference List

(Rev. 1, 10-03-03)

CIM 60-9

The durable medical equipment (DME) list which follows is designed to facilitate the contractor's processing of DME claims. This section is designed to be used as a quick reference tool for determining the coverage status of certain pieces of DME and especially for those items which are commonly referred to by both brand and generic names. The information contained herein is applicable (where appropriate) to all DME coverage determinations discussed in the DME portion of this manual. The list is organized into two columns. The first column lists alphabetically various generic categories of equipment on which national coverage decisions have been made by CMS; and the second column notes the coverage status of each equipment category.

In the case of equipment categories that have been determined by CMS to be covered under the DME benefit, the list outlines the conditions of coverage that must be met if payment is to be allowed for the rental or purchase of the DME by a particular patient, or cross-refers to another section of the manual where the applicable coverage criteria are described in more detail. With respect to equipment categories that cannot be covered as DME, the list includes a brief explanation of why the equipment is not covered. This DME list will be updated periodically to reflect any additional national coverage decisions that CMS may make with regard to other categories of equipment.

When the contractor receives a claim for an item of equipment which does not appear to fall logically into any of the generic categories listed, the contractor has the authority and responsibility for deciding whether those items are covered under the DME benefit.

These decisions must be made by each contractor based on the advice of its medical consultants, taking into account:

The Medicare Claims Processing Manual, Chapter 20, "Durable Medical Equipment, Prosthetics and Orthotics, and Supplies (DMEPOS)."

- Whether the item has been approved for marketing by the Food and Drug Administration (FDA) and is otherwise generally considered to be safe and effective for the purpose intended; and
- Whether the item is reasonable and necessary for the individual patient.

The term durable medical equipment (DME) is defined as equipment which:

- Can withstand repeated use; i.e., could normally be rented, and used by successive patients;
- Is primarily and customarily used to serve a medical purpose;
- Generally is not useful to a person in the absence of illness or injury; and
- Is appropriate for use in a patient's home.

Durable Medical Equipment

Item	Coverage
Air Cleaners	Deny—environmental control equipment; not primarily medical in nature (§1861(n) of the Act).
Air Conditioners	Deny—environmental control equipment; not primarily medical in nature (§1861 (n) of the Act).
Air-Fluidized Bed	(See Air-Fluidized Bed §280.8 of this manual.)
Alternating Pressure Pads, Mattresses and Lambs Wool Pads	Covered if patient has, or is highly susceptible to, decubitus ulcers and the patient's physician has specified that he will be supervising his course of treatment.
Audible/Visible Signal/Pacemaker Monitor	(See Self-Contained Pacemaker Monitor.)
Augmentative Communication Device	(See Speech Generating Devices, §50.1 of this manual.)
Bathtub Lifts	Deny—convenience item; not primarily medical in nature (§1861(n) of the Act).
Bathtub Seats	Deny—comfort or convenience item; hygienic equipment; not primarily medical in nature (§1861(n) of the Act).
Bead Bed	(See §280.8.)
Bed Baths (home type)	Deny—hygienic equipment; not primarily medical in nature ((§1861(n) of the Act).
Bed Lifter (bed elevator)	Deny—not primarily medical in nature ((§1861(n) of the Act).
Bedboards	Deny—not primarily medical in nature ((§1861(n) of the Act).
Bed Pans (autoclavable hospital type)	Covered if patient is bed confined.
Bed Side Rails	(See Hospital Beds, §280.7 of this manual.)
Beds-Lounge (power or manual)	Deny—not a hospital bed; comfort or convenience item; not primarily medical in nature (§1861(n) of the Act).
Beds—Oscillating	Deny—institutional equipment; inappropriate for home use.
Bidet Toilet Seat	(See Toilet Seats.)
Blood Glucose Analyzer—Reflectance Colorimeter	Deny—unsuitable for home use (see §40.2 of this manual).
Blood Glucose Monitor	Covered if patient meets certain conditions (see §40.2 of this manual).
Braille Teaching Texts	Deny—educational equipment; not primarily medical in nature (§1861(n) of the Act).
Canes	Covered if patient's condition impairs ambulation (see §280.2 of this manual).
Carafes	Deny—convenience item; not primarily medical in nature (§1861(n) of the Act).
Catheters	Deny—nonreusable disposable supply (§1861(n) of the Act). (See The Medicare Claims Processing Manual, Chapter 20, Durable Medical Equipment, Prosthetics and Orthotics, and Supplies (DMEPOS)
Commodes	Covered if patient is confined to bed or room.

NOTE: The term "room confined" means that the patient's condition is such that leaving the room is medically contraindicated. The accessibility of bathroom facilities generally would not be a factor in this determination. However, confinement of a patient to his home in a case where there are no toilet facilities in the home may be equated to room confinement. Moreover, payment may also be made if a patient's medical condition confines him to a floor of his home and there is no bathroom located on that floor.

Item	Coverage
Communicator	(See §50.1 of this manual, "Speech Generating Devices.")
Continuous Passive Motion	Continuous passive motion devices are devices Covered for patients who have received a total knee replacement. To qualify for coverage, use of the device must commence within 2 days following surgery. In addition, coverage is limited to that portion of the three week period following surgery during which the device is used in the patient's home. There is insufficient evidence to justify coverage of these devices for longer periods of time or for other applications.
Continuous Positive Airway Pressure (CPAP)	(See §240.4 of this manual.)
Crutches	Covered if patient's condition impairs Ambulation.
Cushion Lift Power Seat	(See Seat Lifts.)
Dehumidifiers (room or central heating system type)	Deny—environmental control equipment; not primarily medical in nature (§1861(n) of the Act.
Diathermy Machines (standard pulses wave types)	Deny—inappropriate for home use (see §150.5 of this manual.)
Digital Electronic Pacemaker Monitor	(See Self-Contained Pacemaker Monitor.)
Disposable Sheets and Bags	Deny—nonreusable disposable supplies (§1861(n) of the Act)

Item	Coverage
Elastic Stockings	Deny—nonreusable supply; not rental-type items (§1861(n) of the Act) (See §270.5 of this manual)
Electric Air Cleaners	Deny—(See Air Cleaners.) (§1861(n) of the Act).
Electric Hospital Beds	(See Hospital Beds §280.7 of this manual.)
Electrical Stimulation for Wounds	Deny—inappropriate for home use. (See §270.1 of this manual)
Electrostatic Machines	Deny—(See Air Cleaners and Air Conditioners.) (§1861(n) of the Act).
Elevators	Deny—convenience item; not primarily medical in nature (§1861(n) of the Act).
Emesis Basins	Deny—convenience item; not primarily medical in nature (§1861(n) of the Act).
Esophageal Dilator	Deny—physician instrument; inappropriate for patient use.
Exercise Equipment	Deny—not primarily medical in nature (§1861(n) of the Act).
Fabric Supports	Deny—nonreusable supplies; not rental-type it (§1861(n) of the Act).
Face Masks (oxygen)	Covered if oxygen is Covered. (See §240.2 of this manual.)
Face Masks (surgical)	Deny—nonreusable disposable items (§1861(n) of the Act)
Flowmeter	(See Medical Oxygen Regulators.) (See §240.2 of this manual.)
Fluidic Breathing Assister	(See Intermittent Positive Pressure Breathing Machines.)
Fomentation Device	(See Heating Pads.)
Gel Flotation Pads and Mattresses	(See Alternating Pressure Pads and Mattresses.)
Grab Bars	Deny—self-help device; not primarily medical in nature (§1861(n) of the Act).
Heat and Massage Foam Cushion Pad	Deny—not primarily medical in nature; personal comfort item (§1861(n) and 1862(a)(6) of the Act).
Heating and Cooling Plants	Deny—environmental control equipment not primary; medical in nature (§1861(n) of the Act).
Heating Pads	Covered if the contractor's medical staff determines patient's medical condition is one for which the application of heat in the form of a heating pad is therapeutically effective.
Heat Lamps	Covered if the contractor's medical staff determines patient's medical condition is one for which the application of heat in the form of a heat lamp is therapeutically effective.
Hospital Beds	(See §280.7 of this manual.)
Hot Packs	(See Heating Pads.)
Humidifiers (oxygen)	(See Oxygen Humidifiers.)
Humidifiers (room or central heating system types)	Deny—environmental control equipment; not medical in nature (§1861(n) of the Act).
Hydraulic Lift	(See Patient Lifts.)
Incontinent Pads	Deny—nonreusable supply; hygienic item (§1861(n) of the Act).
Infusion Pumps	For external and implantable pumps, see §40.2. If the pump is used with an enteral or parenteral nutritional therapy system, see §180.2 for special coverage rules.
Injectors (hypodermic jet)	Deny—not covered self-administered drug supply; pressure powered devices (§1861(s)(2)(A) of the Act) for injection of insulin.
Intermittent Positive Pressure Breathing Machines	Covered if patient's ability to breathe is severely impaired.
Iron Lungs	(See Ventilators.)
Irrigating Kit	Deny—nonreusable supply; hygienic equipment (§1861(n) of the Act).
Lambs Wool Pads	(See Alternating Pressure Pads, Mattresses, and Lamb Wool Pads)
Leotards	Deny—(See Pressure Leotards.) (§1861(n) of the Act).
Lymphedema Pumps	Covered (See Pneumatic Compression Devices, §280.6 of this manual.)
Massage Devices	Deny—personal comfort items; not primarily medical in nature (§1861(n) and 1862(a)(6) of the Act).
Mattress	Covered only where hospital bed is medically necessary. (Separate Charge for replacement mattress should not be allowed where hospital bed with mattress is rented.) (See §280.7 of this manual.)
Medical Oxygen Regulators	Covered if patient's ability to breathe is severely impaired. (See §240.2 of this manual.)
Mobile Geriatric Chair	(See Rolling Chairs.)
Motorized Wheelchairs	(See Wheelchairs (power operated).)
Muscle Stimulators	Covered for certain conditions. (See §250.4 of this manual.)
Nebulizers	Covered if patient's ability to breathe is severely impaired.
Oscillating Beds	Deny—institutional equipment - inappropriate for home use.
Overbed Tables	Deny—convenience item; not primarily medical in nature (§1861(n) of the Act).
Oxygen	Covered if the oxygen has been prescribed for use in connection with medically necessary durable medical equipment. (See §240.2 of this manual.)
Oxygen Humidifiers	Covered if the oxygen has been prescribed for use in connection with medically necessary durable medical equipment for purposes of moisturizing oxygen. (See §240.2 of this manual.)
Oxygen Regulators (Medical)	(See Medical Oxygen Regulators.)
Oxygen Tents	(See §240.2 of this manual.)

Item	Coverage
Paraffin Bath Units (Portable)	(See Portable Paraffin Bath Units.)
Paraffin Bath Units (Standard)	Deny—institutional equipment; in appropriate or home use.
Parallel Bars	Deny—support exercise equipment; primarily for institutional use; in the home setting other devices (e.g., a walker) satisfy the patient's need.
Patient Lifts	Covered if contractor's medical staff determines patient's condition is such that periodic movement is necessary to effect improvement or to arrest or retard deterioration in his condition.
Percussors	Covered for mobilizing respiratory tract secretions in patients with chronic obstructive lung disease, chronic bronchitis, or emphysema, when patient or operator of powered percussor has received appropriate training by a physician or therapist, and no one competent to administer manual therapy is available.
Portable Oxygen Systems	1. Regulated (adjustable Covered under conditions specified in a flow rate). Refer all claims to medical staff for this determination. 2. Preset (flow rate Deny emergency, first-aid, or not adjustable) precautionary equipment; essentially not therapeutic in nature.
Portable Paraffin Bath Units	Covered when the patient has undergone a successful trial period of paraffin therapy ordered by a physician and the patient's condition is expected to be relieved by long term use of this modality.
Portable Room Heaters	Deny—environmental control equipment; not primarily medical in nature (§1861(n) of the Act).
Portable Whirlpool Pumps	Deny—not primarily medical in nature; personal comfort items (§§1861(n) and 1862(a)(6) of the Act).
Postural Drainage Boards	Covered if patient has a chronic pulmonary condition.
Preset Portable Oxygen Units	Deny—emergency, first-aid, or precautionary equipment; essentially not therapeutic in nature.
Pressure Leotards	Deny—non-reusable supply, not rental-type item (§1861(n) of the Act).
Pulse Tachometer	Deny—not reasonable or necessary for monitoring pulse of homebound patient with or without a cardiac pacemaker.
Quad-Canes	(See Walkers.)
Raised Toilet Seats	Deny—convenience item; hygienic equipment; not primarily medical in nature (§1861(n) of the Act).
Reflectance Colorimeters	(See Blood Glucose Analyzers.)
Respirators	(See Ventilators.)
Rolling Chairs	Covered if the contractor's medical staff determines that the patient's condition is such that there is a medical need for this item and it has been prescribed by the patient's physician in lieu of a wheelchair. Coverage is limited to those roll-about chairs having casters of at least 5 inches in diameter and specifically designed to meet the needs of ill, injured, or otherwise impaired individuals. Coverage is denied for the wide range of chairs with smaller casters as are found in general use in homes, offices, and institutions for many purposes not related to the care or treatment of ill or injured persons. This type is not primarily medical in nature. (§1861(n) of the Act).
Safety Roller	(See §280.5 of this manual.)
Sauna Baths	Deny—not primarily medical in nature; personal comfort items (§§1861(n) and (1862(a)(6) of the Act).
Seat Lift	Covered under the conditions specified in §280.4 of this manual. Refer all to medical staff for this determination.
Self Contained Pacemaker Monitor	Covered when prescribed by a physician for a patient with a cardiac pacemaker. (See §§20.8.1 and 280.2 of this manual.)
Sitz Bath	Covered if the contractor's medical staff determines patient has an infection or injury of the perineal area and the item has been prescribed by the patient's physician as a part of his planned regimen of treatment in the patient's home.
Spare Tanks of Oxygen	Deny—convenience or precautionary supply.
Speech Teaching Machine	Deny—education equipment; not primarily medical in nature (§1861(n) of the Act).
Stairway Elevators	Deny—(See Elevators.) (§1861(n) of the Act).
Standing Table	Deny—convenience item; not primarily medical in nature (§1861(n) of the Act).
Steam Packs	These packs are Covered under the same condition as a heating pad. (See Heating Pads.)
Suction Machine	Covered if the contractor's medical staff determines that the machine specified in the claim is medically required and appropriate for home use without technical or professional supervision.
Support Hose	Deny—(See Fabric Supports.) (§1861(n) of the Act).
Surgical Leggings	Deny—non-reusable supply; not rental-type item (§1861(n) of the Act).
Telephone Alert Systems	Deny—these are emergency communications systems and do not serve a diagnostic or therapeutic purpose.
Toilet Seats	Deny—not medical equipment (§1861(n) of the Act).

Item	Coverage
Traction Equipment	Covered if patient has orthopedic impairment requiring traction equipment which prevents ambulation during the period of use (Consider covering devices usable during ambulation; e.g., cervical traction collar, under the brace provision).
Trapeze Bars	Covered if patient is bed confined and the patient needs a trapeze bar to sit up because of respiratory condition, to change body position for other medical reasons, or to get in and out of bed.
Treadmill Exerciser	Deny—exercise equipment; not primarily medical in nature (§1861(n) of the Act).
Ultraviolet Cabinet	Covered for selected patients with generalized intractable psoriasis. Using appropriate consultation, the contractor should determine whether medical and other factors justify treatment at home rather than at alternative sites, e.g., outpatient department of a hospital.
Urinals autoclavable	Covered if patient is bed confined hospital type.
Vaporizers	Covered if patient has a respiratory illness.
Ventilators	Covered for treatment of neuromuscular diseases, thoracic restrictive diseases, and chronic respiratory failure consequent to chronic obstructive pulmonary disease. Includes both positive and negative pressure types. (See also §240.5 of this manual.)
Walkers	Covered if patient's condition impairs ambulation (See also §280.5 of this manual.)
Water and Pressure Pads and Mattresses	(See Alternating Pressure Pads, Mattresses and Lamb Wool Pads.)
Wheelchairs (power operated)	Covered if patient's condition is such and wheelchairs with other that a wheelchair is medically necessary special features and the patient is unable to operate the wheelchair manually. Any claim involving a power wheelchair or a wheelchair with other special features should be referred for medical consultation since payment for the special features is limited to those which are medically required because of the patient's condition. (See §280.9 for power operated and §280.3 for specially sized wheelchairs.)

NOTE: A power-operated vehicle that may appropriately be used as a wheelchair can be Covered. (See §280.9 of this manual for coverage details.)

Item	Coverage
Whirlpool Bath Equipment	Covered if patient is homebound and has a (standard)condition for which the whirlpool bath can be expected to provide substantial therapeutic benefit justifying its cost. Where patient is not homebound but has such a condition, payment is restricted to the cost of providing the services elsewhere; e.g., an outpatient department of a participating hospital, if that alternative is less costly. In all cases, refer claim to medical staff for a determination.
Whirlpool Pumps	Deny—(See Portable Whirlpool Pumps.) (§1861(n) of the Act).
White Cane	Deny—(See §280.2 of this manual.)

Cross-references:

The Medicare Benefit Policy Manual, Chapter 15, "Covered Medical and Other Health Services."

The Medicare Claims Processing Manual, Chapter 20, "Durable Medical Equipment, Prosthetics and Orthotics, and Supplies (DMEPOS)."

Pub 100-3, Section 280.14

Infusion Pumps

THE FOLLOWING INDICATIONS FOR TREATMENT USING INFUSION PUMPS ARE COVERED UNDER MEDICARE:

A. External Infusion Pumps.—

1. Iron Poisoning (Effective for Services Performed On or After 9/26/84).—When used in the administration of deferoxamine for the treatment of acute iron poisoning and iron overload, only external infusion pumps are covered.

2. Thromboembolic Disease (Effective for Services Performed On or After 9/26/84).—When used in the administration of heparin for the treatment of thromboembolic disease and/or pulmonary embolism, only external infusion pumps used in an institutional setting are covered.

3. Chemotherapy for Liver Cancer (Effective for Services Performed On or After 1/29/85).—The external chemotherapy infusion pump is covered when used in the treatment of primary hepatocellular carcinoma or colorectal cancer where this disease is unresectable or where the patient refuses surgical excision of the tumor.

4. Morphine for Intractable Cancer Pain (Effective for Services Performed On or After 4/22/85).—Morphine infusion via an external infusion pump is covered when used in the treatment of intractable pain caused by cancer (in either an inpatient or outpatient setting, including a hospice).

5. Continuous subcutaneous insulin infusion pumps (CSII) (Effective for Services Performed On or After 4/1/2000).—

An external infusion pump and related drugs/supplies are covered as medically necessary in the home setting in the following situation: Treatment of diabetes

In order to be covered, patients must meet criterion A or B:

(A) The patient has completed a comprehensive diabetes education program, and has been on a program of multiple daily injections of insulin (i.e. at least 3 injections per day), with frequent self-adjustments of insulin dose for at least 6 months prior to initiation of the insulin pump, and has documented frequency of glucose self-testing an average of at least 4 times per day during the 2 months prior to initiation of the insulin pump, and meets one or more of the following criteria while on the multiple daily injection regimen:

(1) Glycosylated hemoglobin level (HbAlc) > 7.0 percent

(2) History of recurring hypoglycemia

(3) Wide fluctuations in blood glucose before mealtime

(4) Dawn phenomenon with fasting blood sugars frequently exceeding 200 mg/dl

(5) History of severe glycemic excursions

(B) The patient with diabetes has been on a pump prior to enrollment in Medicare and has documented frequency of glucose self-testing an average of at least 4 times per day during the month prior to Medicare enrollment.

Diabetes needs to be documented by a fasting C-peptide level that is less than or equal to 110 percent of the lower limit of normal of the laboratory's measurement method. (Effective for Services Performed on or after January 1, 2002.)

Continued coverage of the insulin pump would require that the patient has been seen and evaluated the treating physician at least every 3 months.

The pump must be ordered by and follow-up care of the patient must be managed by a physician who manages multiple patients with CSII and who works closely with a team including nurses, diabetes educators, and dietitians who are knowledgeable in the use of CSII.

6. Other uses of external infusion pumps are covered if the contractor's medical staff verifies the appropriateness of the therapy and of the prescribed pump for the individual patient.

NOTE: Payment may also be made for drugs necessary for the effective use of an external infusion pump as long as the drug being used with the pump is itself reasonable and necessary for the patient's treatment.

B. Implantable Infusion Pumps.—

1. Chemotherapy for Liver Cancer (Effective for Services Performed On or After 9/26/84).—The implantable infusion pump is covered for intra-arterial infusion of 5-FUdR for the treatment of liver cancer for patients with primary hepatocellular carcinoma or Duke's Class D colorectal cancer, in whom the metastases are limited to the liver, and where (1) the disease is unresectable or (2) where the patient refuses surgical excision of the tumor.

2. Anti-Spasmodic Drugs for Severe Spasticity.—An implantable infusion pump is covered when used to administer anti-spasmodic drugs intrathecally (e.g., baclofen) to treat chronic intractable spasticity in patients who have proven unresponsive to less invasive medical therapy as determined by the following criteria:

As indicated by at least a 6-week trial, the patient cannot be maintained on noninvasive methods of spasm control, such as oral anti-spasmodic drugs, either because these methods fail to control adequately the spasticity or produce intolerable side effects, and

Prior to pump implantation, the patient must have responded favorably to a trial intrathecal dose of the anti-spasmodic drug.

3. Opioid Drugs for Treatment of Chronic Intractable Pain.—An implantable infusion pump is covered when used to administer opioid drugs (e.g., morphine) intrathecally or epidurally for treatment of severe chronic intractable pain of malignant or nonmalignant origin in patients who have a life expectancy of at least 3 months and who have proven unresponsive to less invasive medical therapy as determined by the following criteria:

The patient's history must indicate that he/she would not respond adequately to non-invasive methods of pain control, such as systemic opioids (including attempts to eliminate physical and behavioral abnormalities which may cause an exaggerated reaction to pain); and

A preliminary trial of intraspinal opioid drug administration must be undertaken with a temporary intrathecal/epidural catheter to substantiate adequately acceptable pain relief and degree of side effects (including effects on the activities of daily living) and patient acceptance.

4. Coverage of Other Uses of Implanted Infusion Pumps .—Determinations may be

made on coverage of other uses of implanted infusion pumps if the contractor's medical staff verifies that:

The drug is reasonable and necessary for the treatment of the individual patient;

It is medically necessary that the drug be administered by an implanted infusion pump; and:

The FDA approved labelling for the pump must specify that the drug being administered and the purpose for which it is administered is an indicated use for the pump.

5.Implantation of Infusion Pump Is Contraindicated.—The implantation of an infusion pump is contraindicated in the following patients:

Patients with a known allergy or hypersensitivity to the drug being used (e.g., oral baclofen, morphine, etc.);

Patients who have an infection;

Patients whose body size is insufficient to support the weight and bulk of the device; and:

Patients with other implanted programmable devices since crosstalk between devices may inadvertently change the prescription.

NOTE: Payment may also be made for drugs necessary for the effective use of an implantable infusion pump as long as the drug being used with the pump is itself reasonable and necessary for the patient's treatment.

THE FOLLOWING INDICATIONS FOR TREATMENT USING INFUSION PUMPS ARE NOTCOVERED UNDER MEDICARE:

A. External Infusion Pumps.—

1. Vancomycin (Effective for Services Beginning On or After September 1, 1996).—Medicare coverage of vancomycin as a durable medical equipment infusion pump benefit is not covered. There is insufficient evidence to support the necessity of using an external infusion pump, instead of a disposable elastomeric pump or the gravity drip method, to administer vancomycin in a safe and appropriate manner.

B. Implantable Infusion Pump.—

1. Thromboembolic Disease (Effective for Services Performed On or After 9/26/84).—According to the Public Health Service, there is insufficient published clinical data to support the safety and effectiveness of the heparin implantable pump. Therefore, the use of an implantable infusion pump for infusion of heparin in the treatment of recurrent thromboembolic disease is not covered.

2. Diabetes—Implanted infusion pumps for the infusion of insulin to treat diabetes is not covered. The data do not demonstrate that the pump provides effective administration of insulin.

Pub. 100-3, Section 280.2

White Cane for Use by a Blind Person
(Rev. 1, 10-03-03)

CIM 60-3

Not Covered

A white cane for use by a blind person is more an identifying and self-help device than an item which makes a meaningful contribution in the treatment of an illness or injury.

Pub. 100-3, Section 280.3

Specially Sized Wheelchairs
(Rev. 1, 10-03-03)

CIM 60-6

Payment may be made for a specially sized wheelchair even though it is more expensive than a standard wheelchair. For example, a narrow wheelchair may be required because of the narrow doorways of a patient's home or because of a patient's slender build. Such difference in the size of the wheelchair from the standard model is not considered a deluxe feature.

A physician's certification or prescription that a special size is needed is not required where the contractor can determine from the information in file or other sources that a specially sized wheelchair (rather than a standard one) is needed to accommodate the wheelchair to the place of use or the physical size of the patient.

To determine the reasonable charge in these cases, the contractor uses the criteria set out in the Medicare Claims Processing Manuals, Chapter 23, "Fee Schedule Administration and Coding Requirements," and Chapter 12, "Physician/ Practitioner Billing," as necessary.

Cross-references:

The Medicare Benefit Policy Manual, Chapter 15, "Covered Medical and Other Health Services," §110.

The Medicare Claims Processing Manual, Chapter 20, "Durable Medical Equipment, Prosthetics and Orthotics, and Supplies (DMEPOS)," §§30.5.3 and 20.2

The Medicare Benefit Policy Manual, Chapter 13, "Rural Health Clinic (RHC) and Federally Qualified Health Center (FQHC) Services," §30.1.

Pub. 100-3, Section 280.4

Seat Lift
(Rev. 1, 10-03-03)

CIM 60-8

Reimbursement may be made for the rental or purchase of a medically necessary seat lift when prescribed by a physician for a patient with severe arthritis of the hip or knee and patients with muscular dystrophy or other neuromuscular disease when it has been determined the patient can benefit therapeutically from use of the device. In establishing medical necessity for the seat lift, the evidence must show that the item is included in the physician's course of treatment, that it is likely to effect improvement, or arrest or retard deterioration in the patient's condition, and that the severity of the condition is such that the alternative would be chair or bed confinement.

Coverage of seat lifts is limited to those types which operate smoothly, can be controlled by the patient, and effectively assist a patient in standing up and sitting down without other assistance. Excluded from coverage is the type of lift which operates by a spring release mechanism with a sudden, catapult-like motion and jolts the patient from a seated to a standing position. Limit the payment for units which incorporate a recliner feature along with the seat lift to the amount payable for a seat lift without this feature.

Cross Reference:

The Medicare Claims Processing Manual, Chapter 20, "Durable Medical Equipment, Prosthetics and Orthotics, and Supplies (DMEPOS)," §90.

Pub. 100-3, Section 280.5

Safety Roller
(Rev. 1, 10-03-03)

CIM 60-15

Effective for Claims Adjudicated On or After June 3, 1985

"Safety roller" is the generic name applied to devices for patients who cannot use standard wheeled walkers. They may be appropriate, and therefore covered, for some patients who are obese, have severe neurological disorders, or restricted use of one hand which makes it impossible to use a wheeled walker that does not have the sophisticated braking system found on safety rollers.

In order to assure that payment is not made for a safety roller when a less expensive standard wheeled walker would satisfy the patient's medical needs, carriers should refer safety roller claims to their medical consultants. The medical consultant determines whether some or all of the features provided in a safety roller are necessary, and therefore covered and reimbursable. If it is determined that the patient could use a standard wheeled walker, the charge for the safety roller is reduced to the charge of a standard wheeled walker.

Some obese patients who could use a standard wheeled walker if their weight did not exceed the walker's strength and stability limits can have it reinforced and its wheel base expanded. Such modifications are routine mechanical adjustments and justify a moderate surcharge. In these cases the carrier reduces the charge for the safety roller to the charge for the standard wheeled walker plus the surcharge for modifications.

In the case of patients with medical documentation showing severe neurological disorders or restricted use of one hand which makes it impossible for them to use a wheeled walker that does not have a sophisticated braking system, a reasonable charge for the safety roller may be determined without relating it to the reasonable charge for a standard wheeled walker. (Such reasonable charge should be developed in accordance with the instructions in the Medicare Claims Processing Manual, Chapter 23, "Fee Schedule Administration and Coding Requirements.")

Cross Reference:

The Medicare Benefit Policy Manual, Chapter 15, "Covered Medical and Other Health Services," §120, and §280.1 of this manual.

Pub. 100-3, Section 280.6

Pneumatic Compression Devices
(Rev. 1, 10-03-03)

CIM 60-16

Pneumatic compression devices consist of an inflatable garment for the arm or leg and an electrical pneumatic pump that fills the garment with compressed air. The garment is intermittently inflated and deflated with cycle times and pressures that vary between devices. Pneumatic devices are covered for the treatment of lymphedema or for the treatment of chronic venous insufficiency with venous stasis ulcers.

PUB 100 REFERENCES

Lymphedema

Lymphedema is the swelling of subcutaneous tissues due to the accumulation of excessive lymph fluid. The accumulation of lymph fluid results from impairment to the normal clearing function of the lymphatic system and/or from an excessive production of lymph. Lymphedema is divided into two broad classes according to etiology. Primary lymphedema is a relatively uncommon, chronic condition which may be due to such causes as Milroy's Disease or congenital anomalies. Secondary lymphedema which is much more common, results from the destruction of or damage to formerly functioning lymphatic channels, such as surgical removal of lymph nodes or post radiation fibrosis, among other causes.

Pneumatic compression devices are covered in the home setting for the treatment of lymphedema if the patient has undergone a four-week trial of conservative therapy and the treating physician determines that there has been no significant improvement or if significant symptoms remain after the trial. The trial of conservative therapy must include use of an appropriate compression bandage system or compression garment, exercise, and elevation of the limb. The garment may be prefabricated or custom-fabricated but must provide adequate graduated compression.

Chronic Venous Insufficiency With Venous Stasis Ulcers

Chronic venous insufficiency (CVI) of the lower extremities is a condition caused by abnormalities of the venous wall and valves, leading to obstruction or reflux of blood flow in the veins. Signs of CVI include hyperpigmentation, stasis dermatitis, chronic edema, and venous ulcers.

Pneumatic compression devices are covered in the home setting for the treatment of CVI of the lower extremities only if the patient has one or more venous stasis ulcer(s) which have failed to heal after a six month trial of conservative therapy directed by the treating physician. The trial of conservative therapy must include a compression bandage system or compression garment, appropriate dressings for the wound, exercise, and elevation of the limb.

General Coverage Criteria

Pneumatic compression devices are covered only when prescribed by a physician and when they are used with appropriate physician oversight, i.e., physician evaluation of the patient's condition to determine medical necessity of the device, assuring suitable instruction in the operation of the machine, a treatment plan defining the pressure to be used and the frequency and duration of use, and ongoing monitoring of use and response to treatment.

The determination by the physician of the medical necessity of a pneumatic compression device must include:

1. The patient's diagnosis and prognosis;

2. Symptoms and objective findings, including measurements which establish the severity of the condition;

3. The reason the device is required, including the treatments which have been tried and failed; and

4. The clinical response to an initial treatment with the device.

The clinical response includes the change in pretreatment measurements, ability to tolerate the treatment session and parameters, and ability of the patient (or caregiver) to apply the device for continued use in the home.

The only time that a segmented, calibrated gradient pneumatic compression device (HCPCS code E0652) would be covered is when the individual has unique characteristics that prevent them from receiving satisfactory pneumatic compression treatment using a nonsegmented device in conjunction with a segmented appliance or a segmented compression device without manual control of pressure in each chamber.

Cross Reference: §280.1.

Pub. 100-3, Section 280.7

Hospital Beds
(Rev. 1, 10-03-03)

CIM 60-18

A - General Requirements for Coverage of Hospital Beds

A physician's prescription, and such additional documentation as the contractors' medical staffs may consider necessary, including medical records and physicians' reports, must establish the medical necessity for a hospital bed due to one of the following reasons:

- The patient's condition requires positioning of the body; e.g., to alleviate pain, promote good body alignment, prevent contractures, avoid respiratory infections, in ways not feasible in an ordinary bed; or

- The patient's condition requires special attachments that cannot be fixed and used on an ordinary bed.

B - Physician's Prescription

The physician's prescription which must accompany the initial claim, and supplementing documentation when required, must establish that a hospital bed is medically necessary. If the stated reason for the need for a hospital bed is the patient's condition requires positioning, the prescription or other documentation must describe the medical condition, e.g., cardiac disease, chronic obstructive pulmonary disease, quadriplegia or paraplegia, and also the severity and frequency of the symptoms of the condition, that necessitates a hospital bed for positioning.

If the stated reason for requiring a hospital bed is the patient's condition requires special attachments, the prescription must describe the patient's condition and specify the attachments that require a hospital bed.

C - Variable Height Feature

In well documented cases, the contractors' medical staffs may determine that a variable height feature of a hospital bed, approved for coverage under subsection A above, is medically necessary and, therefore, covered, for one of the following conditions:

- Severe arthritis and other injuries to lower extremities; e.g., fractured hip - The condition requires the variable height feature to assist the patient to ambulate by enabling the patient to place his or her feet on the floor while sitting on the edge of the bed;

- Severe cardiac conditions - For those cardiac patients who are able to leave bed, but who must avoid the strain of "jumping" up or down;

- Spinal cord injuries, including quadriplegic and paraplegic patients, multiple limb amputee and stroke patients. For those patients who are able to transfer from bed to a wheelchair, with or without help; or

- Other severely debilitating diseases and conditions, if the variable height feature is required to assist the patient to ambulate.

D - Electric Powered Hospital Bed Adjustments

Electric powered adjustments to lower and raise head and foot may be covered when the contractor's medical staff determines that the patient's condition requires frequent change in body position and/or there may be an immediate need for a change in body position (i.e., no delay can be tolerated) and the patient can operate the controls and cause the adjustments. Exceptions may be made to this last requirement in cases of spinal cord injury and brain damaged patients.

E - Side Rails

If the patient's condition requires bed side rails, they can be covered when an integral part of, or an accessory to, a hospital bed.

Pub. 100-3, Section 280.8

Air-Fluidized Bed
(Rev. 1, 10-03-03)

CIM 60-19

Air fluidized beds are covered for services rendered on or after: July 30, 1990.

An air-fluidized bed uses warm air under pressure to set small ceramic beads in motion which simulate the movement of fluid. When the patient is placed in the bed, his body weight is evenly distributed over a large surface area which creates a sensation of "floating." Medicare payment for home use of the air-fluidized bed for treatment of pressure sores can be made if such use is reasonable and necessary for the individual patient.

A decision that use of an air-fluidized bed is reasonable and necessary requires that:

- The patient has a stage 3 (full thickness tissue loss) or stage 4 (deep tissue destruction) pressure sore;

- The patient is bedridden or chair bound as a result of severely limited mobility;

- In the absence of an air-fluidized bed, the patient would require institutionalization;

- The air-fluidized bed is ordered in writing by the patient's attending physician based upon a comprehensive assessment and evaluation of the patient after completion of a course of conservative treatment designed to optimize conditions that promote wound healing. This course of treatment must have been at least one month in duration without progression toward wound healing. This month of prerequisite conservative treatment may include some period in an institution as long as there is documentation available to verify that the necessary conservative treatment has been rendered.

- Use of wet-to-dry dressings for wound debridement, begun during the period of conservative treatment and which continue beyond 30 days, will not preclude coverage of air-fluidized bed. Should additional debridement again become necessary, while a patient is using an air-fluidized bed (after the first 30-day course of conservative treatment) that will not cause the air-fluidized bed to become noncovered. In all instances documentation verifying the continued need for the bed must be available.

- A trained adult caregiver is available to assist the patient with activities of daily living, fluid balance, dry skin care, repositioning, recognition and management of altered mental status, dietary needs, prescribed treatments, and management and support of the air-fluidized bed system and its problems such as leakage;

- A physician directs the home treatment regimen, and reevaluates and recertifies the need for the air-fluidized bed on a monthly basis; and

- All other alternative equipment has been considered and ruled out.

Conservative treatment must include:

- Frequent repositioning of the patient with particular attention to relief of pressure over bony prominences (usually every 2 hours);

- Use of a specialized support surface (Group II) designed to reduce pressure and shear forces on healing ulcers and to prevent new ulcer formation;

- Necessary treatment to resolve any wound infection;

- Optimization of nutrition status to promote wound healing;

- Debridement by any means (including wet to dry dressings-which does not require an occlusive covering) to remove devitalized tissue from the wound bed;

- Maintenance of a clean, moist bed of granulation tissue with appropriate moist dressings protected by an occlusive covering, while the wound heals.

Home use of the air-fluidized bed is not covered under any of the following circumstances:

- The patient has coexisting pulmonary disease (the lack of firm back support makes coughing ineffective and dry air inhalation thickens pulmonary secretions);

- The patient requires treatment with wet soaks or moist wound dressings that are not protected with an impervious covering such as plastic wrap or other occlusive material;

- The caregiver is unwilling or unable to provide the type of care required by the patient on an air-fluidized bed;

- Structural support is inadequate to support the weight of the air-fluidized bed system (it generally weighs 1600 pounds or more);

- Electrical system is insufficient for the anticipated increase in energy consumption; or

- Other known contraindications exist.

Coverage of an air-fluidized bed is limited to the equipment itself. Payment for this covered item may only be made if the written order from the attending physician is furnished to the supplier prior to the delivery of the equipment. Payment is not included for the caregiver or for architectural adjustments such as electrical or structural improvement.

Cross reference:

The Medicare Claims Processing Manual, Chapter 23, "Fee Schedule Administration and Coding Requirements," §§60.

Pub. 100-3, Section 280.9

Power Operated Vehicles That May Be Used as Wheelchairs
(Rev. 1, 10-03-03)

CIM 60-5

Power-operated vehicles that may be appropriately used as wheelchairs are covered under the durable medical equipment provision.

These vehicles have been appropriately used in the home setting for vocational rehabilita-tion and to improve the ability of chronically disabled persons to cope with normal domestic, vocational and social activities. They may be covered if a wheelchair is medically necessary and the patient is unable to operate a wheelchair manually.

A specialist in physical medicine, orthopedic surgery, neurology, or rheumatology must provide an evaluation of the patient's medical and physical condition and a prescription for the vehicle to assure that the patient requires the vehicle and is capable of using it safely. When a durable medical equipment regional carrier (DMERC) determines that such a specialist is not reasonably accessible, e.g., more than one day's round trip from the beneficiary's home, or the patient's condition precludes such travel, a prescription from the beneficiary's physician is acceptable.

The DMERC's medical staff reviews all claims for a power-operated vehicle, including the specialists' or other physicians' prescriptions and evaluations of the patient's medical and physical conditions, to insure that all coverage requirements are met. (See §280.1 and the Medicare Claims Processing Manual, Chapter 20,"Durable Medical Equipment, Prosthetics and Orthotics, and Supplies (DMEPOS)," §§110, 120, 130, 140, 150, 160, and 170.)

Pub. 100-3, Section 280.11

Corset Used as Hernia Support
(Rev. 1, 10-03-03)

CIM 70-1

A hernia support (whether in the form of a corset or truss) which meets the definition of a brace is covered under Part B under §1861(s)(9) of the Act. See the Medicare Benefit Policy Manual, Chapter 15, "Covered Medical and Other Services," §130.

Pub. 100-3, Section 280.12

Sykes Hernia Control
(Rev. 1, 10-03-03)

CIM 70-2

Based on professional advice, it has been determined that the sykes hernia control (a spring-type, U-shaped, strapless truss) is not functionally more beneficial than a conventional truss. Make program reimbursement for this device only when an ordinary truss would be covered. (Like all trusses, it is only of benefit when dealing with a reducible hernia). Thus, when a charge for this item is substantially in excess of that which would be reasonable for a conventional truss used for the same condition, base reimbursement on the reasonable charges for the conventional truss. See the Medicare Benefit Policy Manual, Chapter 15, "Covered Medical and Other Services," §130.

Pub 100-3, Section 300.1

Obsolete or Unreliable Diagnostic Tests

A. Diagnostic Tests (Effective for services performed on or after May 15, 1980).—Do not routinely pay for the following diagnostic tests because they are obsolete and have been replaced by more advanced procedures. The listed tests may be paid for only if the medical need for the procedure is satisfactorily justified by the physician who performs it. When the services are subject to PRO review, the PRO is responsible for determining that satisfactory medical justification exists. When the services are not subject to PRO review, the intermediary or carrier is responsible for determining that satisfactory medical justification exists. This includes:

Amylase, blood isoenzymes, electrophoretic,:

Chromium, blood,:

Guanase, blood,:

Zinc sulphate turbidity, blood,:

Skin test, cat scratch fever,:

Skin test, lymphopathia venereum,:

Circulation time, one test,:

Cephalin flocculation,:

Congo red, blood,:

Hormones, adrenocorticotropin quantitative animal tests,:

Hormones, adrenocorticotropin quantitative bioassay,:

Thymol turbidity, blood,:

Skin test, actinomycosis,:

Skin test, brucellosis,:

Skin test, psittacosis,:

Skin test, trichinosis,:

Calcium, feces, 24-hour quantitative,:

Starch, feces, screening,:

Chymotrypsin, duodenal contents,:

Gastric analysis, pepsin,:

Gastric analysis, tubeless,:

Calcium saturation clotting time,:

Capillary fragility test (Rumpel-Leede),:

Colloidal gold,:

Bendien's test for cancer and tuberculosis,:

Bolen's test for cancer,:

Rehfuss test for gastric acidity, and:

Serum seromucoid assay for cancer and other diseases.

B. Cardiovascular Tests (Effective for services performed on or after January 1, 1997).— Do not pay for the following phonocardiography and vectorcardiography diagnostic tests because they have been determined to be outmoded and of little clinical value. They include:

CPT code 93201, Phonocardiogram with or without ECG lead; with supervision during recording with interpretation and report (when equipment is supplied by the physician),:

CPT code 93202, Phonocardiogram; tracing only, without interpretation and report (e.g., when equipment is supplied by the hospital, clinic),:

CPT code 93204, Phonocardiogram; interpretation and report,:

CPT code 93205, Phonocardiogram with ECG lead, with indirect carotid artery and/or jugular vein tracing, and/or apex cardiogram; with interpretation and report,:

CPT code 93208, Phonocardiogram; without interpretation and report,:

CPT code 93209, Phonocardiogram; interpretation and report only,:

CPT code 93210, Intracardiac,:

CPT code 93220, Vectorcardiogram (VCG), with or without ECG; with interpretation and report,:

CPT code 93221, Vectorcardiogram; tracing only, without interpretation and report, and:

CPT code 93222, Vectorcardiogram; interpretation and report only.

Pub. 100-4, Chapter 1, Section 30.3.5

Effect of Assignment Upon Purchase of Cataract Glasses From Participating Physician or Supp
B3-3045.4

A pair of cataract glasses is comprised of two distinct products: a professional product (the prescribed lenses) and a retail commercial product (the frames). The frames serve not only as a holder of lenses but also as an article of personal apparel. As such, they are usually selected on the basis of personal taste and style. Although Medicare will pay only for standard frames, most patients want deluxe frames. Participating physicians and suppliers cannot profitably furnish such deluxe frames unless they can make an extra (noncovered) charge for the frames even though they accept assignment.

Therefore, a participating physician or supplier (whether an ophthalmologist, optometrist, or optician) who accepts assignment on cataract glasses with deluxe frames may charge the Medicare patient the difference between his/her usual charge to private pay patients for glasses with standard frames and his/her usual charge to such patients for glasses with deluxe frames, in addition to the applicable deductible and coinsurance on glasses with standard frames, if all of the following requirements are met:

A. The participating physician or supplier has standard frames available, offers them for sale to the patient, and issues and ABN to the patient that explains the price and other differences between standard and deluxe frames. Refer to Chapter 30.

B. The participating physician or supplier obtains from the patient (or his/her representative) and keeps on file the following signed and dated statement:

Name of Patient   Medicare Claim Number

Having been informed that an extra charge is being made by the physician or supplier for deluxe frames, that this extra charge is not covered by Medicare, and that standard frames are available for purchase from the physician or supplier at no extra charge, I have chosen to purchase deluxe frames. _____ Signature   Date

C. The participating physician or supplier itemizes on his/her claim his/her actual charge for the lenses, his/her actual charge for the standard frames, and his/her actual extra charge for the deluxe frames (charge differential).

Once the assigned claim for deluxe frames has been processed, the carrier will follow the ABN instructions as described in §60.

Pub. 100-4, Chapter 8, Section 60.4.2

Epoetin Alfa (EPO) Supplier Billing Requirements (Method II) on the Form CMS-1500 and Electronic Equivalent
(Rev 118, 03-05-04)

A. Claims with dates of service prior to January 1, 2004:

For claims with dates of service prior to January 1, 2004, the correct EPO code to use is the one that indicates the patient's most recent hematocrit (HCT) (rounded to the nearest whole percent) or hemoglobin (Hgb) (rounded to the nearest g/dl) prior to the date of service of the EPO. For example, if the patient's most recent hematocrit was 20.5 percent, bill Q9921; if it was 28.4 percent, bill Q9928.

To convert actual hemoglobin to corresponding hematocrit for Q code reporting, multiply the Hgb value by 3 and round to the nearest whole number. For example, if Hgb = 8.4, report as Q9925 (8.4 X 3 = 25.2, rounded down to 25).

One unit of service of EPO is reported for each 1000 units dispensed. For example if 20,000 units are dispensed, bill 20 units. If the dose dispensed is not an even multiple of

1,000, rounded down for 1 - 499 units (e.g. 20,400 units dispensed = 20 units billed), round up for 500 - 999 units (e.g. 20,500 units dispensed = 21 units billed).

Q9920 Injection of EPO, per 1,000 units, at patient HCT of 20 or less

Q9921 Injection of EPO, per 1,000 units, at patient HCT of 21

Q9922 Injection of EPO, per 1,000 units, at patient HCT of 22

Q9923 Injection of EPO, per 1,000 units, at patient HCT of 23

Q9924 Injection of EPO, per 1,000 units, at patient HCT of 24

Q9925 Injection of EPO, per 1,000 units, at patient HCT of 25

Q9926 Injection of EPO, per 1,000 units, at patient HCT of 26

Q9927 Injection of EPO, per 1,000 units, at patient HCT of 27

Q9928 Injection of EPO, per 1,000 units, at patient HCT of 28

Q9929 Injection of EPO, per 1,000 units, at patient HCT of 29

Q9930 Injection of EPO, per 1,000 units, at patient HCT of 30

Q9931 Injection of EPO, per 1,000 units, at patient HCT of 31

Q9932 Injection of EPO, per 1,000 units, at patient HCT of 32

Q9933 Injection of EPO, per 1,000 units, at patient HCT of 33

Q9934 Injection of EPO, per 1,000 units, at patient HCT of 34

Q9935 Injection of EPO, per 1,000 units, at patient HCT of 35

Q9936 Injection of EPO, per 1,000 units, at patient HCT of 36

Q9937 Injection of EPO, per 1,000 units, at patient HCT of 37

Q9938 Injection of EPO, per 1,000 units, at patient HCT of 38

Q9939 Injection of EPO, per 1,000 units, at patient HCT of 39

Q9940 Injection of EPO, per 1,000 units, at patient HCT of 40 or above.

B. Claims with Dates of Service January 1, 2004 and after

The above codes were replaced effective January 1, 2004 by Q4055. This Q code is for the injection of EPO furnished to ESRD Beneficiaries on Dialysis. The new code does not include the hematocrit. See §60.7.

Q4055 – Injection, Epoetin alfa, 1,000 units (for ESRD on Dialysis).

The DMERC shall return to provider (RTP) assigned claims for EPO, Q4055, that do not contain a HCT value. For unassigned claims, the DMERC shall deny claims for EPO, Q4055 that do not contain a HCT value.

DMERCs must use the following messages when payment for the injection (Q4055) does not meet the coverage criteria and is denied:

MSN Message 6.5—English: Medicare cannot pay for this injection because one or more requirements for coverage were not met

MSN Message 6.5—Spanish: Medicare no puede pagar por esta inyeccion porque uno o mas requisitos para la cubierta no fueron cumplidos. (MSN Message 6.5 in Spanish).

Adjustment Reason Code B:5 Payment adjusted because coverage/program guidelines were not met or were exceeded.

The DMERCs shall use the following messages when returning as unprocessable assigned claims without a HCT value:

ANSI Reason Code 16 – Claim/service lacks information, which is needed for adjudication.

Additional information is supplied using remittance advice remarks codes whenever appropriate.

Remark Code M58 – Missing/incomplete/invalid claim information. Resubmit claim after corrections.

Deductibles and coinsurance apply.

Pub. 100-4, Chapter 8, Section 60.4.2.1

Other Information Required on the Form CMS-1500
(Rev 118, 03-05-04)

The following information is required for EPO. Incomplete assigned claims are returned to providers for completion. Incomplete unassigned claims are rejected. The rejection will be due to a lack of a HCT value. Note that when a claim is submitted on paper Form CMS-1500, these items are submitted on a separate document. It is not necessary to enter them into the claims processing system. This information is used in utilization review.

A. Diagnoses - The diagnoses must be submitted according to ICD-9-CM and correlated to the procedure. This information is in Item 21, of the Form CMS-1500.

B. Hematocrit (HCT)/Hemoglobin (Hgb) - There are special HCPCS codes for reporting the injection of EPO for claims with dates of service prior to January 1, 2004. These allow the simultaneous reporting of the patient's latest HCT or Hgb reading before administration of EPO.

The physician and/or staff are instructed to enter a separate line item for injections of EPO at different HCT/Hgb levels. The Q code for each line items is entered in Item 24D.

1. Code Q9920 - Injection of EPO, per 1,000 units, at patient HCT of 20 or less/Hgb of 6.8 or less.

2. Codes Q9921 through Q9939 - Injection of EPO, per 1,000 units, at patient HCT of 21 to 39/Hgb of 6.9 to 13.1. For HCT levels of 21 or more, up to a HCT of 39/Hgb of 6.9 to 13.1, a Q code that includes the actual HCT levels is used. To convert actual Hgb to corresponding HCT values for Q code reporting, multiply the Hgb value by 3 and round to the nearest whole number. Use the whole number to determine the appropriate Q code.

EXAMPLES: If the patient's HCT is 25/Hgb is 8.2-8.4, Q9925 must be entered on the claim. If the patient's HCT is 39/Hgb is 12.9-13.1, Q9939 is entered.

3. Code Q9940 - Injection of EPO, per 1,000 units at patient HCT of 40 or above.

A single line item may include multiple doses of EPO administered while the patient's HCT level remained the same.

Codes Q9920-Q9940 will no longer be recognized by the system if submitted after March 31, 2004. If claims for dates of service prior to January 1, 2004 are submitted after March 31, 2004, then code Q4055 must be used.

C. Units Administered - The standard unit of EPO is 1,000. The number of 1,000 units administered per line item is included on the claim. The physician's office enters 1 in the units field for each multiple of 1,000 units. For example, if 12,000 units are administered, 12 is entered. This information is shown in Item 24G (Days/Units) on Form CMS-1500.

In some cases, the dosage for a single line item does not total an even multiple of 1,000. If this occurs, the physician's office rounds down supplemental dosages of 0 to 499 units to the prior 1,000 units. Supplemental dosages of 500 to 999 are rounded up to the next 1,000 units.

EXAMPLES

A patient's HCT reading on August 6 was 22/Hgb was 7.3. The patient received 5,000 units of EPO on August 7, August 9, and August 11, for a total of 15,000 units. The first line of Item 24 of Form CMS-1500 shows:

Dates of Service	Procedure Code	Days or Units
8/7 – 8/11	Q9922	15

On September 13, the patient's HCT reading increased to 27/Hgb increased to 9. The patient received 5,100 units of EPO on September 13, September 15, and September 17, for a total of 15,300 units. Since less than 15,500 units were given, the figure is rounded down to 15,000. This line on the claim form shows:

Dates of Service	Procedure Code	Days or Units
9/13 – 9/17	Q9927	15

On October 16, the HCT level increased to 33/Hgb increased to 11. The patient received doses of 4,850 units on October 16, October 18, and October 20 for a total of 14,550 units. Since more than 14,500 units were administered, the figure is rounded up to 15,000. Form CMS-1500 shows:

Dates of Service	Procedure Code	Days or Units
10/16 – 10/20	Q9933	15

NOTE: Creatinine and weight identified below are required on EPO claims as applicable.

D. Date of the Patient's most recent HCT or Hgb.

E. Most recent HCT or Hgb level - (prior to initiation of EPO therapy).

F. Date of most recent HCT or Hgb level - (prior to initiation of EPO therapy).

G. Patient's most recent serum creatinine - (within the last month, prior to initiation of EPO therapy).

H. Date of most recent serum creatinine - (prior to initiation of EPO therapy).

I. Patient's weight in kilograms

J. Patient's starting dose per kilogram - (The usual starting dose is 50-100 units per kilogram.)

Pub. 100-4, Chapter 8, Section 70

Payment for Home Dialysis

A3-3644, PRM-1-2706.1.E, PRM-1-2706.2, A3-3169, RO-2 3440.2, B3-4270.1

Home dialysis is dialysis performed by an appropriately trained dialysis patient at home. Hemodialysis, CCPD, IPD and CAPD may be performed at home. For all dialysis services furnished by an ESRD facility, the facility must accept assignment, and only the facility may be paid by the Medicare program. Method II suppliers can receive payment for patients selecting Method II. The Method II supplier must accept assignment. Method II suppliers receive payment for supplies and equipment only.

For purposes of home dialysis, a skilled nursing facility (SNF) may qualify as a beneficiary's home. The services are excluded from SNF consolidated billing for its inpatients. The home dialysis services are billed either by the ESRD facility or the supplier depending on the Method selection made by the beneficiary.

Pub. 100-4, Chapter 8, Section 80

Home Dialysis Method I Billing to the Intermediary

A3-3644.A, PRM-1-2710, PRM-1-2710.4, A3-3169, RDF-318, RO2-3440, B3-4270, B3-4271

If the Medicare home dialysis patient chooses Method I, the dialysis facility with which the Medicare home patient is associated assumes responsibility for providing all home dialysis equipment and supplies, and home support services. For these services, the facility receives the same Medicare dialysis payment rate as it would receive for an in-facility patient under the composite rate system. The beneficiary is responsible for paying any unmet Part B deductible and the 20-percent coinsurance. After the beneficiary's Part B deductible is met, the FI pays 80 percent of the specific facility's composite rate for each in-facility outpatient maintenance dialysis treatment.

Under Method I items and services included in the composite rate must be furnished by the facility, either directly or under arrangement. The cost of an item or service is included under the composite rate unless specifically excluded. Therefore, the determination as to whether an item or service is covered under the composite rate payment does not depend on the frequency that dialysis patients require the item or service, or the number of patients who require it. If the facility fails to provide (either directly or under arrangement) any part of the items and services covered under the rate, the facility cannot be paid any amount for the items and services that it does furnish.

New items or services developed after the rate applicable for that particular year was computed are included in the composite rate payments. As such, ESRD facilities assume the responsibility for providing a dialysis service and must decide whether a particular item or service is medically appropriate and cost effective. Since the composite rate is adjusted, as necessary, based on the most recent cost data available to CMS, the costs of new items and services are taken into account in setting future rates. Similarly, any savings attributable to advancements in the treatment of ESRD accrue to the facility because no adjustment to any individual facility's rate is made.

Pub. 100-4, Chapter 8, Section 90

Method II Billing

A3-3644.A, RO-2-3440.C, B3-4270, B3-4271, B3-4270.1, B3-4270.2, B3-34271, PRM-1-2740, A3-3644.3

Physicians and independent laboratories, must submit claims (Form CMS-1500 or electronic equivalent) to their local carrier for services furnished to end stage renal disease (ESRD) beneficiaries. Suppliers of Method II dialysis equipment and supplies will submit their claims (Form CMS-1500 or electronic equivalent) to the appropriate Durable Medical Equipment Regional Carriers (DMERCs). All ESRD facilities must submit their claims to their appropriate FI.

The amount of Medicare payment under Method II for home dialysis equipment and supplies may NOT exceed $1974.45 for continuous cycling peritoneal dialysis (CCPD) and $1490.85 for all other methods of dialysis.

All laboratory tests furnished to home dialysis patients who have selected payment Method II (see §70.1 above), are billed to and paid by the carrier at the fee schedule, if the tests are performed by an independent laboratory for an independent dialysis facility patient.

If the beneficiary elects to deal directly with a supplier and make arrangements for securing the necessary supplies and equipment to dialyze at home, and chooses Method II, he/she deals directly with a supplier of home dialysis equipment and supplies (this supplier is not a dialysis facility). A supplier other than a facility bills the DMERC. There can be only one supplier per beneficiary, and the supplier must accept assignment. The beneficiary is responsible for any unmet Part B deductible and the 20 percent coinsurance.

Only a supplier that is not a dialysis facility may submit a claim to a DMERC for home dialysis supplies and equipment. Suppliers will submit these claims on Form CMS-1500, or electronic equivalent. Under Method II, beneficiaries may not submit any claims and cannot receive payment for any benefits for home dialysis equipment and supplies.

PUB 100 REFERENCES

The supplier must have a written agreement with a Medicare approved dialysis facility that will provide all necessary support, backup, and emergency dialysis services. The dialysis facility will not receive a regular per treatment payment for a patient who chooses Method II.

However, if the facility provides any support services, backup, and emergency dialysis services to a beneficiary who selects this option, the facility is reimbursed for the items or services it furnishes. Hospital-based facilities are paid the reasonable cost of support services, subject to the lesser of cost or charges provisions of §1833(a)(2)(A) of the Act. Independent facilities are paid on a reasonable charge basis for any home dialysis support services they furnish.

A - Description of Support Services

Support services specifically applicable to home patients include but are not limited to:

  Surveillance of the patient's home adaptation, including provisions for visits to the home in accordance with a written plan prepared and periodically reviewed by a team that includes the patient's physician and other professionals familiar with the patient's condition;

  Furnishing dialysis-related emergency services;

  Consultation for the patient with a qualified social worker and a qualified dietician;

  Maintaining a record-keeping system which assures continuity of care;

  Maintaining and submitting all required documentation to the ESRD network;

  Assuring that the water supply is of the appropriate quality;

  Assuring that the appropriate supplies are ordered on an ongoing basis;

  Arranging for the provision of all ESRD laboratory tests;

  Testing and appropriate treatment of water used in dialysis;

  Monitoring the functioning of dialysis equipment;

  All other necessary dialysis services as required under the ESRD conditions for coverage;

  Watching the patient perform CAPD and assuring that it is done correctly, and reviewing with the patient any aspects of the technique he/she may have forgotten, or informing the patient of modification in apparatus or technique;

  Documenting whether the patient has or has not had peritonitis that requires physician intervention or hospitalization, (unless there is evidence of peritonitis, a culture for peritonitis is not necessary);

  Inspection of the catheter site; and

  Since home dialysis support services include maintaining a medical record for each home dialysis patient, the Method II supplier must report to the support service dialysis facility within 30 days all items and services that it furnished to the patient so that the facility can record this information in the patient's medical record.

The services must be furnished in accordance with the written plan required for home dialysis patients. See the Medicare Benefit Policy Manual, Chapter 15, for coverage of telehealth services, and this manual, Chapter 12 for billing telehealth.

Each of the support services may be paid routinely at a frequency of once per month. Any support services furnished in excess of this frequency must be documented for being reasonable and necessary. For example, the patient may contract peritonitis and require an unscheduled connecting tube change.

B - Reasonableness Determinations

Support services (which include the laboratory services included under the composite rate for in-facility patients) are paid on a reasonable charge basis to independent facilities and a reasonable cost basis to hospital-based facilities, subject to the Method II payment cap (refer to §140). A reasonable cost/charge determination must be made for each individual support service furnished to home patients. With respect to the connecting tube change, facilities may bill Medicare for the personnel services required to change the connecting tube, but must look to the Method II supplier for payment for the connecting tube itself.

The payment cap is not a payment rate that is paid automatically each month. Accordingly, in no case may the FI routinely pay any monthly amount for support services without a claim that shows the services actually furnished.

Pub. 100-4, Chapter 8, Section 90.1

DMERC Denials for Beneficiary Submitted Claims Under Method II

A3-3170.6, A3-3644.3, A3-3644.3.A - E, HO-238.2.C, HO-238.3, HO-238.3.A, B3-2231.3.A and B, B3-2231, B3-4270.1, PRM-1-2709.2.A

Under Method II, beneficiaries may not submit any claims and cannot receive payment for any benefits for home dialysis equipment and supplies. DMERCs must deny unassigned and beneficiary submitted claims with the following MSN messages.

MSN # 16.6: "This item or service cannot be paid unless the provider accepts assignment."

Spanish: "Este artículo o servicio no se pagará a menos de que el proveedor acepte asignación."

MSN # 16.7: "Your provider must complete and submit your claim."

Spanish: "Su proveedor debe completar y someter su reclamación."

MSN # 16.36: "If you have already paid it, you are entitled to a refund from this provider."

Spanish: "Si usted ya lo ha pagado, tiene derecho a un reebolso de su proveedor."

Pub. 100-4, Chapter 8, Section 90.3.2

Home Dialysis Supplies and Equipment HCPCS Codes Used to Bill the DMERC

PM B-01-56, B3-4270 updated 11-16-01(CR 1799)

A - HCPCS Codes

Prior to January 1, 2002, suppliers billed for dialysis supplies using codes describing "kits" of supplies. The use of kit codes such as A4820, A4900, A4901, A4905, and A4914 allows suppliers to bill for supply items without separately identifying the supplies that are being furnished to the patient. Effective January 1, 2002, these kit codes were deleted and suppliers are now required to bill for dialysis supplies using existing and newly developed HCPCS codes for individual dialysis items. Refer to the LMRP for the HCPCS codes for dialysis supplies and equipment that are effective for claims received on or after January 1, 2002.

A4651	A4652	A4656	A4657
A4660	A4663	A4680	A4690
A4706	A4707	A4708	A4709
A4712	A4714	A4719	A4720
A4721	A4722	A4723	A4724
A4725	A4726	A4730	A4736
A4737	A4740	A4750	A4755
A4760	A4765	A4766	A4770
A4771	A4772	A4773	A4774
A4801	A4802	A4860	A4870
A4911	A4913	A4918	A4927
A4928	A4929	A4500	A4510
E1520	E1530	E1540	E1550
E1560	E1570	E1575	E1580
E1590	E1592	E1594	E1600
E1610	E1615	E1620	E1625
E1630	E1632	E1635	E1636
E1637	E1638	E1639	E1699

DMERCs gap-fill reasonable charge amounts for 2002 for all of the applicable codes other than codes A4913 and E1699, the codes used for miscellaneous supplies and equipment that do not fall under any of the other HCPCS codes. The gap-filled amounts should be established using price lists in effect as of December 31, 2000 if available. These gap-filled payment amounts will apply to all claims with dates of service from January 1, 2002, through December 31, 2002.

Codes A4650 - A4927 and E1510 - E1702 may be used only for supplies and equipment relating to home dialysis. In particular, items not related to dialysis should not be included in the supply kit codes (A4820, A4900, A4901, A4905) or listed in the miscellaneous codes (A4910, A4913, E1699). Conversely, supplies and equipment relating to home dialysis should not be billed using other HCPCS codes.

Dialysis supply kits (A4820, A4900, A4901, A4905) billed by an individual supplier must contain the same type and quantity of supplies each time that it is billed. One unit of service would represent the typical amount of supplies needed for one month of dialysis. The content of the kit may not vary from patient to patient or in a single patient from month to month unless the 52 modifier is used (see below). If more than this typical amount of supplies is needed in one month, the excess supplies should be billed using other dialysis supply codes. If significantly less than the usual amount is needed for 1 month, the 52 modifier should be added to the code and the submitted charge reduced accordingly. A listing of the components of each kit billed by a supplier must be available for review by the DMERC.

For items before January 1, 2002, dialysis solutions (A4700, A4705) should not be included in the supply kit but should be separately billed. One unit of service for these codes is for one liter of dialysis solution.

For items before January 1, 2002, items not included in kits must be billed separately, using either a specific code (A4650 - A4927) or miscellaneous code (A4910, A4913, E1699).

Code A4901 and/or E1594 should be billed for each month that the patient receives CCPD.

An EM modifier should be added to a dialysis supply code when it represents emergency reserve supplies over and above the typical monthly amount.

B - Modifiers

Method II suppliers must maintain documentation to support the existence of a written agreement with a Medicare certified support service facility within a reasonable distance from the beneficiary's home.

Effective July 1, 2002, suppliers must use "KX" modifier on the line item level for all Method II home dialysis claims to indicate that they have this documentation on file, and must provide it to the DMERC upon request. As of July 1, 2002, DMERCs must front end reject any Method II claims that do not have the "KX" modifier at the line level. The supplier may correct and resubmit the claim with the appropriate modifier. DMERCs and the shared systems must make all systems changes necessary to reject Method II claims that do not have the "KX" modifier.

The following listed modifiers are frequently used to identify the service/charges billed for Dialysis Supplies.

CC-Procedure code change - Used by the carrier when the procedure code submitted was changed either for administrative reasons or because an incorrect procedure code was filed. Do not use this modifier when filing claims to Palmetto GBA.

EJ-Subsequent Claim (for Erythropoietin Alpha-EPO injection only)

EM-Emergency reserve supply [for End Stage Renal Disease (ESRD) benefit only]

KY-Specific requirements found in the Documentation section of the Medical Policy have been met and evidence of this is available in the supplier's record. Effective July 1, 2002, suppliers must use the "KY" modifier on the line item level for all Method II home dialysis claims.

NU-New Equipment - Used when purchasing new equipment.

RR-Initial Rental - Rental (use the -RR modifier when DME is to be rented).

UE-Used durable medical equipment

ZU-Advance notice of possible medical necessity denial on file (this modifier will be discontinued with the implementation of HIPAA)

ZY-Potentially noncovered item or service billed for denial or at the beneficiary's request (not to be used for medical necessity denials) (this modifier will be discontinued with the implementation of HIPAA)

Pub. 100-4, Chapter 8, Section 120.1

Payment for Immunosuppressive Drugs Furnished to Transplant Patients
PRM-1-2711.5, B3-4471, AB-01-10

A. General

Effective January 1, 1987, Medicare pays for FDA approved self-administered immunosuppressive drugs. Generally, under this benefit, payment is made for self-administered immunosuppressive drugs that are specifically labeled and approved for marketing as such by the FDA, as well as those prescription drugs, such as prednisone, that are used in conjunction with immunosuppressive drugs as part of a therapeutic regimen reflected in FDA approved labeling for immunosuppressive drugs. This benefit is subject to the Part B deductible and coinsurance provision. There is no time limitation on the coverage of these drugs; however, if a beneficiary loses Medicare coverage as a result of the transplant, the drugs are no longer covered. When the beneficiary reaches the age of 65 and becomes entitled, that person can have the drugs covered again. The hospital pharmacy must ask the physician to furnish the patient with a non-refillable 30-day prescription for the immunosuppressive drugs. This is because the dosage of these drugs frequently diminishes over a period of time, and it is not uncommon for the physician to change the prescription from one drug to another because of the patient's needs. Also, these drugs are expensive, and the coinsurance liability on unused drugs could be a financial burden to the beneficiary. Unless there are special circumstances, the FI and carrier do not consider a supply of drugs in excess of 30 days to be reasonable and necessary and limits payment accordingly.

B. Payment

Payment is made on a reasonable cost basis if the beneficiary is the outpatient of a participating hospital. In all other cases, payment is made on an allowable charge basis.

C. FDA Approved Drugs

Some of the most commonly prescribed immunosuppressive drugs are:

Sandimmune (cyclosporine), Sandoz Pharmaceutical (oral or parenteral),

Imuran (azathioprine), Burroughs Wellcome Vial (oral),

Atgam (antithymocyte/globulin), Upjohn (parenteral); and

Orthoclone OKT3 (muromonab - CD3) Ortho Pharmaceutical (parenteral).

Also covered are prescription drugs used in conjunction with immunosuppressive drugs as part of a therapeutic regimen reflected in FDA approved labeling for immunosuppressive drugs.

The payment for the drug is limited to the cost of the most frequently administered dosage of the drug (adjusted for medical factors as determined by the physician).

Consult such sources as the Drug Topics Red Book, American Druggists Blue Book, and Medispan, realizing that substantial discounts are available.

Pub. 100-4, Chapter 8, Section 130

Physicians and Supplier (Nonfacility) Billing for ESRD Services - General
B3-4270 updated with Transmittal 1729

Payment for renal-related physicians' services to ESRD patients is made in either of the following ways:

Under the Monthly Capitation Payment (MCP) (see §140 below for an explanation of the MCP); or

Using the daily codes for ESRD services (CPT codes 90922-90925) with units that represent the number of days services were furnished.

Under the Initial method (IM)

The carrier receives bills (Form CMS—1500 or electronic equivalent) from physicians for services furnished ESRD beneficiaries. DMERCs receive bills for equipment and supplies for Method II beneficiaries. Intermediaries receive bills from ESRD facilities. Lab bills from CLIA certified independent dialysis facilities were billed to the carrier before September 1, 1997, and to the FI beginning on that date. Other certified labs continue to bill the carrier.

Pub. 100-4, Chapter 12, Section 30.4

Echocardiography Services (Codes 93303 - 93350)
B3-15360

Effective October 1, 2000, physicians may separately bill for contrast agents used in echocardiography. Physicians should use HCPCS Code A9700 (Supply of injectable contrast material for use in echocardiography, per study). The type of service code is 9. This code will be carrier-priced.

Pub. 100-4, Chapter 12, Section 70

Payment Conditions for Radiology Services
B3-15022

See Chapter 13 for claims processing instructions for radiology.

Pub. 100-4, Chpater 12, Section 210.1

Application of Limitation
(Rev. 1, 10-01-03)

B3-2472 - 2472.5

A - Status of Patient

The limitation is applicable to expenses incurred in connection with the treatment of an individual who is not an inpatient of a hospital. Thus, the limitation applies to mental health services furnished to a person in a physician's office, in the patient's home, in a skilled nursing facility, as an outpatient, and so forth. The term "hospital" in this context means an institution, which is primarily engaged in providing to inpatients, by or under the supervision of physician(s):

- Diagnostic and therapeutic services for medical diagnosis, treatment and care of injured, disabled, or sick persons;

- Rehabilitation services for injured, disabled, or sick persons; or

- Psychiatric services for the diagnosis and treatment of mentally ill patients.

B - Disorders Subject to Limitation

The term "mental, psychoneurotic, and personality disorders" is defined as the specific psychiatric conditions described in the American Psychiatric Association's (APA) "Diagnostic and Statistical Manual of Mental Disorders, Third Edition - Revised (DSM-III-R)."

When the treatment services rendered are both for a psychiatric condition as defined in the DSM-III-R and one or more nonpsychiatric conditions, separate the expenses for the psychiatric aspects of treatment from the expenses for the nonpsychiatric aspects of treatment. However, in any case in which the psychiatric treatment component is not readily distinguishable from the nonpsychiatric treatment component, all of the expenses are allocated to whichever component constitutes the primary diagnosis.

1. Diagnosis Clearly Meets Definition - If the primary diagnosis reported for a particular service is the same as or equivalent to a condition described in the

PUB 100 REFERENCES

APA's DSM-III-R, the expense for the service is subject to the limitation except as described in subsection D.

2. Diagnosis Does Not Clearly Meet Definition - When it is not clear whether the primary diagnosis reported meets the definition of mental, psychoneurotic, and personality disorders, it may be necessary to contact the practitioner to clarify the diagnosis. In deciding whether contact is necessary in a given case, give consideration to such factors as the type of services rendered, the diagnosis, and the individual's previous utilization history.

C - Services Subject to Limitation

Carriers apply the limitation to claims for professional services that represent mental health treatment furnished to individuals who are not hospital inpatients by physicians, clinical psychologists, clinical social workers, and other allied health professionals. Items and supplies furnished by physicians or other mental health practitioners in connection with treatment are also subject to the limitation. (The limitation also applies to CORF claims processed by intermediaries.)

Carriers apply the limitation only to treatment services. It does not apply to diagnostic services as described in subsection D. Testing services performed to evaluate a patient's progress during treatment are considered part of treatment and are subject to the limitation.

D - Services Not Subject to Limitation

1. Diagnosis of Alzheimer's Disease or Related Disorder - When the primary diagnosis reported for a particular service is Alzheimer's Disease (coded 331.0 in the "International Classification of Diseases, 9th Revision") or Alzheimer's or other disorders coded 290.XX in the APA's DSM-III-R, carriers look to the nature of the service that has been rendered in determining whether it is subject to the limitation. Typically, treatment provided to a patient with a diagnosis of Alzheimer's Disease or a related disorder represents medical management of the patient's condition (rather than psychiatric treatment) and is not subject to the limitation. However, when the primary treatment rendered to a patient with such a diagnosis is psychotherapy, it is subject to the limitation.

2. Brief Office Visits for Monitoring or Changing Drug Prescriptions - Brief office visits for the sole purpose of monitoring or changing drug prescriptions used in the treatment of mental, psychoneurotic and personality disorders are not subject to the limitation. These visits are reported using HCPCS code M0064 (brief office visit for the sole purpose of monitoring or changing drug prescriptions used in the treatment of mental, psychoneurotic, and personality disorders). Claims where the diagnosis reported is a mental, psychoneurotic, or personality disorder (other than a diagnosis specified in subsection A) are subject to the limitation except for the procedure identified by HCPCS code M0064.

3. Diagnostic Services - Carriers do not apply the limitation to tests and evaluations performed to establish or confirm the patient's diagnosis. Diagnostic services include psychiatric or psychological tests and interpretations, diagnostic consultations, and initial evaluations.

   An initial visit to a practitioner for professional services often combines diagnostic evaluation and the start of therapy. Such a visit is neither solely diagnostic nor solely therapeutic. Therefore, carriers deem the initial visit to be diagnostic so that the limitation does not apply. Separating diagnostic and therapeutic components of a visit is not administratively feasible, unless the practitioner already has separately identified them on the bill. Determining the entire visit to be therapeutic is not justifiable since some diagnostic work must be done before even a tentative diagnosis can be made and certainly before therapy can be instituted. Moreover, the patient should not be disadvantaged because therapeutic as well as diagnostic services were provided in the initial visit. In the rare cases where a practitioner's diagnostic services take more than one visit, carriers do not apply the limitation to the additional visits. However, it is expected such cases are few. Therefore, when a practitioner bills for more than one visit for professional diagnostic services, carriers request documentation to justify the reason for more than one diagnostic visit.

4. Partial Hospitalization Services Not Directly Provided by Physician - The limitation does not apply to partial hospitalization services that are not directly provided by a physician. These services are billed by hospitals and community mental health centers (CMHCs) to intermediaries.

E - Computation of Limitation

Carriers determine the Medicare allowed payment amount for services subject to the limitation. They:

- Multiply this amount by 0.625;
- Subtract any unsatisfied deductible; and,
- Multiply the remainder by 0.8 to obtain the amount of Medicare payment.

The beneficiary is responsible for the difference between the amount paid by Medicare and the full allowed amount.

EXAMPLE A

A beneficiary is referred to a Medicare participating psychiatrist who performs a diagnostic evaluation that costs $350. Those services are not subject to the limitation,

and they satisfy the deductible. The psychiatrist then conducts 10 weekly therapy sessions for which he/she charges $125 each. The Medicare allowed amount is $90 each, for a total of $900.

Apply the limitation by multiplying 0.625 times $900, which equals $562.50.

Apply regular 20 percent coinsurance by multiplying 0.8 times $562.50, which equals $450 (the amount of Medicare payment).

The beneficiary is responsible for $450 (the difference between Medicare payment and the allowed amount).

EXAMPLE B

A beneficiary was an inpatient of a psychiatric hospital and was discharged on January 1, 1992. During his/her inpatient stay he/she was diagnosed and therapy was begun under a treatment team that included a clinical psychologist. He/she received post-discharge therapy from the psychologist for 12 sessions, at which point the psychologist administered testing that showed the patient had recovered sufficiently to warrant termination of therapy. The allowed amount for the therapy sessions was $80 each, and the amount for the testing was $125, for a total of $1085. All services in 1992 were subject to the limitation, since the diagnosis had been completed in the hospital and the subsequent testing was a part of therapy.

Apply the limitation by multiplying 0.625 times $1085, which gives $678.13.

Since the deductible must be met for 1992, subtract $100 from $678.13, for a remainder of $578.13.

Determine Medicare payment by multiplying the remainder by 0.8, which equals $462.50.

The beneficiary is responsible for $622.50.

Pub. 100-4, Chapter 13, Section 20

Payment Conditions for Radiology Services
B3-15022

Pub. 100-4, Chapter 13, Section 60

Positron Emission Tomography (PET) Scans – General Information
(Rev. 223, Issued: 07-02-04) (Effective/Implementation: Not Applicable)

Positron emission tomography (PET) is a noninvasive imaging procedure that assesses perfusion and the level of metabolic activity in various organ systems of the human body. A positron camera (tomograph) is used to produce cross-sectional tomographic images which are obtained by detecting radioactivity from a radioactive tracer substance (radiopharmaceutical) that emits a radioactive tracer substance (radiopharmaceutical FDG) such as 2 –[F-18] flouro-D-glucose FDG, that is administered intravenously to the patient.

The Medicare National Coverage Determinations Manual, Chapter 1, §220.6, contains additional coverage instructions to indicate the conditions under which a PET scan is performed.

A – Definitions

For all uses of PET, excluding Rubidium 82 for perfusion of the heart, myocardial viability and refractory seizures, the following definitions apply:

Diagnosis: PET is covered only in clinical situations in which the PET results may assist in avoiding an invasive diagnostic procedure, or in which the PET results may assist in determining the optimal anatomical location to perform an invasive diagnostic procedure. In general, for most solid tumors, a tissue diagnosis is made prior to the performance of PET scanning. PET scans following a tissue diagnosis are performed for the purpose of staging, not diagnosis. Therefore, the use of PET in the diagnosis of lymphoma, esophageal and colorectal cancers, as well as in melanoma, should be rare. PET is not covered for other diagnostic uses, and is not covered for screening (testing of patients without specific signs and symptoms of disease).

Staging and/or Restaging: PET is covered in clinical situations in which (1) (a) the stage of the cancer remains in doubt after completion of a standard diagnostic workup, including conventional imaging (computed tomography, magnetic resonance imaging, or ultrasound) or, (b) the use of PET would also be considered reasonable and necessary if it could potentially replace one or more conventional imaging studies when it is expected that conventional study information is insufficient for the clinical management of the patient and, (2) clinical management of the patient would differ depending on the stage of the cancer identified. PET will be covered for restaging after the completion of treatment for the purpose of detecting residual disease, for detecting suspected recurrence, or to determine the extent of a known recurrence.

Monitoring: Use of PET to monitor tumor response during the planned course of therapy (i.e., when no change in therapy is being contemplated) is NOT covered. Restaging only occurs after a course of treatment is completed, and this is covered, subject to the conditions above.

B - Limitations

For staging and restaging: PET is covered in either/or both of the following circumstances:

Σ The stage of the cancer remains in doubt after completion of a standard diagnostic workup, including conventional imaging (computed tomography, magnetic resonance imaging, or ultrasound); and/or

Σ The clinical management of the patient would differ depending on the stage of the cancer identified. PET will be covered for restaging after the completion of treatment for the purpose of detecting residual disease, for detecting suspected recurrence, or to determine the extent of a known recurrence. Use of PET would also be considered reasonable and necessary if it could potentially replace one or more conventional imaging studies when it is expected that conventional study information is insufficient for the clinical management of the patient.

PET is not covered for other diagnostic uses, and is not covered for screening (testing of patients without specific symptoms). Use of PET to monitor tumor response during the planned course of therapy (i.e. when no change in therapy is being contemplated) is not covered.

Pub. 100-4, Chapter 13, Section 90

Services of Portable X-Ray Suppliers
B3-2070.4, B3-15022.G, B3-4131, B3-4831

Services furnished by portable x-ray suppliers may have as many as four components. Carriers must follow the following rules.

Pub. 100-4, Chapter 16, Section 10

Background
B3-2070, B3-2070.1, B3-4110.3, B3-5114

Diagnostic X-ray, laboratory, and other diagnostic tests, including materials and the services of technicians, are covered under the Medicare program. Some clinical laboratory procedures or tests require Food and Drug Administration (FDA) approval before coverage is provided.

A diagnostic laboratory test is considered a laboratory service for billing purposes, regardless of whether it is performed in:

A physician's office, by an independent laboratory;

By a hospital laboratory for its outpatients or nonpatients;

In a rural health clinic; or

In an HMO or Health Care Prepayment Plan (HCPP) for a patient who is not a member.

When a hospital laboratory performs laboratory tests for nonhospital patients, the laboratory is functioning as an independent laboratory, and still bills the fiscal intermediary (FI). Also, when physicians and laboratories perform the same test, whether manually or with automated equipment, the services are deemed similar.

Laboratory services furnished by an independent laboratory are covered under SMI if the laboratory is an approved Independent Clinical Laboratory. However, as is the case of all diagnostic services, in order to be covered these services must be related to a patient's illness or injury (or symptom or complaint) and ordered by a physician. A small number of laboratory tests can be covered as a preventive screening service.

See the Medicare Benefit Policy Manual, Chapter 15, for detailed coverage requirements.

See the Medicare Program Integrity Manual, Chapter 10, for laboratory/supplier enrollment guidelines.

See the Medicare State Operations Manual for laboratory/supplier certification requirements.

Pub. 100-4, Chapter 16, Section 10.1

Definitions
This section will be updated Jul 04 - Click here for updated section

"Independent Laboratory" - An independent laboratory is one that is independent both of an attending or consulting physician's office and of a hospital that meets at least the requirements to qualify as an emergency hospital as defined in §1861(e) of the Social Security Act (the Act). (See the Medicare Benefits Policy Manual, Chapter 15, for detailed discussion.)

"Physician Office Laboratory" - A physician office laboratory is a laboratory maintained by a physician or group of physicians for performing diagnostic tests in connection with the physician practice.

"Clinical Laboratory" - See the Medicare Benefits Policy Manual, Chapter 15.

"Qualified Hospital Laboratory" - A qualified hospital laboratory is one that provides some clinical laboratory tests 24 hours a day, 7 days a week, to serve a hospital's emergency room that is also available to provide services 24 hours a day, 7 days a

week. For the qualified hospital laboratory meet this requirement, the hospital must have physicians physically present or available within 30 minutes through a medical staff call roster to handle emergencies 24 hours a day, 7 days a week; and hospital laboratory technologists must be on duty or on call at all times to provide testing for the emergency room.

"Hospital Outpatient" - See the Medicare Benefit Policy Manual, Chapter 2.

"Referring laboratory" - A Medicare-approved laboratory that receives a specimen to be tested and that refers the specimen to another laboratory for performance of the laboratory test.

"Reference laboratory" - A Medicare-enrolled laboratory that receives a specimen from another, referring laboratory for testing and that actually performs the test.

"Billing laboratory" - The laboratory that submits a bill or claim to Medicare.

"Service" - A clinical diagnostic laboratory test. Service and test are synonymous.

"Test" - A clinical diagnostic laboratory service. Service and test are synonymous.

"CLIA" - The Clinical Laboratories Improvement Act and CMS implementing regulations and processes.

"Certification" - A laboratory that has met the standards specified in the CLIA.

"Draw Station' - A place where a specimen is collected but no Medicare-covered clinical laboratory testing is performed on the drawn specimen.

"Medicare-approved laboratory - A laboratory that meets all of the enrollment standards as a Medicare provider including the certification by a CLIA certifying authority.

Pub. 100-4, Chapter 16, Section 60

Specimen Collection Fee and Travel Allowance
(Rev. 1, 10-01-03)

Pub. 100-4, Chapter 16, Section 110.4

Carrier Contacts With Independent Clinical Laboratories
B3-2070.1.F

An important role of the carrier is as a communicant of necessary information to independent clinical laboratories. Failure to inform independent laboratories of Medicare regulations and claims processing procedures may have an adverse effect on prosecution of laboratories suspected of fraudulent activities with respect to tests performed by, or billed on behalf of, independent laboratories. United States Attorneys often must prosecute under a handicap or may refuse to prosecute cases where there is no evidence that a laboratory has been specifically informed of Medicare regulations and claims processing procedures.

To assure that laboratories are aware of Medicare regulations and carrier's policy, notification must be sent to independent laboratories when any changes are made in coverage policy or claims processing procedures. Additionally, to completely document efforts to fully inform independent laboratories of Medicare policy and the laboratory's responsibilities, previously issued newsletters should be periodically re-issued to remind laboratories of existing requirements.

Some items which should be discussed are the requirements to have the same charges for Medicare and private patients, to document fully the medical necessity for collection of specimens from a skilled nursing facility or a beneficiary's home, and, in cases when a laboratory service is referred from one independent laboratory to another independent laboratory, to identify the laboratory actually performing the test.

Additionally, when carrier professional relations representatives make personal contacts with particular laboratories, they should prepare and retain reports of contact indicating dates, persons present, and issues discussed.

Pub. 100-4, Chapter 17, Section 80.2

Oral Anti-Emetic Drugs Used as Full Replacement for Intravenous Anti-Emetic Drugs as Part of a Cancer Chemotherapeutic Regimen
(Rev. 1, 10-01-03)

B3-4460, A3-3660.15, PM A-98-5

See the Medicare Benefits Policy Manual ,Chapter 15, for detailed coverage requirements.

Effective for dates of service on or after January 1, 1998, FIs and carriers pay for oral anti-emetic drugs when used as full therapeutic replacement for intravenous dosage forms as part of a cancer chemotherapeutic regimen when the drug(s) is administered or prescribed by a physician for use immediately before, at, or within 48 hours after the time of administration of the chemotherapeutic agent.

The allowable period of covered therapy includes day one, the date of service of the chemotherapy drug (beginning of the time of treatment), plus a period not to exceed two additional calendar days, or a maximum period up to 48 hours. Some drugs are limited to 24 hours; some to 48 hours. The hour limit is included in the narrative description of the HCPCS code.

The oral anti-emetic drug(s) should be prescribed only on a per chemotherapy treatment basis. For example, only enough of the oral anti-emetic(s) for one 24 or 48 hour dosage regimen (depending upon the drug) should be prescribed/supplied for each incidence of chemotherapy treatment. These drugs may be supplied by the physician in the office, by an inpatient or outpatient provider (e.g., hospital, CAH, SNF, etc.), or through a supplier (e.g., a pharmacy).

The physician must indicate on the prescription that the beneficiary is receiving the oral anti-emetic drug(s) as full therapeutic replacement for an intravenous anti-emetic drug as part of a cancer chemotherapeutic regimen. Where the drug is provided by a facility, the beneficiary's medical record maintained by the facility must be documented to reflect that the beneficiary is receiving the oral anti-emetic drug(s) as full therapeutic replacement for an intravenous anti-emetic drug as part of a cancer chemotherapeutic regimen.

Payment for these drugs is made under Part B. Payment is based on the lower of the actual charge on the Medicare claim or 95 percent of the lesser of the median average wholesale price, as reflected in the SDP, for all sources of the generic forms of the drug or lowest priced brand name product. Deductible and coinsurance apply

HCPCS codes shown in §80.2.1 are used.

CWF edits claims with these codes to assure that the beneficiary is receiving the oral anti-emetic(s) as part of a cancer chemotherapeutic regimen by requiring a diagnosis of cancer.

Most drugs furnished as an outpatient hospital service are packaged under OPPS. However, chemotherapeutic agents and the supportive and adjunctive drugs used with them are paid separately.

Pub. 100-4, Chapter 17, Section 80.3.1

Requirements for Billing FI for Immunosuppressive Drugs
(Rev. 1, 10-01-03)

Hospitals not subject to OPPS bill on a Form CMS-1450 with bill type 12x (hospital inpatient Part B) or l3x (hospital outpatient) as appropriate. For claims with dates of service prior to April 1, 2000, providers report the following entries:

- Occurrence code 36 and date in FL 32-35;
- Revenue code 0250 in FL 42; and
- Narrative description in FL 43.

For claims with dates of service on or after April 1. 2000, hospitals report

- Occurrence code 36 and date in FL 32-35;
- Revenue code 0636 in FL 42;
- HCPCS code of the immunosuppressive drug in FL 44; and
- Number of units in FL 46 (the number of units billed must accurately reflect the definition of one unit of service in each code narrative. E.g.: If fifty 10-mg. Prednisone tablets are dispensed, the hospital bills J7506, 100 units (1 unit of J7506 = 5 mg.).

The hospital completes the remaining items in accordance with regular billing instructions.

Pub. 100-4, Chapter 18, Section 50

Prostate Cancer Screening Tests and Procedures
B3-4182, A3-3616

Sections 1861(s)(2)(P) and 1861(oo) of the Act (as added by §4103 of the Balanced Budget Act of 1997), provide for Medicare Part B coverage of certain prostate cancer screening tests subject to certain coverage, frequency, and payment limitations. Effective for services furnished on or after January 1, 2000, Medicare Part B covers prostate cancer screening tests/procedures for the early detection of prostate cancer. Coverage of prostate cancer screening tests includes the following procedures furnished to an individual for the early detection of prostate cancer:

Screening digital rectal examination, and

Screening prostate specific antigen (PSA) blood test.

Each test may be paid at a frequency of once every 12 months for men who have attained age 50 (i.e., starting at least one day after they have attained age 50), if at least 11 months have passed following the month in which the last Medicare-covered screening digital rectal examination was performed (for digital rectal exams) or PSA test was performed (for PSA tests).

Pub. 100-4, Chapter 20, Section 20

Calculation and Update of Payment Rates
(Rev. 1, 10-01-03)

B3-5017, PM B-01-54, 2002 PEN Fee Schedule

Section 1834 of the Act requires the use of fee schedules under Medicare Part B for reimbursement of durable medical equipment (DME) and for prosthetic and orthotic devices, beginning January 1 1989. Payment is limited to the lower of the actual charge for the equipment or the fee established.

Beginning with fee schedule year 1991, CMS calculates the updates for the fee schedules and national limitation amounts and provides the contractors with the revised payment amounts. The CMS calculates most fee schedule amounts and provides them to the carriers, DMERCs, FIs and RHHIs. However, for some services CMS asks carriers to calculate local fee amounts and to provide them to CMS to include in calculation of national amounts. These vary from update to update, and CMS issues special related instructions to carriers when appropriate.

Parenteral and enteral nutrition services paid on and after January 1, 2002 are paid on a fee schedule. This fee schedule also is furnished by CMS. Prior to 2002, payment amounts for PEN were determined under reasonable charge rules, including the application of the lowest charge level (LCL) restrictions.

The CMS furnishes fee schedule updates (DMEPOS, PEN, etc.) at least 30 days prior to the scheduled implementation. FIs use the fee schedules to pay for covered items, within their claims processing jurisdictions, supplied by hospitals, home health agencies, and other providers. FIs consult with DMERCs and where appropriate with carriers on filling gaps in fee schedules.

The CMS furnishes the fee amounts annually, or as updated if special updates should occur during the year, to carriers and FIs, including DMERCs and RHHIs, and to other interested parties (including the Statistical Analysis DMERC (SADMERC), Railroad Retirement Board (RRB), Indian Health Service, and United Mine Workers).

Pub. 100-4, Chapter 20, Section 20.4

Contents of Fee Schedule File
(Rev. 1, 10-01-03)

PM A-02-090

The fee schedule file provided by CMS contains HCPCS codes and related prices subject to the DMEPOS fee schedules, including application of any update factors and any changes to the national limited payment amounts. The file does not contain fees for drugs that are necessary for the effective use of DME. It also does not include fees for items for which fee schedule amounts are not established. See Chapter 23 for a description of pricing for these. The CMS releases via program issuance, the gap-filled amounts and the annual update factors for the various DMEPOS payment classes:

IN	=	Inexpensive/routinely purchased...DME;
FS	=	Frequency Service...DME;
CR	=	Capped Rental... DME;
OX	=	Oxygen and Oxygen Equipment... OXY;
OS	=	Ostomy, Tracheostomy and Urologicals...P/O;
S/D	=	Surgical Dressings...S/D;
P/O	=	Prosthetics and Orthotics...P/O;
SU	=	Supplies...DME; and
TE	=	TENS...DME,

RHHIs need to retrieve data from all of the above categories. Regular FIs need to retrieve data only from categories P/O, S/D and SU. FIs need to retrieve the SU category in order to be able to price supplies on Part B SNF claims.

Pub. 100-4, Chapter 20, Section 40.2

Maintenance and Service of Capped Rental Items

(Rev. 1, 10-01-03)

A3-3629

For capped rental items which have reached the 15-month rental cap, contractors pay claims for maintenance and servicing fees after six months have passed from the end of the final paid rental month or from the end of the period the item is no longer covered under the supplier's or manufacturer's warranty, whichever is later. For example:

Date service begins:	1/5/01
15-month rental period ends:	4/4/02 (1/5/01 + 15 months)
6-month period when no payment is made	
(4/5/02 + 6 months):	4/5/02 - 10/4/02
Date maintenance and servicing payment may begin:	10/5/02
Payment covers all maintenance and servicing through	
(10/5/02 + 6 months):	4/4/03

The maintenance and servicing fee for capped rental items may be paid only once every six months. However, in the event the beneficiary elected to purchase the equipment, maintenance and servicing are paid in accordance with the instructions in §40.1.

Pub. 100-4, Chpater 20, Section 100

General Documentation Requirements

(Rev. 1, 10-01-03)

B3-4107.1, B3-4107.8, HHA-463, Medicare Handbook for New Suppliers: Getting Started, B-02-31

Benefit policies are set forth in the Medicare Benefit Policy Manual, Chapter 15, §§110-130.

Program integrity policies for DMEPOS are set forth in the Medicare Program Integrity Manual, Chapter 5.

See Chapter 21 for applicable MSN messages.

See Chapter 22 for Remittance Advice coding.

Pub. 100-4, Chapter 20, Section 100.2

Certificates of Medical Necessity (CMN)

(Rev. 1, 10-01-03)

B3-3312

For certain items or services billed to the DME Regional Carrier (DMERC), the supplier must receive a signed Certificate of Medical Necessity (CMN) from the treating physician. CMNs are not required for the same items when billed by HHAs to RHHIs. Instead, the items must be included in the physician's signed orders on the home health plan of care. See the Medicare Program Integrity Manual, Chapter 6.

The FI will inform other providers (see §01 for definition pf provider) of documentation requirements.

Contractors may ask for supporting documentation beyond a CMN.

Refer to the local DMERC Web site described in §10 for downloadable copies of CMN forms.

See the Medicare Program Integrity Manual, Chapter 5, for specific Medicare policies and instructions on the following topics:

- Requirements for supplier retention of original CMNs
- CMN formats, paper and electronic
- List of currently approved CMNs and items requiring CMNs
- Supplier requirements for submitting CMNs
- Requirements for CMNs to also serve as a physician's order
- Civil monetary penalties for violation of CMN requirements
- Supplier requirements for completing portions of CMNs
- Physician requirements for completing portions of CMNs

Pub. 100-4, Chapter 20, Section 100.2.2

Evidence of Medical Necessity for Parenteral and Enteral Nutrition (PEN) Therapy

B3-3324, B3-4450

PEN coverage is determined by information provided by the treating physician and the PEN supplier. A completed certification of medical necessity (CMN) must accompany and support initial claims for PEN to establish whether coverage criteria are met and to ensure that the PEN therapy provided is consistent with the attending or ordering physician's prescription. Contractors ensure that the CMN contains pertinent information from the treating physician. Uniform specific medical data facilitate the review and promote consistency in coverage determinations and timelier claims processing.

The medical and prescription information on a PEN CMN can be most appropriately completed by the treating physician or from information in the patient's records by an employee of the physician for the physician's review and signature. Although PEN suppliers sometimes may assist in providing the PEN services, they cannot complete the CMN since they do not have the same access to patient information needed to properly enter medical or prescription information. Contractors use appropriate professional relations issuances, training sessions, and meetings to ensure that all persons and PEN suppliers are aware of this limitation of their role.

When properly completed, the PEN CMN includes the elements of a prescription as well as other data needed to determine whether Medicare coverage is possible. This practice will facilitate prompt delivery of PEN services and timely submittal of the related claim.

Pub. 100-4, Chapter 20, Section 100.2.2.3

DMERC Review of Initial PEN Certifications

B3-4450

In reviewing the claim and the supporting data on the CMN, the DMERC compares certain items, especially pertinent dates of treatment. For example, the start date of PEN coverage cannot precede the date of physician certification. The estimated duration of therapy must be contained on the CMN. This information is used to verify that the test of permanence is met. Once coverage is established, the estimated length of need at the start of PEN services will determine the recertification schedule.

The information shown on the certification must support the need for PEN supplies as billed. A diagnosis must show a functional impairment that precludes the enteral patient from swallowing and the parenteral patient from absorbing nutrients.

Initial assigned claims with the following conditions are denied without development:

Inappropriate or missing diagnosis or functional impairment;

Estimated duration of therapy is less than 90 consecutive days;

Duration of therapy is not listed;

Supplies have not been provided;

Supplies were provided prior to onset date of therapy; and

Stamped physician's signature.

Unassigned claims are developed for missing or incomplete information.

A - Revised Certifications/Change in Prescription

A revised certification is required when:

There is a change in the attending physician's orders in the category of nutrients and/or calories prescribed;

There is a change by more than one liter in the daily volume of parenteral solutions;

There is a change from home-mix to pre-mix or pre-mix to home-mix parenteral solutions;

There is a change from enteral to parenteral or parenteral to enteral therapy; or

There is a change in the method of infusion (e.g., from gravity-fed to pump-fed).

PEN payments are not adjusted unless a revised or renewed certification documents the necessity for the change. Payment levels for the most current certification or recertification may not be changed unless a prescription change is documented by a new recertification.

The DMERC may adjust the recertification schedule as needed.

Pub. 100-4, Chapter 20, Section 130.2

Billing for Inexpensive or Other Routinely Purchased DME

(Rev. 1, 10-01-03)

A3-3629, B3-4107.8

This is equipment with a purchase price not exceeding $150, or equipment that the Secretary determines is acquired by purchase at least 75 percent of the time, or equipment that is an accessory used in conjunction with a nebulizer, aspirator, or ventilators that are either continuous airway pressure devices or intermittent assist devices with continuous airway pressure devices. Suppliers and providers other than HHAs bill the DMERC or, in the case of implanted DME only, the local carrier. HHAs bill the RHHI.

Effective for items and services furnished after January 1, 1991, Medicare DME does not include seat lift chairs. Only the seat lift mechanism is defined under Medicare as DME. Therefore, seat lift coverage is limited to the seat lift mechanism. If a seat lift chair is provided to a beneficiary, contractors pay only for the lift mechanism portion of the chair. Some lift mechanisms are equipped with a seat that is considered an integral part of the lift mechanism. Contractors do not pay for chairs (HCPCS code E0620) furnished on or after January 1, 1991. The appropriate HCPCS codes for seat lift mechanisms are E0627, E0628, and E0629.

For TENS, suppliers and providers other than HHAs bill the DMERC. HHAs bill the RHHI using revenue code 0291 for the 2-month rental period (see §30.1.2), billing each month as a separate line item and revenue code 0292 for the actual purchase along with the appropriate HCPCS code.

Pub. 100-4, Chapter 20, Section 130.3

Billing for Items Requiring Frequent and Substantial Servicing

(Rev. 1, 10-01-03)

A3-3629, B3-4107.8

These are items such as intermittent positive pressure breathing (IPPB) machines and ventilators, excluding ventilators that are either continuous airway pressure devices or intermittent assist devices with continuous airway pressure devices.

Suppliers and providers other than HHAs bill the DMERC. HHAs bill the RHHI.

Pub. 100-4, Chapter 20, Section 130.4

Billing for Certain Customized Items

(Rev. 1, 10-01-03)

A3-3629, B3-4107.8

Due to their unique nature (custom fabrication, etc.), certain customized DME cannot be grouped together for profiling purposes. Claims for customized items that do not have specific HCPCS codes are coded as E1399 (miscellaneous DME). This includes circumstances where an item that has a HCPCS code is modified to the extent that neither the original terminology nor the terminology of another HCPCS code accurately describes the modified item.

Suppliers and providers other than HHAs bill the DMERC or local carrier. HHAs bill their RHHI, using revenue code 0292 along with the HCPCS.

Pub. 100-4, Chapter 20, Section 130.5

Billing for Capped Rental Items (Other Items of DME)

(Rev. 1, 10-01-03)

A3-3629, B3-4107.8

These are DME items, other than oxygen and oxygen equipment, not covered by the above categories. Suppliers and providers other than HHAs bill the DMERC. HHAs bill the RHHIs.

Pub. 100-4, Chapter 32, Section 11.1

Electrical Stimulation

(Rev 124a, 03-19-04)

A - Coding Applicable to Carriers & Fiscal Intermediaries (FIs)

Effective April 1, 2003, a National Coverage Decision was made to allow for Medicare coverage of Electrical Stimulation for the treatment of certain types of wounds. The type of wounds covered are chronic Stage III or Stage IV pressure ulcers, arterial ulcers, diabetic ulcers and venous stasis ulcers. All other uses of electrical stimulation for the treatment of wounds are not covered by Medicare. Electrical stimulation will not be covered as an initial treatment modality.

The use of electrical stimulation will only be covered after appropriate standard wound care has been tried for at least 30 days and there are no measurable signs of healing. If electrical stimulation is being used, wounds must be evaluated periodically by the treating physician but no less than every 30 days by a physician. Continued treatment with electrical stimulation is not covered if measurable signs of healing have not been demonstrated within any 30-day period of treatment. Additionally, electrical stimulation must be discontinued when the wound demonstrates a 100% epithelialzed wound bed.

Coverage policy can be found in Medicare National Coverage Determinations Manual, Chapter 1, Section 270.1 (www.cms.hhs.gov/masnuals/103 cov determ/ncd103index.asp)

The applicable Healthcare Common Procedure Coding System (HCPCS) code for Electrical Stimulation and the covered effective date is as follows:

HCPCS	Definition	Effective Date
G0281	Electrical Stimulation, (unattended), to one or more areas for chronic Stage III and Stage IV pressure ulcers, arterial ulcers, diabetic ulcers and venous stasis ulcers not demonstrating measurable signs of healing after 30 days of conventional care as part of a therapy plan of care	04/01/2003

Medicare will not cover the device used for the electrical stimulation for the treatment of wounds. However, Medicare will cover the service. Unsupervised home use of electrical stimulation will not be covered.

B - FI Billing Instructions

The applicable types of bills acceptable when billing for electrical stimulation services are 12X, 13X, 22X, 23X, 71X, 73X, 74X, 75X, and 85X. Chapter 25 of this manual provides general billing instructions that must be followed for bills submitted to FIs. FIs pay for electrical stimulation services under the Medicare Physician Fee Schedule for hospitals, Comprehensive Outpatient Rehabilitation Facility (CORF), Outpatient Rehabilitation Facility (ORF), Outpatient Physical Therapy (OPT) and Skilled Nursing Facility (SNF).

Payment methodology for independent Rural Health Clinic (RHC), provider-based RHCs, free-standing Federally Qualified Health Center (FQHC) and provider based FQHCs is made under the all-inclusive rate for the visit furnished to the RHC/FQHC patient to obtain the therapy service. Only 1 payment will be made for the visit furnished to the RHC/FQHC patient to obtain the therapy service.

Payment Methodology for Critical Access Hospital (CAH) is payment is made on a reasonable cost basis unless the CAH has elected the Optional Method and pay 115% of the MPFS amount for the HCPCS code.

In addition, the following revenues code must be used in conjunction with the HCPCS code identified:

Revenue Code	Description
420	Physical Therapy
430	Occupational Therapy
520	Federal Qualified Health Center
521	Rural Health Center
977, 978	Critical Access Hospital- method II CAH professional services only

C - Carrier Claims

Carriers pay for Electrical Stimulation services billed with HCPCS codes G0281 based on the MPFS. Claims for Electrical Stimulation services must be billed on the CMS 1500 or the electronic equivalent following instructions in Chapter 12 of this manual (www.cms.hhs.gov/manuals/104_claims/clm104index.asp)

D - Coinsurance and Deductible

The Medicare contractor shall apply coinsurance and deductible to payments for ABPM services except for services billed to the FI by FQHCs. For FQHCs, only co-insurance applies.

Pub. 100-8, Chapter 5, Section 5.1.1.2.1

Written Orders Prior to Delivery

(Rev. 71, 04-09-04)

A written order prior to delivery is required for: pressure reducing pads, mattress overlays, mattresses, and beds; seat lift mechanisms; TENS units; and power operated vehicles. DMERCs and DMERC PSCs may identify other items for which they will require a written order prior to delivery.

For these items, the supplier must have received a written order that has been both signed and dated by the treating physician and meets the requirements of Section 5.1.1.2 before dispensing the item.

If a supplier bills for an item without a written order, when the supplier is required to have a written order prior to delivery, the item will be denied as not meeting the benefit category (see the MCM, Section 12000 for more information on appeals).

APPENDIX 5 — HCPCS CODES FOR WHICH CPT CODES SHOULD BE REPORTED

CPT (HCPCS Level I)	PM/Transmittal	Source	HCPCS Level II
21077			L8042
21087			L8040
21088			L8041, L8042, L8044, L8046
27096	A-02-129		G0259
36400-36405, 36415-36416, 36420-36425	AB-02-163		G0001
38210-38213 replaced deleted code 86915	AB-02-163		G0267
45300-45387 (mutually exclusive)		CCI	Comprehensive code G0105
45300-45387, 46604, 46608, 46614 (mutually exclusive)		CCI	Comprehensive code G0104
46947	R290CP	Pub 100-04	C9717
55859, 77776-77778, 77781-77784 should not be reported in addition to G0261	A-02-129		G0261
55859, 77776-77778, 77781-77784, should not be reported in addition to G0256	A-02-129		G0256
69210 for non-medicare only	A-02-129		G0268
71555		Medicare Claims Processing Manual, Ch. 13, Sec. 40.1.2 (Rev. 10/1/03)	C8909-C8911
72198	A-03-051	Medicare Claims Processing Manual, Ch. 13, Sec. 40.1.2 (Rev. 10/1/03)	C8918-C8920
74270, 74280 (mutually exclusive)		CCI	Comprehensive code G0106
76090	Hospital Manual, Ch. 10, Sec. 458	—	G0206-G0207
76091	Hospital Manual, Ch. 10, Sec. 458	—	G0202-G0205
78491			G0030
78492			G0031
78608	R290CP R278CP	Pub 100-04	G0336
82270	R80CP	Pub 100-04	G0328
82270 (mutually exclusive)		CCI	Comprehensive code G0107
84153, 84154 (mutually exclusive)		CCI	Comprehensive code G0103
85610, 85611, E & M	AB-02-180		G0248
88160-88161		Transmittal 800, CCI	Comprehensive code P3000
88174	AB-02-163		G0144
88175	AB-02-163		G0145
88240	AB-02-163		G0265
88241	AB-02-163		G0266

CPT (HCPCS Level I)	PM/Transmittal	Source	HCPCS Level II
90471-90472	B-03-001		G0008, G0009, G0010
90723 is allowable with G0010		1788 (2-3-2003)	Q code was deleted.
90740 is allowable with G0010		1788 (2-3-2003)	Q code was deleted.
90743 is allowable with G0010		1788 (2-3-2003)	Q code was deleted
90744 is allowable with G0010		1788 (2-3-2003)	Q code was deleted
90746 is allowable with G0010		1788 (2-3-2003)	Q code was deleted
90747 is allowable with G0010		1788 (2-3-2003)	Q code was deleted
90748 is allowable with G0010		1788 (2-3-2003)	Q code was deleted
90782			G0008, G0009, G0010
90919, 90920, 90921		68FR63216	G0308-G0327
99183 (carrier requires) hyperbaric oxygen therapy)	AB-702-183		C1300 (report for hospital outpatient)
Included in E & M code 99201-99456 & 99499		CCI	G0102

New, Changed, and Deleted Codes

APPENDIX 6 — NEW, CHANGED, DELETED, AND REINSTATED HCPCS CODES FOR 2005

NEW CODES

A4223	A4349	A4520	A4605	A7040	A7041	A7045
A7527	A9152	A9153	A9180	B4102	B4103	B4104
B4149	B4157	B4158	B4159	B4160	B4161	B4162
C1093	C1721	C2634	C2635	C2636	C9206	C9211
C9212	C9218	C9220	C9221	C9222	C9399	C9400
C9401	C9402	C9403	C9404	C9405	C9410	C9411
C9413	C9414	C9415	C9417	C9418	C9419	C9420
C9421	C9422	C9423	C9424	C9425	C9426	C9427
C9428	C9429	C9430	C9431	C9432	C9433	C9435
C9436	C9437	C9438	C9439	C9704	C9713	C9716
C9718	C9719	C9720	C9721	C9722	D0416	D0421
D0431	D0475	D0476	D0477	D0478	D0479	D0481
D0482	D0483	D0484	D0485	D2712	D2794	D2915
D2934	D2971	D2975	D5225	D5226	D6094	D6190
D6194	D6205	D6214	D6624	D6634	D6710	D6794
D7283	D7288	D7311	D7321	D7511	D7521	D7953
D7963	D9942	E0118	E0190	E0240	E0247	E0248
E0463	E0464	E0637	E0639	E0640	E0769	E0849
E1039	E1229	E1239	E1841	E2205	E2206	E2291
E2292	E2293	E2294	E2368	E2369	E2370	E2601
E2602	E2603	E2604	E2605	E2606	E2607	E2608
E2609	E2610	E2611	E2612	E2613	E2614	E2615
E2616	E2617	E2618	E2619	E2620	E2621	E8000
E8001	E8002	G0110	G0111	G0112	G0113	G0114
G0115	G0116	G0260	G0308	G0309	G0310	G0311
G0312	G0313	G0314	G0315	G0316	G0317	G0318
G0319	G0320	G0321	G0322	G0323	G0324	G0325
G0326	G0327	G0328	G0329	G0330	G0331	G0336
G0337	G0338	G0339	G0340	G0341	G0342	G0343
G0344	G0345	G0346	G0347	G0348	G0349	G0350
G0351	G0353	G0354	G0355	G0356	G0357	G0358
G0359	G0360	G0361	G0362	G0363	G0364	G0365
G0366	G0367	G0368	G9013	G9014	G9017	G9018
G9019	G9020	G9021	G9022	G9023	G9024	G9025
G9026	G9027	G9028	G9029	G9030	G9031	G9032
G9034	G9035	G9036	G9037	J0128	J0135	J0180
J0878	J1457	J1931	J2357	J2469	J2794	J3110
J3246	J3396	J7304	J7343	J7344	J7518	J7611
J7612	J7613	J7614	J7616	J7617	J7674	J8501
J8565	J9035	J9041	J9055	J9305	K0628	K0629
K0630	K0631	K0632	K0633	K0634	K0635	K0636
K0637	K0638	K0639	K0640	K0641	K0642	K0643
K0644	K0645	K0646	K0647	K0648	K0649	K0669
L1932	L2005	L2232	L4002	L5685	L5856	L5857
L6694	L6695	L6696	L6697	L6698	L7181	L8515
L8615	L8616	L8617	L8618	L8620	L8622	Q4054
Q4055	S0109	S0116	S0117	S0158	S0159	S0160
S0161	S0162	S0164	S0166	S0167	S0168	S0194
S0196	S0257	S0515	S0618	S2082	S2083	S2152
S2215	S2348	S3890	S4042	S8093	S8301	S9097
S9482	S9976	S9977	S9988	T2049	T4521	T4522
T4523	T4524	T4525	T4526	T4527	T4528	T4529
T4530	T4531	T4532	T4533	T4534	T4535	T4536
T4537	T4538	T4539	T4540	T4541	T4542	V2702

CHANGED CODES

A4222	A4332	A5119	B4150	B4152	B4153	B4154
B4155	C1716	C1717	C1718	C1719	C1720	C2616
C2633	D0350	D0415	D0480	D2710	D2910	D3332
D4210	D4211	D4240	D4241	D4260	D4261	D4273
D4276	D4341	D4381	D6056	D6057	D7111	D7286
D7287	D7490	D7955	E0450	E0461	E0625	E0951
E0952	E0955	E0956	E0957	E0958	E0959	E0961
E0966	E0967	E0972	E0973	E0974	E0978	E0986
E0990	E0992	E0995	E1010	E1011	E1014	E1019
E1021	E1038	E1225	E1226	G0008	G0009	G0010
G0173	G0244	G0275	G0278	G0295	J0150	J0152
J1564	J2324	L0430	L1820	L2035	L2036	L2037
L2038	L2039	L2320	L2330	L2755	L2800	L4040
L4045	L4050	L4055	L6890	L6895	L7180	S2150
S9363	T2005	V2745				

DELETED CODES

A4324	A4325	A4347	A4521	A4522	A4523	A4524
A4525	A4526	A4527	A4528	A4529	A4530	A4531
A4532	A4533	A4535	A4536	A4537	A4538	A4609
A4610	B4151	B4156	C1088	C9109	C9124	C9125
C9207	C9208	C9209	C9210	C9213	C9214	C9215
C9216	C9217	C9219	C9408	C9412	C9416	C9434
C9701	C9703	C9712	C9714	C9715	C9717	D2970
D6020	D7281	E0176	E0177	E0178	E0179	E0192
E0454	E0962	E0963	E0964	E0965	E1012	E1013
G0001	G0292	J3245	J3395	J7618	J7619	J7621
K0023	K0024	K0059	K0060	K0061	K0081	K0114
K0115	K0116	K0627	K0650	K0651	K0652	K0653
K0654	K0655	K0656	K0657	K0658	K0659	K0660
K0661	K0662	K0663	K0664	K0665	K0666	K0667
K0668	L0476	L0478	L0500	L0510	L0515	L0520
L0530	L0540	L0550	L0560	L0561	L0565	L0600
L0610	L0620	L2435	L5674	L5675	L5846	L5847
L5989	L8490	Q0182	Q0183	S0115	S0163	S0165
S2085	S2113	S2130	S2131	S2211	S2255	S8182
S8183	T1500					

REINSTATED CODES

A4644	A4645	A4646	C1080	C1081	C1082	C1083
C1713	C1714	C1715	C1722	C1724	C1725	C1726
C1727	C1728	C1729	C1730	C1731	C1732	C1733
C1750	C1751	C1752	C1753	C1754	C1755	C1756
C1757	C1758	C1759	C1760	C1762	C1763	C1764
C1766	C1767	C1768	C1769	C1770	C1771	C1772
C1773	C1776	C1777	C1778	C1779	C1780	C1781
C1782	C1784	C1785	C1786	C1787	C1788	C1789
C1813	C1815	C1816	C1817	C1819	C1874	C1875
C1876	C1877	C1878	C1879	C1880	C1881	C1882
C1883	C1885	C1887	C1891	C1892	C1893	C1894
C1895	C1896	C1897	C1898	C1899	C2615	C2617
C2619	C2620	C2621	C2622	C2625	C2626	C2627
C2628	C2629	C2630	C2631	C9205	G0027	